Communications in Computer and Information Science 373

Constantine Stephanidis (Ed.)

HCI International 2013 – Posters' Extended Abstracts

International Conference, HCI International 2013
Las Vegas, NV, USA, July 21-26, 2013
Proceedings, Part I

Springer

Volume Editor

Constantine Stephanidis
Foundation for Research and Technology - Hellas (FORTH)
Institute of Computer Science (ICS)
N. Plastira 100, Vassilika Vouton
70013 Heraklion, Crete, Greece
and
University of Crete
Department of Computer Science, Crete, Greece
E-mail: cs@ics.forth.gr

ISSN 1865-0929 e-ISSN 1865-0937
ISBN 978-3-642-39472-0 e-ISBN 978-3-642-39473-7
DOI 10.1007/978-3-642-39473-7
Springer Heidelberg Dordrecht London New York

Library of Congress Control Number: 2013942203

CR Subject Classification (1998): H.5, K.3, K.4, H.3, H.1, J.3, J.4, H.4

Typesetting: Camera-ready by author, data conversion by Scientific Publishing Services, Chennai, India

Printed on acid-free paper

Springer is part of Springer Science+Business Media (www.springer.com)

Foreword

The 15th International Conference on Human–Computer Interaction, HCI International 2013, was held in Las Vegas, Nevada, USA, 21–26 July 2013, incorporating 12 conferences / thematic areas:

Thematic areas:

- Human–Computer Interaction
- Human Interface and the Management of Information

Affiliated conferences:

- 10th International Conference on Engineering Psychology and Cognitive Ergonomics
- 7th International Conference on Universal Access in Human–Computer Interaction
- 5th International Conference on Virtual, Augmented and Mixed Reality
- 5th International Conference on Cross-Cultural Design
- 5th International Conference on Online Communities and Social Computing
- 7th International Conference on Augmented Cognition
- 4th International Conference on Digital Human Modeling and Applications in Health, Safety, Ergonomics and Risk Management
- 2nd International Conference on Design, User Experience and Usability
- 1st International Conference on Distributed, Ambient and Pervasive Interactions
- 1st International Conference on Human Aspects of Information Security, Privacy and Trust

A total of 5210 individuals from academia, research institutes, industry and governmental agencies from 70 countries submitted contributions, and 1666 papers and 303 posters were included in the program. These papers address the latest research and development efforts and highlight the human aspects of design and use of computing systems. The papers accepted for presentation thoroughly cover the entire field of Human–Computer Interaction, addressing major advances in knowledge and effective use of computers in a variety of application areas.

This volume, edited by Constantine Stephanidis, contains extended abstracts of posters addressing the following major topics:

- HCI Design Approaches, Methods and Techniques
- Usability Methods, Techniques and Studies
- Universal Access and eInclusion
- Multimodal and Ambient Interaction
- Cognitive and Psychological Aspects of Interaction

- Perception and Interaction
- Ergonomic and Human Modelling Issues
- Capturing Gaze, Biosignals and Brainwaves
- Development Environments
- Product Design, Marketing and Advertisement

The remaining volumes of the HCI International 2013 proceedings are:

- Volume 1, LNCS 8004, Human–Computer Interaction: Human-Centred Design Approaches, Methods, Tools and Environments (Part I), edited by Masaaki Kurosu
- Volume 2, LNCS 8005, Human–Computer Interaction: Applications and Services (Part II), edited by Masaaki Kurosu
- Volume 3, LNCS 8006, Human–Computer Interaction: Users and Contexts of Use (Part III), edited by Masaaki Kurosu
- Volume 4, LNCS 8007, Human–Computer Interaction: Interaction Modalities and Techniques (Part IV), edited by Masaaki Kurosu
- Volume 5, LNCS 8008, Human–Computer Interaction: Towards Intelligent and Implicit Interaction (Part V), edited by Masaaki Kurosu
- Volume 6, LNCS 8009, Universal Access in Human–Computer Interaction: Design Methods, Tools and Interaction Techniques for eInclusion (Part I), edited by Constantine Stephanidis and Margherita Antona
- Volume 7, LNCS 8010, Universal Access in Human–Computer Interaction: User and Context Diversity (Part II), edited by Constantine Stephanidis and Margherita Antona
- Volume 8, LNCS 8011, Universal Access in Human–Computer Interaction: Applications and Services for Quality of Life (Part III), edited by Constantine Stephanidis and Margherita Antona
- Volume 9, LNCS 8012, Design, User Experience, and Usability: Design Philosophy, Methods and Tools (Part I), edited by Aaron Marcus
- Volume 10, LNCS 8013, Design, User Experience, and Usability: Health, Learning, Playing, Cultural, and Cross-Cultural User Experience (Part II), edited by Aaron Marcus
- Volume 11, LNCS 8014, Design, User Experience, and Usability: User Experience in Novel Technological Environments (Part III), edited by Aaron Marcus
- Volume 12, LNCS 8015, Design, User Experience, and Usability: Web, Mobile and Product Design (Part IV), edited by Aaron Marcus
- Volume 13, LNCS 8016, Human Interface and the Management of Information: Information and Interaction Design (Part I), edited by Sakae Yamamoto
- Volume 14, LNCS 8017, Human Interface and the Management of Information: Information and Interaction for Health, Safety, Mobility and Complex Environments (Part II), edited by Sakae Yamamoto
- Volume 15, LNCS 8018, Human Interface and the Management of Information: Information and Interaction for Learning, Culture, Collaboration and Business (Part III), edited by Sakae Yamamoto

- Volume 16, LNAI 8019, Engineering Psychology and Cognitive Ergonomics: Understanding Human Cognition (Part I), edited by Don Harris
- Volume 17, LNAI 8020, Engineering Psychology and Cognitive Ergonomics: Applications and Services (Part II), edited by Don Harris
- Volume 18, LNCS 8021, Virtual, Augmented and Mixed Reality: Designing and Developing Augmented and Virtual Environments (Part I), edited by Randall Shumaker
- Volume 19, LNCS 8022, Virtual, Augmented and Mixed Reality: Systems and Applications (Part II), edited by Randall Shumaker
- Volume 20, LNCS 8023, Cross-Cultural Design: Methods, Practice and Case Studies (Part I), edited by P.L. Patrick Rau
- Volume 21, LNCS 8024, Cross-Cultural Design: Cultural Differences in Everyday Life (Part II), edited by P.L. Patrick Rau
- Volume 22, LNCS 8025, Digital Human Modeling and Applications in Health, Safety, Ergonomics and Risk Management: Healthcare and Safety of the Environment and Transport (Part I), edited by Vincent G. Duffy
- Volume 23, LNCS 8026, Digital Human Modeling and Applications in Health, Safety, Ergonomics and Risk Management: Human Body Modeling and Ergonomics (Part II), edited by Vincent G. Duffy
- Volume 24, LNAI 8027, Foundations of Augmented Cognition, edited by Dylan D. Schmorrow and Cali M. Fidopiastis
- Volume 25, LNCS 8028, Distributed, Ambient and Pervasive Interactions, edited by Norbert Streitz and Constantine Stephanidis
- Volume 26, LNCS 8029, Online Communities and Social Computing, edited by A. Ant Ozok and Panayiotis Zaphiris
- Volume 27, LNCS 8030, Human Aspects of Information Security, Privacy and Trust, edited by Louis Marinos and Ioannis Askoxylakis
- Volume 29, CCIS 374, HCI International 2013 Posters Proceedings (Part II), edited by Constantine Stephanidis

I would like to thank the Program Chairs and the members of the Program Boards of all affiliated conferences and thematic areas, listed below, for their contribution to the highest scientific quality and the overall success of the HCI International 2013 conference.

This conference could not have been possible without the continuous support and advice of the Founding Chair and Conference Scientific Advisor, Prof. Gavriel Salvendy, as well as the dedicated work and outstanding efforts of the Communications Chair and Editor of HCI International News, Abbas Moallem.

I would also like to thank for their contribution towards the smooth organization of the HCI International 2013 Conference the members of the Human–Computer Interaction Laboratory of ICS-FORTH, and in particular George Paparoulis, Maria Pitsoulaki, Stavroula Ntoa, Maria Bouhli and George Kapnas.

May 2013

Constantine Stephanidis
General Chair, HCI International 2013

- Volume 10, LNAI 8019, Engineering Psychology and Cognitive Ergonomics: Understanding Human Cognition (Part I), edited by Don Harris
- [illegible]

Organization

Human–Computer Interaction

Program Chair: Masaaki Kurosu, Japan

Jose Abdelnour-Nocera, UK
Sebastiano Bagnara, Italy
Simone Barbosa, Brazil
Tomas Berns, Sweden
Nigel Bevan, UK
Simone Borsci, UK
Apala Lahiri Chavan, India
Sherry Chen, Taiwan
Kevin Clark, USA
Torkil Clemmensen, Denmark
Xiaowen Fang, USA
Shin'ichi Fukuzumi, Japan
Vicki Hanson, UK
Ayako Hashizume, Japan
Anzai Hiroyuki, Italy
Sheue-Ling Hwang, Taiwan
Wonil Hwang, South Korea
Minna Isomursu, Finland
Yong Gu Ji, South Korea
Esther Jun, USA
Mitsuhiko Karashima, Japan
Kyungdoh Kim, South Korea
Heidi Krömker, Germany
Chen Ling, USA
Yan Liu, USA
Zhengjie Liu, P.R. China
Loïc Martínez Normand, Spain
Chang S. Nam, USA
Naoko Okuizumi, Japan
Noriko Osaka, Japan
Philippe Palanque, France
Hans Persson, Sweden
Ling Rothrock, USA
Naoki Sakakibara, Japan
Dominique Scapin, France
Guangfeng Song, USA
Sanjay Tripathi, India
Chui Yin Wong, Malaysia
Toshiki Yamaoka, Japan
Kazuhiko Yamazaki, Japan
Ryoji Yoshitake, Japan
Silvia Zimmermann, Switzerland

Human Interface and the Management of Information

Program Chair: Sakae Yamamoto, Japan

Hans-Jorg Bullinger, Germany
Alan Chan, Hong Kong
Gilsoo Cho, South Korea
Jon R. Gunderson, USA
Shin'ichi Fukuzumi, Japan
Michitaka Hirose, Japan
Jhilmil Jain, USA
Yasufumi Kume, Japan
Mark Lehto, USA
Hiroyuki Miki, Japan
Hirohiko Mori, Japan
Fiona Fui-Hoon Nah, USA
Shogo Nishida, Japan
Robert Proctor, USA
Youngho Rhee, South Korea
Katsunori Shimohara, Japan

Michale Smith, USA
Tsutomu Tabe, Japan
Hiroshi Tsuji, Japan
Kim-Phuong Vu, USA
Tomio Watanabe, Japan
Hidekazu Yoshikawa, Japan

Engineering Psychology and Cognitive Ergonomics

Program Chair: Don Harris, UK

Guy Andre Boy, USA
Joakim Dahlman, Sweden
Trevor Dobbins, UK
Mike Feary, USA
Shan Fu, P.R. China
Michaela Heese, Austria
Hung-Sying Jing, Taiwan
Wen-Chin Li, Taiwan
Mark A. Neerincx, The Netherlands
Jan M. Noyes, UK
Taezoon Park, Singapore
Paul Salmon, Australia
Axel Schulte, Germany
Siraj Shaikh, UK
Sarah C. Sharples, UK
Anthony Smoker, UK
Neville A. Stanton, UK
Alex Stedmon, UK
Xianghong Sun, P.R. China
Andrew Thatcher, South Africa
Matthew J.W. Thomas, Australia
Rolf Zon, The Netherlands

Universal Access in Human–Computer Interaction

Program Chairs: Constantine Stephanidis, Greece, and Margherita Antona, Greece

Julio Abascal, Spain
Ray Adams, UK
Gisela Susanne Bahr, USA
Margit Betke, USA
Christian Bühler, Germany
Stefan Carmien, Spain
Jerzy Charytonowicz, Poland
Carlos Duarte, Portugal
Pier Luigi Emiliani, Italy
Qin Gao, P.R. China
Andrina Granić, Croatia
Andreas Holzinger, Austria
Josette Jones, USA
Simeon Keates, UK
Georgios Kouroupetroglou, Greece
Patrick Langdon, UK
Seongil Lee, Korea
Ana Isabel B.B. Paraguay, Brazil
Helen Petrie, UK
Michael Pieper, Germany
Enrico Pontelli, USA
Jaime Sanchez, Chile
Anthony Savidis, Greece
Christian Stary, Austria
Hirotada Ueda, Japan
Gerhard Weber, Germany
Harald Weber, Germany

Virtual, Augmented and Mixed Reality

Program Chair: Randall Shumaker, USA

Waymon Armstrong, USA
Juan Cendan, USA
Rudy Darken, USA
Cali M. Fidopiastis, USA
Charles Hughes, USA
David Kaber, USA
Hirokazu Kato, Japan
Denis Laurendeau, Canada
Fotis Liarokapis, UK
Mark Livingston, USA
Michael Macedonia, USA
Gordon Mair, UK
Jose San Martin, Spain
Jacquelyn Morie, USA
Albert "Skip" Rizzo, USA
Kay Stanney, USA
Christopher Stapleton, USA
Gregory Welch, USA

Cross-Cultural Design

Program Chair: P.L. Patrick Rau, P.R. China

Pilsung Choe, P.R. China
Henry Been-Lirn Duh, Singapore
Vanessa Evers, The Netherlands
Paul Fu, USA
Zhiyong Fu, P.R. China
Fu Guo, P.R. China
Sung H. Han, Korea
Toshikazu Kato, Japan
Dyi-Yih Michael Lin, Taiwan
Rungtai Lin, Taiwan
Sheau-Farn Max Liang, Taiwan
Liang Ma, P.R. China
Alexander Mädche, Germany
Katsuhiko Ogawa, Japan
Tom Plocher, USA
Kerstin Röse, Germany
Supriya Singh, Australia
Hsiu-Ping Yueh, Taiwan
Liang (Leon) Zeng, USA
Chen Zhao, USA

Online Communities and Social Computing

Program Chairs: A. Ant Ozok, USA, and Panayiotis Zaphiris, Cyprus

Areej Al-Wabil, Saudi Arabia
Leonelo Almeida, Brazil
Bjørn Andersen, Norway
Chee Siang Ang, UK
Aneesha Bakharia, Australia
Ania Bobrowicz, UK
Paul Cairns, UK
Farzin Deravi, UK
Andri Ioannou, Cyprus
Slava Kisilevich, Germany
Niki Lambropoulos, Greece
Effie Law, Switzerland
Soo Ling Lim, UK
Fernando Loizides, Cyprus
Gabriele Meiselwitz, USA
Anthony Norcio, USA
Elaine Raybourn, USA
Panote Siriaraya, UK
David Stuart, UK
June Wei, USA

Augmented Cognition

Program Chairs: Dylan D. Schmorrow, USA, and Cali M. Fidopiastis, USA

Robert Arrabito, Canada
Richard Backs, USA
Chris Berka, USA
Joseph Cohn, USA
Martha E. Crosby, USA
Julie Drexler, USA
Ivy Estabrooke, USA
Chris Forsythe, USA
Wai Tat Fu, USA
Rodolphe Gentili, USA
Marc Grootjen, The Netherlands
Jefferson Grubb, USA
Ming Hou, Canada
Santosh Mathan, USA
Rob Matthews, Australia
Dennis McBride, USA
Jeff Morrison, USA
Mark A. Neerincx, The Netherlands
Denise Nicholson, USA
Banu Onaral, USA
Lee Sciarini, USA
Kay Stanney, USA
Roy Stripling, USA
Rob Taylor, UK
Karl van Orden, USA

Digital Human Modeling and Applications in Health, Safety, Ergonomics and Risk Management

Program Chair: Vincent G. Duffy, USA and Russia

Karim Abdel-Malek, USA
Giuseppe Andreoni, Italy
Daniel Carruth, USA
Eliza Yingzi Du, USA
Enda Fallon, Ireland
Afzal Godil, USA
Ravindra Goonetilleke, Hong Kong
Bo Hoege, Germany
Waldemar Karwowski, USA
Zhizhong Li, P.R. China
Kang Li, USA
Tim Marler, USA
Michelle Robertson, USA
Matthias Rötting, Germany
Peter Vink, The Netherlands
Mao-Jiun Wang, Taiwan
Xuguang Wang, France
Jingzhou (James) Yang, USA
Xiugan Yuan, P.R. China
Gulcin Yucel Hoge, Germany

Design, User Experience, and Usability

Program Chair: Aaron Marcus, USA

Sisira Adikari, Australia
Ronald Baecker, Canada
Arne Berger, Germany
Jamie Blustein, Canada
Ana Boa-Ventura, USA
Jan Brejcha, Czech Republic
Lorenzo Cantoni, Switzerland
Maximilian Eibl, Germany

Anthony Faiola, USA
Emilie Gould, USA
Zelda Harrison, USA
Rüdiger Heimgärtner, Germany
Brigitte Herrmann, Germany
Steffen Hess, Germany
Kaleem Khan, Canada
Jennifer McGinn, USA
Francisco Rebelo, Portugal
Michael Renner, Switzerland
Kerem Rızvanoğlu, Turkey
Marcelo Soares, Brazil
Christian Sturm, Germany
Michele Visciola, Italy

Distributed, Ambient and Pervasive Interactions

Program Chairs: Norbert Streitz, Germany, and Constantine Stephanidis, Greece

Emile Aarts, The Netherlands
Adnan Abu-Dayya, Qatar
Juan Carlos Augusto, UK
Boris de Ruyter, The Netherlands
Anind Dey, USA
Dimitris Grammenos, Greece
Nuno M. Guimaraes, Portugal
Shin'ichi Konomi, Japan
Carsten Magerkurth, Switzerland
Christian Müller-Tomfelde, Australia
Fabio Paternó, Italy
Gilles Privat, France
Harald Reiterer, Germany
Carsten Röcker, Germany
Reiner Wichert, Germany
Woontack Woo, South Korea
Xenophon Zabulis, Greece

Human Aspects of Information Security, Privacy and Trust

Program Chairs: Louis Marinos, ENISA EU, and Ioannis Askoxylakis, Greece

Claudio Agostino Ardagna, Italy
Zinaida Benenson, Germany
Daniele Catteddu, Italy
Raoul Chiesa, Italy
Bryan Cline, USA
Sadie Creese, UK
Jorge Cuellar, Germany
Marc Dacier, USA
Dieter Gollmann, Germany
Kirstie Hawkey, Canada
Jaap-Henk Hoepman, The Netherlands
Cagatay Karabat, Turkey
Angelos Keromytis, USA
Ayako Komatsu, Japan
Ronald Leenes, The Netherlands
Javier Lopez, Spain
Steve Marsh, Canada
Gregorio Martinez, Spain
Emilio Mordini, Italy
Yuko Murayama, Japan
Masakatsu Nishigaki, Japan
Aljosa Pasic, Spain
Milan Petković, The Netherlands
Joachim Posegga, Germany
Jean-Jacques Quisquater, Belgium
Damien Sauveron, France
George Spanoudakis, UK
Kerry-Lynn Thomson, South Africa

Julien Touzeau, France
Theo Tryfonas, UK
João Vilela, Portugal
Claire Vishik, UK
Melanie Volkamer, Germany

External Reviewers

Maysoon Abulkhair, Saudi Arabia
Ilia Adami, Greece
Vishal Barot, UK
Stephan Böhm, Germany
Vassilis Charissis, UK
Francisco Cipolla-Ficarra, Spain
Maria De Marsico, Italy
Marc Fabri, UK
David Fonseca, Spain
Linda Harley, USA
Yasushi Ikei, Japan
Wei Ji, USA
Nouf Khashman, Canada
John Killilea, USA
Iosif Klironomos, Greece
Ute Klotz, Switzerland
Maria Korozi, Greece
Kentaro Kotani, Japan
Vassilis Kouroumalis, Greece
Stephanie Lackey, USA
Janelle LaMarche, USA
Asterios Leonidis, Greece
Nickolas Macchiarella, USA
George Margetis, Greece
Matthew Marraffino, USA
Joseph Mercado, USA
Claudia Mont'Alvão, Brazil
Yoichi Motomura, Japan
Karsten Nebe, Germany
Stavroula Ntoa, Greece
Martin Osen, Austria
Stephen Prior, UK
Farid Shirazi, Canada
Jan Stelovsky, USA
Sarah Swierenga, USA

HCI International 2014

The 16th International Conference on Human–Computer Interaction, HCI International 2014, will be held jointly with the affiliated conferences in the summer of 2014. It will cover a broad spectrum of themes related to Human–Computer Interaction, including theoretical issues, methods, tools, processes and case studies in HCI design, as well as novel interaction techniques, interfaces and applications. The proceedings will be published by Springer. More information about the topics, as well as the venue and dates of the conference, will be announced through the HCI International Conference series website: http://www.hci-international.org/

General Chair
Professor Constantine Stephanidis
University of Crete and ICS-FORTH
Heraklion, Crete, Greece
Email: cs@ics.forth.gr

Table of Contents – Part I

HCI Design Approaches, Methods and Techniques

Usability Methods, Techniques and Studies

Universal Access and eInclusion

Multimodal and Ambient Interaction

Cognitive and Psychological Aspects of Interaction

Perception and Interaction

Ergonomic and Human Modelling Issues

Capturing Gaze, Biosignals and Brainwaves

Development Environments

Product Design, Marketing and Advertisment

Health and Medicine

Media, Art and Culture

Transport

Web and Social Media

Information Search and Retrieval

Work, Collaboration and Creativity

Text and Storytelling

Agents, Avatars and Robots

Smart Environments

Virtual and Mixed Environments

Security and Privacy

Part I

HCI Design Approaches, Methods and Techniques

User Driven Service Design and Innovation Platforms

Birgitta Bergvall-Kåreborn[1] and Mikael Wiberg[2]

[1] Social Informatics, Luleå University of Technology, Sweden
Birgitta.Bergvall-Kareborn@ltu.se
[2] Informatics, Umeå University, Sweden
Mikael.Wiberg@informatik.umu.se

Abstract. Integrating consumers into the design and development process of IT is a promising strategy for companies. To stimulate this co-production of IT through end-user programming specific user platforms for innovation have been developed. In this paper we illustrate how end-user programming and configurations has been a successful practice throughout the history of the PC – from the early stationary computers in the 80s, via the development of the web, to recent toolkits for end-user configuration of mobile hardware. While this trend has been stable this paper illustrate how corresponding support for end-user programming of mobile applications is still missing. To address this need this paper presents the SATIN platform and its underlying design concepts. We view this as a contribution for advancing the development of innovation platforms and as an illustration of how concept design can help in envisioning the next step in user-driven service design.

Keywords: Concept design, Innovation Platforms, User-driven service design.

1 Introduction

Integrating consumers into the design and development process is a promising strategy for companies as they struggle with a growing individualization of consumer demands. To stimulate and facilitate user service design technical platforms for innovation have been developed. Platforms are defined as a set of user-friendly design tools that makes it easier for the user to design a product or service through a trial and error process [3, 8]. During the last years the interest in technical platforms for third-party development has increased significantly [9] and some authors even argue that that software platforms are emerging as a dominant model for software development and software-based services [7]. As Tiwana, Konsynski and Bush [7] states "Unlike traditional soft-ware development, these services leverage the expertise of a diverse developer community –with skills and an appreciation of user needs that platform owners might not posses- to creatively develop new capabilities unforeseeable by the platform's original design" (p. 675). However, within the filed of software development there is still a lack of available platforms that enables user-driven software design on a broad level. One main obstacle to achieve this is the existing toolkit languages. Taking this lack as a point of departure this paper present a

C. Stephanidis (Ed.): Posters, Part I, HCII 2013, CCIS 373, pp. 3–7, 2013.

prototype of a platform for user-driven software design for non-programmers. The aim is to use this platform as a stimuli material for discussions related to the vision, form, and function of this type of platform.

2 The History of User Driven Design

There are many different approaches for defining and categorizing platforms. In this paper we use these as an inspiration/base for our categorization where we aim to illustrate in what sectors end-user programming has a history and where there are empty fields that needs exploring and development.

In our illustration of how end-user programming has been enabled through the history of personal computing we have organized this development along two axises (see the 3'4 matrix in table 1). Along the horizontal axis we trace support for end-user programming chronologically from the development of the desktop computer, via the web into contemporary developments in the mobile IT segments. Further on, we trace this development vertically along this timeline in an attempt to reflect how end-user programming has been made possible on both hardware and software. In doing so we adopt the basic structure behind this matrix from earlier work conducted by Bosch [1] in which they have demonstrated how system ecologies nowadays include several platforms (desktop, web and mobile) and how these platforms support end-user programming to different extents. Further on, as our illustration will show the trend has been quite clear. In pushing the technological envelope forward support for end-user programming has followed. Taking this logic as a point of departure our illustration will show that while the most recent developments in IT platforms brings IT to its users in mobile forms support for end-user programming has not yet been made available to the public masses of users. Accordingly, our proposal of the SATIN platform as a tool for end-user programming of mobile applications comes in timely in the current development in our field.

Table 1. End-user programming and configurations (table structure adopted after Bosch 2009)

	80s -	**90s -**	**2000 - today**
Software	From excel to Linux	Yahoo! Pipes, Scratch, Google mashup editor	Still lacking
Hardware	Peripherals, Chip, Memory, Power, Mother-board, CPU, PC	Router, blue tooth connections, (internet of things)	Configurations of mobile hardware (e.g. Arduino)
	Desktop	**Web**	**Mobile**

As illustrated in table 1. even the early version of the desktop computer presented to the public eye in the mid 80s provided support for simple end-user programming at the level of its hardware architecture. The end-user could through quite simple steps attach preferable peripherals to the computer to customize it for different personal needs. More advanced user-enabled configurations of the machine included a range of activities from easy exchange of memory cards and chips to the more complex activity of assembling a complete PC including integration of power, motherboard, CPU, memory/ hard drive, etc. The architecture of the PC allowed for end-user configurations at the hardware level. Further on, the PC was deliberately designed to allow for end-user programming at the software level of the architecture as well. This possibility for end-user programming stretched from simple possibilities like designing scripts in Excel to more complex programming via Basic, Pascal, Linux, etc for more advanced end-users. In a similar way the development of the web has been followed by a trend of end-user programming and development – hardware wise in how end-users can easily add routers and other network hardware (including wifi, blueooth, etc) to configure the internet hardware infrastructure for different purposes. Ultimately, we view this as only the beginning of a much wider trend of end-user programming in the development of the Internet of Things. Software wise, tools (including Yahoo Pipes, Scratch, Google mashup editor) are now rapidly being developed and made available for end-users to enable people to program their own web based services. Most recently we can now witness that this trend continues as we ex-tend IT platforms into the mobile domain. On the hardware side end-user programming has already picked up pace through open source initiatives like Arduino which enable end-users to build their own net-worked mobile devices with simple modules of electronics. However, while all of this is now constantly being developed there is still very little support available in support of end-user programming of mobile devices. While e.g. most smart phones allow for the organization of information and apps on the device there is still little support for pro-gramming or configuring the functionality of the phone. We see the SATIN platform as presented in this paper as an important contribution to this lack and as a first sign to a movement in this direction.

3 Research Methodology

The research reported in this paper follows the method of concept-driven design research. In relation to this we found good methodological support for our project since the concept-driven approach is a well-suited method when:

1. The point of departure is conceptual/theoretical rather than empirical.
2. The research furthers conceptual and theoretical explorations through hands-on design and development of artifacts.
3. The end result—that is, the final design—is optimized in relation to a specific idea, concept, or theory rather than to a specific problem, user, or a particular use context [6, p.98].

In the next section we present our concept design (the SATIN platform) followed by a description of how this method was applied in our project.

4 The Design Concept – The SATIN Platform

The SATIN platform (www.satinproject.eu) aims at offering a tool for non-programmers to create applications using modern web-tools, which are to be consumed in a mobile setting. It is based on visual programming using drag-and-drop, see figure 1. For more detailed information about the platform see Davoli and Kuenen [2].

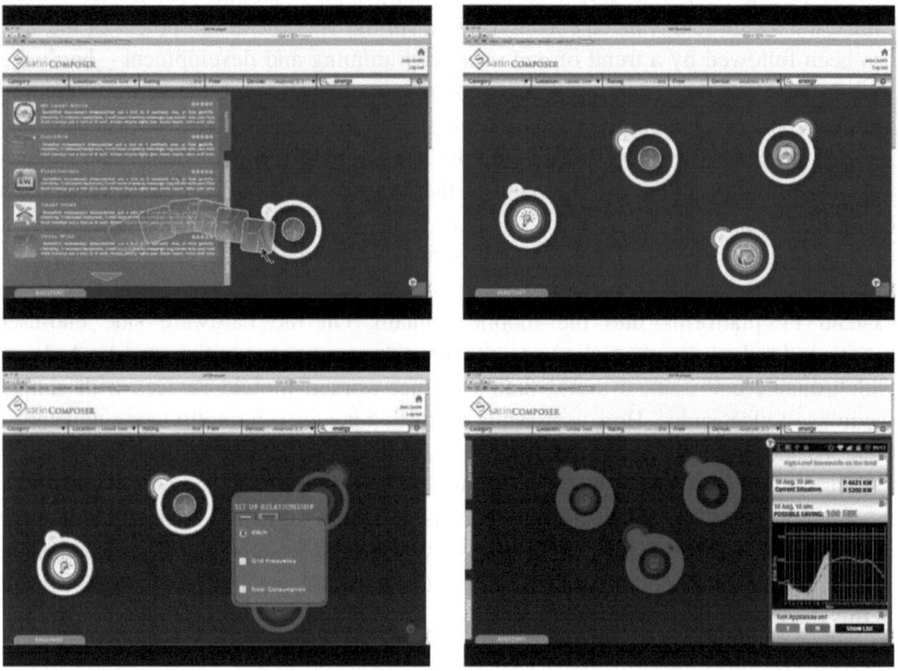

Fig. 1. The SATIN platform

From a methodological perspective we have since October 2009 worked back and forth between concept development and design of the SATIN platform. Methodologically we have 1) taken a point of departure in the concepts of user-driven service design and end-user programming 2) elaborated on these concepts through a process of concept development and design of the SATIN platform, and 3) seek to optimized the SATIN platform in terms of how it can support the idea of a platform for mobile app development for non-programmers. As to further situate our conceptual design work we have undertaken a literature study in which we have anchored the core concepts of user-driven de-sign and innovation platforms in the existing body of research.

5 Discussion and Conclusion

In this paper we have presented the concept design of the SATIN platform. We view this as an important contribution for advancing user –driven innovation for mobile devices. We also notice how our concept-driven design of the SATIN platform also brings with it some theoretical contributions. While some authors focus on the more technical components and processes of a platform such as the codebase of soft-ware-based systems [4, 7] other take a broader view and also include knowledge, people, and relationships into the fundamental assets of a platform [5]. Our work adds to this broader view and we illustrate how our proposed design also brings with it potential not only to include people and knowledge, but also the (mobile) contexts of the people enabling anyone to form their own mobile IT environment. Accordingly, we suggest that future research on platform development should focus not only at technology and people, but also on innovation processes – whether in front of the desktop computer or out there in the field.

References

1. Bosch, J.: From Software Product Lines to Software Ecosystems. In: The 13th International Software Product Line Conference (SPLC 2009), San Francisco, CA, USA (2009)
2. Davoli, L., Kuenen, S.: New Participative Tools Require New Foundations. The Experience of Satin: programming for non-programmers. In: Crafting The Future, European Academy of Design Conference, Gothenborg, Sweden, April 17-19 (2012)
3. Franke, N., Keinz, P., Schreier, M.: Complementing Mass Customization Toolkits with User Communities: How Peer Input Improves Customer Self-Design. Journal of Product Innovation Management 25, 546–559 (2008)
4. Ghazawneh, A., Henfridsson, O.: Balancing Platform Control and External Contribution in Third-Party Development: The Boundary Resources Model. Information Systems Journal (2012)
5. Robertson, D., Ulrich, K.: Planning for Product Platforms. Sloan Management Review 39, 19–31 (1998)
6. Stolterman, E., Wiberg, M.: Concept-driven Interaction Design Research. Human Computer Interaction (HCI) 25 (2010)
7. Tiwana, A., Konsynski, B., Bush, A.A.: Platform Evolution: Coevolution of Platform Architecture, Governance, and Environmental Dynamics. Information Systems Research 21, 675–687 (2010)
8. Von Hippel, E.: Perspective: User Toolkit for Innovation. The Journal of Product Innovation Management 18, 247–257 (2001)
9. Yoo, Y., Henfridsson, O., Lyytinen, K.: The New Organizing Logic of Digital innovation: An Agenda for Information Systems Research. Information Systems Research 21, 724–735 (2010)

Affective Service Design Considered Informational Assimilation of Layout Factors

Youngil Cho[1] and SuKyoung Kim[2]

[1] Hiroshima Kokusai Gakuin University, Nakano 6-20-1, Aki-ku, Hiroshima-shi, Hiroshima-ken 739-0321

[2] Hiroshima City University, 3-4-1 Ozukahigashi, Asaminami-ku, Hiroshima-shi, Hiroshima-ken 731-3166

cho@hkg.ac.jp

Abstract. While the changes in the focus and characters of service design have been complicated, its qualities regarding intuitively preferred factors, have not been investigated enough. This study shows how design factors affect user's intuitive preference and what make a user's attention focused on informational assimilation. Through the experiment, the layout factors and its values are verified. It was investigated (1) which layout factors arouse a user's attention, (2) how much uers were satisfied with the verified factors. The results shows that (1) elaborate images are the most important layout factor among five considerable factors, to arouse user's attentions, (2) the elaborate figures affect significantly all affective evaluation values, which were proved its relationship between user's attentions and the evaluation values through previous study; preference, aesthetic, and pleasure.

Keywords: affective, empathy, and design.

1 Introduction

According to Johnson et al. [1], new service development comprises four major phases: design, analysis, development, and full launch. Although the new service development process cycle might represent a progression of planning, analysis, and activity execution, the process is iterative and nonlinear in nature [2]. Instantly, the design stage involves formulation of new services objectives, strategies, idea generation, screening, and concept development and testing. However, the design stage does not involve its general process, such as in hospitals. Doctors make a diagnosis; nurses support doctors' works; and patients follow their directions." Typical top-down process is. Patients are not the beneficiaries of medical services. This study purpose an approach to human-centered service design considered "the user".

As one of the essential components in the new service development process, service design focuses on the operational basics of the development work. It involves understanding and planning the interaction of a variety of physical, electronic, and human elements [3]. On the hand, other definitions include "the idea to design high quality into the service system from the outset, and to consider and respond to

C. Stephanidis (Ed.): Posters, Part I, HCII 2013, CCIS 373, pp. 8–12, 2013.

customer expectations in designing each element of the service [4]", the concretization of the service concept in drawing flowcharts [5], and "the work of specifying an idea about a new service in drawings and specifications [6]". This study adopt both of considerations, understanding and planning the interaction of a variety of inset and the idea from the outset.

The purpose of this study is twofold. First, it shows affective layout factors arouse of people attentions. Second, it presents a conceptual framework for information based layout design. *Kansei* can contribute to understand how the present study approach to the purpose of the first stage. By the definition of *Kansei* [Fig. 1], [7], *Kansei* postulates individual as a subjective innate filter considering the variety of subjectivity. By subjective innate filter, inner and outer separated. When human captors (eyes, hear, nose…) receive a stimulus as an external feature from outer, the sensor data gathered in *Kansei* (repository). *Kansei* (repository) contains full data acquired by subjective innate filter (human sensors); the information synthesizes through in the brain *Kansei* process); and comes out as reaction such as emotion or intuition (Kansei information). Decision is a result of 'understanding.' In other words, data in Kansei (as repository) is assimilated (*Kansei* process), and is sent to understanding process (as *Kansei* information). *Kansei* presents as two types of outcome: emotion or intuition as Kansei information per se; decision as a result of understanding. Hence, individual's subjective perspectives can be investigated by understanding their *Kansei* information.

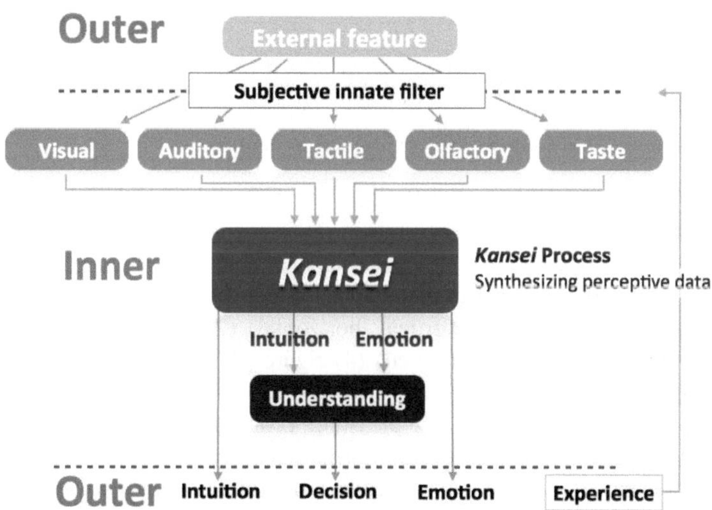

Fig. 1. It shows the definition of *Kansei* and how individuals modify their subjective filter

2 Method

To investigate individual's intuitive and emotional responses considered *Kansei* information process, three significant evaluation values were used in the experiment; preference, aesthetic, and pleasure [8]. Regarding the previous study conducted by Kim et al. showed the relationship between well-designed uninominal layouts and the evaluation values (preference, aesthetic, and pleasure). Considering the findings of the previous study as mentioned, it hypothesize that if a uninominal layout shows statistical significances in the all evaluation values, its layout designed well.

2.1 Subjects

Fifteen subjects participated in the experiment. The age range of the subjects is from twenty to fourty. No subjects have taken part in any kind of a similar experiment.

2.2 Stimuli

Forty-eight stimuli were used in the experiment considering five factors of its layout; (1) contents axis (vertical, horizontal) (2) contents positioning (default, modified) (3) font (default, modified) (4) figure (default, modified) (5) information type (three various contents layout). Based on the five factors and the two (or three) levels, forty-eight stimuli were prepared.

2.3 Procedure

The subjects were given directions firstly. And they evaluated on three evaluation factors, preference, aesthetic, and pleasure, with nine scales from strongly disagree to strongly agree. "Don't know" was explained as neutral.

3 Analysis and Results

One-way ANOVA was used in the analysis. Independent values were five factors of its layout; (1) contents axis (vertical, horizontal) (2) contents positioning (default, modified) (3) font (default, modified) (4) figure (default, modified) (5) information type (three various contents layout), and dependent values were the three evaluation values; preference, aesthetic, and pleasure. From the results, two factors showed statistical significances in figure and information type.

It shows statistical significances between the figure factors (default, modified) and the three evaluation values (less than .0001* in preference and pleasure, .0002* in aesthetic) [Fig. 2]. Also, the information type shows in statistical significances in aesthetic and pleasure values, does not show in preference [Fig. 3], [Table 1]. Aesthetic (p value = .0464*) and pleasure (p value = .0141*) evaluation values show statical significances in the information type factor. Fig. 3 shows that T3 was evaluated more aethetical and preferred information than T1 and 2.

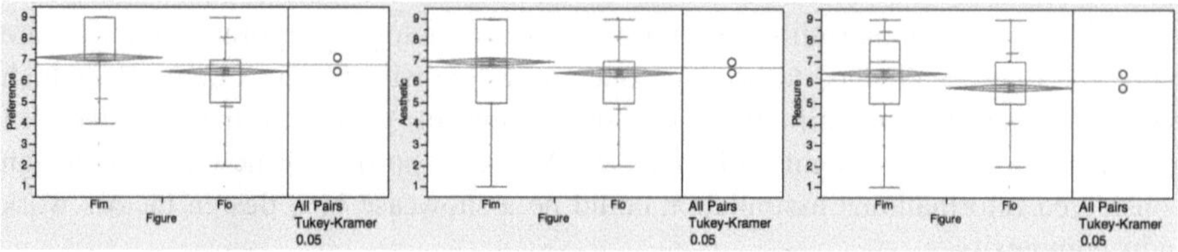

Fig. 2. "Fim" shows the results of modified figures. "Fio" shows the results of default figures.

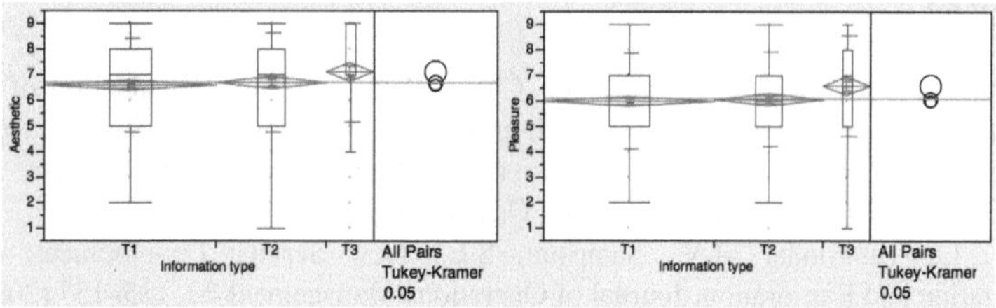

Fig. 3. "T1" shows the results of the information type 1. "T2" and "T3" shows the same pattern.

Table 1. It is the results that did not show statistical significances of the experiment and the p values

Evaluation value	Layout factor	P value
Preference	Contents axis	.2412
	Contents positioning	.3339
	Font	.2944
	Information type	.0530
Aesthetic	Contents axis	.3872
	Contents positioning	.2084
	Font	.3455
Pleasure	Contents axis	.8273
	Contents positioning	.4874
	Font	.3309

4 Conclusions

From the results, it shows that (1) elaborate images are the most important layout factor among five considerable factors, to arouse people attentions, (2) the elaborate images affect significantly all intuitive evaluation values (preference, aesthetic, and pleasure). Furthermore, information type shows its influence on aesthetic and pleasure evaluations in layout design. It can be including preference due to its p value. It is not far away .05 [Table 1]. It means, more attractive figure arouse peoples attention, and the attention affect their evaluation in preference, aesthetic, and pleasure. The findings are worthy to understand more effective design factors, which involves its affective consequences.

In this age of globalization and information technology, corporate strategies are more and more challenged to bring production in line with complex demands, which requires a substantial shift from the production of goods to the provision of knowledge-intensive systemic solutions [9]. And this approach to new service design considered informational assimilation could be a showcase how design factors work in its complexity.

References

1. Johnson, S.P., Menor, L.J., Roth, A.V., Chase, R.B.: A Critical Evaluation of the New Service Development Process: Integrating Service Innovation and Service Design. In: Fitzsimmons, J.A., Fitzsimmons, M.J. (eds.) New Service Development: Creating Memorable Experiences. Sage, Thousand Oaks (2000)
2. Menor, L., Tatikonda, M.V., Sampson, S.E.: New Service Development: Area for Exploitation and Exploration. Journal of Operations Management 20, 135–157 (2002)
3. Edvardsson, B., Thomasson, B., Øvretveit, J.: Quality of Service. Making It Really Work. McGraw-Hill, London (1994)
4. Zeithaml, V.A., Berry, L.L., Parasuraman, A.: Delivering Quality Service. Balancing Customer Perceptions and Expectations, p. 157. Free Press, New York (1990)
5. Gummesson, E.: Service Management: An Evaluation and the Future. International Journal of Service Industry Management 5(1), 77–96 (1994)
6. Norling, P., Edvardsson, B., Gummesson, E.: Tjänsteut - veckling och tjänstekonstruction. Research Report, Service Research Center, University of Karlstad, Sweden 92(5) (1992)
7. Kim, S.K., Cho, Y.I., Niki, K., Yamanaka, T.: The Influence of Holistic View Impression in Product Evaluation by an Approach in Kansei. In: Proceedings of International Conference on Kansei Engineering and Emotion Research, pp. 945–952 (2012)
8. Kim, S.K., Cho, Y.I., Niki, K., Yamanaka, T.: The Relationship between Preference and Kansei Values. Kansei Engineering International Journal 11(4), 1–8 (2012)
9. Pilat, D.: Innovation and Productivity in Services. State of the Art, Sydney (2000)

The Question Concerning Technology as Art

HyunKyoung Cho and Chang-Soo Park

GIST, Cultural Technology Institute, Korea
{hkcho,csp}@gist.ac.kr

Abstract. This paper presents that politics and the aesthetic meet in creative tensions between art, technology and humanities. The coincidence of politics and the aesthetic comes from the doubleness of technology performed by collaborative action of "We" human-and-technology. The way of technology posing the pairing of politics and the aesthetic in contemporary art opens a new way of understanding of relationships of humans and technology in collaborative action rooted in interdependent perspective.

Keywords: "We" human-and-technology, collaborative action, doubleness, politics, art, technology.

1 Introduction

Enlightenment asks enlightenment. Truth is Circe's poison [1]. Can the poison that transformed man into swine change the swine into man? Enlightenment that answers 'yes' or 'no' is a fraud. The quintessence of enlightenment is in the events in which firm belief in the universality of spirit and science, ensuring this solidly, becomes suddenly fluid, evaporating into air [2].

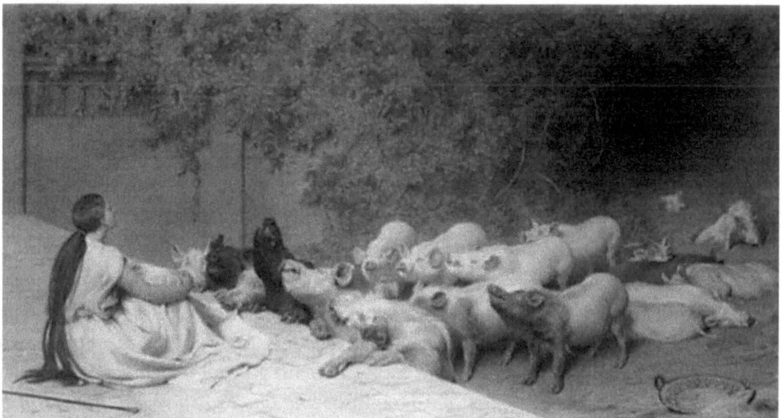

Fig. 1. Circe *and her Swine* (1871) by Briton Riviere (1840-1920), Hand-printed etching, 53 x 84 cm, Manchester Art Gallery

C. Stephanidis (Ed.): Posters, Part I, HCII 2013, CCIS 373, pp. 13–16, 2013.

The interventions between and consilience of technology, man, and industry is part of the Enlightenment. The question here is, is the industrialization of cutting-edge technology-art based on an art of capitalist politics, or politicization of capitalist art? If the question concerning technology reveals enlightenment within enlightenment, is cutting-edge technology-art with commodity value in exhibition a business skill, dedicated to improving capitalistic productivity from an instrumental perspective? Or is this a new way of knowing the enlightening nature of spirit?

2 The Collaborative Action of "We" Human-and- Technology

Technology more than represents human thought and action. A computer with high intelligence and sensibility can think and act like man. Artificial intelligence and life-technology with an indigenous principle solves problems man cannot. In human-computer interaction and interface, computer technology can respond to human action with autonomy.

The reality and condition of technology today is that technology does not simply respond to human action but naturally reacts to them, or leads human action. Technology and we humans here are a pair of dancers performing on stage; collaborators sharing an objective and process; two performers in equality. When humans and technology communicate through collaborative action, as in a relationship between humans, they become "we," in a multi-dimension network, beyond "I" of a one-dimensional relationship.

Cutting-edge technology-based art composed of human-technology and collaborative action intervenes in issues beyond art, like knowledge-power relations, bringing an instrumental perspective questioning this relation. This perspective prioritizes human-subject-thinking, bringing an organic relation between man, technology, subject, object, thought and action in a binary frame, encouraging mutual degradation. Technology-object-behavior deteriorates to a means for objectives, and an organic relation is reduced and distorted to appearance, or inversed to the physical. Through criticism of the instrumental perspective, cutting-edge technology-based art underlines the importance of an action-based context-interdependent perspective, imprinting the politics of collaborative action of humans and technology [3][4].[1]

3 Doubleness of Technology

In his *The* Question *Concerning Technology*, Martin Heidegger argues technology is not technology, and knowing or understanding technology as a tool covers the nature of our

---

[1] The point of this essay, a criticism of and distinction between the rule-based and experience-based behavior, and context-dependent and independent-perspective, is applied with the Dreyfus Model, formalized by Hubert and Stuart Dreyfus for the phenomenological analysis of human learning. See, Hubert and Stuart Dreyfus, *Mind and Machine: The Power of Human Intuition and Experience in the Era of the Computer* (New York: Free Press, 1986). On the methodology of natural science and social science for this analysis, refer to Bent Flyvbjerg, *Making Social Science Matter: Why Social Inquiry Fails and How It Can Succeed Again* (Cambridge: Cambridge University Press, 2001).

The Role of Knowledge Management in Agile Software Development

Broderick Crawford[1,2], Claudio León de la Barra[1], Ricardo Soto[1,3], Mario Dorochesi[4], and Eric Monfroy[5]

[1] Pontificia Universidad Católica de Valparaíso, Chile
FirstName.Name@ucv.cl
[2] Universidad Finis Terrae, Chile
[3] Universidad Autónoma de Chile, Chile
[4] Universidad Técnica Federico Santa María, Chile
FirstName.Name@usm.cl
[5] Université de Nantes, France
FirstName.Name@univ-nantes.fr

Abstract. A software engineering project depends significantly on team performance, software is created by people for people involving human cooperation. In the last years, the tradicional software development approaches are changing and agile methods have received considerable appreciation. Among other attributes, the agilists claim that knowledge sharing is one of the keys to response to common problems and challenges of software development today. The agile principles and values have emphasized the importance of collaboration and interaction in the software development and, by other hand, creative work commonly involves collaboration in some form and it can be understood as an interaction between an individual and a sociocultural context. Agile methods had attained worldwide fame for its ability to increase the productivity of software teams by several magnitudes through empowering individuals, fostering a team-oriented environment, and focusing on project transparency and results. Particularly relevant are the team structure (creative and agile roles) and its functioning (creative techniques used).

Keywords: Knowledge Management, Software Engineering, Agile Development, Creativity, Creative teams.

1 Introduction

Knowledge management and associated processes have been incorporated progressively to frameworks of reference and organizational practices related to software development. These developments–more broadly–reach up topics related to organizational learning, complex systems, the individual and his personality [5,6].

One of the fundamental aspects in knowledge management is creation of knowledge and transformation of tacit knowledge into explicit knowledge (epistemological aspect); this process emerges and is performed person to person and group to group (ontological aspect) [14,9,16,18].

C. Stephanidis (Ed.): Posters, Part I, HCII 2013, CCIS 373, pp. 17–21, 2013.

Considering the time spent since the publication of the Agile Manifesto [2] and the development of knowledge management, is especially relevant the research about mature development teams in order to reinforce creativity and productivity in software development [5,11,15,16].

2 Fundamental Aspects of Creative Teams

For this purposes it is necessary to consider that a team, particularly creative and productive, must present three fundamental aspects:

- The ordination and regulation criteria related to the dynamic structure of the team, which shows of how people prepare and order for ideation (generation of a new software), and elements (resources) they use.
- The practical criteria related with the team operation, which indicates the dynamics of action that people establish and develop for the ideation, and finally.
- The teleological criteria, referring to the purposes, it means, the objectives of the group of people (both individuals as such). The group itself and its future viability, and effectiveness in achieving the purpose for which they were established [1].

3 Creative Roles in Software Development

Considering that the purpose of team is to develop software, it becomes relevant the criteria related to the structure of the team and its operation.

Regarding the first criterion, the evidence indicates that the definition of the roles established by the main Agile methodologies (Extreme Programming, SCRUM, ...) corresponds to various creative/innovative roles advisable in high performance teams. This correspondence is not seen in the traditional methodologies or taylorians of software development, as these more traditional approaches point to the high standardization, extensive documentation and roles that do not privilege enough the relationship with others (for example, with the client), this traditional view contrasts to creativity itself, which favors dialogue and the interaction between roles in a flexible method (understanding, agile) and sometimes also contradicts with the productivity, in the extent that the developed software does not respond to the requirements and needs of the client.

Particularly in Extreme Programming (XP) roles are the Customer, who writes the requirements and functional testing; the programmer who maintains the code as simple as possible and helps the client to write the functional tests; the Tester, who runs the functional tests; the Tracker, who tracks the estimates made by the team, the coach, who is responsible for the global process; the consultant who has specific expertise and, finally, the Manager, who is a link between the client and the programmers.

Lumsdaine and Lumsdaine [13] have proposed the detective that collects a big quantity of information related to a problem or situation in startup; Explorer, who tries to perceive the problem or situation in a broader sense, defining it more precisely and anticipating changes in a relevant context; the artist, who generates new ideas to solve the problem or to face the situation; the Engineer, who evaluates the generated ideas; the judge, who decides which idea will be implemented and, finally, the producer, who is responsible for implementing selected idea.

Trías de Bes and Kotler [17] in their model A-F to foster creativity, innovation and change in organizations have proposed the Activators roles, those who start the process of innovation; the browsers, who are the specialists in search for information, to generate new ideas and to their implementation; the Creators, who generate new ideas; the Developers, who turn ideas into products and/or specific service; the Executors, who implement and execute ideas in the institution and finally; the Facilitators, who approve the necessary resources for the innovation process and facilitate that the process develops properly.

The equivalence between these different typologies has been developed, concluding a high parallelism between the Agilists roles and the creative roles [3,12,7,8].

4 Operation of the Software Creative Team

Moreover, regarding the performance of team of software development, agile methods propose a series of practices that indicate how the team should develop. Particularly in XP practices are: game planning, 40 hours weekly, small deliveries, metaphors, customer on site, tests, simple design, coding standards, refactoring, pair programming, collective ownership, continuous integration, just the rules and open workspaces.

In our opinion, such practices show the operation of the team and what is expected of people in general, emphasizing what should ensure the software development process, but do not deepen on how are generated the specific proposals in the new software, through specific techniques. This aspect is crucial to consider in mature teams, as it seeks to further enhance their performance and ensure their future viability in other software development projects.

For this purpose, it is possible to use what it has been present in the theory of creativity [4], in which it is argued that it is imperative that new ideas (understanding, new software or new code) are stimulated properly, and to do this, it is required that the process of ideation start from an "specific" product (a software that "preexists" in the customer's mind and surely shows a software problem or an "ideal" software in the mind of the programmer, coach or consultant ...), where constant modifications are made agreeing with the client. These modifications will constitute, in short, the new software.

To this end, a technique widely used is the SCAMPER [10] which proposes seven basic modification operations: substitution, which involves taking one or more elements of the initial "specific" product and change it with new ones; the combination, in which it is added one or more elements or new characteristics to the initial "specific" product ; amplification, which is exaggerated in ascending way one or more characteristics (elements) of the initial "specific" product; minimization, which refers–to the reverse of the previous operation–to reduce one or more characteristics, passing to another use, which consists in altering substantially any characteristic of the initial "specific" product, to such an extent that the final product will present another utility (unrelated to the original); the elimination, in which it is removed one or more characteristics (elements) of initial "specific" product and, finally, the reordering (re inverse), which refers to change the order or the sequence of one or more characteristics (elements) of the initial "specific" product.

5 Conclusions

We considered that a deepening and formalization of this type, both in the comparative study of Agilists roles and creative roles, as in the operation more subtle of the development team at the moment when generating new software, is fundamental, because it allows- in practice- to ensure that tacit knowledge of all team members is effectively results into explicit knowledge and shared.

In mature agile software development teams it is necessary to enhance the support of its operation. In this sense, creative techniques like SCAMPER and the use of initial points such as "preexisting" or "ideal" software can be useful to agilists.

References

1. Aranda, E., Aranda Muñoz, E.: Manual de la creatividad: Aplicaciones prácticas. Vicens Vives (2000)
2. Beck, K.: Agile alliance (2001), `http://agilemanifesto.org`
3. Crawford, B., de la Barra, C.L.: Enhancing creativity in agile software teams. In: Concas, G., Damiani, E., Scotto, M., Succi, G. (eds.) XP 2007. LNCS, vol. 4536, pp. 161–162. Springer, Heidelberg (2007)
4. de Bono, E., Arnau, A.: El pensamiento lateral práctico. In: Biblioteca Edward De Bono. Ediciones Paidós (2008)
5. Dingsøyr, T., Nerur, S.P., Balijepally, V., Moe, N.B.: A decade of agile methodologies: Towards explaining agile software development. Journal of Systems and Software 85(6), 1213–1221 (2012)
6. Drury, M., Conboy, K., Power, K.: Obstacles to decision making in agile software development teams. Journal of Systems and Software 85(6), 1239–1254 (2012)
7. Glass, R.: Software creativity. Prentice-Hall, USA (1995)
8. Gu, M., Tong, X.: Towards hypotheses on creativity in software development. PROFES 3009, 47–61 (2004)
9. Jabar, M.A., Sidi, F., Selamat, M.H.: Tacit knowledge codification. Journal of Computer Science 6(10), 1170 (2010)
10. Kotler, P., Trías de Bes, F.: Marketing Lateral. Editorial Pearson/Prentice Hall, Spain (2004)
11. Layman, L., Williams, L., Damian, D., Bures, H.: Essential communication practices for extreme programming in a global software development team. Information & Software Technology 48(9), 781–794 (2006)

12. de la Barra, C.L., Crawford, B.: Fostering creativity thinking in agile software development. In: Holzinger, A. (ed.) USAB 2007. LNCS, vol. 4799, pp. 415–426. Springer, Heidelberg (2007)
13. Lumsdaine, E., Lumsdaine, M.: Creative Problem Solving: Thinking Skills for a Changing World. McGraw-Hill, New York (1995)
14. Nonaka, I., Takeuchi, H.: The Knowledge Creating Company. Oxford University Press (1995)
15. Stankovic, D., Nikolic, V., Djordjevic, M., Cao, D.-B.: A survey study of critical success factors in agile software projects in former yugoslavia it companies. Journal of Systems and Software (2013)
16. Sung, S.Y., Choi, J.N.: Effects of team knowledge management on the creativity and financial performance of organizational teams. Organizational Behavior and Human Decision Processes 118(1), 4–13 (2012)
17. Trías de Bes, F., Kotler, P.: Winning at Innovation: The A-to-F Model. Palgrave Macmillan (2011)
18. Wang, L.: The multi-dimension spiral model of the knowledge-based corporation - theoretical thinking of beijing future advertising corporation. JSW 4(5), 469–477 (2009)

Issues and Understandings for Rural HCI Systems Development: Agile Approaches "In the Wild"

Mark Davies, Alan Chamberlain, and Andy Crabtree

University of Nottingham, Jubilee Campus, Wollaton Road, Nottingham
{first name.last name}@nottingham.ac.uk

Abstract. HCI system design has largely been focused towards urban areas, the technology and the infrastructure of such environments. Researchers are often unaware of the local, real-word context and the restraints that this can have upon the both the interactional possibilities and use of their systems in rural-settings. Over the past decade, new developments in mobile and ubiquitous computing now make it possible for users to move beyond the urban fringes and into areas that are 'on the edge' of connectivity. Many modern systems take advantage of the Internet capabilities and being "always connected" to provide rich dynamic content, which sits within this always on and always connected model. Systems where data connectivity is relied upon can become redundant in rural spaces, where often, mobile signal is weak and connectivity unreliable. Popular digital services such as Google Maps work well in urban areas however, such services lack the detailed information required for use in rural areas and expect the user to have a good level of connectivity. This paper draws upon our research in HCI, system development and the issues relating to understanding the design and development of rural systems with real-world communities. We focus our research in this rural setting in order to provide appropriate interaction and reliable methods for improving mapping in rural spaces. We highlight the features of our research through outlining a set of principles and discussing an online and mobile solution to allow people to create mobile digital books, made up with rich multimedia, about the places they visit and activities they engage in.

1 Introduction

In this paper we outline the issues and understandings for developing HCI systems for a real-world setting and how agile methodologies and working with communities of people influence the design process when developing systems "in the wild". We discuss how we engaged and worked with a local community of people in a rural setting to design a digital solution that could help map rural spaces better. The core focus of this paper discusses the approaches and methods taken to building a system "in the wild" within a rural community and what are the issues to developing real-world systems in rural settings. We begin our paper by first discussing the methodology that we used throughout the process - an agile methodology. We then discuss what the benefits were in using this methodology for working with a community in a rural setting and how it influenced the design of our system – Placebooks (www.placebooks.org).

C. Stephanidis (Ed.): Posters, Part I, HCII 2013, CCIS 373, pp. 22–26, 2013.

2 Agile

Agile is a software development method that focuses on iterative or incremental approaches, collaborative effort (within the development team and between the team and stakeholders/clients) and is highly flexible (agile) in being able to meet the changing needs of the stakeholders. Agile methodologies are not only for software development, but can also be applied to user-centred design (1) and do not demand the over-documentation of the development process. Beck, et al (2) outline four key priorities over traditional software development strategies:

- Individuals and interactions over processes and tools
- Working software over comprehensive documentation
- Customer collaboration over contract negotiation
- Responding to change over following a plan (3).

Using Agile methodologies for in the wild settings works very well, being able to quickly adapt to new and emerging requirements is very important in order to keep people engaged and to enable the system to evolve. We found that within our project we were rarely dealing with a static set of requirements. The requirements for such projects were often in a state of flux, so an agile approach was needed in order to deal with these circumstances. More often than not the requirements that surface during the life of the project, as Greenberg and Buxton write (4), can lead to "innovation along new trajectories". Agile methods also, as we have seen, focus on individuals and interactions, "most practitioners already know that people matter more than process" (5). It is this focus that enabled the research team to come together and quickly respond to the ongoing and evolving requirement, without having to focus on large amounts of paperwork and planning. The team knew what they were capable of and what skills needed to be employed to carry out the work quickly and efficiently, and having people in-situ meant that we were able to pass information between the community and research team. This was often done using short iterations. When we combine this with our rapid, flexible approach, it is clear that this is what enabled us to deal with any issues that cropped up. Traditional design/implement/test software development methods (as can be seen in Sommerville (6) are often not flexible and have a very segmented, defined structure, in terms of the development process and the allocation of work. This happens on one level and often cannot deal with a series of parallel workflows as often happened when working in the wild. As Greenberg and Buxton (4) propose, "…the design/implement/test loop, if done naively, encourages the sequential evolution/refinement of ideas rather than the multiple parallel solutions that characterize most traditional design disciplines". This agile approach meant that we were able to rapidly construct prototypes with beta level functionality without having to spend too much time planning, over-documenting and following set processes/procedures.

Of course when using the Agile approach one has to be wary of the limitations of such approaches. One such limitation noted was that it can force prioritization in a research-based context. By this we mean that if something is suggested during the design process and the team decides to follow that design route (prioritize) then this can affect stakeholder participation, this can lead to systems that are developed that are not wanted or understood. The interaction between stakeholders, users, researchers and the role that prioritization is yet to be fully understood in relation to the development of systems using agile approaches. Indeed we would also go as far as to say that there needs to be an appreciation of the software development methods used when working with communities and the development of HCI-based systems/understandings. To further illustrate this point we would like to give an example. At the start of the project there was a push from groups involved in the project that what was needed was a variety of different technologies. A geo-sensor-based system, 3D maps, and whole range of situated display technologies, and for a short time we examined these as possibilities, prioritizing them as elements that would be part of, or the whole system. It wasn't until we engaged with more people that it became clear that this isn't what the stakeholders wanted, used, or for that matter understood. To avoid this sort of prioritsation we adopted an approach related adapted from CRA (Context Resource Approach) (7), in which we could quickly discuss and evaluate and develope the system through pooling our collective competences, both at a stakeholder level and from within the design team itself.

3 Understanding the Rural Setting

The setting of our work was based in rural West Wales, in the small coastal villages of Borth and Ynyslas. This area attracts a lot of business and tourism during the summertime, the peak season, and offers numerous activities for visitors to engage in. However, there is a paucity of quality maps on digital services such as Google Maps, with many public footpaths, business services and even a national nature reserve being unmapped. It's not only this area but many rural spaces suffer from a lack of online presence and remain digitally unexplored, making it more difficult for people to discover interests and information in general when in rural areas. Recent developments in mobile and ubiquitous computing allow people to move beyond the urban fringes and into rural spaces. However data connectivity and data coverage cannot always be guaranteed. In order to develop a dependable system, it is key to understand the setting in which the system will be located. From spending time being sited in the rural area at the start of the project, testing mobile coverage, connectivity and exploring the area as visitors, we discovered these issues of accessing information and having a reliable connection before we started to think about designing a system (figure 1 shows us exploring the place and testing connectivity). The context of the connectivity was mapped. This meant that we were able to identify some barriers early on, which prevented us from falling into an in situ-incompatibility trap a further down the line.

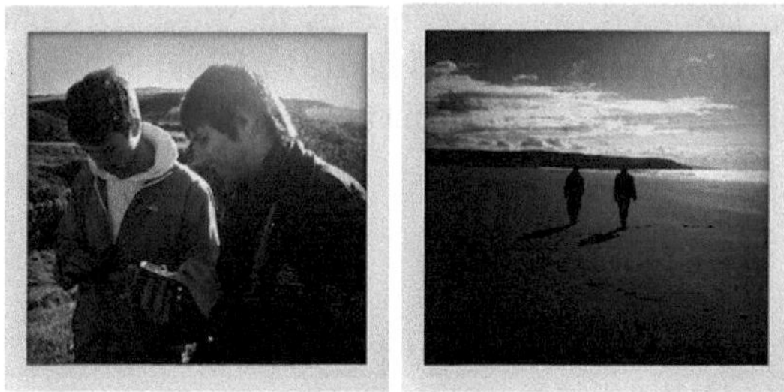

Fig. 1. Initial exploration of the situated rural area (Borth and Ynyslas) mapping network and data connectivity

4 Designing with a Real-World Community of People

Before engaging with the community in the rural setting, based on prior research experience, that it would not be realistic to engage with communities without first spending a considerable amount of time in order to understand the social 'lie of the land' (8). This meant going into the area to visit on a regular weekly basis and developing trust within these relationships with the locals and business owners of the area. Once a level of trust was gained, we could then begin to successfully recruit volunteers in the community to participate in our research and for them to provide the input to 'drive' the innovation of a broad socio-technical rural system. We worked directly with a rural community group, made up from individuals, to business owners, to ramblers, to windsurfers, to Countryside Council for Wales volunteers. This community group had a range of diverse interests so one of the first design issues we encountered was: how do we implement agile approaches with a community of varying diverse needs? Designing the system in-situ and working with people helped us understand the needs more speedily and in a more appropriate manner, allowing us to report back to the lab to refine our design, often on a weekly basis. Taking an agile approach and working in iterative bursts (design/evaluate/refine), we noticed that not only did it keep the community participants involved and interested but their interest also grew by them seeing a perceived benefit based on design progression from their input.

5 Conclusion

This paper has given a brief discussion about the development of a real-world system for a rural context through agile methodologies and has highlighted some of the issues surrounding rural system development. We acknowledge that this is just a snapshot of a project, but would like to think in offering some of the insights as we have done here that we would enable researchers to further think about the issues related to the building, design and development of systems in rural settings. In carrying out work in other settings, such as farmers markets (9) and small rural towns we are developing an appreciation of the issues that exist for many researchers trying to understand the complexity of using agile approaches, in particular within the field of HCI and the use of agile systems with communities.

Acknowledgments. This work was supported by the Research Councils UK Bridging the Rural Divide (RCUK) [grant number EP/I001816/1] and Scaling the Rural Enterprise [grant number EPSRC EP/J000604/1 & grant number EPSRC EP/J000604/2].

References

1. Sy, D.: Adapting Usability Investigations for Agile User-centered Design. Journal of Usability Studies 2(3) (2007)
2. Beck, K., et al.: Manifesto for Agile Software Development. Agile Alliance (2001), http://agilemanifesto.org (retrieved September 6, 2012)
3. Crabtree, A., Rouncefield, M., Tolmie, P.: Doing Design Ethnography. Springer (2012)
4. Greenberg, S., Buxton, B.: Usability Considered Harmful (Some of the Time). In: Proceedings of the 2008 ACM Conference on Human Factors in Computing Systems, CHI 2008, pp. 111–120 (2008)
5. Glass, R.: Agile Versus Traditional: Make Love, Not War. Cutter IT Journal (December 2001)
6. Sommerville, I.: Software Engineering, 8th edn. Addison – Wesley (2007)
7. Ehn, P., Kyng, M.: The Collective Resource Approach to Systems Design. In: Bjerknes, G., Ehn, P., Kyng, M. (eds.) Computers and Democracy - A Scandinavian Challenge, pp. 17–58. Avebury, Aldershot (1987)
8. Chamberlain, A., Crabtree, A., Davies, M., Greenhalgh, G., Rodden, T., Valchovska, S., Glover, K.: Fresh and local: the rural produce market as a site for co-design, ubiquitous technological intervention and digital-economic development. In: ACM Conference Mobile and Ubiquitous Multimedia, Ulm, Germany (2012)
9. Chamberlain, A., Crabtree, A., Davies, M.: Community Engagement for Research: Contextual design in rural CSCW system development. In: The 6th International Conference on Communities and Technology, C&T 2013, Munich, Germany (2013)

A Study on the Prototype of Focusing on the Operability for Requirement Acquisition

Yusuke Emori[1], Yusuke Kishiyama[2], and Tsutomu Konosu[2]

[1] Department of Management Science, Chiba Institute of Technology
[2] Department of Project Management, Chiba Institute of Technology
2-17-1, Tsudanuma, Narashino-shi, Chiba, 275-0016, Japan
s1291002SJ@it-chiba.ac.jp

Abstract. The purpose of this study is to propose the effective usage of the prototype of focusing on operability. As a result, participants indicated the design aspects and operability aspects when using the High-fidelity prototype more than Medium and Low-fidelity prototype. Also, participants indicated the function aspects when evaluating the Low-fidelity prototype more than High and Medium-fidelity prototype. The results suggested that a High-fidelity prototype is suitable for evaluating design aspects and operative aspects. In this study, the effective usage of prototype was proposed based on the experiments. It is possible to decrease the additional demand in the later phase of the project.

Keywords: prototype, requirement acquisition, operability, protocol analysis.

1 Introduction

It is difficult to complete the whole users demands at the early phase of the software development project. The lack of communication leads to vague specification of the demand definition of users. It is important to grasp the user's real needs in the early stage of the project. The prototype is useful for user's demand acquisition, it will be able to assume the products image. According to the previous work, the developer can obtain much functional demand when Low-fidelity prototype was used [1]. And it was also useful to obtain much design demand by High-fidelity prototype. In the experiment, the prototype of focusing on operability was used. This experiment was conducted with the stimulus varied the quantity of color information and quantity of graphical information. This contains the sum quantity of cognitive selective and brightness information.

2 Objective

The purpose of this study is to propose the effective usage of the prototype of focusing on operability. Two kinds of experiment were conducted in this study.

C. Stephanidis (Ed.): Posters, Part I, HCII 2013, CCIS 373, pp. 27–30, 2013.

3 Experiment 1

Overview

In this experiment, the employed prototype was divided into 3 types, low fidelity, medium fidelity and high fidelity. A subject's utterance was recorded and analyzed.

3.1 Method

(a) Experiment procedure

Three kinds of stimuli (High, Medium, and Low fidelities) were given to each participant. The protocol of each participants were measured and analyzed.

(b) Stimulus

The High-fidelity prototype was close to the actual usage. Color information was not included for the Medium-fidelity prototype. Color information and graphical information was not include for the Low-fidelity prototype. This prototype based on the 7steps model Norman (1986) [2]. This prototype was developed by Axure RP 6.0.

(c) Participants

Participants were 14 students (male: 13, female: 1) of Chiba Institute of Technology. Each participant were with normal visual performance, and their binocular vision was 0.7 or better.

3.2 Results

Participants talked the design aspects and operability aspects when evaluating the High-fidelity prototype more than Medium and Low-fidelity prototype. Participants talked the function aspects when evaluating the Low-fidelity prototype more than

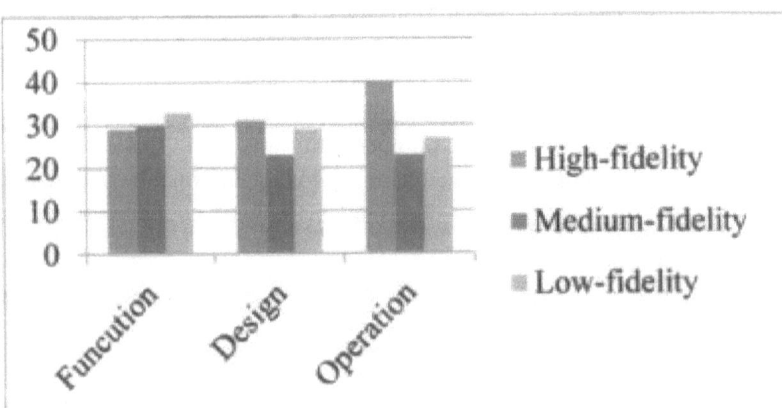

Fig. 1. Comparison of protocol analysis data 1

High and Medium-fidelity prototype. Frequency of protocol was different. High-fidelity prototype was 100 times. Medium-fidelity prototype was 76 times. Low-fidelity prototype was 89 times.

The results suggested that a High-fidelity prototype is suitable for evaluating design aspects, and suitable for evaluating operative aspects. A Low-fidelity prototype is suitable for acquiring function requirements. As a result, the effective usage of prototype was proposed based on the experiments. It is possible to decrease to the additional demand in the later phase of the project.

4 Experiment 2

Overview

In the experiment 1, the user's demands were divided into functional, design and operational demands. In the experiment 2, the design demands were clarified as "color and scheme", "lay out", "form", "arrangement", "operational design elements" and "feedback".

4.1 Method

The participants of this experiment were 10 students of the department of Chiba Institute of Technology. In this experiment, the employed prototype was divided into 3 types, low fidelity, medium fidelity, and high fidelity. The protocol of each participants were recorded and analyzed. The utterance data obtained in the experiment was classified into the functional elements design elements and operability. The amount of utterance was measured by each fidelity.

4.2 Results

The prototype of lower fidelity is effective for acquiring functional demand. The cognitive level differed by design elements. Such as "The operation method" and "feedback". In some elements contained in a design element, there were some in which a cognitive level differs from other things. They are the operation method and feedback. It is necessary to pay attention for the low design element of cognitive level than the other design elements.

Figure 2 show the utterance frequency for each design elements. From this figure, it is suggested that Low fidelity prototype is effective for accruing functional demands. This is the same tendency as experiment 1. Also, High fidelity prototype was effective for acquire the design elements such as "color and scheme", "Lay out", "Form", "Arrangement", "Operational design elements", and "Feedback". On the contrary, there were Low frequency of utterance on "the operational demand" and "feedback". It is assumed that this kinds of elements required higher cognitive information processing than the other design elements. When acquiring such "the operational design elements" and "feedback", the more careful approach is required.

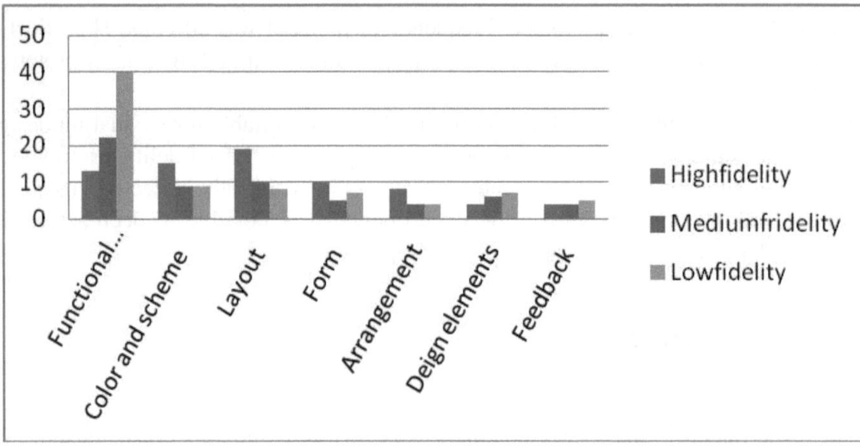

Fig. 2. Comparison of protocol analysis data 2

5 Conclusion

For acquire user's demands effectively, it is important to use prototype properly based on the purpose. Low-Fidelity Prototype is effective to acquire functional demands. Low-Fidelity Prototype is effective to acquire functional design and operational demands. Especially, when acquire cognitive difficult design elements, such as "the operational design elements"; "feedback" the more careful approach is required.

References

1. Nagasue, K., Takaishi, S., Kimura, T., Ishii, H., Takahashi, R., Konosu, T.: A Study on the Relationship between Prototype's Fidelity and Design Process for the Initial Phase of Software Development Project. In: 13th International Conference on Human-Computer Interaction (2009)
2. Jakob, N.: Usability Engineering, Academic Press (1999); (Translation Kaoru MIYOSI: Usability engineering theory, pp. 21–28. Capital electricity university press (2006)

Employing Creative Practice as a Research Method in the Field of Wearable and Interactive Technologies

Tania Raune Frankjaer[1], Patricia Jean Flanagan[2], and Daniel Gilgen[1]

[1] University of Applied Sciences Trier, Department of Design, Trier, Germany
[2] Hong Kong Baptist University, Academy of Visual Arts, Hong Kong SAR, P.R.C.
raune@frankjaer.de, tricia@triciaflanagan.com,
gilgen@hochschule-trier.de

Abstract. With the emergence of relatively accessible programmable microcontrollers, artistic use and designer application of wearable technologies have increased significantly over the last decade. This paper suggests these creations are more than a mere implementation of emerging technologies for creative practitioners to extend their artistic expression, but a method applicable within research and development. Creative practitioners generally approach their subject matter intuitively and holistically and are therefore capable of facilitating insights where rational approaches may not. Working on the periphery of computer science has the advantage of an outsider perspective, which can result in un-thought of solutions to previously unresolved problems. In this paper we discuss the merits of this approach within wearable and interactive research and describe one such procedure on the basis of a wearable device.

Keywords: Creative practice, alternative research methods, wearable technologies, interactive technologies, Arts Based Research, insight, outsiders perception, Bamboo Whisper, perception of communication.

1 Introduction

In recent years, technological development of relatively accessible programmable microprocessors and programming platforms has seen a surge in artistic use and designer application of wearable technologies. The results range from pragmatic gadgetry, in some way augmenting its wearer, through to aesthetically enhanced fashion and the more whimsical artistic creations, which to a greater or lesser extent seem best described by their lack of usability. Assuming research to be a process concerned with the creation of knowledge and of knowing, we suggest these latter creations to be more than artistic expression of emerging technologies by tech-savvy creative people, but also possessing an inherent quality that is applicable as a method for research and development of interactive and wearable technologies [1], [2]. Arts-based research is defined by Eliot W. Eisner as 'an effort to extend beyond the limiting constraints of discursive communication in order to express meanings that would otherwise be ineffable' [3]. Philosopher Michael Polanyi speaks of tacit knowledge, knowledge that exists beyond the boundaries of language [4]. Outside the limitations of linguistics,

C. Stephanidis (Ed.): Posters, Part I, HCII 2013, CCIS 373, pp. 31–35, 2013.

the creative practitioner has an aesthetic awareness and a refined sense of perception combined with an ability to find form articulated through the affordances of shapes, haptics, lights and sounds to facilitate comprehension and knowledge transfer.

2 Applying Creative Strategies in Problem Solving

Problem solving generally involves one of the following strategies: analytical processing: methodological and conscious search, or insight: sudden awareness of the solution to a problem with little or no conscious access to the processing. Insight is a key aspect of creative thought and associated with a propensity toward diffuse rather than focused attention, resulting in ineffective filtering and enhanced awareness of peripheral environmental stimuli, which trigger remote association [5]. Phenomena like serendipity, hunches and sudden insights play a considerable part in scientific discovery. Often perceived as luck or coincidence, these occurrences are not accidental but denote an ability to combine hitherto disparate parts and create an environment fertile for the unexpected to manifest [6]. This is a skill regularly taught and developed as part of the curriculum in arts and design schools.Creative practitioners have the liberty to explore new technologies in unanticipated ways, uninhibited by the computer science tradition of Human Computer Interaction (HCI) and free from market demands for profitable research [7]. Experts operating on the margin of their field are known to achieve great results by creating and engaging in unique projects[1].

3 Research Focus

Wearable technology has traditionally been regarded as a subcategory to ubiquitous computing and consequently the main concern within research has been on technological development, work tasks and usability. However, wearables signify a break away from the computer as a cognitive and rational device augmenting our brains and constitute a convergence point of a multitude of disciplines. As such, our concern is not with the technology itself but aims to deconstruct the narratives created by market-oriented research into a humanistic and cultural perception of the agents involved [2].

4 Applied Methods

Leaning on the principles of grounded theory, the research case study cited below began without a preconceived hypothesis or anticipated results. Rather, the process is more like one of reverse engineering a hypothesis that begins with a trial and error method of praxis-based experiments; the results of which constitute primary data collection that inform a second set of experiments. This process continues as

[1] In crowd-sourcing initiatives focusing on scientific problem-solving, a thirty per cent resolution rate has been observed when handing over problems to experts outside their respective fields [8].

categories of interest become apparent, in this case a deeper understanding of human communication and the effects of alteration and augmentation thereof. Key to this methodology is an openness to embrace discovery and remain free of expectations of what will be found or precisely how to get there [9]. Furthermore, direct experiences, being the emerging notions perceived whilst creating the project, constitute inductive and deductive thinking through phenomenological experience of materials and forms. Following an arts-based approach, the authors initiated the creation of Bamboo Whisper, two wearable communication devices, each consisting of a felted garment with a conical bamboo headdress. Both devices incorporate an electronic system and a micro-processor, translating the voices into movement of the protruding bamboo sticks and vibration in the other wearers' device. The design of the headdress encloses the head, thereby directing the wearer's vision forward and limiting their peripheral vision, amplifying somatic immediate proprioception and limiting distraction. Unlike arts-based research, we consider the creative result a vehicle for approaching our subject matter as opposed to it constituting the research in itself [3]. For example, this device generates patterns of information in the form of rhythmic percussive structures which represent the source bio-data in new forms. Anomalies can become apparent that were previously invisible. Another implication identified is the user experience of haptic interfaces and their implications in HCI. The wealth of experiential capacity of the body informs what the authors identify as 'interface aesthetics' [10].

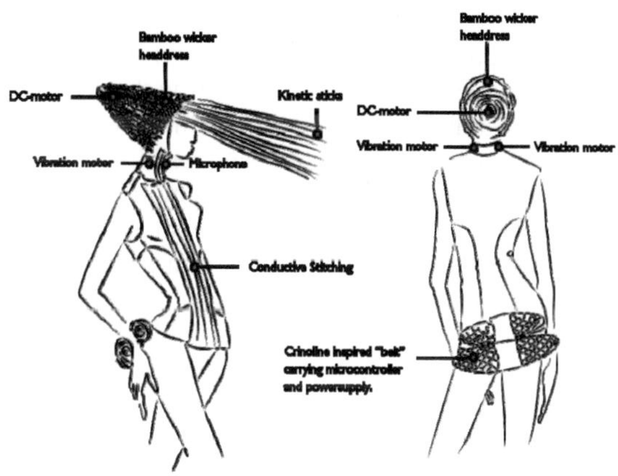

Fig. 1. The Bamboo Whisper devices, powered by Arduino Lilypads. Integrated microphones capture the vocal input. The data is send via Xbee Radios to the other wearers device in real-time to drive the DC- and vibrating motors, causing the kinetic movement and haptic feedback.

5 Observations

The sensory system constitutes a fundamental source of cognition [11]; so when working through the senses one gains an understanding of the affordances, properties and limitations of a medium that are difficult to explain or learn by means other than practical application. The occurrence of insight is inherent in the process. It is probable that this effect can be attributed to the interplay between the brain entering a resting or meditative state due to the monotonous work processes involved and the associations evoked by the haptic feedback of the materials. The entire project found its shape step-by-step within this process. The aural aspect created by the movement only became apparent when testing revealed an unintended delay in the code. This led to the discovery of the bonnet "talking back". Subsequently the project was adapted to an initial prototype that enabled the bonnet to "talk" directly to the public. This approach sits in contrast to conducting experiments in controlled laboratory environments that easily trigger preconceived cognitive patterns or reactions: behavior is not the same as it would be in a natural setting. Therefore, presenting Bamboo Whisper in a performative, public setting is a strategy and effective research technique to gauge and observe underlying attitudes toward the design of wearables [12].When the prototype was exhibited, visitors usually suspected motion-detection was triggering the hats' movement and paced about in front of the mannequin wearing the device. Unable to produce a controllable response, they disregarded the reaction as being random and lost interest. They only continued to play if they established a working relationship with the bamboo. One observer associated the clacking sticks with human echolocation, a technique applied by a minority of blind people to orient themselves within objects, working similarly to the sonar of several animal species.

6 Discussion/Results

When applying creative practice in research, the process starts with the recognition of an interesting aesthetic phenomenon and combines it with seemingly unrelated fields of interest. In the case of Bamboo Whisper, the fascinating appearance and physical properties of a traditionally woven basket is transformed into an instrument to explore extended capacities of human communication. The intuitive approach of the creative practitioner to a subject leads to unforeseen results which do not need an interpretation as such. Instead the crafted product is placed in a performative setting, opening up for the possibilities of spontaneous interaction with the public. Observing reactions and evaluating interpretations can facilitate new insights. Avoiding traditional methods such as representative user groups and controlled settings, in combination with the strong presentation aesthetics, allows for extreme and normally overlooked aspects to emerge. One example of this is the association of echolocation with the clacking of the moving sticks. Confidence in both the value of the process and that the means will ultimately lead to the goal negates a concept of failure, a prerequisite to maintaining the receptive state of mind paramount to achieving results.

7 Future Development

A congruent next step will be to expand the project to encompass a swarm of devices in a large network, engaging the wearers in a collective experience shaping a bizarre yet common space defined by new modes and parameters of interaction. Likewise, introducing new testing devices which are controlled by the public and enhance public engagement in the haptic experience will add another angle to the experiment.

Further, the responses to the audible aspect and potentials of Bamboo Whisper, are encouraging development of evolutionary designs, catering directly for use as echolocation devices, investigating the possibility of creating artificially induced multi-modal transfer. In this regard selecting user-groups with abnormal sensory development could provide new and extraordinary insights to the project.

Acknowledgements. Bamboo Whisper was developed as part of Haptic InterFace 2012, with support from the Wearables Lab at the AVA HKBU, Seeed Studios, Woolmark Company and the Medienförderung Rhineland-Palatinate. Flanagan was supported with funding from HKBU RC-NACADFLANAGAN PJ 38-40-006, Frankjaer from the PROMOS program of the DAAD.

References

1. Eisner, E.: Does Arts-Based Research Have a Future? Inaugural Lecture for the First European Conference on Arts-Based Research: Belfast. Northern Ireland (June 2005); Studies in art education 48(1), 9–18 (2006)
2. Inouye, A.S., Mitchell, W.J., Blumenthal, M.S. (eds.): Beyond productivity: Information technology, innovation, and creativity, pp. 96–117. National Academy Press (2003)
3. Barone, T., Eisner, E.W.: Arts based research, p. 1. SAGE Publications, Inc. (2011)
4. Sen, A.: The Tacit Dimension. University of Chicago Press (2009)
5. Kounios, J., Fleck, J.I., Green, D.L., Payne, L., Stevenson, J.L., Bowden, E.M., Jung-Beeman, M.: The origins of insight in resting-state brain activity. Neuropsychologia 46(1), 281–291 (2008)
6. Kounios, J., Beeman, M.: The Aha! Moment The Cognitive Neuroscience of Insight. Current Directions in Psychological Science 18(4), 210–216 (2009)
7. Wilson, S.: Information arts: Intersections of art, science, and technology, p. 28. The MIT Press (2002)
8. Lakhani, K.R., Jeppesen, L.B., Lohse, P.A., Panetta, J.A.: The Value of Openess in Scientific Problem Solving. Division of Research, Harvard Business School (2007)
9. Cairns, P., Cox, A.L.: Research methods for human-computer interaction, pp. 138–157. Cambridge University Press (2008)
10. Flanagan, P.: Haptic Interface Aesthetics - HCII 2013 Conf. Proc. Springer LNCS of LNAI series (2013)
11. Gallese, V., Lakoff, G.: The brain's concepts: The role of the sensory-motor system in conceptual knowledge. Cognitive Neuropsychology 22(3-4), 455–479 (2005)
12. Garabet, A., Mann, S., Fung, J.: Exploring design through wearable computing art (ifacts). In: CHI 2002 Extended Abstracts on Human Factors in Computing Systems, pp. 634–635. ACM (2002)

Task-Oriented M-Commerce Interface Design

Eugenia Y. Huang[1], Yu-Ju Lin[1], and Travis K. Huang[2]

[1] National Chengchi University, Department of Management Information Systems, Taiwan
[2] Ling Tung University, Department of Information Management, Taiwan
{huang.eugenia,frank78525,travisk.huang}@gmail.com

Abstract. As pocket-size mobile devices are equipped with relatively small screen, when displaying web pages which are designed for personal computers and laptops, viewing poses a great challenge. Due to the limited space, items or components on the screen of pocket-size mobile devices should be much more intuitive so that users can interact with the interface more quickly. Thus, the study posits that m-commerce mandates a completely different approach, namely scenario-based design, to interface design which is task-oriented rather than functional-oriented. The result can be further summarized and compared with prior research which focused on a list of design factors.

Keywords: m-commerce, scenario-based design, interface design.

1 Introduction

Advances of technology has enabled much more satisfying internet surfing experience, as compared with almost two decades ago when World Wide Web just emerged and quickly became the widely accepted platform for e-commerce. Nowadays, being present on WWW is no longer a novel move, but a necessity for business survival. Further, with the tremendous penetration speed of pocket-size mobile devices, such as smart phones and mini pads, online experience has now extended to the tether-less world. Surfing the internet on the go is rapidly becoming a preferred life style and often a necessity of life for many people. Yet smooth transition from e-commerce to m-commerce requires that businesses recognize a major paradigm shift in web interface design.

As pocket-size mobile devices are equipped with relatively small screen, when displaying web pages and previous design procedure were deeply influenced by traditional methodologies. It is necessary to create a mobile vision of web interface with better considering the characteristics of pocket-size mobile devices.

The objective of the study is to identify critical tasks while designing web interface for pocket-size mobile devices based on a task-oriented methodology, namely scenario-based design. Due to the complexity of scenario-based design, all the design phases should be taken into consideration. Thus, three rounds of focus groups will be held in order to collect ideas and opinions from participants. In the future, the result will be summarized and compared with prior research which focused on a list of design factors, to demonstrate the feasibility of a scenario-based design for m-commerce user interface.

C. Stephanidis (Ed.): Posters, Part I, HCII 2013, CCIS 373, pp. 36–40, 2013.

2 Literature Review

2.1 Design Factors for E-Commerce Website

In the field of interface design, researchers have made much effort to identify critical design factors. For example, Cyr [1] found that website navigation design, website visual design, and website information design had positive effects on website satisfaction. Javenpaa and Todd [5] summarized four aspect of functional factors, including product perception, shopping experience, customer service and consumer risks. Wan [14] proposed four categories of factors that affected website quality, namely information, friendliness, responsiveness, and reliability. Furthermore, Zhang & von Dran [15], Liang & Lai [9], Huang & Fu [4] utilized Herzberg's two factor theory [2] to improve websites, to attract customers and even to make customers to revisit the websites by identifying hygiene and motivation factors [13,15]. While hygiene factors refer to the necessary functionality and increase the degree of customer's willingness to visit the website, motivation factors motivate users to revisit the website.

Besides, Zhang and von Dran [16] stated that different types of websites should pay attention to different factors, and that some factors which are critical to one type of website may not be suitable for another. Whether a design factor is critical or not may depend on the website type. For instance, the top five factors of e-commerce website are data security, easy to navigate, appropriate explanation, search tools, and the price of product and service, respectively.

2.2 The Framework of Mobile Commerce Interface

With the bloom of mobile telephony, people gradually get used to browsing websites with mobile devices. However, the interface of traditional website which was designed for PC or laptops does not fit the small screen of mobile devices. Thus, using pocket-size mobile devices to browse traditional e-commerce websites will encounter difficulties. As the study of interface design for mobile commerce was just emerging, Lee and Benbasat [8] summarized previous research and proposed the framework of mobile commerce interface, in which seven design elements of the framework were presented, including context, content, community, customization, communication, connection, and commerce.

Basically, a "commerce" interface or website must provide a safe purchasing environment. "Context" and "connection" indicate that designers should put appropriate links to let customer navigate smoothly and achieve their goals easily. "Content" and "customization" refer to the web page should provide the nearby users with specific information. "Community" represents that it is necessary to provide a way for people to exchange information in m-commerce interface. Finally, "communication" is the feedback between customers and organizations. Thus, according to the feedback, organizations can improve services, and customers can get useful offerings or promotions.

2.3 Scenario-Based Design

With the tremendous progress of information technology, the interactive systems become more and more popular. Designers have paid more and more attention to users' real requirements and preference. However, in interactive systems, some requirements are not definite enough and it is difficult to acquire those requirements in the early stages. In this regard, the focus is shifted to the system usability, which includes the concepts of ease of learning, ease of use, and user satisfaction [12]. Besides functional requirements, there are still some non-functional requirements such as portability, reliability, and maintainability that will finally influence system usability. On the other hand, factor-based design concepts described above seem to follow the traditional system development life cycle. Users are not highly-involved until prototype system is implemented. Once users are not satisfied with the prototype system, designers need to adjust or even come back to redesign the system. Consequently, in order to improve this phenomenon, scenario-based design is a better methodology to conduct our research and to identify appropriate tasks which can be integrated into m-commerce websites.

Scenarios are just like stories and emphasize the coordination of information resources and data. Besides, scenarios have several significant elements including setting, agents or actors, goals or objectives, and a plot. The framework of scenario-based design is consisted of five steps, including developing problem scenarios, designing activity scenarios, designing information scenarios, designing interaction scenarios, and evaluating prototype. First of all, by analyzing requirements appropriately, a problem scenario, which describes the practical activities that need to be revised and improved, will be proposed. Second, activity design will be developed based on the problem scenario. More specifically, designers need to develop a proper and specific solution to improve current activities and utilize information technology wisely. The objective of activity design is focusing on system capability including both functional and non-functional requirements rather than user interface design. Third, information design includes general data on the interface and visual elements such as dialog boxes, icons or menus. Also, Designers should make a good arrangement of elements on the screen, and confirm the meanings of all objects' representation. Whereas the focus of information design is to present all design elements on the screen clearly, the objective of interaction design is to help people execute their tasks smoothly. Finally, in order to evaluate the design idea, a prototype system will be implemented and verified. Although many design elements are not well-defined yet, users can evaluate the design by using both the scenarios and prototype. According to the result of evaluation, designers get an opportunity to further improve their design.

3 Research Method

The study intends to apply a task-oriented approach, namely scenario-based design, to identify critical subtasks while designing m-commerce interface for pocket-size mobile devices. Numerous potential issues should be considered in designing user interface, including synergism, stimulation, security, spontaneity, and snowballing

[3]. To make sense of what issues matter the most in helping users accomplish tasks, this research employs three rounds of focus group studies [7] to conduct each phase of design.

Participants should be familiar with the use of pocket-size mobile device and have shopping experience on the e-commerce website, because experienced users can easily comprehend the problem and propose more ideas for the revision of the design in each step of scenario-based design. In addition, as Morgan [11] suggested, a small group is more efficient and effective for complex problems. Due to the complexity of the scenario-based design, we use a small group design process. There are nine members in the focus group. This is in accordance to Merton, Fiske, and Kendall's [10] suggestion. In order to allow full discussion, two to three hours are allocated for each round of focus group study.

Topic and question approach are two important portions to generating focus group questions [6]. The study tries to develop detailed questions regarding scenarios in order to handle the whole process perfectly and to analyze easily. Also, our questions should stay away from technical language, be brief and specific [7]. In the study, there are five types of focus group questions, including opening questions, introductory questions, transition questions, key questions, and concluding questions [7].

The study will focus on four steps of scenario-based design. However, because presentation and execution frequently happen simultaneously, information design and interaction design will be conducted in the same session. Therefore, as each step has its specific objective, our study will conduct three rounds of focus group to obtain detailed information corresponding to four steps of scenario-based design.

In the first session of focus group, the focus is requirements analysis. The study will conduct the focus group to generate problem scenarios and claims by asking all participants questions, observing their reactions, and even drawing diagrams. Problem scenarios refer to the detail descriptions of current activities, while claims are the advantages and disadvantages.

In the second round of focus group, the study intends to conduct activity design which includes functional and non-functional features. By referencing problem scenarios and claims, participants can specify their design ideas deliberately with appropriate information technologies. Metaphors and useful information technologies will be identified in this step. The output of this session includes activity scenario and claims.

In the last round of focus group, information design and interaction design will be conducted simultaneously. While the purpose of information design is to arrange appropriate elements on the screen for enhancing user's perception, interpretation, and making sense of what they see, the goal of interaction design is to construct a list of user interaction and system response step by step. Interaction design will focus on how to use and operate the system. Participants can combine these design ideas to construct both information scenarios and interaction scenarios. Besides, claims will be improved synchronously in order to help the study to retain advantages and remove disadvantages.

After summarizing the findings in three sessions of focus group, the result will be further compared with prior research which focused on a list of design factors.

References

1. Cyr, D.: Modeling Website Design across Cultures: Relationships to Trust, Satisfaction, and E-Loyalty. Journal of MIS 24, 47–72 (2008)
2. Herzberg, F., Bermard, M., Synderman, B.: The Motivation to Work. Wiley, New York (1959)
3. Hess, J.M.: Group Interviewing. In: King, R.L. (ed.) New Science of Planning. American Marketing Association, Chicago (1968)
4. Huang, T.K., Fu, F.L.: Understanding User Interface Needs of E-Commerce Web Sites. Behavior & Information Technology 28, 461–469 (2009)
5. Jarvenpaa, S.L., Todd, P.A.: Consumer Relations to Electronic Shopping on the World Wide Web. IJEC 1, 59–88 (1996)
6. Kruger, R.A.: Developing Questions for Focus Groups (Focus Group Kit), vol. 3. Sage Publications, Thousand Oaks (1998)
7. Krueger, R.A., Casey, M.A.: Focus group: A Practical Guide for Applied Research, 3rd edn. Sage Publications, London (2000)
8. Lee, Y.E., Benvasat, I.: A Framework for the Study of Customer Interface Design for Mobile Commerce. IJEC 8, 79–102 (2004)
9. Liang, T.P., Lai, H.J.: Effect of Store Design on Consumer Purchases: An Empirical Study of On-Line Bookstores. Information & Management 39, 431–444 (2002)
10. Merton, R.K., Fiske, M., Kendall, P.L.: The Focus Interview. The Free Press, New York (1990)
11. Morgan, D.L.: Planning Focus groups (Focus Group Kit), vol. 2. Sage Publications, Thousand Oaks (1998)
12. Rosson, M.B., Carroll, J.M.: Usability Engineering: Scenario-Based Design Development of Human-Computer Interaction, 1st edn. Morgan Kaufmann, San Francisco (2001)
13. Valacich, J.S., Parboteeah, D.V., Wells, J.D.: The Online Consumer's Hierarchy of Needs. CACM 50, 84–90 (2007)
14. Wan, H.A.: Opportunities to Enhance a Commercial Website. Information & Management 38, 15–21 (2000)
15. Zhang, P., von Dran, G.M.: Satisfiers and Dissatistiers: A Two-Factor Model for Website Design and Evaluation. JASIST 51, 1253–1268 (2000)
16. Zhang, P., von Dran, G.M.: User Expectations and Ranking of Quality Factors in Different Web Site Domains. IJEC 6, 9–33 (2011)

Towards Exploring Web Interface Sign Ontology: A User Study

Muhammad Nazrul Islam

Turku Centre for Computer Science (TUCS)
Department of Information Technologies
Åbo Akademi University, 20520 Turku, Finland
nazrulturku@gmail.com

Abstract. The smallest elements of web user interface (UI) like navigation links, buttons, icons, labels, thumbnails, symbols, etc. are defined in this paper as interface signs.The term Ontology is referred to the set of concepts and skills a user should own in order to understand the meaning of an interface sign. Designer should aware of web interface sign ontology to design user-intuitive web interface signs to get an idea what kind of presupposed knowledge end users hold to interpret the web interface signs. The objective of this research is to reveal the set ontologies available in web UI and the complexity associated with different ontological signs to interpret the meaning of web interface sign from semiotics perspective. Towards achieving the research goals a user study was replicated with 26 participants. So far, a preliminary analysis has performed on 13 participants' data and reports the preliminary outcomes in this work-in-progress paper.

Keywords: Semiotics, web usability, user interface design, web sign ontology.

1 Introduction

The content and functions of web applications are usually directed by interface signs to provide the system's logic to the end users. For instance, (i) to access the admission information, a prospective student should click on 'Admissions' sign of a university website, (ii) to submit an online application form a user should click on the 'Submit' button, and the like. Designing intuitive interface signs is vital to achieve the goal of communicability, user satisfaction, learn ability, effective and efficient use, etc… i.e., the usability standards of web applications[1],[2],[3],[4],[5]. The interface sign design principles are semiotics by nature as semiotics is considered as the doctrine of signs [6]. A complete definition of semiotics can be defined as "the study of signs, signification, and signifying systems" [7]. Speroni [2] defined the term 'ontology' as the set of concepts and skills that a user should own for understanding the referential meaning of an interface sign. From the users' perspective, ontology is the knowledge or concepts that are needed to understand and properly interpret the meaning of an interface sign. From the designers' perspective, it is the knowledge or concepts presupposed and pointed by an interface sign. UI designers need to know what kind of

C. Stephanidis (Ed.): Posters, Part I, HCII 2013, CCIS 373, pp. 41–45, 2013.

presupposed knowledge end users hold to interpret web interface signs. For example, if a sign 'inbox' in email application is designed well in terms of representation, position, etc. but if a user don't know the concept it refers to then this sign will not make any sense to him/her to interpret its meaning. The set of ontologies to interpret interface signs lead designers to understand the paradigm of users' interpretations of interface signs. Again, the concept of interpretation complexities associated to different ontological signs help a designer to design user-intuitive interface signs. According to Speroni [2], the most common ontologies used in many websites are: Inter Locutor/Institution Ontology, Internet Ontology, Website Ontology, Commonsense Ontology, Web Domain Ontology, Topic Ontology, and Context Ontology. Speroni's [2] concept and definition of Ontology are used as background theory in this paper. Speroni [2] presents these ontologies as an example list of most common ontologies used in information intensive web UI. He also stated that the set of ontologies might be varying depending on different websites. Again a number of studies were conducted to observe the interpretation complexity associated to each of these ontologies for different websites, for instance [8], [9], [10], [11]. These studies were conducted mainly by expert inspection. Therefore, few important issues raise such as (i) what kind of ontologies may exist web user interfaces in general, rather than only in information intensive web user interfaces, (ii) how much complexity are associated with different ontological signs, (iii) what kind of ontological signs are comparatively more intuitive to interpret, and the like. Therefore two questions for this research are formulated as which ontologies are available in web user interfaces in general? How interpretation difficulties are associated to each ontological signs to interpret the meaning of interface signs?

2 Research Method

A user study following a semi structured user interview research method was conducted to attain the research objective. The fundamental objective of this study was to reveal the factors of users' interpretations of interface signs. However, the scope of this paper is limited to a specific objective, which is a part of the fundamental objective. Indeed, the objective of this study is to find the set of ontologies in web UI and the interpretation complexities associated to each ontological signs. The study was replicated with 26student participants at usability test laboratory in Finland.A total 72 Interface signs were selected from user interfaces of two web application domains (online calendar and email application) and two web domains (university and museum websites). Selected interface signs were presented them in a different form (i.e., sign without context and with context). Participants were not allowed to click on the signs, they were only supposed to response to a number of questions for each interface sign such as what could be the referential meaning of this sign?Why do you think this (user's response for the first question) as the meaning of this sign? How much complicacy or difficulty do you feel to interpret this sign (score: 1(very easy) – 7(extremely difficult))? How certain or confident are you that you are right in your interpretation (score: 1(very low) – 7(very high))? The methodology is discussed more comprehensively in [13].

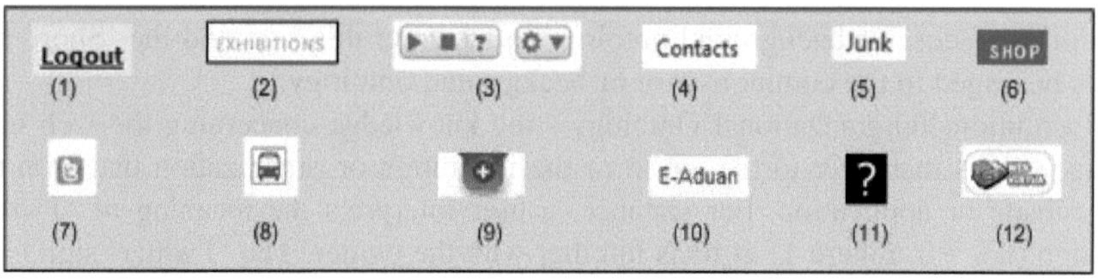

Fig. 1. A list of example interface signs selected for this user test

3 Preliminary Results and Conclusions

So far, data for the 13 test-participants are transcribed, summarized and synthesized. The preliminary results observed that the following ontologies are available in web user interfaces in general:

1. Internet Ontology – this ontology refers to the knowledge of the world of web, web browsing and its concepts and conventions. For instance, as a basis of interpreting the 'Logout' sign (no. 1 in Figure 1) a user responses as "…All kind of web application has this sign. Underline refers to hyperlink since the 19s internet…" That means the user uses his internet ontology to interpret this sign and the 'Logout' sign is belonged to internet ontology.
2. System's Real World Ontology - this ontology refers to the knowledge of the system's real world, its functionalities and concepts. For instance, a user never visit museum websites but experienced (visited) real world museum. He interprets the sign 'Exhibition' (no. 2 in Figure 1) properly based on his museum's real world ontology.
3. Computer Ontology - the knowledge concerning the world of computer and computer uses. This mainly concerns the web interface signs which are common in computer OS and applications (e.g., windows OS, MS word, etc.). For instance, a user interprets the sign number 3 in Figure 1 based on his familiarity with windows media player.
4. Mobile Ontology - the knowledge concerning the world of mobile and mobile application uses. This mainly concerns the web interface signs which are common in mobile phones and also in mobile applications. For instance, a user interprets the 'Contact' sign (no. 3 in Figure 1) based on his familiarity with mobile phone uses.
5. Web Domain Ontology - the knowledge concerning the web interface signs which are specific enough to a particular web domain (e.g., educational web domain, email application domain, etc.). For instance, as a basis of interpreting the 'Junk' sign (no. 5 in Figure 1) a user responses as "my previous knowledge of using email application". That means the user uses his web domain ontology to interpret this sign and the 'Junk' sign is belonged to the web domain ontology.
6. Common-Sense/Background Ontology- the knowledge concerning concepts belonging to common background of users and uses common sense. For instance, as a basis of interpreting the 'Shop' sign (no. 6 in Figure 1) a user responses as"…interpret based on the word meaning…" That means the user uses his

commonsense or background ontology to interpret this sign and the 'Shop' sign is belonged to the commonsense or background ontology.

7. Institutional/Organizational Ontology - the knowledge concerning the web interface signs that refer to the world of the institution or organization that won that website or application. For instance, a user interprets the meaning of 'Twitter' sign (no. 7 in Figure 1) as he is familiar with the twitter. The 'Twitter' sign is belonged to the institutional/organizational ontology.
8. Real World Ontology - this ontology refers to the knowledge of the real world experiences and concepts. For instance, a user interprets the meaning of 'Bus' sign (no. 8 in Figure 1) in a museum website since he is familiar with the bus sign in real life at every bus stops.
9. Cultural/Environmental Ontology - the knowledge concerning the web interface signs which are specific enough to a particular cultural or environmental context. For instance, a user interprets the meaning of 'red color plus' sign (no. 9 in Figure 1) as a museum hospital or medical help centre at museum based on her experience in a specific country context, where red color plus sign refers to the hospital or medical help. The actual meaning of this sign was to expand a menu list in a museum website.
10. Website Ontology - the knowledge concerning the web interface signs which are specific enough to a particular website, e.g., a specific sign could be used in a university website to represent the departments and this could be intuitively understandable only to the users who are familiar with this particular website. For instance, as a basis of interpreting the 'E-aduan' sign (no. 1 in Figure 1) a user responses as"…I never seen this word before…".The user was unable to interpret this sign due to the lack of his knowledge of website ontology as he never visits the websites that hold this sign.
11. Topic Ontology - the knowledge concerning the particular subject or topic the website talks about. For instance, '?' (No. 11 in Figure 1) is actually stands for providing information about a topic (an exhibition) in spy museum. A user knows that this sign stands for providing information about a topic but he failed to understand the topic properly. One of the reasons for this was the lack of familiarity with this topic (topic ontology) to interpret its meaning properly.

It is important to mention here that the ontology number 1, 5-7, 10 and 11 were stated by Speroni in [2]. Preliminary results also observed that the level of complexity experienced in interpreting the meaning of interface signs varied depending on different ontological signs.To interpret the meaning of interface signs properly end user experiences comparatively-

- Higher level of difficulty with signs belongs to Website Ontology.
- Above average level of difficulty with signs belong to Institutional/Organizational Ontology, Cultural/Environmental Ontology, and Topic Ontology.
- Average level of difficulty with signs belongs to System's Real World Ontology, Web Domain Ontology, and Real World Ontology.
- Lower level of difficulty with signs belongs to Internet Ontology, Computer Ontology, Mobile Ontology, and Common Sense / Background Ontology.

An interface sign may belong to multiple ontologies rather than sign ontology. In other word, a user may use multiple ontologies to interpret an interface signs. For instant, a user interprets the 'Web Virtua' sign (no. 12 in Figure 1) by using website ontology, cultural/environment ontology and web domain ontology, i.e., this sign belong to multiple ontologies. Further research is needed to observe the interpretation complexities for interface signs that belongs to multiple ontologies or interpreted by using multiple ontologies.

However, this work-in-progress paper reports the preliminary outcomes, where half of the test-participants data were considered. Author is intended to conduct a rigorous analysis considering the complete set of study data to provide a complete set of web interface sign ontology and the complexity associated with different ontological signs to interpret the meaning of web interface sign will depict more evidently.

References

1. DeSouze, C.S.: The Semiotic Engineering of Human-Computer Interaction. The MIT Press, Cambridge (2005)
2. Speroni, M.: Mastering the Semiotics of Information-Intensive Web Interfaces. Unpublished doctoral dissertation, Faculty of Communication Sciences, University of Lugano, Switzerland (2006)
3. Islam, M.N.: A Systematic Literature Review of Semiotics Perception in User Interfaces. Journal of Systems and Information Technology (JSIT) 15(1), 45–77 (2013)
4. Islam, M.N., Tetard, F.: Integrating Semiotics Perception in Usability Testing to Improve Usability Evaluation. In: Garcia-Ruiz, M.A. (ed.) Cases on Usability Engineering: Design and Development of Digital Products, pp. 145–169. IGI Global, USA (2013)
5. Islam, M.N.: A Semiotics Perspective to Web Usability: An Empirical case Study. In: IADIS Interfaces and Human Computer Interaction 2011, pp. 19–28. IADIS (2011)
6. Peirce, C.S.: Collected Writings (8 Vols.). Hartshorne, C., Weiss, P., Burks, A. (eds.), vol. 1-8. Harvard University Press (1931-1952)
7. Robert, S., Robert, B., Sandy, F.L.: New Vocabularies in Film Semiotics: Structuralism, Post-Structuralism and Beyond. Taylor & Francis, London (1992)
8. Islam, M.N., Ali, M., Al-Mamun, A., Islam, M.: Semiotics Explorations on Designing the Information Intensive Web Interfaces. International Arab Journal of Information Technology 7(1), 45–54 (2010)
9. Islam, M.N.: Semiotics of the Web Interface: Analysis and Guidelines. Journal of Computer Science and Technology (JCS&T) 8(3), 166–167 (2008)
10. Islam, M.N.: Towards Designing Users' Intuitive Web Interface. In: 6th International Conference on Complex, Intelligent, and Software Intensive Systems (CISIS 2012), pp. 513–518. IEEE Computer Society (2012)
11. Islam, M.N.: Semiotics Perception towards Designing Users' Intuitive Web User Interface: A Study on Web Sign Redesign. In: Rahman, H., Mesquita, A., Ramos, I., Pernici, B. (eds.) MCIS 2012. LNBIP, vol. 129, pp. 139–155. Springer, Heidelberg (2012)
12. Stanton, N.S., Young, M.S.: A guide to methodology in Ergonomics. Taylor & Francis, UK (1999)
13. Islam, M.N.: Towards determinants of user-intuitive web interface signs. In: Marcus, A. (ed.) DUXU/HCII 2013, Part I. LNCS, vol. 8012, pp. 84–93. Springer, Heidelberg (2013)

Designing for Culturally Diverse Audiences: Can Automated Attention Analysis Substitute the Eye-Tracking in Website Development?

Tomáš Kincl, Michal Novák, and Michal Charvát

Faculty of Management, University of Economics, Prague. Jarošovská 1117/II, 377 01 Jindřichův Hradec, Czech Republic
{kincl.tomas,charvatmi}@gmail.com, novak@michalnovak.eu

Abstract. Developers use a variety of methods to evaluate user's reactions to the website. Research in neuroscience and natural vision processing resulted in the development of automated methods which simulate human attention and are able to provide similar results to eye-tracking. However robust evidence is still missing.

This study contributes and expands on this debate. Eye-tracking studies on cultural differences confirmed that users from different cultures have different expectations and preferences. This study answers the question whether cultural differences in web design could be revealed also by automated attention analysis. Websites of the largest beer producers from different countries with different cultural background were analyzed through automated attention analysis tool to determine whether there is a difference in the number of potential areas of interest and their size. The study confirms that automated tools can depict cultural differences and thus provide fast and inexpensive results for initial assessment of website interfaces.

Keywords: culture, differences, webdesign, attention analysis, automated tool.

1 Introduction

One of the key components of website development is design testing [1]. Web developers use a variety of methods to evaluate user's reactions to the website [2]. For instance, eye-tracking can be used to determine user's visual attention over objects on the website [3]. However, eye-tracking is usually an extensive resource-consuming exercise and requires highly skilled researchers capable to analyze and interpret research evidence [4]. Research in neuroscience and natural vision processing resulted in the development of automated methods which simulate human attention and thus might be able to provide similar results to eye-tracking studies [5]. Website snapshot can be automatically analyzed on various features to predict consumer's reactions to visual stimuli. The analysis includes several website features such as color, orientation, density, contrast, intensity, size, weight, closure, length, width or

C. Stephanidis (Ed.): Posters, Part I, HCII 2013, CCIS 373, pp. 46–50, 2013.

curve of displayed objects (including skin color and face detection). Developers of those automated detection tools claim 75-90 % correlation with real eye-tracking data, however much debate has evolved around their ability to simulate human perception and robust evidence is missing [6].

The aim of this study is to contribute and expand on this debate. Eye-tracking studies on cultural differences in web design confirmed that consumers from different cultures have different expectations and preferences [7]. This study answers the question whether cultural differences in web design could be revealed also by automated attention analysis. A number of websites of the largest beer producers from six countries (ten largest from each country) with different cultural background were analyzed through automated attention analysis tool to determine whether there is a difference in the number of potential areas of interest and their size. Our study confirms that automated tools can be useful to depict cultural differences and thus could provide fast and inexpensive results for initial assessment of website interfaces.

2 Research Design and Methodology

Market interdependence has stimulated emergence of theories trying to explain differences between markets [8]. With a massive expansion of World Wide Web, web designers also began reflecting user‘s cultural characteristics [9]. Culture impacts on web design as well as on web content [10]. Websites need to be culturally adapted [11] and studies on cultural differences in web design supported the hypothesis that consumers from different cultures have different expectations and preferences about web design [12], [13]. This has been also confirmed by eye-tracking studies [7]. This study answers the question whether cultural differences could be revealed also by automated attention analysis.

Research sample consisted of commercial websites of large beer brands. Beer is popular with consumers across the world and has been the most widespread alcohol drink [14]. Local beer markets offer opportunity to global as well as local brands, whereas brand cultural belongingness is usually well articulated. Beer is also a product with comparable price and societal positioning in most cultures [15]. All selected countries have ranked on top positions in beer consumption and production per capita and have strong beer culture and tradition [16] (but national cultures differ [17]).

The study also included (as a control group) a group of prime international brands with highest worldwide consumption (in the case the brand has been previously selected as a national brand, it was surveyed with the international group only as international brands could speak different than local cultural values). List of all websites included in the study is in Table 1.

Opening introductory web sites (in resolution, which was the most typical at the time of research) were surveyed. Screenshots were then analyzed through Feng-Gui (http://www.feng-gui.com) tool for the number of areas of interest (AOIs) which would be likely the focal points of user eye activity. The number of AOIs was captures as well as the overall area occupied by AOIs (in pixels).

Table 1. List of Surveyed Websites

Czech Republic	Great Britain	Japan
Gambrinus	Carling	Asahi
Radegast	John Smith's	Kirin
Staropramen	Old Speckled Hen	Suntory
Krušovice	Cobra	Sapporo
Pilsner Urquell	Newcastle Brown	Orion
Budějovický Budvar	Fuller's London Pride	Baird
Bernard	Hobgoblin	Taisetsu Ji Bīru
Velkopopovický Kozel	Marston's Pedigree	Okhotsk Bīru
Starobrno	Abbot Alle	Tokachi Bīru
Ostravar	Tanglefoot	Otaru Bīru
Germany	**Brazil**	**International**
Oettinger	Brahma	Snow (China)
Krombacher	Antárctica	Budlight (USA)
Bitburger	Cintra	Budweiser (USA)
Warsteiner	Bohemia	Skol (Brazil)
Beck's	Bavaria	Corona (Mexico)
Hasseröder	Nova Schin	Heineken (Netherlands)
Veltins	Kaiser	Miller Lite (USA)
Paulaner	Xingu	Guiness (UK)
Radeberger	Colonia	Coors (USA)
Erdinger	Stella Artois	Fosters (Australia)

3 Results and Conclusion

Paired similarity in number and area of AOIs was tested through non-parametric Mann-Whitney test [18]. The analysis was performed through SPSS Statistical Software. Table 2 depicts the key findings.

Czech British and German beer sites are similar in terms of number and size of focal points. All three markets are labeled as low context; hence approaching consumers through websites might be similar. All three website groups feature rich and vibrant colors with shades emphasizing trust, tradition or nature. Number of interactive objects is high complemented by rich information content. Number and size of AOIs is different for Czech sites and for the Japanese ones. Japan is considered one of the most high context cultures. Absence of interactive features could be explained through the lens of Japanese cultural distinctiveness. Traditional beer cultures use rich and vibrant colors bringing forward natural and calming impressions, Japanese beer websites utilize plain white color which reduces first-impression attractiveness.

Number of AOIs (but not their size) is different for Brazilian and International brands and for Czech leading beers. Several international brands do not originate from western low-context cultures but from Asia or Latin America featuring fewer interactive qualities less diverse and informative content and are less informative in general. Number of AOIs is different for Great Britain, Japanese, Brazilian and International brands comparison. Representation of non-Western brands from high context cultures which do not have English websites could explain some of the differences. The number of AOIs is higher on Germans websites and they are smaller than on Japanese (Brazilian and International) websites. German websites seems to be on the half way between traditional brewing countries and the other groups.

The number of AOIs is similar on of Japanese and International (and Brazilian) websites. In contrary, there is a difference between AOIs size. International (and Brazilian) websites stand on the verge between East and West. There was no difference in number of AOIs or their size. It may well be that developing or emerging markets seem more promising for international beer brewers. Traditional beer cultures typically host several strong local brands which outperform international brands.

Table 2. The Results

		Great Britain	Japan	Germany	Brazil	International
Czech Republic	AOIs	same	different	same	different	different
	AOIs size	same	different	same	same	same
Great Britain	AOIs		different	same	different	different
	AOIs size		different	same	same	same
Japan	AOIs			same	same	same
	AOIs size			same	different	different
Germany	AOIs				same	same
	AOIs size				same	same
Brazil	AOIs					same
	AOIs size					same

Cultural differences between websites can be deduced not only through demanding resource-consuming user testing or through expert panels. Cultural differences can be diagnosed via automated tools which simulate natural vision processing. Automated tools do not reflect local fluctuations or context and are prone to inappropriate sampling and personal bias. On the other hand, automated approaches offer less rich findings. The results could be also interpreted another way, since the automated tools do not perform testing on the same basis – user testing is based on specified task and eye-tracking results could be different according to different user scenarios. The results are also influenced by prior user experience or task with the website. None of these factors are included in automated attention analysis and automated tools are not suited to depict such contingencies. Nevertheless, automated tools for website assessment have been a recent and increasingly popular phenomenon and have become prominent in other areas of web design. Automated tools can never fully substitute human experts in assessing human-computer interaction or user experience. Automated tools may provide fast and relatively inexpensive results for initial assessment of e commerce and online marketing interfaces. Using initial automated testing may significantly reduce website development cost and contribute to more efficient marketing communications.

References

1. Pressman, R.S., Lowe, D.: Web Engineering. International Journal of Information Technology and Web Engineering 4, 78–80 (2009)
2. Zikmund, W.G., Babin, B.J.: Exploring marketing research. South-Western Pub. (2006)
3. Duchowski, A.T.: A breadth-first survey of eye-tracking applications. Behavior Research Methods 34, 455–470 (2002)
4. Berger, S., Wagner, U., Schwand, C.: Assessing Advertising Effectiveness: The Potential of Goal-Directed Behavior. Psychology and Marketing 29, 411–421 (2012)
5. Mancas, M.: Computational Attention: Modelisation & Application to Audio and Image Processing. TCTS laboratory, Ph.D. thesis. Faculty of Engineering, Mons, Belgium, Mons, Belgium (2007)
6. Harty, J.: Finding usability bugs with automated tests. Communications of the ACM 54, 44–49 (2011)
7. Cyr, D., Head, M., Larios, H.: Colour appeal in website design within and across cultures: A multi-method evaluation. International Journal of Human-Computer Studies 68, 1–21 (2010)
8. Maheswaran, D., Shavitt, S.: Issues and new directions in global consumer psychology. Journal of Consumer Psychology 9, 59–66 (2000)
9. Hsieh, H.C., Holland, R., Young, M.: A Theoretical Model for Cross-Cultural Web Design. In: Kurosu, M. (ed.) HCD 2009. LNCS, vol. 5619, pp. 712–721. Springer, Heidelberg (2009)
10. Blake, B.F., Shamatta, C., Neuendorf, K.A., Hamilton, R.L.: The cross-national comparison of website feature preferences: A practical approach. International Journal of Internet Marketing and Advertising 5, 145–165 (2009)
11. Usunier, J.C., Roulin, N., Ivens, B.S.: Cultural, National, and Industry-Level Differences in B2B Web Site Design and Content. International Journal of Electronic Commerce 14, 41–88 (2009)
12. Callahan, E.: Cultural similarities and differences in the design of university web sites. Journal of Computer-Mediated Communication 11, 239–273 (2005)
13. Goyal, N., Miner, W., Nawathe, N.: Cultural differences across governmental website design, pp. 149–152. ACM (Year)
14. Ferreira, M.P., Willoughby, D.: Alcohol consumption: the good, the bad, and the indifferent. Applied Physiology, Nutrition, and Metabolism 33, 12–20 (2008)
15. Dimofte, C., Zeugner-Roth, K., Johansson, J.: Local or Global Brand Choice: Do Travelers Really Prefer Global Brands? In: Proceedings of the Global Brand Management Q7 Conference (2010)
16. Mäkelä, P., Gmel, G., Grittner, U., Kuendig, H.É., Kuntsche, S., Bloomfield, K., Room, R.: Drinking patterns and their gender differences in Europe. Alcohol and Alcoholism 41, i8 (2006)
17. House, R.J.: Culture, leadership, and organizations: The GLOBE study of 62 societies. Sage Publications, Inc. (2004)
18. Black, K.: Business statistics: Contemporary decision making. Wiley (2009)

Application of Kinect Technology in the Design of Interactive Products for Chinese Senior Citizens

Chor-Kheng Lim

Department of Art and Design, YuanZe University, Taiwan
kheng@saturn.yzu.edu.tw

Abstract. In this study, it is hoped to propose communicative pattern based on Chinese "Filial Piety" that is more intuitive and interactive and to propose the criteria for innovative technology product design to benefit senior citizens and their family members. An interactive product design: *Grass Tone interactive flowerpot*, which using Kinect as input device is proposed.

Keywords: Filial Piety, Kinect technology, interactive design, product design.

1 Introduction

Aging society is becoming a global social issue now and Taiwan is no exception."Filial Piety" is the most prominent characteristics in the Chinese culture. Xiao, Chun-Chung (2002) mentioned that, in certain perspective, the traditional Chinese culture is a culture of Filial Piety. The traditional Chinese society is one built upon it. This concept of being filial is so widely accepted in the Chinese culture that it is even influencing Taiwan's society regardless of various changes to the family structure. It is a widely adopted practice for children to take good care of their parents.

2 Problem and Objective

According to existing literature, the elderly is the focus of current studies on the issues with aging society or technology products developed for their welfare. Very few mainly address the issues of interaction between the elderly and their family members. This study therefore intends to begin with the above mentioned issue which arises from the change to the family structure due to the aging society.

This study aims to propose a more intuitive interaction communication model based on Chinese Filial Piety culture, and a guide in creating technologies that may bring benefits to the elderly and family members. Finally the life of the elderly in the future will be simulated in various scenarios, with product concept designed for the interaction between the elderly and their children based on Chinese Filial Piety culture.

C. Stephanidis (Ed.): Posters, Part I, HCII 2013, CCIS 373, pp. 51–55, 2013.

3 Concept of Filial Piety

The main purpose of the traditional Filial Piety is summarized through related studies on classical Chinese scriptures and stories, from which the communication model for the elderly and their children is derived through the understanding of this culture.

The inspiration for the product design comes from well-known poems and classical Chinese literature regarding Filial Piety:

> *Make the hearts of parents glad, without violating their wishes; make sound and sights pleasant to their ears and eyes, and make their living places comfortable. -*
> -- “孝子之養老也，樂其心不違其志，樂其耳目，安其寢處.”

Based on this concept, design guidelines for the product design as below:

-- Product which enable children to accompany elderly for his/her interest leisure activities (communication)
-- Product which can integrate with the behavior of daily life (interaction)
-- Product which related to body gesture and music (interaction)
-- Health care and daily care (communication)

4 Design Prototype: *Grass Tone* Interactive Flowerpot Design

The product for interaction and communication between the elderly and their children was designed based on the concept Filial Piety. The technologies are covered and provided for by physical interactive devices with more intuitive input model today. Kinect is the design platform.

Scenario:
It is expected to capture the movements of the elderly with physical movement input technology Kinect while they are doing gardening and exercising (Figure 1). The movements are then transformed into musical rhythm which expresses their moods,

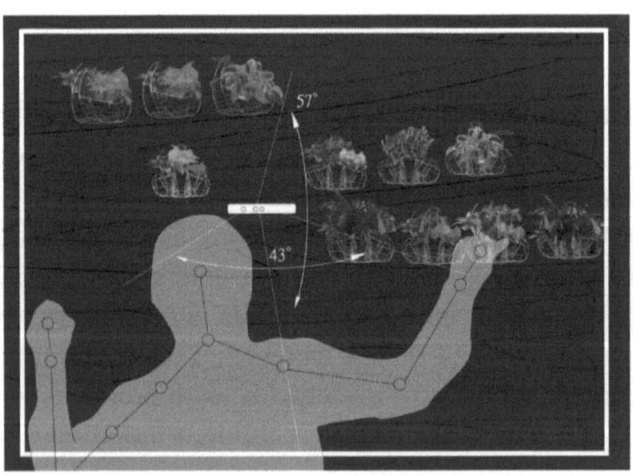

Fig. 1. Kinect capture the movements of the elderly while exercising

weather, or conditions of the plant. The interactive flowerpot will react and interact (caring and gardening also stimulate senses of hearing and sight) to please the elderly while doing gardening. During interaction, the transformed rhythm, image, or text is sent to their children via cell phone or email. This allows the children to feel what their parents feel when doing gardening and to show their care and concern. Though they are separated by long distance, children can still plant with their parents as if they are nearby.

Interactive Elements with Chinese Culture:
Grass Tone is an interactive flowerpot design for elderly, which engage elderly to do gardening and exercising to reach their healthcare and family communication. The interactive elements of this design derived from Chinese culture:

In the ancient times, Chinese people had profound knowledge of the relationship between music and emotion and body organs, which is known as the theory of the five notes (do, re, mi, so, la)"五音", five elements (metal, wood, water, fire and earth) "五行, and five zang-organs (liver, heart, spleen, lung, kidney) "五臟". These theories are interrelated as figure 2.

表一、五味、五色、五音及五行與人體五臟相對應表[3]

自然界 Nature						5 elements	人體 Body				
flavors 五味	colors 五色	notes 五音	weather 氣候	season 季節	position 方位	五行	organs 臟	腑	features 五官	五體	emotions 五志
酸	青	宮 do	風	春	東	木	肝 liver	膽	眼	筋	怒
苦	赤	商 re	暑	夏	南	火	心 heart	小腸	舌	脈	喜
甘	黃	角 mi	濕	長夏	中	土	脾 spleen	胃	口	肉	思
辛	白	徵 so	燥	秋	西	金	肺 lung	大腸	鼻	皮毛	悲
鹹	黑	羽 la	寒	冬	北	水	腎 kidney	膀胱	耳	骨	恐

Fig. 2. Relationship between music, emotion and body organs

Figure 3.shows the relationship between interactive elements of flowerpot design. First, flowerpots sense the weather condition as input data, and play the corresponding music. Elderly follow the music rhythm and does related exercise. Kinect capture the body movement and gestures, and then trigger the watering system and LED light on the flowerpots. Data of the weather condition and body movement capture by Kinect will send via internet to the children side after parents finish their exercise (figure 4).

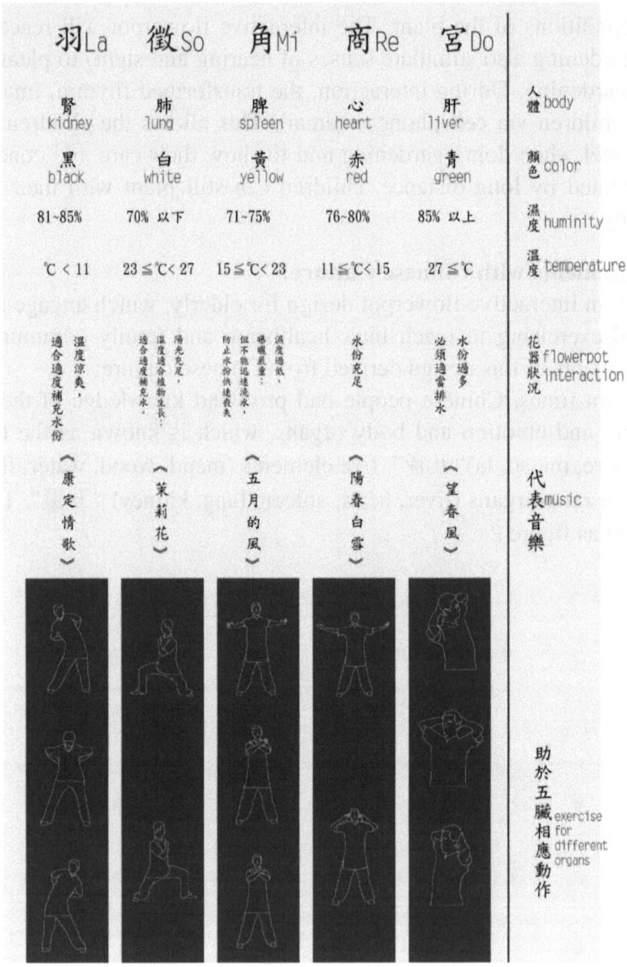

Fig. 3. Relationship between interactive elements

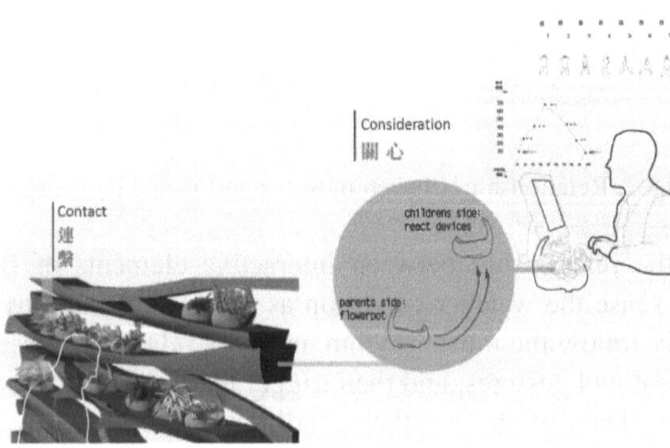

Fig. 4. Grass Tone interactive flowerpots act as communication devices

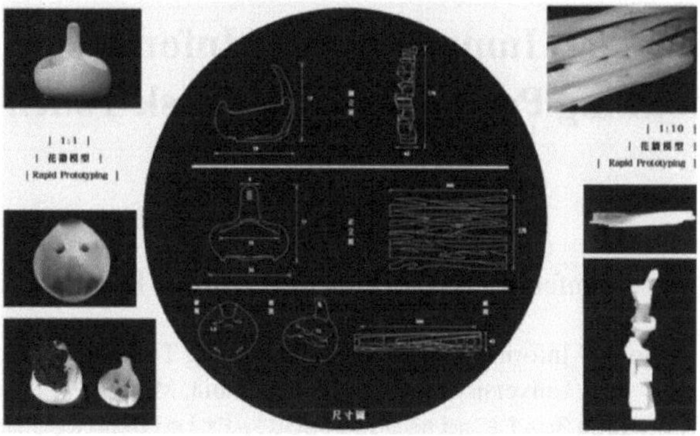

Fig. 5. Grass Tone interactive flowerpots prototype models

5 Conclusion

Through carrying out concept design and producing design prototype, the design guides for technology products combining the merit of Filial Piety in Chinese culture and suitable for the elderly to interact with their family members are therefore concluded as follows:

1. The application of the technology products for the elderly must fit in their daily life, leisure activities or interests.
2. The technology product for the elderly must be very intuitive and simple in operation, and can be used by user without additional training.
3. The added values of the technology products for the elderly must be taken into consideration so as to please the elderly and meet their mental and physical needs.
4. Communication should happen naturally and easily, but not compellingly so the children may be more motivated to express their concerns for their parents and perform their filial duty.
5. If the elderly may feel the concerns from their family members through the product, they will be less resistant to using it.

Factors and Cues Impacting User Information Selection and Processing Performance in Kiosk Touch Screen Interfaces

Yanfei Ma, Wanli Xing, and Cathryn Friel

School of Information Science and Learning Technologies,
University of Missouri, Columbia, MO
{ymyp6,wxdg5}@mail.missouri.edu, FrielC@missouri.edu

Abstract. Designing kiosk touch screen interfaces challenges our basic knowledge of human-computer interaction. Touch screens are used by people of all ages and educational levels for a wide variety of applications. An empirical study on a kiosk touch screen design was conducted to test the cues and factors influencing user performance by examining design elements and principles from a designer's perspective and implementing usability testing to investigate end user satisfaction. Using cue-summation theory and simplicity theory as theoretical frameworks, this paper presents the main factors and cues required in designing kiosk touch interfaces with the goal to test user performance and satisfaction.

Keywords: kiosk touch screen interface, cue-summation theory, simplicity theory, usability testing.

1 Introduction

A touch screen kiosk provides a user-friendly interface for performing a variety of simple routine functions. For example, it can help visitors find their way around with interactive maps, site photographs, or links to more information. Touch screens are used by people of all ages and educational levels in a wide variety of applications. A well-designed informational touch screen interface can be an effective and efficient method for visitors to obtain information quickly and easily. However, designing touch screen interfaces challenges basic knowledge of human-computer interaction because of the restrictive physical size of the systems, the operating system used on the device and the diversity of users [2].

A building directory touch screen kiosk was selected and tested in this study. The touch screen kiosk is currently in use in a complex building at a Midwestern university. The primary purpose of the kiosk is to provide visitors with directory information and listings of scheduled events. This study examined how the information cues: location, color, text notation and navigation relate to user information selection and processing performance. Using cue-summation theory and simplicity theory as theoretical frameworks, the authors investigated the main factors

C. Stephanidis (Ed.): Posters, Part I, HCII 2013, CCIS 373, pp. 56–60, 2013.

and cues required in designing kiosk touch interfaces with the goal to test user information selection and processing performance. Usability testing was conducted with nine users to test user performance and satisfaction. Additional information was obtained by interviewing the lead designer of the kiosk touch screen interface. This paper discusses the essential findings; limitations and implication of this research on kiosk touch interface design.

2 Background

According to Karvonen [1], both experienced users and novices require the same kind of user interface design to satisfy their needs, that is, a simple design. From a usability perspective, "simplicity" means that users are able to easily obtain what they need. Karvonen [1] further augured that simplicity is also a notion of aesthetic considerations, which affects the user's experience and interpretation of the design.

Cue-summation theory proposes that multiple cues presented both across and within media/channels can improve information processing and learning performance [3]. The usability of any interaction design depends on the relationship between interaction style and input device [4]. Interaction styles represent ways in which the specific input from these devices is translated and used by the computer application such as direct manipulation, command language or menu selection. While a lot of effort is being made towards the development of new input devices and the design of large graphical interfaces, additional research is needed on the design of kiosk touch interfaces to improve user information selection and processing performance.

3 Purpose of Study

This study seeks to understand what design elements and principles are vital in the design. Of particular interest was the determination if color cues, location cues and texture cues impact user performance. Since color and location cues play a significant role in user information processing and selection, the cue-summation theory was applied to categorize main cues of this kiosk touch screen interface. The simplicity principle was the guiding principle in the design of the kiosk touch screen interface and was applied the study to examine how the simplicity attribute contributes to the user's information processing. Selected users interacted with the interface to find information about department events and conduct a lookup in a department directory. This study investigated which design elements and principles were vital during the design process. Additionally, the researchers were interested in determining if color, location, and text cues and simple navigation can impact user performance.

4 Methodology

An empirical study on a kiosk touch screen design was conducted to test how simple navigation and color cue, location cue and text cue would impact user information selection and processing performance. A usability study was performed to evaluate the design of the kiosk touch screen interface. Researchers were interested in determining if users can accomplish common tasks and easily find information using this application and how they perceive the cues and factors while they were implementing the tasks. An interview with the lead designer was conducted to identify what design elements and principles were used during the design of the kiosk touch screen interface.

4.1 Participants

Nine participants identified as potential users of the kiosk touch screen and a lead designer participated in this study. Of the nine participants of the usability study, four were male and five were female with diverse backgrounds and experience. All nine of the participants had prior experience using a touch screen kiosk but none had used the particular touch screen kiosks employed in this study. The lead designer of the kiosk touch screen interface participated in an interview to identify the design elements and principles employed in the development of this touch screen kiosk.

4.2 Data Collection and Analysis

Nine usability tests were conducted using two separate but identical kiosk touch screen devices in situ. During the usability study session, participants were asked to complete four tasks (understand the purpose of the kiosk touch screen; start to use the application; find a designated person; find the schedule of events) by using the kiosk touch screen. As participants completed the tasks, members of the research team observed and took notes. Positive and negative attributes were identified, which impact user information selection and processing performance on the kiosk. After the tasks were completed, the participants were interviewed based on their experience with the touch screen interface. Information obtained during an interview with the lead designer was used to better understand the design choices.

5 Results

5.1 Color Cues

Through the interview with the lead designer it was determined that simplicity was the primary design principle guiding the development of the kiosk touch screen navigation. Color was not a big part of this design process. This did not seem to effect user satisfaction with the interface as six of the nine users indicated that they were satisfied with the color schemes. However, more than half of the participants complained navigation bar background and navigation buttons was too similar in color and there needed to be greater contrast between the two. One participant commented that gray color of the background body text was unattractive and wanted to see a more color in that area.

5.2 Text Cues

Text cue are important indicators but can sometimes be confusing on touch screen devices. All participants indicated that the text was simple and clear, especially on the touchable buttons. Three participants thought that homepage was too busy making it difficult to distinguish between which areas are touchable and which are not. Eight out of nine participants expressed that the instructions for starting the touch screen were too vague and small with regards to font size. In tasks related to finding events on the kiosk, two participants complained about the timeframe limitation of the events schedule, which only covers one week at a time.

5.3 Location Cues

Location cues can refer to the physical location of the device and the location of button and text within the touch screen. The kiosks were in two visible locations on the first floor of the building. Two participants felt the kiosk would be better served if more centrally located in the floor lobby. Three participants did not initially understand the purpose of the kiosk. Two of the three suggested that signage near the kiosk would assist visitors in understanding the purpose of the kiosk.

5.4 Navigation Cues

Overall, participants found the navigation of the system to be very easy and straightforward with the navigations making sense to them. Two participants pointed out that there was no home or back button on any of the screens. Another participant found it hard to figure out how to start the application. One additional problem found by the participants is the similarity in looks between touchable and not touchable areas on the screen leading to confusion in navigation for some.

6 Discussion

The results of this study provide basic recommendations for designers of touch screen interfaces. Basic navigation improvements for this device include: adding a Home or Back button to each page to ease navigation. Devices need an obvious indicator as to how the device or application should be started. Participants indicated that some of the text and area on the screen looked touchable but some were not. Clear indicators should exist if a particular area on the screen is touchable. Suggestions for color include using a more vibrant colors for the body color and a more distinctive color contrast should exist between the navigation bar and buttons. As more and more devices incorporate touch screens, it is important that human-computer interface models adjust to assist designers in helping users interact with them more easily and effectively.

Acknowledgements. We would like to express our greatest gratitude to the people who have helped & supported us throughout this study. We are grateful to Dr. Gail Fitzgerald for her continuous support of this study, from her initial advice in the early stages and her ongoing encouragement.

References

1. Karvonen, K.: The beauty of simplicity. In: Thomas, J. (ed.) Proceedings on the 2000 Conference on Universal Usability (CUU 2000), pp. 85–90. ACM, New York (2000), doi:10.1145/355460.355478, `http://doi.acm.org/10.1145/355460.355478` (retrieved)
2. Maquire, M.C.: A review of user-interface design guidelines for public information kiosk systems. Int. J. Human-Computer Studies 50, 263–286 (1999)
3. McNab, A.L., Hess, T.J., Valacich, J.S. (2009). Designing Interfaces for Faster Information Processing: Examination of the Effectiveness of Using Multiple Information Cues. In: Proceedings of AMCIS 2009, Paper 699 (2009)
4. Kjedskov, J., Skov, M.B.: Interaction design for handheld computers. In: Proceedings of the 5th Asian Pacific Conference on Human-Computer Interaction, APCHI 2002. Science Press (2002)

Automa-Persona: A Process to Extract Knowledge Automatic for Improving Personas

Andrey Araujo Masiero[1], Ricardo de Carvalho Destro[1,2], Otávio Alberto Curioni[3], and Plinio Thomaz Aquino Junior[1]

[1] FEI University Center
Av. Humberto A. Castelo Branco, 3972
09859-901, S. Bernardo Campo, SP, Brazil
[2] Volans Informatica Ltda.
Av. Dr. Cardoso de Melo, 1470, Cj. 907
04548-005, Sao Paulo, SP, Brazil
[3] Department of Head and Neck Surgery, Heliopolis Hospital
Rua Conego Xavier, 276
04231-030, Sao Paulo, SP, Brazil
{amasiero,destro,plinio.aquino}@fei.edu.br, curioni@usp.br

Abstract. During the development of a product, it is necessary for a designer to attempt the special needs of devices and also the target users. To help designers with the problem to attend users' needs, a technique called Personas is applied during the project. Usually, the Personas creation process is manual, lengthy and also it doesn't have a attendance during the project. With this objective in mind, this paper presents a process to automatize and to address the users needs through Personas during the whole project.

Keywords: Knowledge Extraction, Q-SIM, Clustering, User Modeling, Personas.

1 Introduction

Designers need to identify which kind of devices will access and who are the users for the systems they are creating. Devices and users identification are important to comply with particular requirements for the project. To meet all devices needs is a hard task due to lots of different types of these devices. This task becomes harder when designer has to identify particular features for each target users. The users' diversity is wide and to analyze each one is a task that spends a lot of effort and time from the professionals.

An alternative to analyze users' needs is clustering into groups with similar features or characteristics. Thus, the designer's analysis becomes easier. Jung [7] presents a technique called Personas, where he says that each person assumes a role according to an inserted scenario. Cooper [2] popularized Personas to generate a user model which is capable to represent a users' group. This model was defined as hypothetical archetypes of actual users, in other words, despite

C. Stephanidis (Ed.): Posters, Part I, HCII 2013, CCIS 373, pp. 61–64, 2013.

it represents real users of the system, the Persona is not real, it is a fictitious character as defined by Aquino Junior [1].

To adopt this technique in the FINEP PEAP-PMPT project, telemedicine field, we found another problem. How could be possible to create Personas in an automatic way to improve constantly the system and more, to apply this knowledge into future projects.

Therefore we create a process to apply in the project such is possible automatized the improving of Personas. The process presented in section 2 uses the clustering technique to group users information. The clustering technique search for identifying in a finite data set some features to form groups, where elements inside a group are more similar to the outside of the group [10].

Next sections are discussed the algorithms tested and the process applied on this work.

2 Automatized Improving of Personas Process

This section will present the process to improve Personas in a automatized way and also to compare the clustering algorithm used during this work to construct the process. Figure 1 presents the process proposed in this paper.

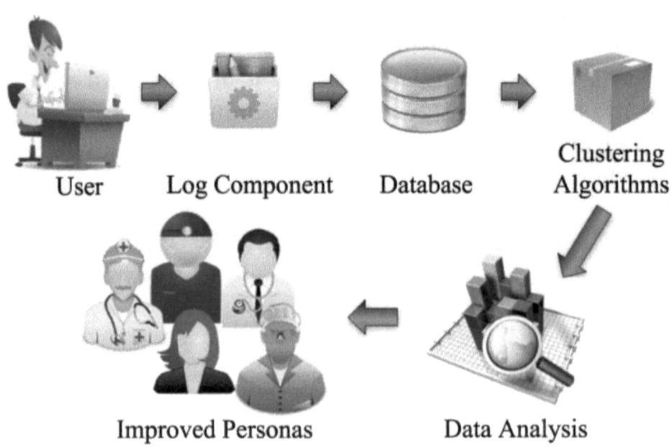

Fig. 1. Process to improve Personas automatized

First step of the process is capture information of the system's use through the log component. This information is important for designer identifies which difficult users have during the system's use and what is he real computational experience. All this data is stored into a database to the clustering algorithm work after. The information capture in PEAP-PMPT project was: (I) Time to fill a text field; (II) Type speed; (III) Percentage of Backspace use; (IV) Errors during fill a form; (V) Relapse errors in a form; (VI) Double click; and (VII) Wrong clicks.

With the information collected and stored into the database, it is necessary to execute the clustering algorithm to obtain the group of similar users and so to improve the Personas acquired in the begin of the project. Algorithms present in table 1 were studied to identify which present better results.

Table 1. Clustering Algorithms studied

Algorithm	Parameter / Property
k-means	k_*: number of groups
DBSCAN	ϵ: distance between two points
Affinity Propagation	θ: threshold of similarity
RObust Clustering using linKs (ROCK)	k_*: number of groups
QROCK (Quick ROCK)	θ: threshold of similarity
Q-SIM (Quality Similarity Clustering)	Q: similarity desired

ROCK and QROCK algorithms [3] were created to perform with categorical data, in other words, text data. This feature exclude them of the comparison because the user data can contain different kind of data like categorical or numerical.

K-means [6] needs that the designer informs the number of clusters that he wants. This parameter becomes the process imprecisely because designer doesn't have how to analyze generated groups and he also doesn't know how many groups exist into database.

DBSCAN [4] present some good results but when database has density information it returns bigger groups and sometimes only one group for the entire database. This kind of result is not good for a user scenario due to the generalized result. To represent a big size population with only one group is almost impossible.

Next algorithm analyzed was Affinity Propagation [5], despite it works with similar measure between the elements in database its methods have some problems. Usually, Affinity Propagation creates some big groups and another small groups due to this features some groups are generalized or specific.

The last algorithm tested was Q-SIM [9]. It demonstrates a better result during the tests, because the designer only needs to inform the similarity degree that he desires and Q-SIM will find the number of groups keeping the quality of similarity between elements' group. Therefore, we use Q-SIM algorithm to create the cluster and to support the improving of Personas features.

With groups created, we need to find a central point that represent the information of each variable in the group. To perform this task, a method present by Masiero et al.[8] is applied. This method applies a dispersion measure in each variable of the elements. These measures are mean, median or mode.

Values obtained in this process are analyzed and then inputted into the Personas description in a narrative way. It helps the designer to identify if appears new Personas and improve new features into old ones. This improvement helps to update the system's interaction. Thus, the process is complete and it is possible to improve the Personas automatically without using interviews or questionnaires with the users.

3 Conclusion

In the end of this research, we identify the related techniques of data mining to support a new process to improve Personas automatically using history data of use's systems. This new process is part of a research to create a new clustering algorithm to support creation and improving of Personas automatically [9].

This process is important due to facility the identification of user needs which turns possible the update of the system and application of this knowledge into future projects.

Beyond that, the mechanism was important to capture the information about computational experience of the doctors of PEAD-PMPT project. It turns easy to acquire the information about them because the process is automatically and they don't have much time to give us interviews and make many tests.

It also was identified a set of variables that allows to know computational experience and some difficult faced by the user during the interaction of the system. As a future work, we are studying the evolution of Personas during the lifecycle of the system.

Acknowledgment. To CNPq Scholarship 383677/2011-4 and PEAP-PMPT project, ref. 1465/10, In- stitutional Process number 01.10.0765.00, MCT/FINEP/ SAUDE TELESAUDE E TELEMEDICINA No - 1/2010 and FAPESP funding process number 2013/07837- 3.

References

1. Aquino Jr., P.T.: Picap: padroes e personas para expressao da diversidade de usuarios no projeto de interacao. uSP Digital Library (2008)
2. Cooper, A.: The Inmates Are Running the Asylum. Macmillan Publishing Co., Inc., Indianapolis (1999)
3. Dutta, M., Mahanta, A.K., Pujari, A.K.: Qrock: A quick version of the rock algorithm for clustering of categorical data. Pattern Recogn. Lett. 26(15), 2364 (2005)
4. Ester, M., Peter Kriegel, H., Sander, J., Xu, X.: A density-based algorithm for discovering clusters in large spatial databases with noise, pp. 226–231. AAAI Press (1996)
5. Frey, B.J., Dueck, D.: Clustering by passing messages between data points. Science 315(5814), 972–976 (2007), `http://www.sciencemag.org/content/315/5814/972.abstract`
6. Jain, A.K.: Data clustering: 50 years beyond k-means. Pattern Recogn. Lett. 31(8), 651–666 (2010)
7. Jung, C.: The archetypes and the collective unconscious (1991)
8. Masiero, A.A., Leite, M.G., Filgueiras, L.V.L., Aquino Jr., P.T.: Multidirectional knowledge extraction process for creating behavioral personas. In: Proceedings of the 10th Brazilian Symposium on on Human Factors in Computing Systems and the 5th Latin American Conference on Human-Computer Interaction, IHC+CLIHC 2011, pp. 91–99. Brazilian Computer Society, Porto Alegre (2011)
9. Masiero, A.A., Tonidandel, F., Aquino Jr., P.T.: Similar or not similar: That is a parameter question. In: Yamamoto, S. (ed.) HIMI/HCII 2013, Part I. LNCS, vol. 8016, pp. 484–493. Springer, Heidelberg (2013)
10. Witten, I.H., Frank, E., Hall, M.A.: Data Mining: Practical Machine Learning Tools and Techniques, 3rd edn. Morgan Kaufmann Publishers Inc., San Francisco (2011)

Document Analysis (DA) as a Sociotechnical Design Framework for HCI: A Novel Tele-psychiatric Service as a Case Study

Bernt Ivar Olsen[1], Peter M. Yellowlees[2], Alberto Odor[2], Niels Windfeld Lund[3], and Gunnar Hartvigsen[1]

[1] Department of Computer Science, University of Tromsø
[2] Department of Health Informatics, UC Davis
[3] Documentation- and Media Studies, University of Tromsø Norway
bernt-ivar.olsen@uit.no

Abstract. We present a novel sociotechnical analysis framework; a document model and a first attempt at utilizing it in an information systems design context. We argue document analysis (DA) to be a holistic framework that encompasses technical, cognitive and social aspects of the system and may act as boundary objects to communicate the system model effectively between stakeholders, designers and engineers.

Keywords: Analysis and design methods, Sociotechnical Systems, Document- and Information Theory, Telepsychiatry.

1 Introduction - Motivation

Human Computer Interaction is a field of study ripe with powerful concepts, frameworks and techniques [1] to study and analyze human information behavior and our interaction with information systems with the goal of designing ever better and more useful systems with hassle free interaction. Although studies show that Usability and Interaction Design seem to be perceived as integrated in the same software engineering process today (which is sort of good news), there seems to be (still) a mismatch between an intention of wanting to include concepts such as usability into the product development and what is realized in projects [2, 3]. Furthermore, there seems to be agreement that a gap exists between the developers and the users [4, 5]. Several proposed solutions to amend this gap revolve around the issue of how to integrate usability or human factors analysis into systems design (i.e. [6]). At the center of this process we find the usability expert/consultant or user experience designer who is more or less supposed to build this bridge, communicating with both prospective users and developers/designers and also management [7].

As a field with a rich selection of methods, models and frameworks that, at least in sum – more than adequately facilitates detailed scrutiny of almost any human interaction with information systems – HCI is not in dire need for "yet another" framework.

C. Stephanidis (Ed.): Posters, Part I, HCII 2013, CCIS 373, pp. 65–68, 2013.

However, it seems like – despite this richness of tools and frameworks something is still lacking in order to fully integrate HCI in systems design. What can be argued to be missing in this context are communication artifacts that can be used across several or all levels of the hierarchy of design of systems [8]; artifacts that are both structured and specific when needed and that also can 'paint' a more loosely description of the system and the parts, components and pieces of it – in order to create a coherent view and (mental) model of the system. These kinds of artifacts are commonly denoted "boundary objects" [9]. This idea of using boundary objects in this regard has been proposed by several [10, 11] and i.e. lately in Eriksson [12]. Our proposal is to suggest conceiving these artifacts as documents or document-analysis, on the basis of a broad and complementary document model. Our aim is that they may act as such communicators of a common or at least a converging model of a system to be built that will safely guide both expectations of the system (from the principal(s) of the system and all related stakeholders) and design of the system accordingly.

2 The S&F Telepsychiatric Service Case Study

We have used a proposed novel telepsychiatric service as a case study for applying the document model to a real world problem. A store-and-forward psychiatry system is based on the concept of asynchronous medical services, where an information system is utilized in order to describe a problem (an illness) of a patient and to request a specialist opinion (service). In other words, information about the patient and the illness is first collected before it is stored within the system and transferred to a remote site for evaluation by a human agent (psychiatric specialist) – who in turn evaluates the patient and the problem based on the available (provided) information and issues a response when the evaluation is finished [13].

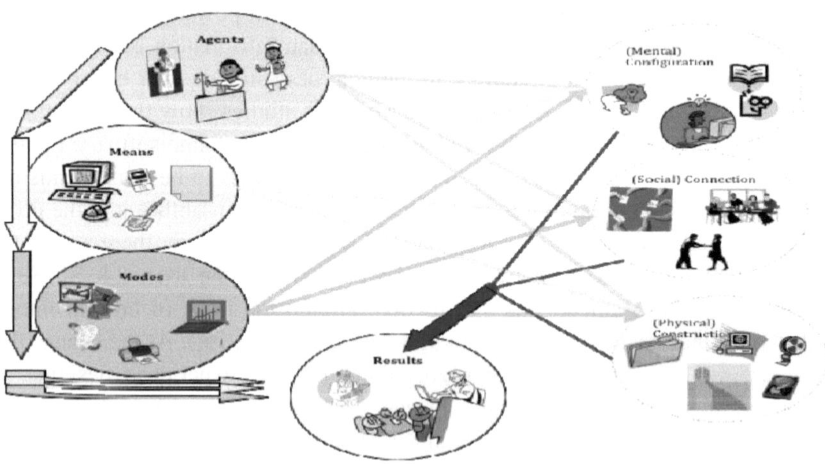

Fig. 1. The Document Model

In Figure 1 we present an illustration of the current document model, conceived from the last couple of decades of research and discourses of what constitutes a document [14]. This document model is a very broad and complementary model that encompasses many "objects", both digital and physical that contemporary interpretation of "a document" does not, especially after the digitization of many documents.

We have created a document analysis of the system, which – in turn was used as input into the modeling process. In the analysis of the S&F system we have modeled this into a system of 2 documents: (1) the MD-doc created at the primary care giver on the basis of a standardized psychiatric interview and (2) the Psych-doc created by the psychiatric specialist.
The Psych-doc is created based on the videotaped (and possibly edited-) interview contained within the MD-doc and provides diagnostic information, treatment details as well as follow up plans for the patient. Both documents in this system are analyzed with respect to the 7 constituents of the document model: (1) Agents: who creates (authors) the documents; (2) Means: what means are used to create the document; (3) Modes: in which ways are the means used (combined) to create the document. These 3 basic "attributes" (or collections of attributes) are subsequently scrutinized in 3 complementary ways: (4) Configuration: the cognitive perspective – how the document is perceived by [users] (5) Connection: the social and cultural perspective (who relates how to this document) and, finally (6) the physical Construction of the document.

The first 3 constituents of the DM constitute sort of a "casting mold" for "classes" (groups) of similar documents while the latter 3 (4-6) identify the specific document in question. The seventh (7) constituent is the Resulting (and physically manifesting-) document and may be regarded the sum- or product of the 6 first constituents. The complete analysis may be obtained in [15] (pp. 136-156).

3 Discussion

What can be argued from the preliminary analysis of the S&F system is that the document model is a holistic approach to systems analysis. It has for years been applied to projects within the science of the Arts and within the Humanities and ours is the first attempt at gathering the concepts and model into one in order to utilize it for analysis of information systems (or rather – documentation systems).

From what we have learned it encompasses all four levels of sociotechnical systems design [16]: (1) Algorithms and (2) software containing algorithms in (1); (3) Humans interacting with computers and; (4) Social systems in which humans interact. Level (1) and (2) are contained within the conceptual model's "means", "modes" and "construction", while levels (3) and (4) are covered within the "Agents", "Configuration" and "Connection" part of the Document Model. The document analysis provides a holistic view of the system and the parts of the system, along with the processes that need to be analyzed and accommodated in order to fulfill the consequential requirements to 'support the documentation process. Future and remaining work includes expanding the analysis of the system and applying it to design of a technical system.

References

1. Carroll, J.M. (ed.): HCI Models, Theories and Frameworks: Toward A Multidisciplinary Science. Morgan Kaufman, New York (2003)
2. Bygstad, B., Ghinea, G., Brevik, E.: Software development methods and usability: Perspectives from a survey in the software industry in Norway. Interacting with Computers 20, 375–385 (2008)
3. Majid, R.A., Noor, N.L.M., Adnan, W.A.W., Mansor, S.: A survey on HCI considerations in the software development life cycle: from practitioner's perspective. In: Proceedings of the 2nd International Conference on Interaction Sciences: Information Technology, Culture and Human, pp. 21–24. ACM, Seoul (2009)
4. Borgholm, T., Madsen, K.H.: Cooperative usability practices. Communications of the ACM 42, 91–97 (1999)
5. Grudin, J.: Interactive systems: Bridging the gaps between developers and users. Computer 24, 59–69 (1991)
6. Goransson, B., Gulliksen, J., Boivie, I.: The usability design process-integrating user-centered systems design in the software development process. Software Process: Improvement and Practice 8, 111–131 (2003)
7. Gulliksen, J., Boivie, I., Göransson, B.: Usability professionals—current practices and future development. Interacting with Computers 18, 568–600 (2006)
8. Walenstein, A.: Finding Boundary Objects in SE and HCI: An Approach Through Engineering-oriented Design Theories. In: Bridging the Gaps Between Software Engineering and Human-Computer Interaction (2003)
9. Star, S.L.: Institutional Ecology,Translations' and Boundary Objects: Amateurs and Professionals in Berkeley's Museum of Vertebrate Zoology, 1907-1939. Social Studies of Science 19, 387 (1989)
10. John, B.E., Bass, L., Kazman, R., Chen, E.: Identifying gaps between HCI, software engineering, and design, and boundary objects to bridge them. In: Conference on Human Factors in Computing Systems (2004)
11. Fischer, G., Giaccardi, E., Eden, H., Sugimoto, M., Ye, Y.: Beyond binary choices: Integrating individual and social creativity. International Journal of Human-Computer Studies 63, 482–512 (2005)
12. Eriksson, J.: Supporting the cooperative design process of end-user tailoring, Ph.D Dissertation. Department of Interaction and System Design, School of Engineering. Doctor of Philosophy, p. 310. Blekinge Institute of Technology, Karlskrona, Sweden (2008)
13. Butler, T., Yellowlees, P.: Cost analysis of store-and-forward telepsychiatry as a consultation model for primary care. Telemed. J. E Health 18, 7 (2012)
14. Olsen, B.I., Lund, N.W., Ellingsen, G., Hartvigsen, G.: Document theory for the design of socio-technical systems: A document model as ontology of human expression. Journal of Documentation 68, 100–126 (2012)
15. Olsen, B.I.: Display Scale in a 'Document' perspective: size matters. Department of Computer Science, Ph.D, p. 319. University of Tromsø, Tromsø, Norway (2012)
16. Coiera, E.: Putting the technical back into socio-technical systems research. International Journal of Medical Informatics 76, 98–103 (2007)

Developing a Performance-Based Design System with Semantic Interoperability

Jae Wan Park[1] and Yun Gil Lee[2]

[1] Global School of Media, Soongsil University, Korea
jaewan.park@ssu.ac.kr
[2] Department of Architecture, Hoseo University, Korea
yglee@hoseo.edu

Abstract. This paper presents an attempt to develop a performance-based design expert system intended to automate the checking of building code compliance. The proposed system may be used repeatedly throughout the design phase, from the earliest stages of development to the end of the design process, in order to improve the efficiency and quality of the design and to decrease the occurrences of design misapplication. Two of the critical issues in the development of the rule-based expert system presented here were the data modeling of building codes to be used as a knowledge base, and the algorithm for the application of this knowledge base. Both an object-oriented and a constraint-based approach to these issues are discussed in this paper. This paper gives a detailed overview of "CODE-MAVEN" as well as discussing an intelligence-based intuitive and graphical interface for the system that will also contribute to increased feedback on designs.

Keywords: building code, rule-based expert system, data modeling, object-oriented design system.

1 Introduction

This paper discusses an attempt to develop a rule-based expert system for real-time checking of building code compliance. They are legal regulations that have a direct influence on buildings from the very beginnings of an architectural proposal and throughout the phases of architectural planning, design, and construction. In particular, building code compliance must be thoroughly checked in the planning and design phase, if one intends to improve the efficiency and quality of the design and to decrease the occurrence of misapplications (Park, 1993). One may also assume that stringent checks on building code compliance will increase design feedback by offering a variety of alternatives methods. Not surprisingly, research into and development of expert-based systems for the analysis of building code and its compliance has been underway in a variety of places across the globe.

This paper details the development process of the rule-based expert system called CODE-MAVEN. Its particular focus is on establishing knowledge bases, data models, and algorithms for rule-based systems. At the end of this paper, we present

C. Stephanidis (Ed.): Posters, Part I, HCII 2013, CCIS 373, pp. 69–73, 2013.

our successful development of a rule-based expert system for building code compliance checking. The conclusion also includes an outline of the research and development issues to be considered next.

2 System Overview

Despite this recent development and interest, however, systems for building code analysis have not been entirely successful and so the occurrence of real-world industrial applications of rule-based expert systems is still rare (Sinz, 2002). The reason for this scarcity is that these expert systems have generally been developed separately from already existing design tools. Accordingly since these newer systems do not have a sufficient understanding of geometrical shapes as well as semantic meanings, building code checks on various complicated models that also include site details are not completely implemented. To fundamentally resolve this problem, we began by investigating the building data model of an apartment and then developed a data model based on ArchiCAD™ which was designed to be flexible, extensible, and easily applicable. Also important was the classification of building codes for storage in a rational database: building codes were classified by their application procedure and then stored computationally in a relational database that we call a knowledge base, based on the data model for a database. Finally, this knowledge base was connected with a constraint-based system for checking building code compliance that is currently under development, which should, when completed, fulfill the need for an effective analysis tool for compliance checking.

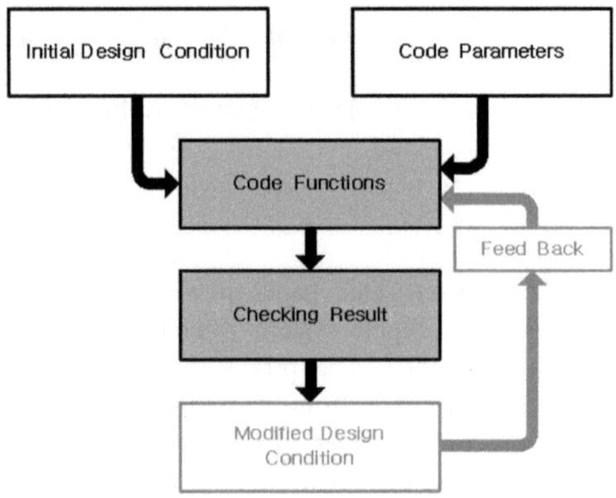

Fig. 1. The architecture of CODE-MAVEN

This system is composed of three parts: the design conditions, the code parameter called the knowledge base, and a rule-based system that includes code functions and results checking. we adopted a rule-based system from the infant phase of Artificial Intelligence as being practically applicable for the analysis of building codes. Figure 1 illustrates the architecture of CODE-MAVEN. The design conditions consist of modeling by ArchiCADTM and the specific conditions for code checking. Checking results will continuously modify the design condition at any level or any time during the design process.

The knowledge of building codes is composed of a set of provisions and relations governing the design of buildings (Yang, 2004). Generally, in Korea, the checklist of building codes for an apartment is classified by the land-use plan, the examination of area, the examination of height, the examination of interval, and so on. This classification is closely related with site planning. The building code provisions and regulations for the apartment are extracted according to the classifications on the checklist.

3 Implementation

To implement our system, we initially entered information about the design conditions. The design conditions for building code compliance checking are divided into two parts: project conditions and specific conditions. Project conditions such as the province, the area, and the circumferential environment are added by defining each condition, while specific conditions such as unit floor plans, parking areas, and outdoor spaces are added by using and customizing the parts library, as well as making new drawings. The functions in the modeling group are used to establish design conditions; those in the code-checking group are used to evaluate building codes. These functions were developed using ArchiCADTM, API, and C++.

After completing an apartment design, the users can perform a building code compliance check on their design. CODE-MAVEN returns results graphically in two- and three-dimensional interfaces to visually represent non-conformity with the building code, as well as providing numerical information. The interface also provides the manifold color necessary for intuitively distinguishing differences, particularly in areas where code checking is related to views and natural light levels. These diverse results are illustrated in Figure 2.

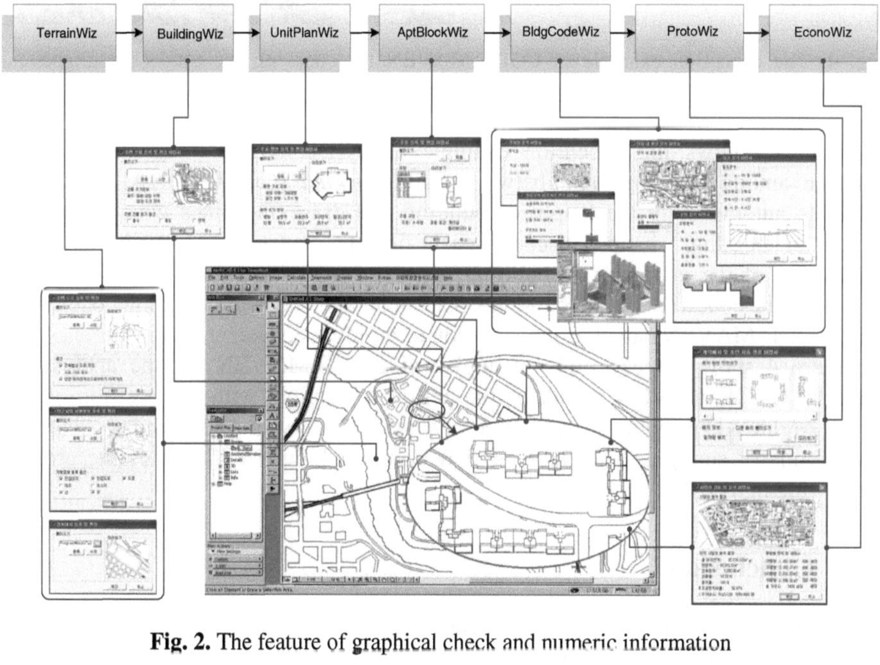

Fig. 2. The feature of graphical check and numeric information

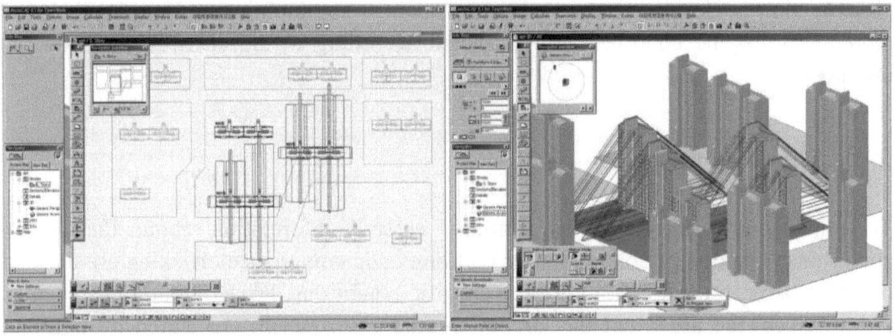

Fig. 3. The execution example of CODE-MAVEN for checking the distance among the buildings

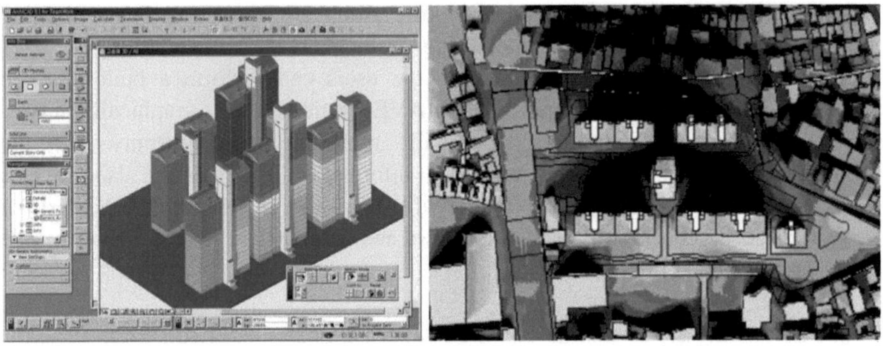

Fig. 4. The execution example of CODE-MAVEN for checking the time of sunlight and shadow

Figure 3 shows the execution example of CODE-MAVEN for checking the distance among buildings and between buildings and road. CODE-MAVEN can calculate automatically the height of building and draw blue lines which show the region of building shadow because each objects of CODE-MAVEN have the parameters of the geometry of building, site, and road. Therefore, the users easily figure out the condition o0066 buildings placement and check the building codes. And also, CODE-MAVEN can alert the violation of building codes.

Figure 4 show the execution examples of CODE-MAVEN for the analysis of sunlight. CODE-MAVEN calculates the period of sunlight with the position of sun which ArchiCAD provides by each time of a day and shows the color index according to the time of sunlight. The figure of left down of Figure 4 illustrates the area of shadowing in a day.

4 Conclusion

In this paper, we presented a rule-based expert system, CODE-MAVEN, which integrates building code compliance checking within the design process in a real-time fashion, and is based on ArchiCADTM, and gave a practical example of the development of the system. In general, many expert systems developed to analyze building codes are separate from the existing CAD engine, in turn limiting the development of systems designed for code compliance checking. This system, however, has been developed specifically with the practical and commercial use of compliance checking in mind. We expect that CODE-MAVEN will be effectively utilized throughout the entire design process, from its earliest stages to its final ones. Architectural designers will be able to generate and then immediately check various design options and alternatives in the schematic phase, which will, we believe, result in a decrease in design misapplication and an increase in design efficiency.

Acknowledgment. This research is supported by the Technology Innovation Program(World Best Software Project, 10040794) funded by the Ministry of Knowledge Economy(MKE, Korea).

References

1. Carrara, G., et al.: Knowledge-Based Computational Support for Architectural Design. Automation in Construction 3, 157–175 (1994)
2. Choi, J.W.: Real-time Management of Spatial Information of Design: A Space-Based Floor Plan Representation of Buildings. In: Israel-Korea Binational Conference on Geometrical Modeling and Computer Graphics, Seoul, pp. 221–234 (2001)
3. Choi, J.W., Park, J.W.: Developing A Building Design Compiler That Frequently Evaluates Building Design Performance within the Design Process. In: Proceedings of the 8th International Conference on Computer-Aided Architectural Design Research in Asia, Thailand, pp. 553–565 (2003)
4. Kalay, Y.E., Khemlani, L., Choi, J.W.: An Integrated Model to Support Distributed Collaborative Design of Buildings. Automation in Construction 7, 177–188 (1998)
5. Korean Ministry of Legislation, http://www.moleg.go.kr
6. Korean Ministry of Construction & Transformation, `http://www.moct.go.kr`
7. Nicholson-Cole, D.: The GDL Cookbook. Marmalade (2002)
8. The National Assembly of the Republic of Korea, `http://www.assembly.go.kr`
9. Park, J.B., Lee, Y.M., Cho, M.S., Lee, B.H.: A study on the Systematization of Building Regulations Related to a Mass Housing Site Planning. Journal of the Architectural Institute of Korea 9(3), 3–10 (1993)
10. Park, J.W., Choi, J.W.: A computational Approach to Evaluate Physical Requirement and Spacial Managements of Apartment Unit Floor Plans. Journal of Asian Architecture and Building Engineering 2(2), 103–109 (2003)
11. Sinz, C., Lumpp, T., Schneider, J., Kuchlin, W.: Detection of Dynamic Execution Errors in IBM System Automation's Rule-Based Expert System. Information and Software Technology 44, 857–873 (2002)
12. Yang, Q.Z., Xu, X.: Design Knowledge Modeling and software Implementation for Building Code Compliance Checking. Building and Environment 39, 689–698 (2004)
13. Yessios, C.I.: The Computability of Void Architectural Modeling. In: Proceedings of Symposium on Computer-Aided Design, Suny Buffalo, New York (1986)

Introducing Need Items – A Basis for Understanding User Experience Centered Product Requirements for Web Products

Katrin Schulze and Heidi Kroemker

Institute of Media Technology, Ilmenau University of Technology, Ilmenau, Germany
{Katrin.Schulze,Heidi.Kroemker}@TU-Ilmenau.de

Abstract. This paper presents a study to understand which psychological needs require to be fulfilled to elicit positive experiences with web products. We therefore conducted in-depth interviews with website users to understand which needs are to be fulfilled with five of the most frequently used websites in Germany. The interviews helped to inductively extract 56 need items. These need items were related to established need categories according to [8] and therefore help to specify relevant psychological needs in the area of web products. Results aim to provide a basis for practitioners to understand product requirements as part of user experience centered software engineering.

Keywords: Need items, user experience, product requirements, user experience engineering, human centered product development.

1 Introduction

In academia and business the importance to develop human centered products that enhance human well-being is becoming more and more central. Within this context, User eXperience (UX) is nowadays an established component of product quality. However, the transformation of the UX concept into practical software engineering is still in early stages [see e.g. 1 and 2]. Therefore, the present work aims to provide a basis for understanding human-centered product requirements based on specified psychological needs for the area of web products.

2 User Experience (UX)

A common understanding of UX provides the norm DIN EN ISO 9241-210 by defining UX as "*a person's perceptions and responses that result from the use and/or anticipated use of a product, system or service*" [3]. This definition describes the concept of UX phenomenologically, however, it is considered too abstract for practical product development. The question in product development is to understand how to develop for UX.

C. Stephanidis (Ed.): Posters, Part I, HCII 2013, CCIS 373, pp. 74–78, 2013.

Looking at developing for UX deeper requires investigating desired product quality. However, different existing approaches to user centered product quality of interactive products appear difficult to apply [4-6]. Saying that, they do not provide a relation between perceived product quality and underlying human motives in order to understand the drivers that constitute positively perceived product quality and, correspondingly, a positive user experience. In order to understand underlying human motives, [7] suggest referring to psychological needs as they are assumed to be particular qualities of experiences that all people require to drive [8].

3 UX Framework

To connect both worlds – product quality and psychological needs – for understanding their influence on perceived product quality, we proposed an early UX framework. The framework included the needs for *autonomy – independence, competence – effectance, relatedness – belongingness, security – control, pleasure – stimulation and influence – popularity* [9 and 10] as well as the product qualities usability and attractiveness as they were shared by all product quality approaches within the context of user experience.

The next logical step was to make the framework applicable. Therefore, the abstract psychological needs require to be specified according to the product context.

An evaluation of the framework with the mobile social media service *LiveShare* by *Cooliris* has shown that the process to specify needs was only marginally applicable in practical software engineering as a result of its time- and resource consuming procedure. The framework itself was considered to be useful [10].

Based on the study results, we draw the conclusion that applicable support to develop for UX requires a pre specified framework for a specific product area.

That said, the goal of this work was to understand *which psychological needs lead to satisfying experiences in web product usage* by identifying specified needs for the area of web products. We subsume these specified needs under *need items*.

4 Study Approach

To answer the research question, a qualitative approach was chosen in order to understand underlying concepts of meaning. This is, to *inductively improve the early UX framework* by identifying psychological needs that are central for eliciting positive experiences as well as to *deductively prove the existence of the proposed psychological needs by [8] within the area of web products*. Therefore, we conducted problem-centered semi-structured episodic interviews according to [11] with 31 individual website users of about 45 minutes for each interview. During the interviews, we asked funnel questions from general (open) to specific (closed) for assuring induction and deduction. We furthermore emphasized to think aloud and followed a question style as proposed in the Valence Method by [12].

Study objects were the five websites *Facebook.de, Ebay.de, Amazon.de, Google.de* and *Spiegel Online*. The selection is based on the 20 most frequently used websites in

Germany according to Nielsen/Statista 2012. A broad selection aims at understanding psychological needs in different fields of web (desktop) products. The selected websites cover Social Network, eCommerce, Search, Email and News/Information. Each interviewee used two of these websites during the interview.

Study participants were selected according to thematical sampling [13, p.402]. Of the 31 participants, 13 were female and 18 male, they used the Internet for at least 5-15 hours a week, knew all evaluated websites and had strong experience in usage of at least two of the five study object websites. The sampling helped to collect at least 10 interviews for each website and to exclude invalid interviews.

5 Results – Revised Framework

The research was successful in inductively deriving 56 *need items* from user statements that specify relevant psychological needs in the area of web products. We classified these need items into 24 more general *need categories*. Mapping these 24 need categories with the top-ten *psychological needs by [8]* has shown that the psychologists need concept is appropriate in the area of web products and, more influential on the previous work, that the *need for self-esteem – self-respect adds to the earlier proposed framework* in [10]. Figure 1 displays the revised framework for the area of web products.

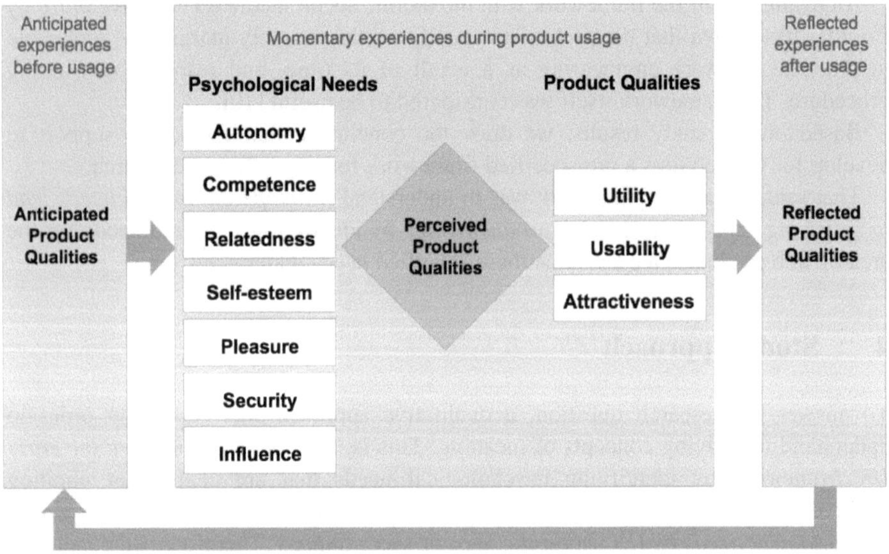

Fig. 1. UX Framework in the Area of Web Products

6 Results – Need Items

Table 1 shows the 56 need items and 24 need categories, related to the model of psychological needs from [8].

Table 1. Need Categories and Need Items in the Area of Web Products

Psychological Need [12]	Need Category	Need Item (To be...)	
Autonomy – Independence	Freedom of Choice	• Self-dependent	• Self-determined
	Freedom of Opinion	• Honest • Profound	• Informative
	Independency	• Uncommitted	• Unrestricted
Competence – Effectance	Success	• Successful • Capable	• Effective
	Planning	• Tactical	• Prepared
	Knowledge	• Educated • Experienced	• Informed • Up-to-date
Relatedness – Belongingness	Exchange	• Involved	• Available
	Altruism	• Inspiring • Selfless	• Generous • Helpful
	Participation	• Participating	• Existent
Self-esteem – Self-respect	**Approval**	• **Approved** • **Accepted**	• **Appreciated** • **Respected**
	Individuality	• **Individual**	
Pleasure – Stimulation	Excitement	• Playful	• Excited
	Curiosity	• Gawping • Curious	• Attentive
	Inspiration	• Explorative	• Inspired
	Creativity	• Imaginative	• Artistic
	Distraction	• Entertained • Amused	• Relaxed
	Surprise	• Surprised	
Security – Control	Overview	• Structured	• Oriented
	Self-control	• Self-controlled	• Prudent
	Certainty	• Safe • Certain	• Protected
	Ease	• Assured	• Carefree
	Trust	• Confident	• Trusting
Influence – Popularity	Reputation	• Influential	• Exemplary
	Presence	• Regarded	

7 Summary and Conclusion

The paper presented a study that aimed to understand which psychological needs require to be fulfilled to elicit positive experiences in web products. A qualitative research design was chosen to inductively answer this research question and to deductively prove an earlier proposed UX framework which relates psychological needs as put forward by [8] with product qualities.

The study was successful in extracting 56 need items and defining 24 overall need categories that specify relevant psychological needs in the area of web products. Results aim to support practitioners in engineering human-centered web products.

However, there are still many more steps to go to make this research topic more valuable in practical software engineering. These first research results open up a spectrum of future research, such as:

- Reproducing the findings by conducting, *firstly*, other qualitative studies to derive need categories or, *secondly*, applying a quantitative research design that aims at proving the resulting 24 need categories within the area of web products.
- Understanding the prioritization of presented need categories for different product contexts, different life areas, and if applicable, for the different life stages of humans.

References

1. Hassenzahl, M., Tractinsky, N.: User experience – a research agenda. Behaviour & Information Technology (2006)
2. Roto, V., Rantavuo, H., Väänänen-Vainio-Mattila, K.: Evaluating User Experience of Early Product Concepts. In: International Conference on Designing Pleasurable Products and Interfaces (2009)
3. ISO 9241-210, I. Ergonomics of human- system interaction–Part 210: Human-centred design for interactive systems. International Organization for Standardization (ISO), Switzerland (2010)
4. Hassenzahl, M.: The thing and i: understanding the relationship between user and product. Funology from usability to enjoyment, 31–42 (2003)
5. Mahlke, S.: Factors influencing the experience of website usage. In: CHI 2002 Extended Abstracts on Human Factors in Computing Systems, pp. 846–847 (2002)
6. Van der Heijden, H.: Factors influencing the usage of websites: the case of a generic portal in the Netherlands. Information & Management, 541–549 (2003)
7. Hassenzahl, M., Diefenbach, S., Göritz, A.: Needs, affect, and interactive products–facets of user experience. Interacting with Computers, 353–362 (2010)
8. Sheldon, K., Elliot, A., Kim, Y., Kasser, T.: What is satisfying about satisfying events? Testing 10 candidate psychological needs. Journal of Personality and Social Psychology, 325–339 (2001)
9. Schulze, K., Krömker, H.: A Framework to Measure User Experience of Interactive Online Products. In: Proceedings of Measuring Behavior 2010, Eindhoven, pp. 261–264 (2010)
10. Schulze, K., Krömker, H.: Extracting user experience centered product requirements for mobile social media applications. In: Proceedings of 14th International Conference on Human-Computer Interaction with Mobile Devices and Services (2012)
11. Witzel, A.: Das problemzentrierte Interview. Qualitative Forschung in der Psychologie. Grundfragen, Verfahrensweisen, Anwendungsfelder, 227–255 (1989)
12. Burmester, M., Mast, M., Jäger, K., Homans, H.: Valence method for formative evaluation of user experience. In: Proceedings of the 8th ACM Conference on Designing Interactive Systems, pp. 364–367 (2010)
13. Flick, U.: Qualitative Sozialforschung: Eine Einführung, 4, vol. 55694. Rowohlt Taschenbuch Verlag (2011)

A Review on Emotional Evaluations for Smart Phone

Amaka Mercy Udengwu, Tek Yong Lim, and Soon-Fatt Cheong

Faculty of Computing and Informatics, Multimedia University, Jalan Multimedia, 63100 Cyberjaya, Selangor, Malaysia
lyamy2001@yahoo.com, {tylim,sfcheong}@mmu.edu.my

Abstract. Human Computer Interaction (HCI) has become progressively more concerned with user experience and emotions. A variety of what experience and emotions is has been expressed in modern years which propose an amount of vital insights but it is unclear on how they inform design. The aim of this paper is to gain a deeper understanding on the techniques to collect and evaluate emotional responses conducted by other researchers. Four evaluation methods were reviewed, namely valence method, self-reported method, experiment method and semantic differential method.

Keywords: Emotional Design, Smart Phone, Evaluation.

1 Introduction

Recently, emotion is playing an important role in customer interaction with the products [1].The evaluation of customers experiences help to determines various perspectives. In this regard, Kansei engineering proposed by [2, 3] is one of the consistent and practical methodologies in dealings with customer's emotional needs.

Emotional situations are frequently incorporated in the explanation of customer requirements and evaluations. Products that reflect on emotion responses and inducing positive emotions tend to draw customers. Thus, emotional design model has been proposed to integrate customer's emotional requirements into design elements to convey customer emotional satisfaction [4].

Emotional design model proposed that design elements can be associated to three different levels of emotional responses, namely visceral, behavioral and reflective. Visceral responses are concerned with aesthetic measures. Behavioral responses are related to the usability and effectiveness of use. Reflective responses are simulated by the rationalization and intellectualization of a product. Besides that, product also can evoke a wide range of emotions, both negative and positive. Negative emotions stimulate individuals to reject or withdraw from the object while a positive emotion stimulates individuals to accept the object.

2 Literature Review

This paper reviews different methods used by other researchers to elicit and analyze emotional responses from users while interacting with an interactive product such as smart phone.

C. Stephanidis (Ed.): Posters, Part I, HCII 2013, CCIS 373, pp. 79–82, 2013.

2.1 Valence Method

Valence method was developed to gather customer experience during evaluations. It was able to elicit every possible detail, extract aspect of product that causes good and bad customer experience [5]. It is significant for designers to recognize which design aspects have caused a good (positive) or bad (negative) experience. This method involved two phases, namely exploration phase and retrospective interview phase.

In the exploration phase, users explored product in whichever way that they like best. There was no pre-defined task given to users. Whenever customers experienced positive and negative emotions, their feelings were spotted by pressing colored button on remote control (either a green button for positive feelings or red button for negative feelings). The button presses were recorded as valence markers with time stamps in a video recording.

In the retrospective interview phase, two main aspects were investigated: (1) product attribute design that caused setting of the valence marker and (2) the underlying customer needs. Each valence marker is discussed in order to recognize the design aspect of a product causing the experience, its meaning to customer and customer's underlying needs. The outcome of this phase was a verbal protocol for each marker with the following properties: attribute design, meaning for the customer and underlying customer needs.

2.2 Self-reported Method

The self-reported method adopted both verbal and non-verbal scales for gathering information about user's emotions [6]. The advantage of this method is that researchers do not need to be present. Three variations of self-reported method were identified, namely experience clip, expressing emotions and experiences (3E), and feedback app.

Experience clip was introduced by [7]. In this method, two friends would work together to evaluate a product where one person would capture a short video clip of his/her friend using the product. Since the video clip was taken by a friend, user can express his/her emotion easier. This method also enabled them to share and compare experiences with each other after they switched roles during the evaluation.

3E was a controlled way of expressing user emotions by scribbling in a diary. It can be a drawing, written expression or combination of both. However, it can be very challenging for researchers to analyze these outputs because each symbolizes user inner feelings. Thus, each user was interviewed in order to understand the diary content. In other words, this semi-structured interview allowed researchers to get deeper information of what users have drawn and written in diary.

Feedback app was a mobile application used to capture user emotions at different times, especially straight away after an interaction being completed. This is also known as experience sampling method (ESM). In this app, users would be prompted using a predefined question and choose one of the nine emoticons as their emotions. This method also integrated both application to be tested and emotion gathering instrument on the same device.

2.3 Experiment Method

Attractiveness of a product appearance can influence perceive usability and [8] carried out an experiment method to investigate the effect of attractiveness, effectiveness, and efficiency on perceived usability. Participants were asked to use mobile phones to perform nine different tasks such as place a call, change assigned ringer and others. Then, they rated each mobile phone with respect to usability and attractiveness. The result revealed that participants who can use a phone effectively and efficiently to complete common phone tasks, tend to rate the phone high in usability whereas participant who cannot, tend to rate the phone low in usability. In short, attractive products were rated high in usability than unattractive products.

2.4 Semantic Differential Method

User's first choice is one of the vital user requirements. Therefore, it becomes a difficult job for product designers to convey user's unspoken first choice into detailed design specification [9]. The semantic differential method examined the association between user's first choice impression of mobile phones and design element. The semantic differential method is comprised of two steps, namely (1) build a measurement scale for preference study, and (2) measure the image perception and user's preference.

The goal of first step was to derive a set of image words to be used as measurement scale. Thus, experienced designers were selected to evaluate forty mobile devices and eleven pairs of image words were obtained. The second step was to determine the relationship between user preference and product design element. 102 participants were asked to assess 26 mobile devices using the eleven pairs of image words. The result showed that participants preferred soft and compact mobile phone.

3 Discussion and Conclusion

Self-reported method, valence method, experiment method and semantic differential method are various ways of eliciting user emotion in different circumstances. Our future work will use web-based questionnaire to elicit emotional response from participants in three different levels of emotional design model [1]. Visceral level will be conducted through exploration, whereby participants are expected to see and feel the smart phones, and required to enter their first impression. Behavioral level will be measured through perceived usability of the smart phones. Participants are also required to enter their emotional response after performing some tasks such as place a call and send a text message. In reflective level, participants are expected to make purchase decision by using laddering techniques.

Acknowledgement. This work is supported by Malaysian Ministry of Higher Education (MOHE) under the Fundamental Research Grant Scheme (FRGS/2/2010/SG/MMU/03/4).

References

1. Norman, D.A.: Preface. In: Schifferstein, H.N.J., Hekkert, P. (eds.) Product Experience, pp. xix–xx. Elsevier, San Diego (2008)
2. Nagamachi, M.: Perspectives and the New Trend of Kansei/Affective Engineering. TQM Journal 20(4), 290–298 (2008)
3. Nagamachi, M.: Kansei Engineering: A New Ergonomic Consumer-Oriented Technology For Product Development. International Journal of Industrial Ergonomics 15(1), 3–11 (1995)
4. Norman, D.A.: Emotional Design: Why Do We Love (Or Hate) Everyday Things. Basic Books, New York (2004)
5. Burmester, M., Mast, M., Jager, K., Homans, H.: Valence Method for formative evaluation of user experience. In: Proceedings of the 8th ACM Conference on Designing Interactive Systems, Stuttgart, Germany, pp. 364–367 (2010)
6. Isomursu, M., Tahti, M., Vainamo, S., Kuutti, K.: Experimental evaluation of five methods for collecting emotions in field settings with mobile applications. International Journal of Human-Computer Studies 65(4), 404–418 (2009)
7. Isomursu, M., Kuutti, K., Väinämö, S.: Experience Clip: Method For User Participation and Evaluation of Mobile Concepts. In: Proceedings of the Participatory Design Conference, pp. 83–92 (2004)
8. Quinn, J.M., Tran, T.Q.: Attractive phones don't have to work better: independent effects of attractiveness, effectiveness and efficiency on perceived usability. In: Proceedings of the SIGCHI Conference on Human Factors in Computing Systems, Atlanta, GA, USA, pp. 353–362 (2010)
9. Chuang, M.C., Chang, C.C., Hsu, S.H.: Perceptual factors underlying user preferences towards product form of mobile phones. International Journal of Industrial Ergonomics 27(4), 247–258 (2001)

HCI in S&T Foresight by Korean Government

Seung-Kyu Yi

Technology Foresight Division, Korea Institute of S&T Evaluation and Planning (KISTEP), Seoul, South Korea
skyist@kistep.re.kr

Abstract. HCI is expected as one of significant technological tools for improving quality of life and solving social issues in the future. This was verified in the 'The 4th Korean Technology Foresight (2020~2035)' conducted by the KISTEP and National Science and Technology Commission of Korean government last year. In foresight, 652 future technologies were predicted to be developed and practically used until 2020 or 2035, and 40 technologies among them were related to HCI. The aim of this paper is to briefly review HCI technologies from this report, and to find policy implications for national R&D. Characteristics and R&D strategies will be drawn from reviewing the report in terms of different index about technical completion, social propagation, technology level, importance, negative impact, type of R&D agents, domestic and international research collaboration, R&D strategery, and necessity of government investment. The study will provide R&D strategies for R&D and practical implication toward future HCI technologies.

Keywords: S&T foresight, Korean government, R&D strategery, HCI.

1 Introduction

If the change of trends and needs in the future can be predicted, countries can establish efficiently/effectively the national strategies and policies for measures to resolving uncertainty and not missing opportunities in the future. Considering important role of science and technology in the national/social innovation, innovative future technologies can be the important measures for the future needs. Above all, HCI will be one of main technical tools providing us different benefit in the future environment where is expected to be full of electronic instruments. This was verified in the 'The 4th Korean Technology Foresight (2020~2035)' conducted by the KISTEP and National Science and Technology Commission of Korean government last year [1]. By the way, Korean government conducted technology foresight 4 times since the 1st foresight survey in 1997. 652 future technologies of the 4th Foresight were predicted to be developed and practically used until 2020 or 2035 [1], and 40 technologies from 5 technical fields among totally 8 fields were related to HCI. Considering the 3 rd foresight result was directly reflected on Framework Act on Science and Technology of the last Government [1], HCI can be expected to be reflected on next R&D policy.

C. Stephanidis (Ed.): Posters, Part I, HCII 2013, CCIS 373, pp. 83–87, 2013.

< 40 HCI-related future technologies in 'The 4th Korean Technical Foresight (2020~2035)'>

Field 1. Machinery/Manufacture/Aircraft/Aerospace/Astronomy (7 technologies)
10. LVC(Live, Virtual, Constructive) training system technology that enables land/sea/air joint-training by utilizing the weapon system in the actual, simulation and virtual reality 15. Wearable robot available for utilization in the accident site and disaster site with being designed so as to demonstrate power beyond limitation of human being 16. Manufacturing robot understanding common expressions(natural language and behavior knowledge) of the human workers, detecting movement of the human and change of factory status, and avoiding dangerous situation by themselves, such as collision, with prediction 18. Biologically combined robot combined with parts(brain, sensory system, arms, legs) of living organisms (animals, insects) to improve performance 26. CAx technology using 3D hologram 57. Aircraft control technology using brain signal of the pilot 76. Automobile available for emergency parking by itself, if necessary, or warning with checking status of drivers (drowsy driving, heart attach)
Field 2. Agriculture and Forestry/Fisheries (1 technology)
130. Wearable robot technology for agricultural work or forestry work that can perform work promptly, accurately, and conveniently, by wearing agricultural and forestry worker
Field 3. Urban/Construction/Transport (6 technologies)
189. Technology of operating customized interior equipment based on human sensibility ergonomics 190. Senior citizen-friendly house that can remove space that can be a barrier to the senior citizen, provide bilateral medical service, and monitoring emergency situation 191. Housing technology that can provide educational, shopping, and medical support based on 3D image and control house-keeping robot's activities 194. Wearable or ride-on assisting robot to make construction easy 199. Small construction equipment technology to be adjusted by long-distance worker motion remote 256. BIM(Building Information Modeling) 용용 용용용용용용용 Integrated design system using BIM(Building Information Modeling) available for designing, modeling, and production
Field 4. Life/Medical (13 technologies)
267. Optimized medication notification system for patients with chronic diseases through measuring drug concentration 268. Medical treatment and medical science simulation technology with using virtual reality 270. Smart pills technology that can sending information related to functional abnormality by wireless with moving gastro-intestinal tract. 273. Fine treatment robot that can process treatment after diagnosing abnormal areas with roaming around various organs and blood vessels by using bio-mass energy. 274. Nano-antibody robot that can detect and neutralize/destruct specific viruses with direct input inside the human body 281. Technology of clarifying recognition, memories, perception, learning, and sensory function of brain with using high resolution brain map imaging technology 287. Bilateral thought recognition interface technology between machinery and human body 290. Brain scan technology for recording memory 291. Brain implant technology for memory loss with using chip/ substitute 306. Technology of developing customized sport outfits interlocking with real time biometric data monitoring system 314. Instrument that can assist activities by monitoring biometrics of the aged who have difficult in normal activities in real time 315. Technology of designing and manufacturing human nerve connecting type cochlear implantation, prosthetic leg, prosthetic hand 316. Artificial intelligent eye technology
Field 7. Information/Electronics/Communication (13 technologies)
517. High precision augmented reality technology for Industry or in the medical field 518. Virtual reality technology using human senses 519. Holographic technology to deliver texture to virtual object such as clothing 521. Holographic mobile terminal technology 525. Multi-modal interface technology which can change input method for the environment and conditions of user to movement, facial expressions and brain waves 547. Technology to transfer smell and taste in real-time by analyzing and synthesizing. 551. Technology which can express movement(3D motion recognition) such as sign language with character 552. Speaker-independent voice recognition technology with more than 95% accuracy 559. Personal life log technology which can make database by saving personal life with sound and image data 561. Korean Automatic Ontology Generation Technology 562. Technology which provide service considering current condition and emotions by synthesizing personal Physiological information, history, and preferences through installed sensors and devices 564. Customized interactive advertising services 568. Technology which simulate the environment change for the external factors with global weather, ocean, environment, ecosystems, infectious diseases, economic, movement of people based on real time data

2 Review of HCI in the 4th Korean Technology Foresight

The 4th technology foresight was processed for the purpose of providing the basic index related to national S&T/R&D policy, such as technical completion time and social distribution time of the future technologies, importance, necessity of governmental investment and priority enforcement measures, portfolio of R&D agent and necessity of collaboration, etc., through Delphi survey for experts in science & technology [1]. The main results are as following [1].

- (Related trends) average 1.8 trends each technology, and totally 15 trends from 22 mega-trends
- (Technical Completion) average time of Korea is 2021, world is 2018
- (Social Propagation) average time of Korea is 2024, world is 2021
- (Tech. Level) average level of Korea is 61.8% compared to World-best countries, such as U.S. (best in 34 technologies), Japan (best in 6 technologies), and Germany (best in 1 technology).
- (Government priority invested technology) 2 priority invested technologies (No. 316, 561) and 12 nominee technologies (No. 10, 16, 18, 274, 281, 291, 314, 315, 316, 517, 518, 552, 561)

3 Approach

To find national R&D strategery about HCI technologies for the future, some results of the 4th Foresight was compared to similar index of present R&D activities. If there is a significant difference between future foresight and present status, measures to bridge the gap can be the trigger to make better the related policy or to plan the new one.

National Science and Technology Statics (FY2011) as the result of governmental R&D survey are used [2]. From this data, the recent R&D status information related to 40 HCI technologies in the 4th Technology Foresight was gotten through the process consisting of keyword-search, S&T classification-comparing, and expert-check. Used Statics is about R&D activities in FY2011, when the 4th Foresight began.

Only one index is found to compare the 4th Foresight and present R&D. Both data contained the ratio in 3 kinds of R&D Agent, university, governmental research institute (GRI), industry. All types of agent have unique roles in national R&D, and import play in the policy flow. Additionally, R&D status in terms of collaboration and Technical Life Cycle (TLC) was analyzed, and conducted comprehensive analysis through integration with agent related analysis results.

4 Results

4.1 R&D Agents

The result of comparing analysis shows decreasing of ratio of university, and increasing of ration of GRI and industry. This result means necessity of strengthen policy for GRI and industry.

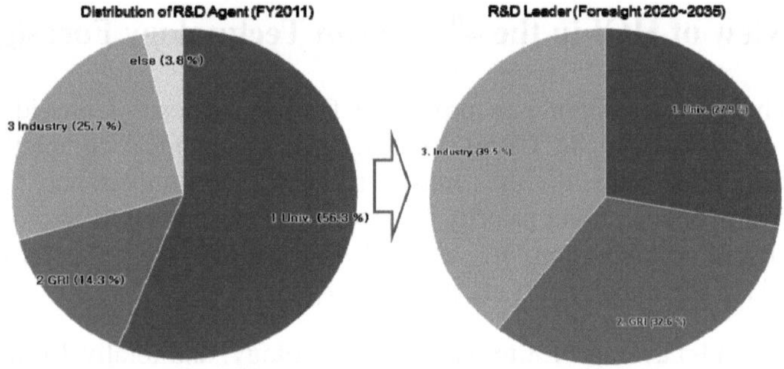

Fig. 1. Comparing R&D leadership on HCI tech R&D

4.2 R&D Collaboration

The result of comparing analysis shows increasing of necessity of international collaboration on HCI R&D in the future.

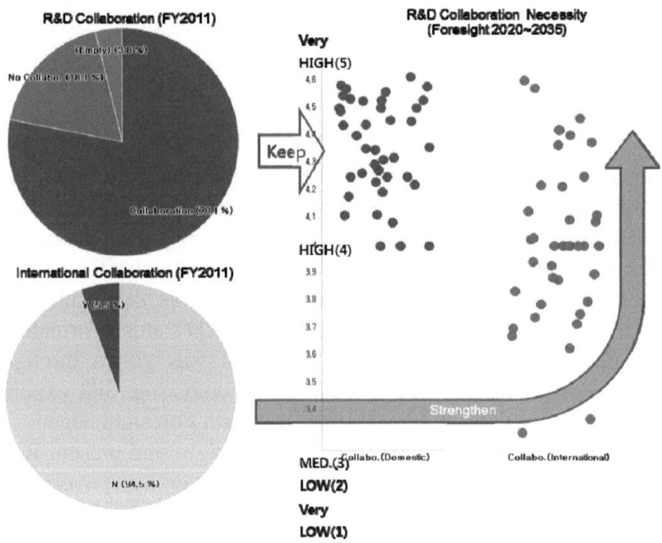

Fig. 2. Comparing R&D collaboration on HCI tech R&D

4.3 TLC Analysis

The analysis result suggest considering necessity to strengthen R&D in higher TLC stage by GRI and industry in the future.

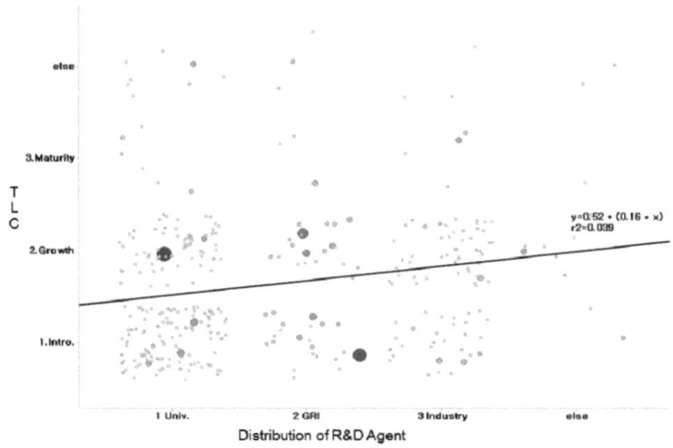

Fig. 3. TLC analysis of each R&D agent

5 Conclusion

HCI is one of important future technology field. 14 technologies selected as 'Government priority invested technology analyses through the 4th Korean Technology Foresight can be reflected importantly on government's policy in Korea. In addition, as appears by review and analysis results in this study, some change should be considered in the planning of HCI related R&D policy for future. Comparing analysis of 'technology foresight-present R&D result' shows that supporting GRI and industry could be an important way. To put it concretely, strengthening their R&D by governmental R&D investment or other institutional benefits, activation of international collaboration and advancement of time to enter the in higher TLC stage could be effective way to catch up with world-best level countries, such as U.S., Japan, Germany.

References

1. National S&T Commission, Korea Institute of S&T Planning and Evaluation, The 4th Korean Technology Foresight (2020-2035) (May 2012) (written in Korean)
2. National Science and Technology Information Service, `http://www.ntis.go.kr`

Part II
Usability Methods, Techniques and Studies

Usability and User Acceptance of University Web Portal Interfaces: A Case of South African Universities

Vathiswa M. Booi and George E. Ditsa

Department of Computer Science
Tshwane University of Technology
Pretoria, South Africa
{BooiVM,DitsaGE}@tut.ac.za

Abstract. There are growing concerns over the user friendliness and other usability issues of South African Universities Web Portal Interfaces (UWPIs), which obviously will negate the user acceptance of the UWPIs. The main objective of this study is to select and use appropriate usability and user acceptance criteria to evaluate South African web portal interfaces for their usability and user acceptance and to suggest improvement on them. The study applied a triangulation of Ubiquitous computing Evaluation Areas (UEAs) and Technology Acceptance Model (TAM) as a theoretical research model for this study. Multiple regression and stepwise regression analysis were used. The results suggest that Interaction and Invisibility of UWPIs are the most important measures, which have a huge impact on user acceptance and usability respectively. The results of the study will provide guidelines for the development and design of UWPIs to meet their usability and user acceptance standards or needs.

Keywords: Technology Acceptance Model, Ubiquitous computing Evaluation Areas, Usability, User Acceptance, University Web Portal Interfaces.

1 Introduction

Computers are playing a vital role and continue to play this role in our daily existence. For more than two decades computers have grown to such a point where they are present anywhere, anytime and in almost every facet of life. Usability and user acceptance of Computer System Websites and Interfaces attract many researchers from different domains such as psychology, human factors, human computer interaction and management because of usability and user acceptance problems associated with them.

Currently web portal interfaces, including South African UWPIs, suffer from a number of weaknesses such as technical difficulties, user friendliness and other usability issues, and there are growing concerns over the usability of South African UWPIs. These concerns will obviously negate the user acceptance of the UWPIs. Different methods have been recommended in the literature to solve the problems of usability and user acceptance of Computer System Websites and Interfaces.

In South Africa, there are 23 universities, which consist of 11 traditional universities, 6 comprehensive universities and 6 universities of technology. All these universities

C. Stephanidis (Ed.): Posters, Part I, HCII 2013, CCIS 373, pp. 91–95, 2013.

have one major objective: to provide quality information and knowledge to students; staff and the general public to sustain their competitive advantage locally and globally. With the functions and services offered by universities to provide the variety of information and services, the question to be asked is: are users happy about what they are getting in terms of portal interface usability, information content, as well as their functionalities? This question raises some concerns; hence it is justifiable to evaluate South African UWPIs for their usability and user acceptance to make ratings and recommendations for their improvement.

User participation studies were used in this study and the research model for the study was derived using constructs from both TAM and the UEAs framework. Questionnaire based on the research model was used in conducting the evaluation of the interfaces. Data collected for the main survey was analysed using SPSS. The results indicate that Interaction, Invisibility, Application robustness and Appeal of South African UWPIs give rise to the usability of the interfaces which subsequently lead to user acceptance of the portals. This study provides guidelines for the development and evaluation of South African UWPIs for their usability and user acceptance.

2 Theoretical Underpinning of the Study

Technology Acceptance Model (TAM) is regarded as the most noticeable model describing the acceptance of computer technology [1]. Research had identified TAM as a cost effective tool for predicting user acceptance of systems [2]. Davis[1] further argues that the goal of TAM is to provide an explanation of the determinants of computer acceptance that is general, capable of explaining user behaviour across a broad range of end-user computing technologies and user populations, while at the same time being both economical and theoretically.

Scholtz and Consolvo [3] incorporated ideas of usability evaluation from different researchers such as Freidman et al. [4], Bellotti et al. [5] and etc. With these incorporated ideas, a framework called Ubiquitous computing Evaluation Areas (UEAs) was formulated. The UEAs presents numerous metrics and conceptual measures. These metrics and conceptual measures help in comparing the technology under evaluation to the users' normal environment.

TAM was selected for this study based on the fact that all usability and user acceptance aspects are covered in the model. The UEAs were adopted for this study because of the conceptual measures which best complements the main objective of the study, which is to select and use the appropriate usability and user acceptance criteria to evaluate South African University Web Portal Interfaces for their Usability and User Acceptance.

The research model for this study was derived by the triangulation of TAM and the UEAs framework. The following constructs were selected from TAM and are used in this study: the actual system use; perceived ease of use; perceived usefulness and external variables. The external variables used in the study, which fed into TAM were taken from UEAs constructs - Interaction; Appeal; Application Robustness and Invisibility. All the identified constructs were used in this study to form the research model. Based on the research model, the following hypotheses were formulated:

H1: Interaction positively impacts usability of ubiquitous web portal interfaces
H2: Appeal positively impacts usability of ubiquitous web portal interfaces.
H3: Application robustness positively impacts usability of ubiquitous web portal interfaces.
H4: Invisibility positively impacts usability of ubiquitous web portal interfaces
H5: Usability of ubiquitous web portal interfaces positively impacts user acceptance of ubiquitous web portal interfaces

3 Research Design and Methodology

3.1 Research Design

The research design for this study will be based on the guidelines provided by Babbie [6], which describes the important research design and methodology aspects employed in the study. The research design includes aspects such as: nature of the research; unit of analysis; time dimension; research methodology and data collection method.

The nature of this research is exploratory and explanatory [6]. It is exploratory because it is generally developed to initial rough understanding of the some phenomenon; and also explanatory because the research is conducted in a way that will discover and report some relationship among different aspects of the phenomenon under study. In this study the unit of analysis is the individual existing students in the institutions, students seeking information, staff members, the public, employers and job seekers. There are two options in terms of time dimension: cross-sectional and longitudinal dimensions. In cross-sectional study, the unit of analysis is observed at one point in time whilst in longitudinal, the unit study is observed over a long period of time. In this study cross-sectional dimension is the most appropriate and feasible.

3.2 Research Methodology

Two major methodologies for usability testing, which are laboratory studies (user participation) and field studies were identified in the work of [7]. Interface design process involves user participation and it has been considered as the best practice in the HCI domain and it was used in this study. User participation or laboratory studies have been considered to be the most appropriate methodology for this problem, because the individuals such as staff, students and the general public are the ones interacting with the university portals and will be involved in the evaluation and rating of the portals. Using the user participation or laboratory studies is considered to be very helpful to usability studies that which emphasis on comparing multiple interface designs or data input mechanism for ubiquitous computing applications.

3.3 Data Collection

Questionnaire based on the research model formulated for this study was used in conducting the evaluation of the interfaces. A pre-test and pilot test of the questionnaire was conducted and data collected was analysed manually.

A representative sample was drawn from the traditional universities, comprehensive universities and universities of technology for the main survey. A total of 200 questionnaires were administered and the primary data collected was analysed using SPSS. The results of the main study are presented in the section below.

4 Results of the Study

A total number of 200 questionnaires were distributed and 180 returned. Of the total 180 returned, only 118 questionnaires were suitable for analysis. Pearson's product-moment correlation matrix was used to analyse the degree of the relationship or association amongst variables. The results of the Pearson's Product-moment correlations indicated that the majority of correlations were statistically significant. The highest correlation reported was between Invisibility of the UWPIs and usability of UWPIs (H4, $r = 0.720$).

In order to identify the variables that were relatively important in determining Usability leading to User Acceptance of UWPIs, Multiple Regression analysis was performed. In this study's analysis, a variable was not entered into regression model unless the p-value for that variable was less than or equal to 0.05. The same level was also set for removal of variables. A stepwise regression was used by allowing addition and removal of variables at various steps in progressively building the regression model.

The results of the analysis indicate that all hypothesized relationships were supported. However, the results indicate that there is a low positive correlation between Usability and User Acceptance. This proves Dillon's [8] explanation that there are no guarantees that the web portals will be acceptable despite the fact that they may be highly usable. The research questions which were addressed using multiple regression analysis and the stepwise regression analysis showed that Appeal, Application Robustness and Invisibility constructs from the UEAs have no significant contribution towards User Acceptance. It is also suggested that invisibility and interaction of South African UWPIs have a great impact on user usability and acceptance respectively.

5 Significance of the Study

The significance of the study is twofold: theoretical and practical. Theoretically, the study is significant in providing a framework for research into UWPIs usability and user acceptance. Practically, the results of this study will provide guidelines for designers/developers, particularly in South Africa, by creating better understanding on how to plan and design UWPIs that are usable and acceptable to users.

6 Conclussion

This study reported the evaluation of South African UWPIs for usability and user acceptance. The study applied a triangulation of UEAs and TAM as a theoretical framework for the evaluation of the web portal interfaces. Based on the findings presented, the overall conclusion that can be drawn for this study is that: Interaction, Appeal, Application Robustness and Invisibility measures represent important variables that explain how the UWPIs are evaluated as well as the criteria which users use for evaluating UWPIs. Their importance from the most influential to the least influential is Invisibility, Interaction, Appeal and Application Robustness. Once these are taken into account designers/developers can use these as guidelines when designing, developing and evaluating the UWPIs.

7 Future Work

This study did not include all constructs of the UEAs framework. A further study may be necessary to include all the constructs. Also perceived usefulness and perceived ease of use constructs of TAM were conceptualized as usability in this study. It may be necessary to use these TAM constructs as they are in a further study.

Based on the results of the study a prototype needs to be developed to validate the results. The results of this study needs to be used as proper guidelines for the prototype, and the prototype needs to be evaluated against the results. Future studies should therefore concentrate on the implementation of the prototype and also aim at including more variables in the research model. This may assist in explaining the variances in the usability leading to user acceptance.

References

1. Davis, F.D.: Perceived Usefulness, Perceived Ease of Use, and User acceptance. MIS Quarterly 13(3), 319–340 (1989)
2. Dillon, A., Morris, M.G.: User Acceptance of Information Technology. Theories and Models. In: Williams, M. (ed.) Annual Review of Information Science and Technology, Information Today, Medford (1996)
3. Scholtz, J., Consolvo, S.: Applications towards a framework for evaluating ubiquitous computing applications. Pervasive Computing, 82–88 (April-June 2004)
4. Friedman, B., Kahn Jr., P.H., Borning, A.: Value Sensitive Design: Theory and Methods, Tech. report 02-12-01, Univ. Washington (Decmeber 2003)
5. Bellotti, V., Back, M., Edwards, W.K., Grinter, R.E., Henderson, A., Lopes, C.: Making Sense of Sensing Systems: Five Questions for Designers and Researchers. In: Proc. Conf. Human Factors in Computing Sys. ACM Press (2002)
6. Babbie, E.: The Practice of Social Research, 9th edn. Wadsworth (2001)
7. Zhang, D., Adipat, B.: Challenges, methodologies, and issue in usability testing of mobile applications: I. International Journal of Human Computer Interaction 18(3) (2005)
8. Dillon, A.: User Acceptance of Information Technology. In: Karwoski, W. (ed.) Encyclope dia of Human factors and Ergonomics, Taylor and Francis, London (2001)

Calculating Website's Usability Metrics Using Log File Information

Marcus Vinicius Cerrato and Marcelo Morandini

School of Arts, Science and Humanities, University of São Paulo, São Paulo, Brazil
{mcerrato,m.morandini}@usp.br

Abstract. Log files are interesting.

Keywords: usability, evaluation, log file, metrics.

1 Introduction

Usability describes how a system is easy to be used. It is the quality of a system that allows its users, in a given context of use, to get specific objectives in an efficient and effective manner, while promoting satisfaction.[1] Usability may be a matter of survival, because users will prefer not to use systems that present difficulties to be learned or that do not permit an easy achieving of specific goals.[2] This is particularly true in the context of websites.

Usability evaluation is increasingly becoming part of software development process. As long as technology evolves, users are becoming more exigent and demand more frequent system's updates. The product of this updates may be new interfaces which should be evaluated to verify whether the changes made to the system were efficient and efficacious.

Log files are text files where all interactions with a website are kept. Using web server log files to evaluate a website is a remote evaluation method. This is a practice and costless way to evaluate a website's usability, and helps the gathering of usability metrics.[3]

This method has the advantage of not interfering in the common use of the website. Users will not feel part of the evaluation process this way. Evaluators will not even conduct the evaluation process at the same time the system is being used.

On the other hand, this process has its own problems, so that, for example, sometimes it will not be possible to know if the user found what he was looking for or what action the user was intending to do. This happens because web server log files only have results of interactions with websites, but they don't have the purpose of such interactions neither their objectives. And as we are using a remote evaluation method, we have only log file information to use.

---

[1] ISO 9241 (1997)
[2] Nielsen (2000)
[3] Ivory & Hearst (2001)

C. Stephanidis (Ed.): Posters, Part I, HCII 2013, CCIS 373, pp. 96–99, 2013.

Although accessing and analyzing the log files should not provide meaningful answers, they can give us an approach of which areas of the website need a further evaluation. Other more expensive evaluation methods should be used in these cases to analyze these areas.

Doing this way we are promoting a quick evaluation with the information we have at hand, to evaluate with more details later only in the problematic points. It is important to mention that log file analysis give us only a tip of what area should be further evaluated and don't take the place of other evaluation methods, specially the qualitative ones as questionnaires and checklists. We suggest a methodology of how this can be done with a website.

We have chosen Apache as the web server model to our research, because it has almost 55% of the whole market.[4] As Apache log files have their information in two standard formats and most people don't change it, we know exactly what information we will find and in what order.

The process of evaluating a website using the analysis of the web server log files should be automated, because log files have a lot of information to be analyzed. Our tool makes use of Regular Expressions (a special set of texts to describe a search pattern) to separate small significant pieces from the log file lines, so that we can get relevant and meaningful information to be compared.

The standard formats of Apache log files are:

```
LogFormat "%h %l %u %t \"%r\" %»s %b" common
LogFormat "%h %l %u %t \"%r\" %»s %b \"%{Referer}i\"
\"%{User-agent}i\""
combined
```

The common type is included in the combined type. The information contained in such formats are: remote server, remote logname, remote user, moment of request receiving, request first line, request status, answer size in bytes, browser and operating system that make the request, and the request properly. Request status may have the following values: success, redirecting, client error, and server error.

Apache log files also have some other information that are not essential resources in order to describe what users have been doing while using the website.

We used a PHP parser in order to obtain the parts of the Apache log file parts by regular expression. The code line to do this is:

```
preg_match("/^(\S+) (\S+) (\S+) \[([^:]+):(\d+:\d+:\d+)
([^\]]+)\] \"(\S+) (.*?) (\S+)\" (\S+) (\S+) (\".*?\")
(\".*?\")$/", $line, $matches); // pattern to format the
line
```

Initially we must identify all the web pages of the website being analyzed. The job of finding the best task mapping for the website is the most important of all the process and affects the final result.

[4] Netcraft (2013)

After that we map the tasks of the website that we would like to analyze. In other words, we select the sequences of web pages that characterize the independent actions that are possible to be done in the website and that we would like to analyze. Only the lines of the log file which describe the tasks possible to be done with the web site are important in this analysis. Filtering the entries of the log file helps to achieve a more accurate result.

As log files are such big text files, we must take from the web server only the ones which correspond to the dates we would like to analyze. Besides that, we may filter only some IPs or take the whole file. This is done by a command from the operational system. We present examples of the commands in Windows and in Linux.

```
cat default_access.log.3 | grep 127.0.0.217 » teste.log
cat default_access.log.3 | egrep
'127.0.0.217|127.0.0.218' » teste.log
```

[Example of command line to filter by IP in Linux]

```
type default_access.log.3 | findstr 127.0.0.217 >
teste.log
type default_access.log.3 | findstr "127.0.0.217
127.0.0.218" > teste.log
```

[Example of command line to filter by IP in Windows]

Our tool will look inside the selected and filtered log files, and compare each entry with the tasks previously registered. The time difference will be calculated also. After collecting the rates related with the completed tasks and the times for doing that, metrics will be calculated.

Our main interest is collecting metrics to quantify the usability of the web site. The metrics we calculate are based on some rates that were chosen because they are closely related to usability. The rates collected are:

- Hit Rate: it counts every URL that were contempled by the search conditions, for example dates interval, beginning and ending times;
- Task Complete Rate: it counts how many times a certain task was completed, in other words, all its URLs were hited, from first to last, without interruption and in the specified order;
- Task Incomplete Rate: it make us know how many times a task was initiated but not completed for such reason (not in the order, not from first to last);
- No Task Rate: it indicates the moments where the URL found is not part of any task being analysed; for great values we suggest the inclusion of other tasks or the splitting of the existing ones, so that the conditions can be fitted;
- Agent Change Rate: it may indicate moments in which the user couldn't continue using the browser or the operating system because of some problem between this resource and the web site;

- Long Time Rate: it may indicate a problem in using the web site, because a long time has passed without internet activity, but it is not conclusive because the user could go out for a cup of water or was in a telephone conversation.

The metrics are calculated by the division of the rates for the first one. This way we obtain values which help in a usability website evaluation that is remote and automated. For each task this metrics get how the use of the functionalities of the website is.

References

1. ISO/DIS 9241. Dialogue Principles in Guiding the Evaluation of User Interfaces - Guidance on Usability (1997)
2. Ivory, M.Y., Hearst, M.A.: The State of the Art in Automating Usability Evaluation of User Interfaces. ACM Computing Surveys 33(4), 470–516 (2001)
3. Netcraft News, `http://news.netcraft.com/archives/2013/` (accessed, February 2013)
4. Nielsen, J.: Designing Web Usability. New Riders, California (2000)

The Design and Usability Testing of a Mobile Application to Aid in Child-to-Adult-Care Transition

Jeremy Dixon[1], Josh Dehlinger[1], and Shannan DeLany Dixon[2]

[1] Department of Computer and Information Sciences Towson University, Towson, MD
[2] Department of Pediatrics University of Maryland - School of Medicine, Baltimore, MD
jdixon6@students.towson.edu, jdehlinger@towson.edu,
smdixon@som.umaryland.edu

Abstract. As mobile devices become more central in our lives, accessibility and utility for users becomes essential. The widespread availability of mobile devices introduces a number of challenges to traditional software engineering including: 1. mobile user interfaces differ from traditional interfaces; and, 2. the diversity of mobile platforms. As part of a larger research effort, this poster presents the design, implementation and initial testing of a mobile application aimed at helping the child-to-adult-care transition process for children with chronic disease. Based on recommendations from the American Academy of Pediatrics, the application will help guide patients through four main components of transition: 1. assess transition readiness; 2. plan the transition; 3. implement the transition; and, 4. help document the transition. The design, implementation and testing of a mobile application may ease the transition process. By leveraging modern cross-compilation tools, this application can be implemented on multiple mobile platforms. This will lead to a variety of users, including those who may be differently-abled, to have a more fluid transition to their new health care providers.

Keywords: mobile applications, human-computer interaction, accessibility.

1 Introduction

As mobile application usage has grown, user accessibility and utility for those who are differently-abled has become essential [1]. A large portion of the differently-abled population must undergo process of medical transition. Medical transition is defined as the process of an individual taking complete control of their medical care and transferring care from a pediatric focused medical team to one based in adult medicine. The transition from pediatric care to adult care occurs most commonly in an individual when they are in their late teens or early twenties [2]. Transition is an important step in the healthcare of a young adult and a failed or incomplete transition may cause physical and/or mental health issues for adolescents with chronic conditions [3]. Medical transition for patients with chronic diseases from pediatric-based care to adult-based care is one that has been studied, developed and implemented for a number of years; recently, it has become a top priority in

C. Stephanidis (Ed.): Posters, Part I, HCII 2013, CCIS 373, pp. 100–104, 2013.

healthcare [2]. Due to the complexities of the transition process, a well-designed, intuitive mobile application should improve the standardization and ease of care for these patients. The significance of this applied research is to bring needed attention to the evaluation and necessity of a mobile application that assists with pediatric-to-adult transition which is considered to be a critical issue in healthcare today.

The application is designed to help with the transition process by leading the patient through the four main components recommended by the American Academy of Pediatrics [2]. First, the application will illustrate key questions to help decide if a patient is ready to initiate the transition process. These questions will help the patient to assess their knowledge of the disorder, their personal patient information, their ability to complete daily activities, and an assessment of communication practices. If a patient is not ready to start the transition process, the application will provide guidance as to what tasks need to be established prior to starting the transition.

Second, the application will help patients plan the transition process. It will provide suggestions for goals to complete along with realistic timelines. Goals include: understanding the importance of obtaining medical records, identifying current and future care team members, demonstrating the ability to communicate a working knowledge of the genetic disorder as well as places to identify disease based information and understanding the complexities of management of the disorder. The main purpose of this phase is to help educate a patient as to what is involved in a successful transition.

Third, the application will help initiate patient transition. The primary goal of the implementation phase is to educate all involved parties regarding the plan for transition. In many cases, this will require the patient, caregivers, family members and the healthcare team to be educated as to a patient's condition, the expectations of care, and the timeline for completion. The application will provide a list of resources, a task completion checklist and talking points to help with the implementation phase but will not provide any disease-specific resources. The talking point section will include lists of questions to ask current and future care providers, insurance companies, and pharmacies [2]. Additionally, a list of talking points will be provided to the patient within the mobile application to help initiate and engage their family and care providers in open and honest conversations.

Finally, the application will help document important aspects of the transition process, such as important insurance information, contact information for the healthcare team, and checklists to help ensure that nothing is missed [4]. The complete application will be able to be emailed or printed so that the patient may provide this information to their care providers to add to their medical record.

2 Application Design

Designing the application so that it meets the needs of the transition plan can be complex as each patient is different. As the goal is to complete the four transition plan components, it is important for the application to meet each of those needs.

Additionally, the application will store important information about both the patient and their medical care team. Finally, the application needs to provide both assistance for the user interface and any required usability enhancements. The application is being built using the Sencha Touch 2 mobile framework. Importantly, Sencha Touch allows developers to create HTML5 based mobile apps that work on Android, iOS and Blackberry devices [4].

The first step is to assess transition readiness [2]. The transition readiness evaluations often look like a checklist or a series of questions. For example, a question might be, "I understand my health care needs, and disability and can explain my needs to others" [5]. If these questions are yes/no questions, Sencha Touch includes a list with a checkbox option. If the question requires options such as, "Yes", "I want to do this", "I need to learn how", or "Someone else will have to do this - Who?" then a dropdown can be employed with a comment section. The comment section will provide detailed explanations of the task itself to help patients minimize any confusion. Figure 1 shows an example of the option boxes in Sencha.

The second phase involves planning the transition [2]. This phase includes developing a timeline for the transition, identifying responsibilities, and developing a skill list. From an application implementation standpoint, this phase has some of the components related to the previous phase with the exception that the list of caregivers will be documented. In order for the patient to record their current caregiver information, a series of forms were generated that document important contact information and comments regarding each person on the team. This will be very important when seeking new caregivers in the next phase. As in the previous phase, this section of the application will also contain drop down boxes, which will provide descriptions of the services that each type of physician provides. Figure 2 shows an example of the interface that will allow new information to be stored in the application. In this case, the information is patient related.

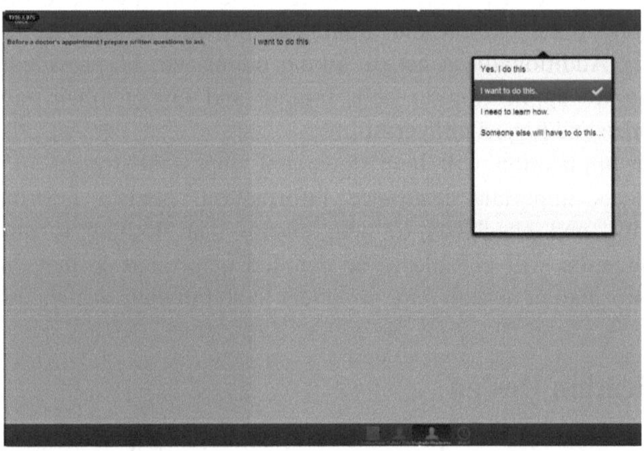

Fig. 1. Example of Option Boxes in Sencha (as viewed in Chrome)

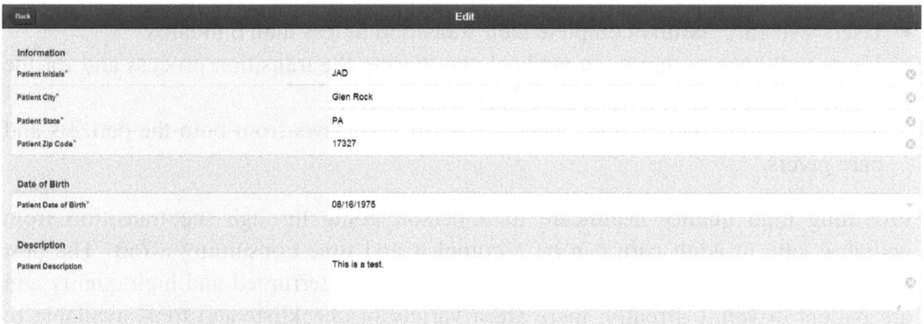
Back
Edit
Information
Patient Initials*
JAD
Patient City*
Glen Rock
Patient State*
PA
Patient Zip Code*
17327
Date of Birth
Patient Date of Birth*
08/16/1975
Description
Patient Description
This is a test.

Fig. 2. Example of Editable Form in Sencha (as viewed in Chrome)

The third phase involves implementing the plan through education and goal achievement [2]. This phase will provide the user with a variety of goals related to the transition process. For example, in this phase, the user may be provided with a goal of scheduling an interview with a prospective doctor in order to discuss their diagnoses. The application will also provide an important topic list to discuss with the prospective doctor and how to make sure that they will be an appropriate fit for care of the patient. From an implementation standpoint, this phase requires checklists with a number of forms. The checklists and forms are generated from a thorough review of the literature and discussions with various transition clinics.

The fourth phase involves documenting the transition process. As the patient continues through the transition process, it is important to know what areas have been completed and what areas still need to be worked on to complete the process. This part of the application will review the information already reported and generate a summary of additional steps to be completed. From an application implementation standpoint, this phase will query to database to see what aspects of the transition have not been completed. It will list all of the sections that need to be worked on including links to the appropriate part of the application. In many ways, this is a dashboard that shows the user's progress through the transition.

3 Conclusion

In order to ensure the best transition experiences, it is important for this application to guide the patient in order to ensure that the care is uninterrupted and of high quality. The design, implementation and testing of a mobile application may significantly help with the transition process. By leveraging modern cross-compilation tools, the application can be implemented on multiple mobile operating systems so that a variety of users, including those who may be differently-abled, to have a fluid transition to their new health care providers. The application's success will be measured in three ways:

- Users will successfully complete their transition in less than 6 months.
- Users will have no lapses in medical care during the transition process and for the six months after the transition has been completed.
- The application will receive generally positive reviews from both the patients and care givers.

Providing high quality healthcare to a person going through the transition from pediatric care to adult care can be a complex and time consuming effort. The best transition experiences are those where the care is uninterrupted and high quality and are patient driven. Currently, there are a variety of checklists and tools available to help people who are going through the transition period to complete the process however are not provided in a centralized location and have varying results.

Advances in medical knowledge and skills are helping children and young adults with chronic conditions live much longer than in previous generations. Due to this, the population of people going through the transition process is increasing. By designing a mobile application framework that helps with the transition process, the efforts required to successfully complete this may be improved. Once the application is developed and validated, it may be distributed to a broader patient base throughout the medical system to determine effectiveness to a global patient population.

Acknowledgements. We would like to acknowledge New York Mid Atlantic Consortium for Genetics and Newborn Screening Services (NYMAC) for their support and funding of this project.

References

1. Dehlinger, J., Dixon, J.: Mobile Application Software Engineering: Challenges and Research Directions. In: Mobile Software Engineering Workshop, MobiCase 2011, Santa Monica (2011)
2. American Academic of Pediatrics, Supporting the Transition from Adolescence to Adulthood in the Medical Home. Pediatrics, 182–200 (2011)
3. Binks, J.A., Barden, W.S., Burke, T.A., Young, N.L.: What Do We Really Know About the Transition to Adult-Centered Health Care? A Focus on Cerebral Palsy and Spina Bifida. Archives of Physical Medicine Rehabilitation 88, 1064–1073 (2007)
4. Sencha Inc., Sencha Touch (Feburary 2013), `http://www.sencha.com/products/touch/`
5. New England Consortium of Metabolic Programs, Transition Toolkit (August 2010), `http://newenglandconsortium.org/for-families/transition-toolkit/`

Verification of the Questionnaire for the Level of Mental Models Building

Toshihisa Doi[1], Keisuke Ishihara[1], and Toshiki Yamaoka[2]

[1] Wakayama University Graduate School of Systems Engineering
930, Sakaedani, Wakayama-Shi, Wakayama, 640 8510, Japan
[2] Wakayama University Faculty of Systems Engineering
930, Sakaedani, Wakayama-Shi, Wakayama, 640 8510, Japan
info@toshihisadoi.com, k.ishihara62@gmail.com,
yamaoka@ja2.so-net.ne.jp

Abstract. In this study, the verification of the questionnaire for the level of mental model building was examined from viewpoint of the actual users' operation. The user testing is conducted to grasp the level of mental model building. The validity of the questionnaire was investigated in terms of (a) operation time of the digital camera, (b) operation errors of the digital camera and (c) Structural model / Functional mode (the test result for measurement the level of mental model building after the operation). Then, the correlation between the score of the user testing and the questionnaire score was calculated. As the result, the significant correlation is confirmed between each score and the questionnaire score. Then, we believed the proposed questionnaire can be measured the users' mental model building level in the user-interfaces operation.

Keywords: Mental model, Questionnaire, Usability testing.

1 Background

In user-interface design, the examination of users' mental model is important. However, we don't think that mental model is examined enough in design development process because mental model cannot be easily examined. Therefore, we proposed the questionnaire items for measurement of the level of mental model building which can examine easily in the previous study. The reliability and validity of this questionnaire is shown based on the questionnaire development methods. However, the relationship between the questionnaire and the actual users' operation still is not clarified by experiments.

2 Objective

The goal of this study is the verification of the questionnaire from viewpoint of the actual users' operation. We verified the questionnaire to use this mental model examining method for design development.

C. Stephanidis (Ed.): Posters, Part I, HCII 2013, CCIS 373, pp. 105–108, 2013.

3 Questionnaire for the Level of Mental Models Building [1]

The questionnaire for the level of mental models building is proposed by our previous study to estimate users' mental model building level quantitatively. This questionnaire consists of 36 items based on the elements for structuring mental model. This questionnaire is conducted using a 5-point scale (e.g., 5: strongly agree to 1: strongly disagree).

This questionnaire was made by questionnaire survey to 726 people. Besides, the reliability and validity are certificated based on questionnaire development method. However, this qualification method is the method which be used for psychological scale development. Our proposed questionnaire should be investigation method for usability and design development. So, we should show the relativity with users' operation to confirm the utility and the validity as usability investigation method.

4 Methods

In this experiment, (1) digital camera operation task, (2) Mental model measurement task of the digital camera, and (3) the proposed questionnaire were conducted to 24 people. The participants are the students (age: 21-25, ave: 23.21, SD: 1.10). Besides, the utility and the validity were considered in terms of (a) task complete time, (b) operation error, (c) mental model measurement task after operation.

4.1 Digital Camera Operation Task

Firstly, the mental model of the participants for the digital camera operation was constructed by 5 tasks of digital camera operation. Next, 4 tasks were conducted for the measurement of task complete time and operation error score.

4.2 Mental Model Measurement Test

The level of mental model structuring for the digital camera operation was investigated. This test was conducted in terms of Functional model and Structural model [2]. Functional model is the model regarding to understanding the contexts and the functions to understand "how to use it?" Structural model is the model regarding to understanding the structure and the principle to understand "how it works?" In this study, the test for the level of understanding the button function is conducted as the function model measurement [3]. In this test, the participants replay the operation procedure of the 4 tasks. The test for the level of understanding the hierarchy structure is conducted as the structural model measurement [3]. In this test, the participants conduct the card sorting of the card which is wrote each function of the digital camera. Then, the each scale is calculated to estimate the level of mental model structuring.

4.3 Proposed Questionnaire

After all tasks, the participants answered the proposed questionnaire for the digital camera. Then, correlation coefficient was calculated between the questionnaire scale and the score which are gotten from each test.

5 Results

The correlation coefficient between the questionnaire scale and 4 items (task complete time, operation error score, Functional model score, and Structural model score) were calculated. Firstly, we explain the score of each item.

- Task complete time score

This score is sum of 4 tasks operation times.

- Operation error score

This score detail is as below. This score use 5 level scale; 4: correct operation to 0: not complete.

- 4: Correct operation
- 3: Not smooth operation; Stop for a moment, dither for a moment, cheap mistake, etc.
- 2: Error operation; Stop, more noticeable error that 3, etc.
- 1: Critical error operation; clear error, repeating error, accidental complete, etc.
- 0: Not complete

- Structural model test

The scoring for structural model was conducted by the point deduction method. Correct hierarchy structure is perfect score (68 points).

- Functional model test

The scoring for functional model was also conducted by the point deduction method. The correct procedure is perfect score (36 points).

Table 1 shows the correlation analysis result between these 4 items and the questionnaire score. The significant correlation was confirmed with all 4 items.

Table 1. Correlation analysis result

Experiment items	Questionnaire score		
	Pearson correlation coefficient	p	
Operation error	0.6664	p < 0.01	**
Complete time	-0.4666	p < 0.05	*
Structural model	0.5919	p < 0.01	**
Functional model	0.4174	p < 0.05	*

**: p<0.01, *: p<0.05

6 Discussion

We confirmed the significant correlation between the questionnaire score and each item regarding to the level of mental model structuring. So, the questionnaire for mental model can estimate the users' mental model building level in user-interface operation. We think the questionnaire has the validity to measure users' mental model for user-interface operation. Besides, this questionnaire can quantitatively estimate the level of mental model structuring. We believe that the quantitative investigation for users' mental model is helpful to usability survey and user-interface design. This questionnaire can investigate usability in terms of mental model easily.

References

1. Doi, T., et al.: Fundamental Consideration of the Level of Constructing the Mental Model Measurement Scale in User Interface'. In: 13th JSKE Annual Conf. (2011)
2. Preece, J., et al.: Human-Computer Interaction, pp. 123–139. Addsion-Wesley Publishing Company (1994)
3. Doi, T., et al.: Analysis of Users' Knowledge Structures and Mental Models by the Difference of Attitude to Electrical Appliances. Transactions of Japan Society of Kansei Enginieering 9(4), 611–619 (2010)

Towards Usable and Secure Natural Language Processing Systems

Yasser M. Hausawi and Liam M. Mayron

Department of Computer Sciences
Florida Institute of Technology
Melbourne, FL 32901, USA
{yhausawi@my.,lmayron@}fit.edu

Abstract. Natural Language Processing (NLP) systems must be both secure and usable, but this remains an elusive objective. This work considers the relationship between usability and security in NLP systems. Development and lifecycle practices are discussed with the goal of a more integrated, comprehensive process for NLP system development.

Keywords: Natural Language Processing, Security, Usability, Artificial Intelligence, Human-Computer Interaction.

1 Introduction

Natural Language Processing (NLP) systems are used with increasing frequency by a growing number of people. Such systems interpret text or voice that is generated by a human in a manner interpretable by a machine. They employ a variety of machine learning methods in order to determine the meaning of the original material. Scenarios for usage of NLP systems range from the automated extraction of entities from text or speech and translation to determining the emotion of a human or the relationships between people. In this work, we consider the effectiveness of NLP systems in the context of their usability and security. Despite the widespread usage and potential applications of NLP systems, investigations into their usability are scarce. Furthermore, the security implications of NLP systems merit additional investigation. Perhaps most interesting is the intersection of usability, security, and the capabilities of NLP systems. In terms of usability, an NLP system must be able to satisfy metrics of effectiveness, efficiency, and satisfaction. Security requirements include confidentiality, integrity, and availability. Security and usability requirements can sometimes be in opposition [4], but work towards bridging this gap has been undertaken [7].

2 Usability and Security for NLP Systems

NLP occurs in five main stages: user interface (for example, the input from a microphone or text), recognition and conversion, segmentation and parsing, matching, and processing (Figure 1). In the case of audio input, an Automatic

C. Stephanidis (Ed.): Posters, Part I, HCII 2013, CCIS 373, pp. 109–113, 2013.

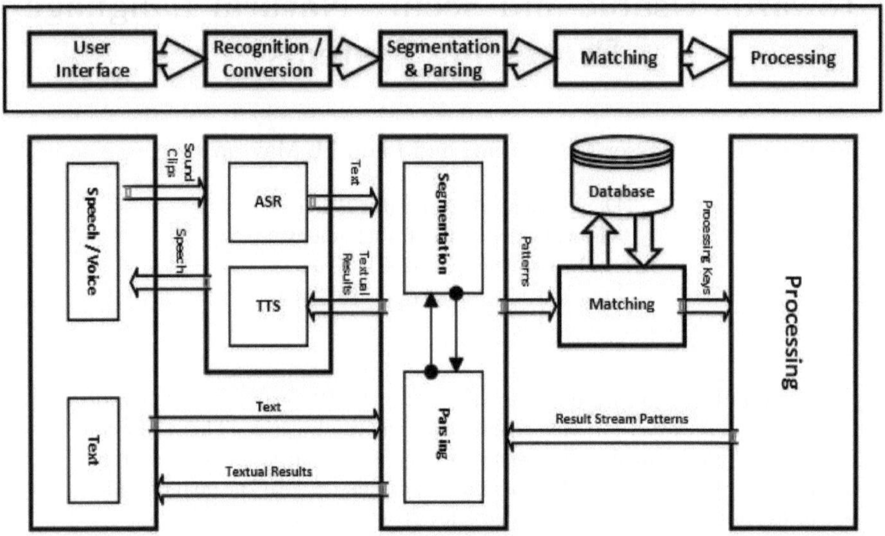

Fig. 1. NLP system architecture

Speech Recognition (ASR) subsystem can be used to recognize sound and covert to textual patterns. After processing, the resulting text is converted back to audio through a Text-to-Speech (TTS) system if the response is to be presented as speech. If the system uses only textual input, the recognition and conversation stage can be eliminated.

The term usability is defined by the International Standard Organization (ISO) as the range in which a product can be operated by legitimate users to satisfactorily perform specific tasks in an effective, efficient, and specified way [6]. The assessment of an NLP system's usability must consider these three factors (efficiency, effectiveness, and satisfaction). An NLP system can only be considered as effective if its users are able to achieve their goal of operating it. An efficient NLP system must complete specific task or process to reach a particular goal within an acceptable amount of time. For a NLP system to be satisfactory, both the vendors and the users must be happy with the system (as determined by their willingness to rely on and reuse the system). Evaluating satisfaction can be challenging due to the difficulty of measuring it. The best way to evaluate system satisfaction is through vendor and user questionnaires, surveys, and interviews [7].

System security is a set of methods and techniques applied to prevent weaknesses from being exploited. At a high level, there are three main security objectives: confidentiality, integrity, and availability [8]. NLP systems, like all other computer systems, have vulnerabilities that need to be discovered and remedied.

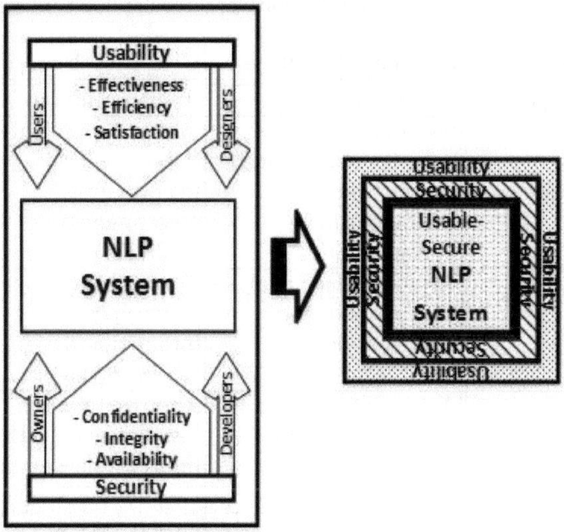

Fig. 2. Usability and security in NLP systems

In order for a NLP system to be considered confidential, it must limit access to its features and services solely to authorized users. Integrity requires that a system protects its contents from unauthorized alteration. Finally, a system must be available for use when needed by authorized users for legitimate purposes.

The interaction between usability and security in NLP systems is illustrated in Figure 2.

3 Developing Secure and Usable NLP Systems

Building a NLP system using the standard waterfall model of software development tends to be linear [9], following the Software Development Lifecycle (SDLC). NLP system development starts from the pre-development planning phase. Subsequently, the requirements phase establishes objectives for the project. The design phase details the requirements and develops a system architecture. Implementation consists of programming and creating functionality. The testing phase evaluates and validates the system. During deployment, the system is delivered and configured. The maintenance phase keeps the system in working order.

Although the SDLC can satisfy functional requirements, the implementations of security and usability benefit from their own processes that occur within the SDLC [1,2,3,5,9,10]. This alignment is shown in Table 1. It can be used as guidance by software engineers in achieving both a usable and secure development process.

Table 1. Usability and security during the software development lifecycle [1,2,3,5,9,10]

Phase	Security Practice	Usability Practice
Planning	Security training	Human-centered
Requirements	Security objectives Security requirements Quality gates Risk assessment Specifications	Context specification Usage scenarios User analysis Task analysis Usability specifications
Design	Attack surface analysis Threat modeling Design review	Concept development Prototypes Interaction design Design review
Implementation	Approved tools Security patterns Static analysis Code review	Approved tools User interface patterns Interface development User interface review
Testing	Dynamic analysis Attack surface review	Expert review Usability evaluation Acceptance testing
Deployment	Incident response plan Security review Release Archive	Surveys and interviews
Maintenance	Incident plan	Usability review

4 Conclusion

NLP has a significant impact on human-computer interaction. There is a strong relationship between NLP systems, usability, and security, as NLP systems must be both usable and secure in order to engender the trust of both users and vendors. NLP systems can be evaluated in terms of both usability and security, and enhanced as needed.

References

1. Costabile, M.F., et al.: Usability in the software life cycle. Handbook of Software Engineering and Knowledge Engineering 1, 179–192 (2001)
2. Cranor, L., Garfinkel, S.: Security and usability: designing secure systems that people can use. O'Reilly Media, Incorporated (2005)
3. Ferre, X.: Integration of usability techniques into the software development process. In: International Conference on Software Engineering (Bridging the Gaps between Software Engineering and Human-Computer Interaction), pp. 28–35 (2003)
4. Fléchais, I.: Designing Secure and Usable Systems. Ph.D. thesis, Citeseer (2005)
5. Howard, M., Lipner, S.: The security development lifecycle. Microsoft Press (2009)
6. ISO, W.: 9241-11, Ergonomic requirements for office work with visual display terminals (vdts). The international organization for standardization (1998)

7. Kainda, R., Flechais, I., Roscoe, A.: Security and usability: Analysis and evaluation. In: International Conference on Availability, Reliability, and Security, ARES 2010, pp. 275–282. IEEE (2010)
8. Pfleeger, C.P., Pfleeger, S.L.: Security in computing. Prentice Hall PTR (2006)
9. Preece, J., Rogers, Y., Sharp, H., Benyon, D., Holland, S., Carey, T.: Human-Computer Interaction. Addison - Wesley (1994)
10. Shneiderman, B., Plaisant, C.: Designing the user interface: Strategies for effective human-computer interaction. Pearson Education (2005)

Variables of Usability

James Helfrich

219 Austin Building, Rexburg, ID 83460 - 1015
HelfrichJ@byui.edu

Abstract. Though many have proposed heuristics, maximums, and guidelines to describe the various aspects of heuristic usability analysis, none offer a comprehensive variable set that is both valid and reliable. This paper proposes an eight-variable criteria-set through which usability inspections can be performed. Each variable will be compared with prior work and a precise definition through which each variable can be identified will be proposed.

Keywords: Usability engineering, usability inspection, heuristic analysis.

1 Introduction

Usability inspection is the process of evaluating a user interface to identify usability issues [23]. There are many methods for conducting such an inspection, including the empirical method, an expert analysis, and heuristic evaluation [5]. Empirical evaluation involves creating experiments where qualitative and quantative data is collected through observations of users. Expert analysis involves an expert giving an opinion of the design based on his or her experiences and judgment. The final method, heuristic evaluation, involves using a structured critique by means of a set of heuristics or variables [23]. This paper will focus on the third method: heuristic evaluation.

The quality of a heuristic evaluation methodology, as is true with all evaluation instruments or methodologies, is a function of two properties: validity (measuring the right thing) and reliability (the lack of error in the measurement) [8]. Though a large number of heuristic evaluation methodologies have been described in the literature [5, 9, 13, 18, 21, 23, 25, 27, 29], each is based on variable set exhibiting validity or reliability challenges. This paper will identify a new variable set based on those previously defined to allow for more valid and reliable heuristic evaluation.

2 Variables Set

For a variable set to be valid, it must cover all aspects of usability and nothing else. Currently there does not exist a variable set covering all the components of usability identified in the literature. For a variable set to be reliable, it needs to produce similar results with reevaluation. This requires it to be as objective as possible while not resorting to false metrics resulting in validity challenges. Stemming from these constraints and based on work of previous researchers, a new variable set is proposed: Efficiency, Learnability, Familiarity, Simplicity, Mapping, Motivation, Trust, and Visibility.

C. Stephanidis (Ed.): Posters, Part I, HCII 2013, CCIS 373, pp. 114–118, 2013.

2.1 Efficiency

The term and concept of Efficiency has been a focus of human factors research since 1903 [30]. Though Efficiency has been identified by many researchers [1, 29], possibly Raskin [26] put it best: "A computer shall not waste your time or require you do to more work than is strictly necessary." Efficiency is defined as the amount of effort or time required to perform a task, is an important variable in usability because it sets the limit on a user's productivity. It can be influenced by many factors, including flexibility [9, 24], directness of action [9, 23], and speed to perform the task [9, 21]. Though most measurements of Efficiency (such as time to completion, work throughput, mouse movements, processing requirements, etc.) lend themselves to absolute measures, Efficiency from the HCI perspective is fundamentally a relative measure: it compares the time or effort of a user against some norm or standard.

2.2 Learnability

The term "Learnability" was first applied to the context of HCI by Licklider [17] though the term can be traced to 1959 when it was originally used in the field of linguistics. Learnability has been identified in many variable sets [4, 5, 16, 21], though at present there is no generally accepted definition [12]. There are, however, reoccurring themes and ideas in the various definitions.

Learnability is the path to becoming proficient, largely a function of the number and size of inductive leaps the user must make to master the system. It is not the amount that needs to be learned (Simplicity) nor how pleasurable may be the journey (Motivation). Instead, the Learnability is a function of the difficulty of the learning process. The goal of managing Learnability is to maximize the level of proficiency achieved by the target user with as little user-effort as possible.

2.3 Familiarity

"Familiarity" was first applied both in term and in concept to HCI in 1983 [3] and has been identified directly as a variable of usability by many researchers [9, 21]. There are two main components of Familiarity: Consistency and Compatibility. Consistency is a measure of how one part of a system's interface is similar to another. Compatibility, on the other hand, is how much one system's interface resembles other systems performing similar functions. Both relate to the degree in which the design resembles other designs the user may have encountered before [9, 13, 16].

2.4 Simplicity

Though the concept of Simplicity has been applied to HCI and human factors from the beginning, there does not appear to be a consensus on the definition. Definitions vary from the complexity of the interface [6], the amount of distractions to the user [23], and how streamlined the interface is [22]. Simplicity, in simplest terms, is a measure of how much the user needs to know to operate the system. A more precise definition is the size and complexity of the minimally consistent mental model. Because perceptions of Simplicity are inherently subjective, any measurement of Simplicity must similarly have a degree of judgment built in. Also, discussions of the size and complexity of a user's mental model are intrinsically relative: it is only meaningful to compare two mental models rather than make absolute statements about one.

2.5 Mapping

The concept of Mapping was first described by Gibson [11], though the term entered common use in the context of usability inspections by Norman [24]. Other names have been used to describe all or part of the concept of Mapping, include Task Match [16], Directness [9], "Product Compatibility and User Compatibility" [21], and Affordance [11, 24]. Though a large number of definitions for Mapping exist [10, 13, 16, 24, 25], two essential components are present in all: the user's mental model and the system model. Mapping consists of cues within the design encouraging the user to form a consistent mental model of the system. While Simplicity is a measure of the size of the mental model, Mapping is about how well the interface communicates the intended model. It is important to note that the user is ultimately responsible for his or her own mental model; the best the interface can do is to encourage the user to form a consistent one and to discourage an inconsistent one. No research has been done to measure Mapping, in part due to the nature of the variable; while it is possible to accurately and completely describe a system model, it is impossible to directly measure a user's mental model. Possibly for this reason there have also been no metrics offered to quantify Mapping; indirect evidence and judgment will always be part of the equation.

2.6 Motivation

Motivation addresses the users' desire to use the system, encompassing both internal and external sources. Though Motivation has been described by many, Keller [14] provided the most widely acceptable framework in his ARCS (Attention, Relevance, Confidence, and Satisfaction) model. Motivation has been described through external sources (how the user is compelled to use the system) [13] and internal sources (how rewarding, aesthetically appealing, and how fun the interface is) [2, 9, 16, 25].

Some of the best usability examples are successful because their level of fun overshadows problems with Efficiency or Familiarity. Users tend to try harder, be more forgiving, and be more patient when their Motivation levels are higher [15, 31]. Because Motivation lies in the affective domain [7], it is impossible to directly measure. However, like Mapping, indirect evidence can be collected and often a certain amount of judgment is required.

2.7 Trust

Trust, defined by Kavonen as "the user's willingness to commit any transaction," has also been called safety [9, 13] and control [9, 21, 25]. Trust is the amount of confidence the user has when using the system, being a function of how much the system encouraging the user feel in control and how little the system behaves in an unexpected way. The variable of Trust encompasses both measures of user's perceived control over the system and avoidance of trust-compromising experiences. In both cases, poor Trust often results in poor Motivation and poor Efficiency.

2.8 Visibility

Visibility was first described as a HCI design constraint by [3] when building the XEROX Star system. Galitz [9] defined Visibility as "indications of status, possible actions that can be taken, and the results of actions once they are performed." Heim [13] offers a similar definition: "making the user aware of the system's components and processes, including all possible functionality and feedback from user actions."

Many researchers break Visibility into several components: reachability (any state can be reached from any other state) [5, 9], observability (visibility of data) [5], Discoverability (the probability the user will find the information or functionality he or she needs), and Precedence (the degree of prominence a desired piece of data or functionality is on a given display interface). Each definition has the common component: the degree of availability of the functionality and the data of the system to the user when he or she needs it. Thus any metric describing Visibility must include the user and his scenario.

3 Conclusion

Through the last two decades, there have been many heuristic evaluation frameworks proposed, including AIDE [28], MUSiC [20], PUTS [19], Dix's adaptation of Nielsen's heuristic scale [5], and QUIM [29]. It is the hope of this researcher that each of these frameworks can be improved through the adaptation of a more valid and reliable variable set. This will enable heuristic evaluation methodologies to be a more practical and useful tool in the design process, classroom, and usability lab.

References

1. Bailey, R.W.: Performance vs. preference. In: Human Factors and Ergonomics Society Annual Meeting Proceedings, pp. 282–286 (1993)
2. Barber, W., Badre, A.: Culturability: The merging of culture and usability. In: Proceedings of the 4th Conference on Human Factors & the Web (1998)
3. Bewley, W., Roberts, T., Schroit, D., Verplank, W.: Human factors testing in the design of Xerox's 8010 "Star" office workstation In. In: CHI 1983, pp. 72–77 (1983)
4. Brown, A., Chung, L., Patterson, D.: Including the human factor in dependability benchmarks. In: Workshop on Dependability Benchmarking, pp. 9–14 (2002)
5. Dix, A., Finlay, J., Abowd, G.D., Beale, R.: Human-Computer Interaction, 3rd edn. Pearson Education Limited, Essex (2004)

6. Dourish, P., Herrmann, T., Kellogg, W., Kunau, G.: Discussion report: Simplicity and appropriation. In: International Reports on Socio-Informatics, pp. 113–116 (2005)
7. Gagné, R.M.: Learning Hierarchies (1968)
8. Gagné, R.M., Wager, W.W., Golas, K.C., Keller, J.M.: Principles of Instructional Design, 5th edn. Thomson Learning, Belmont (2005)
9. Galitz, W.O.: The Essential Guide to User Interface Design: An Introduction to GUI Design Principles and Techniques, 3rd edn. Wiley Publishing, Inc., Indianapolis (2007)
10. Gaver, W.: Technology affordances. In: Proceedings of the CHI 1991 Conference on Human Factors in Computing Systems, pp. 79–84 (1991)
11. Gibson, J.J.: The Ecological Approach to Visual Perception. Lawrence Erlbaum (1979)
12. Grossman, T., Fitzmaurice, G., Attar, R.: A survey of software learnability: Metrics, methodologies, and guidelines. In: CHI 2009, pp. 649–658 (2009)
13. Heim, S.: The Resonant Interface. Addison-Wesley, San Francisco (2007)
14. Keller, J.M.: The systematic process of motivation design. Performance and Instruction 108 (1987)
15. Kurosu, M., et al.: Apparent usability vs. inherent usability. In: CHI 1995, pp. 292–293 (1995)
16. Leventhal, L.M., Barnes, J.A.: Usability Engineering: Process, Products, and Examples. Pearson Prentice Hall, Upper Saddle River (2008)
17. Licklider, J.C.: User-oriented interactive computer graphics. In: Proceedings of the ACM/SIGGRAPH Workshop on User-Oriented Design, Pittsburgh, PA, pp. 89–96 (1976)
18. Lidwell, W., Holden, K., Butler, J.: Universal Principles of Design. Rockport (2003)
19. Lin, H., Choong, Y., Salvendy, G.: A proposed index of usability. In: Behavior & Information Technology, pp. 267–278 (1997)
20. Macleod, M., Bowden, R., Bevan, N., Curson, I.: The MUSiC performance method. In: Behavior and Information Technology, pp. 279–293 (1997)
21. Mayhew, D.J.: Principles and Guidelines in Software User Interface Design. Prentice-Hall, Inc., Upper Saddle River (1992)
22. Mollerup, P.: Simplicity. In: Design Research Quarterly, pp. 7–15 (2006)
23. Nielsen, J., Mack, R.L.: Usability Inspection Methods. John Wiley & Sons (1994)
24. Nielsen, J.: Ten Usability Heuristics (2001), `http://www.useit.com/papers/heuristic/`
25. Preece, J., Rogers, Y., Sharp, H.: Interaction Design: Beyond Human-Computer Interaction. John Wiley & Sons, Inc., New York (2002)
26. Raskin, J.: The Humane Interface. Addison-Wesley, Reading (2000)
27. Rorres, R.J.: Practitioner's Handbook for User Interface Design and Development. Prentice-Hall, Inc., Upper Sandle River (2002)
28. Sears, A.: AIDE: A step toward metric-based interface development tools. In: UIST 1995, pp. 101–110. ACM Press, Pittsburgh (1995)
29. Seffah, A., Donyaee, M., Kline, R., Padda, H.: Usability measurement and metrics: A consolidated model. Software Quality Journal, 159–178 (2006)
30. Taylor, F.W.: Shop management. American Society of Mechanical Engineers (1903)
31. Tractinsky, N.: Aesthetics and apparent usability: Empirically assessing cultural and methodological issues. In: CHI 1997, pp. 115–121 (1997)

The Convergence of Security and Usability: Defining a Framework for Mobile Design

Ann-Marie Horcher and Gurvirender Tejay

Nova Southeastern University
horcher@nova.edu

Abstract. Security and usability have traditionally been at odds in the design process [1]. In spite of this, the usability of security is widely recognized as a key component of security effectiveness[2-4] Design principles for good security have been designed by security experts [5]. Similarly principles for designed usability have also been created by usability experts [6-8]. In both cases the design principles were defined for the traditional workstation environment, instead of the mobile environment. This study examines both security and usability design principles for conflict or convergence, specifically in relation to a mobile environment. The resulting framework of combined security-usability principles identifies which design principles are critical for success in the mobile environment.

Keywords: usability, security, mobile devices, design principles.

1 Introduction

Security and usability design principles have been articulated for the traditional workstation environment. In contrast to the workstation environment, mobile devices have significant differences in the interaction of users, and the availability of resources [9]. These realities call for a revised set of design principles that address the limitations of a mobile environment to achieve both security and usability. Unlike desktop workstations, every micrometer of internal space, every inch of screen real estate, and every amp of power is at a premium [10] on a mobile device. From environmental information to e-government services to phone directories, information delivery and interaction has shifted from print to exclusively electronic [11]. E-only delivery makes technology a necessity for all instead of a non-essential luxury item [12]. Increasingly mobile devices have moved from companion devices [13] to the primary or stand-alone device for digital information access [14]. Computer crime, already a problem on the traditional workstation [15, 16], has followed computer users to the mobile platform [17]. A mobile computing platform provides challenges in security that differ from the traditional computing workstation [9], and the structured work environment [18]. To effectively design these principles for usability and security in mobile devices, attention must be paid to the following:

C. Stephanidis (Ed.): Posters, Part I, HCII 2013, CCIS 373, pp. 119–123, 2013.

- The effort required of the user to follow security protocols [19]
- appropriate security for the value of the information
- resource constraints of the devices in terms of physical form factors [20] and device capabilities [21] .

2 Security versus Usability Design Principles

Systems designed with both security and usability principles remain more secure, because the users do not circumvent security for functionality [22]. System design can turn in a tug-of-war between the twin priorities, with many systems designers choosing to trade off usability for security and vice versa [23]. A combined framework removes the conflicting priorities.

Table 1. Combined Principles of Usability and Security

Saltzer & Schroeder [5]	Shneiderman [7]	Nielsen [6]	Garfinkel [24]
Psychological Acceptability	Internal locus of control Shortcuts for experience Easy reversal of actions	User control and freedom Flexibility and efficiency of use Match between system and the real world	Least Surprise
Complete Mediation	Dialog to Closure Informative Feedback	Visibility of system status Error prevention Help and documentation	Consistent Meaningful Vocabulary
Least Common Mechanism	Consistency	Consistency and standards	Consistent Controls and Placement
Economy of Mechanism	Reduce short-term memory load	Recognition rather than recall Aesthetic and minimalist design	No External Burden
Failing Secure	Simple Error Handling	Help users recognize, diagnose, and recover from errors	Provide standard security policies
Reluctance to Trust Promote Privacy Never Assume Secrets are Safe Principle of Least Privilege Separation of Privilege/duty	Not mentioned	Not mentioned	Good Security Now

To articulate the concept of secure design Saltzer & Schroeder (1975) created ten principles. At least half of the secure design principles relate directly to the interface with the user. Consequently "good" security design, or design created according to the principles, already includes guidance about the usability of the interface. Similar to the security principles created by Saltzer & Schroeder [5], the usability practitioners have the two seminal sets of heuristics or principles for design. The Golden Eight from Shneiderman [7] and ten more from Jakob Nielsen [6] form the core of usability design. Mapping the Shneiderman's Golden Eight Principles for usability [7] and Nielsen's Ten Heuristics for User Interface Design [6] to Saltzer & Schroeder's security design principles [5] yields an interesting result. Usability principles are not in conflict with secure design principles. Looking at the chart shows that for all the principles that address the user interface for security there is a parallel usability principle or principles stated for the same concept in both Shneiderman's Golden Eight Principles for Usability Design and Nielsen's Ten Heuristics for User Interface Design. Furthermore, Garfinkel [24] suggests design patterns as concrete examples of solutions to common security-usability problems. Design patterns leverage the best practices of a more skilled practitioner to compensate for the lack of skill in lesser experienced designer [25].

3 Security-Usability Design Principles for Mobile

Mobile devices have resource constraints that further impact the design of usable security The current security-usability framework described above does not address the resource constraints upon mobile devices. Creating a framework of combined security-usability principles that address the constraints yields principles more relevant to the mobile device platform. Simply transferring security practices from desktop to mobile has not yielded satisfactory usability and user acceptance [9]. The reality is that in the traditional workstation environment of a business or research organization ignoring certain security-usability principles has minor consequences [26]. In risk management assessment of information, the vulnerabilities are weighed against the probability of the occurrence, and the loss potentially incurred from the occurrence [27]. In the resource-constrained mobile device ignoring the consequences will compromise the practical functionality of the device.The three major resource constraints of the mobile device platform are power, form factors, and user expertise. To be mobile, the devices must run from a portable and renewable power source, such as a battery [28]. Security design drains battery life reduces the usability of the device. To be convenient mobile devices must be small enough and light enough to carry easily [29]. The screens must be big enough to use but small enough to fit in pocket or purse [30] and manipulated for information gathering in a variety of settings [31]. In the absence of a formal organization to compensate for individual user deficiencies, the applications must reduce complexity [30].

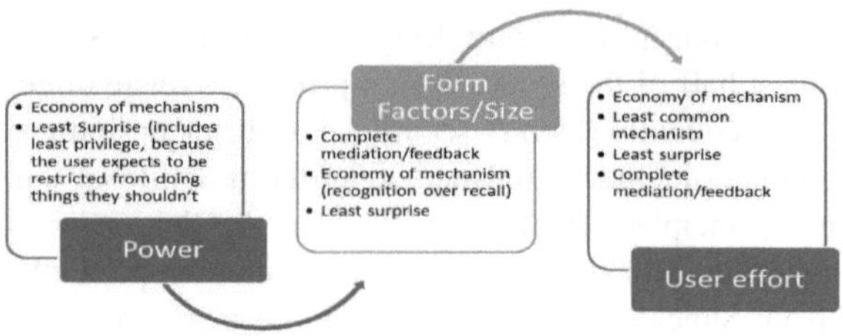

Fig. 1. Security-usability principles addressing resource constraints of mobile devices

Based on this analysis, the combined security-usability principles that address the resource constraints are:

- Economy of mechanism
- Least surprise
- Complete mediation and feedback

The result of mapping resource constraints to the combined design principles is a framework that prioritizes conservation of resources. The framework also provides a common set of design principles that put security designers and usability designers on the same page instead of on opposing sides.

References

1. Braz, C., Robert, J.-M.: Security and usability: the case of the user authentication methods. In: Proceedings of the 18th International Conference of the Association Francophone d'Interaction Homme-Machine, ACM, Montreal (2006)
2. Theofanos, M.F., Pfleeger, S.L.: Shouldn't All Security Be Usable? IEEE Security & Privacy 9(2), 12–17 (2011)
3. Cranor, L.F., Garfinkel, S.L.: Security and Usability: Designing Secure Systems that People Can Use. O'Reilly and Assoc. (2005)
4. Ka-Ping, Y.: Aligning security and usability. IEEE Security & Privacy 2(5), 48–55 (2004)
5. Saltzer, J.H., Schroeder, M.D.: The protection of information in computer systems. Proceedings of the IEEE 63(9), 1278–1308 (1975)
6. Nielsen, J.: Traditional dialogue design applied to modern user interfaces. Communications of the ACM 33(10), 109–118 (1990)
7. Shneiderman, B., et al.: Designing the user interface: Strategies for effective human-computer interaction, 5th edn. Addison-Wesley, Reading (2009)
8. Norman, D.A.: THE WAY I SEE IT: Systems thinking: a product is more than the product. Interactions 16(5), 52–54 (2009)
9. Oberheide, J., Jahanian, F.: When mobile is harder than fixed (and vice versa): Demystifying security challenges in mobile environments. In: Proceedings of the Eleventh Workshop on Mobile Computing Systems Applications, vol. 38, pp. 43–48 (2010)
10. Rahmati, A., Zhong, L.: Human-battery interaction on mobile phones. Pervasive and Mobile Computing 5(5), 465–477 (2009)

11. Kirk, C.P., Chiagouris, L., Gopalakrishna, P.: Some people just want to read: The roles of age, interactivity, and perceived usefulness of print in the consumption of digital information products. Journal of Retailing and Consumer Services (2011)
12. Kim, E., Lee, B., Menon, N.M.: Social welfare implications of the digital divide. Government Information Quarterly 26(2), 377–386 (2009)
13. Myers, B.A.: Using handhelds for wireless remote control of PCs and appliances. Interacting with Computers 17(3), 251–264 (2005)
14. West, J., Mace, M.: Browsing as the killer app: Explaining the rapid success of Apple's iPhone. Telecommunications Policy 34(5-6), 270–286 (2009)
15. Brenner, S.W.: History of computer crime. In: De Karl, L., Jan, B. (eds.) The History of Information Security, pp. 705–721. Elsevier Science B.V., Amsterdam (2007)
16. Lawton, G.: Web 2.0 Creates Security Challenges. Computer 40(10), 13–16 (2007)
17. Salerno, S., Sanzgiri, A., Upadhyaya, S.: Exploration of Attacks on Current Generation Smartphones. Procedia Computer Science 5(0), 546–553 (2011)
18. Green, A.: Management of security policies for mobile devices. In: Proceedings of the 4th Annual Conference on Information Security Curriculum Development, pp. 1–4 (2007)
19. Yuan, Y., et al.: Identifying the ideal fit between mobile work and mobile work support. Information & Management (2010) (in Press, corrected proof)
20. Mittal, A., Sengupta, A.: Improvised layout of keypad entry system for mobile phones. Computer Standards & Interfaces 31(4), 693–698 (2009)
21. Shih, H.-C., Wang, K.: An adaptive hybrid dynamic power management algorithm for mobile devices. Computer Networks (2011)
22. Albrechtsen, E., Hovden, J.: The information security digital divide between information security managers and users. Computers & Security 28(6), 476–490 (2009)
23. Faily, S., Flechais, I.: To boldly go where invention isn't secure: applying security entrepreneurship to secure systems design. In: Proceedings of the 2010 Workshop on New Security Paradigms, pp. 73–84 (2010)
24. Garfinkel, S.L.: Design principles and patterns for computer systems that are simultaneously secure and usable, p. 1. Massachusetts Institute of Technology (2005)
25. Hertzum, M., Clemmensen, T.: How do usability professionals construe usability? International Journal of Human-Computer Studies 70(1), 26–42 (2012)
26. Botha, R.A., Furnell, S.M., Clarke, N.L.: From desktop to mobile: Examining the security experience. Computers & Security 28(3-4), 130–137 (2008)
27. Azer, M.A., El-Kassas, S.M., El-Soudani, M.S.: Security in Ad Hoc Networks: From Vulnerability to Risk Management. In: Proceedings of 2009 Third International Conference on Emerging Security Information, Systems and Technologies, pp. 203–209 (2009)
28. Economides, A.A., Grousopoulou, A.: Students' thoughts about the importance and costs of their mobile devices' features and services. Telematics and Informatics 26(1), 57–84 (2009)
29. Haverila, M.: What do we want specifically from the cell phone? An age related study. Telematics and Informatics (2011) (in Press, corrected proof)
30. Churchill, D., Hedberg, J.: Learning object design considerations for small-screen handheld devices. Computers & Education 50(3), 881–893 (2008)
31. McGibbon, T., et al.: Use of Mobile Technology for Information Collection and Dissemination (2011)

Fundamental Study for New Evaluation Method Based on Physical and Psychological Load in Human Movement

Hiroaki Inoue and Shunji Shimizu

Tokyo University of Science, SUWA, Japan
jgh12701@ed.suwa.tus.ac.jp, shun@rs.suwa.tus.ac.jp

Abstract. Recently, Japan (also world-wide countries) has become aged society, and wide variety welfare device and system have been developed. But evaluation of welfare system and device are limited only stability, intensity and partial operability. So, evaluation of usefulness is insufficient. Therefore, we will attempt to establish the standard to evaluate usefulness for objectively and quantitatively on the basis of including non-verbal cognition. In this paper, we measure load of sitting and standing movement to use EMG (Electoromyogram) and 3D Motion Capture and set a goal to establish objective evaluation method. We think that establishing objective evaluation method is necessity to develop useful welfare device. We examined possibility of assessing load and fatigue from measuring brain activity to use NIRS (Near Infra-Red Spectoroscopy).

Keywords: Evaluation, Movement, Exercise, 3D Motion Capture, NIRS, EMG, Care, Welfare Technology, Evaluation method.

1 Introduction

As increasing aging population in Japan and world-wide countries, welfare systems and device are rapidly developing, and various devices are manufactured based on the increased popularity of welfare device and system. Also the market of welfare device and system are expanding. However, the evaluation method is limited respectively to stability, strength and a part of operability for individual system or device. It means that evaluation methodology for usefulness of them was not established. Therefore, we will attempt to establish the standard to evaluate usefulness for objectively and quantitatively on the basis of cognition such as physical load, reduction of fatigue and postural stability. Especially, in considering universality, it is necessary to measure human movement and brain activity in daily life. Also, we looked into the possibility of quantitative evaluation of tiredness and load on the basis of brain activity using NIRS. Also, we consider that physical and psychological load are linked to cognition including non-verbal cognition. In this paper, the purpose of experiments is to evaluate motion focusing on sitting and standing movement which is usually done in our life by using NIRS. We consider that human feel physical and psychological load during life motion. We tried to measure non-verbal cognition about psychological load by using NIRS.

C. Stephanidis (Ed.): Posters, Part I, HCII 2013, CCIS 373, pp. 124–128, 2013.

2 Experimental Method

We measured brain activity during motion with the purpose of establishing evaluation method based on generality (Fig. 1). Subjects were six males aged twenties. They were asked to read and sign an informed consent regarding the experiment too. Measurement apparatus was NIRS (SHIMADZU CO. Ltd products-FOIRE3000). Measurement region was at right and left prefrontal cortex.

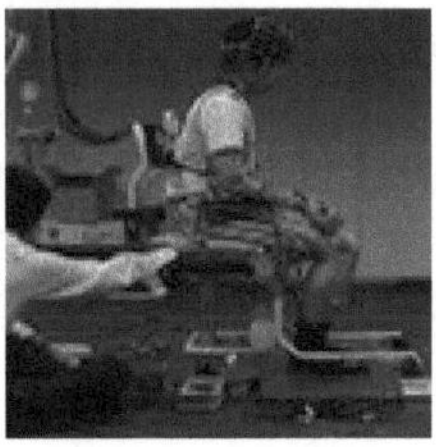

Fig. 1. Experimental view of NIRS

Measuring Brain Activity during Transfer with Standing Position (task1). At this measurement, subject used welfare device to perform transferring in a standing position. In this measurement, subject sat on seating face of welfare device appeared on the top of chair after raising hip until kneeling position. Also, subject performed inverse transferring from seating face to chair. Time design was rest (5 seconds) - task (10 seconds) - rest (5 seconds). This time design was repeated 30 times.

Measuring Brain Activity during Transfer with Half-Crouch Position (task2). At this measurement, subject used welfare device to perform transferring in a half-crouch position. In this measurement, subject sat on seating face of welfare device appeared on the top of chair after raising hip until kneeling position. Also, subject performed inverse transfer from seating face to chair. Time design was rest (5 seconds) - task (10 seconds) - rest (5 seconds). This time design was repeated 30 times. In experiments of task1 and task2, operation of welfare device was performed by operator other than subject. Before this measuring, subjects adjusted to transferring by use of welfare device.

Measuring Brain Activity during Keeping Half-Crouch Position (task3). Subjects performed two tasks at this measurement. During task3-1, they sat on seating face of welfare device with eyes open. During task3-2, they kept a half-crouch position. Subjects alternated task3-1 and task3-2. Also, subjects took resting time between two types of motion with eyes close. Therefore time design was rest (5 seconds) - task3-1(10 seconds) - rest (5 seconds) - task3-2(10 seconds) - rest (5 seconds). This time design was repeated 15 times.

3 Experimental Result

As common result of all subjects, oxy-Hb tended to increase during task and to decrease in resting state. Therefore, it was thought that change of hemoglobin density due to task was measured. Fig. 2, 3 and 4 shows trend of the channel in which significant different was shown. Analysis was performed via one-sample t-test by a method similar to previous researches [1,2,3,4,5]. In this analysis, it was necessary to remove other than change of blood flow due to fatigue. So, our method was mainly focused on resting state to compare with the 1st trial and other trials of brain activity. In task1 1 and 2, each of sample data for analysis was 4 seconds after the task. In task 3, sample data was 4 seconds during task. In the t-test of the same task, we performed t-test with first time trial and other trial which was from second times to thirty times, and examined relationship the number of trials and significant differences.

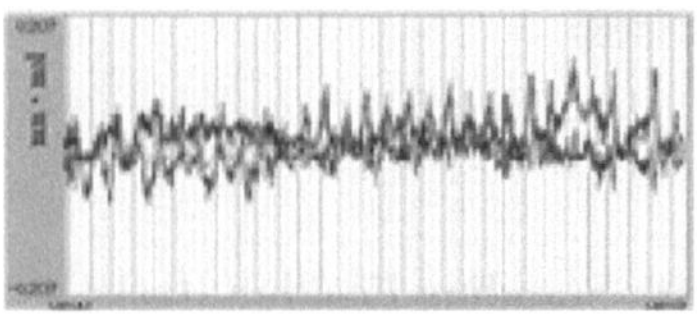

Fig. 2. Measuring Result of Task1

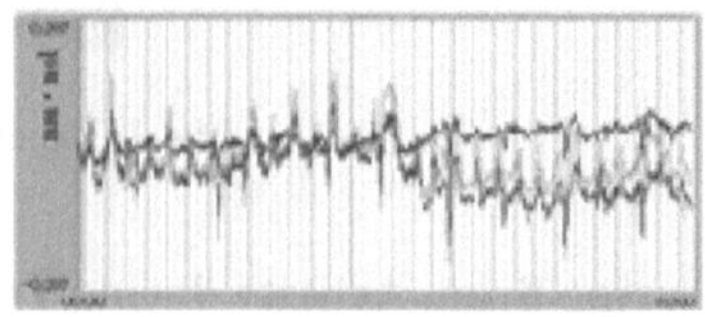

Fig. 3. Measuring Result of Task2

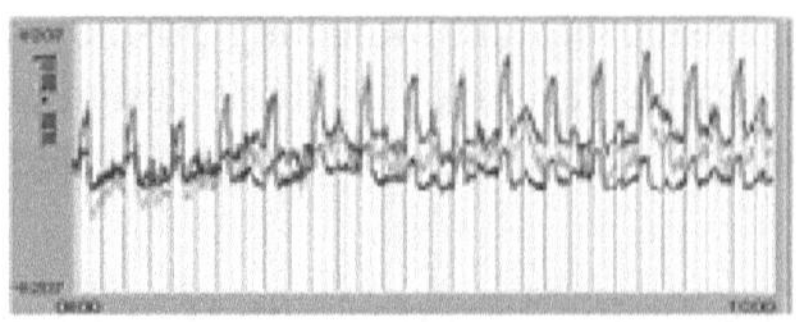

Fig. 4. Measuring Result of Task3

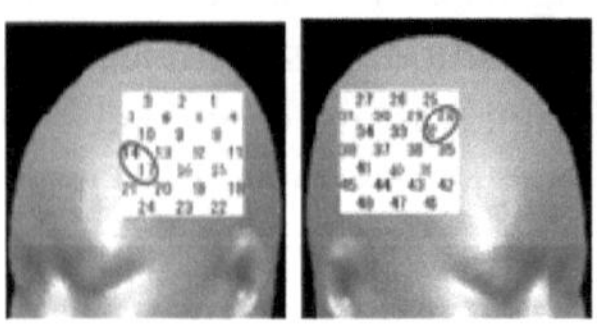

Fig. 5. Significant Difference of task1

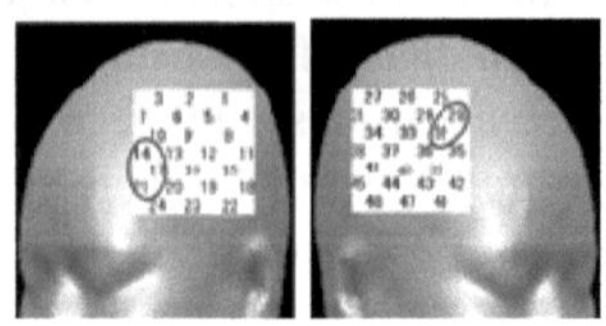

Fig. 6. Significant Difference of task2

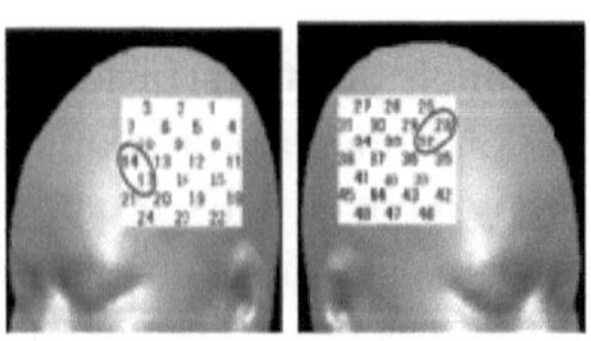

Fig. 7. Significant Difference of task1 and 2

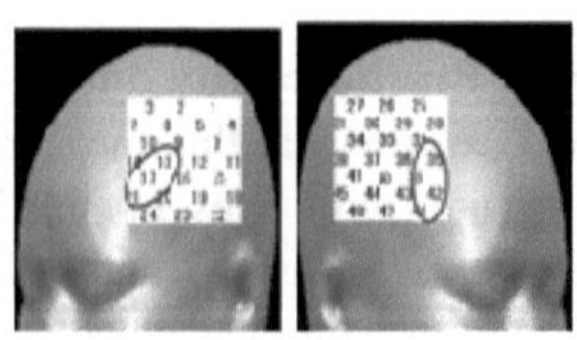

Fig. 8. Significant Difference in sitting position

In task 1, significant different could be found from the about 10th trials. Fig. 4 show region confirmed significant different. In task 2, significant different could be found from the about 10th trials too. Fig. 5 show region confirmed significant difference. Next, we performed t-test with case of standing position (task 1) and half-crouch position (task 2). In this analysis, significant different could be found at prefrontal area (14ch, 17ch, 28ch and 32ch). Fig. 6 show region confirmed significant difference.

Also, two type of motion which was sitting and keeping a half-crouching position were repeated alternatively in task 3. At first, we performed t-test using 4 seconds during first trial and 4 seconds during other trials which were from second to fifteenth in same position. Regarding to analysis result using sample data during sitting position and half-crouching position, there were significant different at Prefrontal area. Fig.7 show region confirmed significant difference.

4 Results and Verification Experiments

In this experiment, we tried to measure quantitatively the physical and psychological strain on the basis of brain activity. Also, we think that brain activity disclose human cognitive including non-verbal. As a result, it was shown that there were differences at brain activity due to number of trials and postural. In this time, analysis was performed via one-sample t-test using sample of brain activity in resting state during task or after task. Hence, analysis method was to remove disturbance such as body motion and angular variation of neck to the extent possible although there was the possibility to measure skin blood flow. Therefore, it was thought that strain due to tasks was quantitatively measured by being recognized significant differences.

Also, in previous research, it was reported to decrease in activity in the brain around #10, 11 [6] as the result of measuring brain activity during Advanced Trial Making Test using PET(Positron Emission Tomography) [7]. Therefore, this result came out in support of previous research in no small part.

Of course, it is necessary to increase number of subject at the present stage. In addition, there are problems associated with experiment, number of subject, method and measured region. However, in terms of being recognized significant differences at brain activity due to movement, it was thought to show useful result in evaluating quantitatively daily movements.

5 Conclusion and Future Work

We tried to measure physical and psychological load quantitatively on the basis of brain activity. And there were significant differences due to number of trials, holding position. In this experiment, analysis method was to remove disturbance such as body motion and angular variation of neck to the extent possible by using measurement result in resting state as sample. Therefore, it was thought to show useful result in evaluating quantitatively load due to movement task by being recognized difference in brain activity caused by number of trials, substance of task and holding position.

Main purpose in this study is to evaluate physical load and fatigue quantitatively. So, we tried to evaluate change of muscle load due to difference of motion by simultaneous measuring with 3D motion analysis System and EMG quantitatively. However, evaluation of psychological load is necessary, too. In terms of using welfare device, prolonged use must be taken into account. In this case, it is important to consider not only physical load but also psychological load due to prolonged use from standpoint of developing welfare device and keeping up surviving bodily function. And, in previous research, separation between physical and psychological load has been performed. But, our view is that there is correlation with physical and psychological load. So, we tried to measure psychological load including physical one based on brain activity and quantitatively evaluate both load. For the future, our aim is to establish method of discussing useful of welfare device by evaluating load involved in other daily movements with increasing number of subjects.

References

1. Takahashi, N., Shimizu, S., Hirata, Y., Nara, H., Miwakeichi, F., Hirai, N., Kikuchi, S., Watanabe, E., Kato, S.: Fundamental Study for a New Assistive System during Car Driving. In: Proc. of International Conferrence on Robotics and Biomimetics, China (2010)
2. Takahashi, N., Shimizu, S., Hirata, Y., Nara, H., Inoue, H., Hirai, N., Kikuchi, S., Watanabe, E., Kato, S.: Basic study of analysis of human brain activities during car driving. In: Smith, M.J., Salvendy, G. (eds.) HCII 2011, Part I. LNCS, vol. 6771, pp. 627–635. Springer, Heidelberg (2011)
3. Shimizu, S., Takahashi, N., Nara, H., Inoue, H., Hirata, Y.: Fundamental study for human brain activity based on the spatial cognitive task. In: Hu, B., Liu, J., Chen, L., Zhong, N. (eds.) BI 2011. LNCS, vol. 6889, pp. 218–225. Springer, Heidelberg (2011)
4. Shimizu, S., Takahashi, N., Nara, H., Inoue, H., Hirata, Y.: Basic Study for Human Brain Activity Based on the Spatial Cognitive Task. In: The Third International Conference on Advanced Cognitive Techonologies and Applications, Italy (2011)
5. Shimizu, S., Takahashi, N., Inoue, H., Nara, H., Miwakeichi, F., Hirai, N., Kikuchi, S., Watanabe, E., Kato, S.: Basic Study for a New Assitive System Based on Brain Activity associated with Spatial Perception Task during Car driving. In: Proc. International Conferrence on Robotics and Biomimetics, Thailand (2011)
6. Watanabe, Y.: Molecular/neural mechanisms of fatigue and the way to overcome fatigue. Folia Pharmacological Japonica 129, 94–98 (2007)
7. Kuratsune, H., Yamaguti, K., Lindh, G., Evengard, B., Hagberg, G., Matsumura, K., Iwase, M., Onoe, H., Takahashi, M., Machii, T., Kanakura, Y., Kitani, T., Langstrom, B., Watanage, Y.: Brain Regions Involved in Fatigue Sensation: Reduced Acetylcarnitine Uptake in to the Brain. Neuroimage 17, 1256–1265 (2001)
8. Maruta, K.: The influence of Seat Angle on Forward Trunk Inclination During Sit-to-Stand. Jounal of Japanese Physical Therapy Association 31(1), 21–28 (2004)

A Two-Step Click Interaction for Mobile Internet on Smartphone*

Kihyo Jung** and Jinah Jang

School of Industrial Engineering, University of Ulsan, Ulsan 680-749, South Korea
kjung@ulsan.ac.kr, orange1787@hanmail.net

Abstract. Mobile Internet gains popularity due to the increasing use of smartphones having wireless network capabilities. However, the current click interaction method (hereafter, *CC*) hinders user experience when the size of the target hyperlink to be selected is small. The present study developed a two-step click interaction method (called *Press and Flick;* hereafter *PF*) for smartphone and evaluated its effectiveness by GOMS model. GOMS results indicate that the PF has a substantial benefit compared to the CC when a click error is occurred. The PF can enhance usability and user experience (UX) by reducing click error and providing a joyful interaction.

Keywords: Press and Flick, Two-step Click Interaction, Mobile Internet, Smartphone.

1 Introduction

With the increasing use of smartphones having wireless network capabilities (e.g., 4G and Wi-Fi), mobile Internet access becomes daily life. The percentages of smartphone users in South Korea and North America have reached about 63% (Korea Communications Commission, 2013) and 50% (Wikipedia, 2013), respectively. In South Korea, the 88% of smartphone users are regularly accessing to mobile Internet, and the 87% of them connects to it at least once a day (KISA, 2011). Especially, the 51% of mobile Internet users are willing to access Internet through smartphone even if there is a personal computer nearby. This survey results indicate that Internet access through smartphone becomes daily life among smartphone users.

User interaction methods commonly used in a smartphone for website navigation can be divided into 3 types: 1) press, 2) flick, and 3) tap. The press interaction is to click a hyperlink on the touch screen of a smartphone. The flick interaction is to scroll up or down the touch screen. Lastly, the tap interaction is to zoom in or out by touching the touch screen twice. The aforementioned interactions can strongly enhance both usability and user experience (UX) of a smartphone.

---

* This research was supported by Basic Science Research Program through the National Research Foundation of Korea (NRF) funded by the Ministry of Education, Science and Technology (2012-011373).

** Corresponding author.

C. Stephanidis (Ed.): Posters, Part I, HCII 2013, CCIS 373, pp. 129–133, 2013.

The press interaction for click hinders user experience when the size of target hyperlink is small. Not only the current press interaction provides no feedback for the recognition of click error before touch, but also allows no mean to recover a click error. The only way to correct a click error is to press the Back button on the lower part of a smartphone. Therefore, the current press interaction can cause unhappy experience to users; otherwise, to avoid a click error, it requires elaborative effort in precise press.

The present study developed a two-step click interaction for website navigation on a smartphone. Based on the analysis of mobile users' behavior, a two-step (Press and Flick) interaction was developed. The initial interaction of press is for click a target hyperlink; the post interaction of flick is for recovery of a click error if necessary. The present study evaluated the effectiveness of the new click interaction by GOMS model.

2 Development of a Two-Step Interaction Method

The present study developed a two-step click interaction by 3 steps: 1) users' behavior observation, 2) interaction characteristic analysis, and 3) new interaction development. In the first step, a visual observation was conducted while users surfed mobile websites for about 10 min. Ten mobile users (female: 5, male: 5) were asked to surf mobile websites with their own smartphone without any restriction. Mean age of the users was 23 (SD: 2) and their dominant hand was all right-side.

In the second step, three characteristics for click interaction were identified by the visual observation conducted in the first step. First, click errors tended to increase as the size of a target hyperlink displayed on a touch screen decreased. Second, time required for a click interaction tended to delay as the size of a target hyperlink decreased because a small hyperlink requires precise interaction. Lastly, click errors were commonly occurred by pressing a neighbor hyperlink of the target hyperlink.

In the last step, the press and flick interaction (hereafter, PF) was developed which reduces both click errors and psychological burden caused by precise touch of a small target hyperlink. The PF consists of two-step interactions of press and flick. The initial interaction is to press a target hyperlink with the index finger. If the target hyperlink is not successfully selected by the initial interaction, the post interaction of flick with the index finger while pressing down is followed. The post interaction allows a user to reselect the target hyperlink by flicking the index finger upward, downward, leftward, or rightward. Therefore, the post interaction can be an effective remedy when a user mistakenly pressed a neighbor hyperlink of the target hyperlink.

3 Performance Evaluation

3.1 GOMS Model

The GOMS operators used in the present study (Table 1) can be divided into 3 types: 1) physical operator, 2) mental operator, and 3) system operator. The physical operator includes Position (P), Keystroke (K), and Movement (M) which are related to finger interactions. The mental operator includes Attention Shift (S) and Mental Act (A). Lastly, the system operator includes Smartphone Response (R) which is an idle status of a user while waiting for system's response.

Time for the operators was determined by referring to existing studies (Card et al., 1983; Chi and Chung, 1996; Kieras, 1999; Holleis et al, 2007; Oyewole and Haight, 2011) except for smartphone response and mental act. The existing studies did not provide time for smartphone response because it relies on system's performance (Kieras, 1999). Therefore, the present study measured transition time between webpages in a smartphone using a stopwatch and determined smartphone's response time (1 sec) as their average value. In addition, the existing studies used different time for mental act (Holleis et al, 2007). For example, Oyewole and Haight (2011) and Dunlop and Crossan (2000) applied the original value of 1.35 sec for mental act; however, Mori et al. (2003) and Myung (2004) used 0.38 sec and 0.57 sec, respectively. This difference seems to rise due to difference in context (Holleis et al, 2007). The present study determined time for mental act as 0.22 sec by summation of two median values of perceptual process time (median = 0.125 sec, range = 0.05 sec ~ 0.2 sec) and cognitive process time (median = 0.098 sec, range = 0.025 ~ 0.17 sec) reported in Card et al. (1983). This study used a smaller value for mental act because the mental act in this study is simple to detect whether a click error exists or not after press interaction.

The GOMS model of the current click interaction method (hereafter, CC) consisted of two goals (click and undo) as shown in Table 2.a. The first goal of click is achieved through three operators (P-K-K) in relation to click interaction. The second goal of undo is conditionally conducted when the target hyperlink is not successfully clicked by the first goal. The second goal is achieved by six operators (R-A-M-K-K-A) associated with going back to the original webpage to recover a click error.

The GOMS model of the PF consisted of two goals (press and flick) as shown in Table 2.b. The first goal of press is achieved by four operators (P-K-A-K). The last operator, K, is conditionally included in the first goal when the target hyperlink is successfully selected by the first goal. The second goal of flick is conditionally conducted when the target hyperlink is not selected by the first goal. The second goal is achieved by two operators (A-K) associated with flicking the index finger toward the target hyperlink.

3.2 Analysis Results

Completion time (hereafter, Time) of the CC without a click error was estimated as 0.43 sec (Table 3); however, Time of the CC with a click error significantly increased

Table 1. GOMS operators for mobile interactions

Type	Code	Name	Description	Time(sec)	Reference
Physical operator	P	Position	Position the index finger above a target hyperlink	1.10	Card et al. (1983), Chi and Chung (1996), Oyewole and Haight (2011), Kieras (1999)
	K	Keystroke	Press or release a hyperlink with the index finger	0.10	Card et al. (1983), Oyewole and Haight (2011), Kieras (1999)
	M	Movement	Move the index finger	0.23	Holleis et al. (2007)
Mental operator	S	Attention shift	Shift display-to-hotkey	0.14	Holleis et al. (2007)
	A	Mental act	Detect an error	0.22	Card et al. (1983)
System operator	R	Smartphone response	Wait for smartphone's response	1.00	Measured in this study

Table 2. GOMS models for click interaction

(a) Current click method

Goal	Method	Operator	Time (sec)	Total (sec)
Click	Point to the target link	P	0.23	0.43
	Press the target link	K	0.10	
	Release the target link	K	0.10	
Undo	Wait smartphone's response	R	1.00	1.71
	Shift attention from display to hotkey	A	0.14	
	Move to the hotkey back	M	0.23	
	Press the hotkey back	K	0.10	
	Release the hotkey back	K	0.10	
	Shift attention from hotkey to display	A	0.14	

(b) Press and flick method

Goal	Method	Operator	Time (sec)	Total (sec)
Press	Point to the target link	P	0.23	0.65
	Press the target link	K	0.10	
	Judge whether the target link clicked	A	0.22	
	(conditional*) Release the target link	K	0.10	
Flick	Decide flick direction	A	0.22	0.32
	Conduct flick	K	0.10	

* This operator is conditionally included when the hyperlink is selected by the goal of press.

Table 3. Completion time estimated by GOMS models

Method	Condition	Time (sec)
Current	No error	0.430
	One error	2.570
Press and flick	No error	0.650
	One error	0.870

to 2.57 sec (click time 0.43 sec + undo time 1.71 sec + re-click time 0.43 sec). Therefore, the CC can deteriorate usability and user experience because Time and number of the interactions required drastically increase when a click error occurs.

Times of the PF with or without an error were not significantly different. Time of the PF without an error was 0.65 sec, and Time with an error was 0.87 sec (click time 0.65 sec – release time 0.1 sec + flick time 0.32 sec). Mean difference between with and without an error was only 0.22 sec.

Time of the PF without an error (0.65 sec) delayed 0.22 sec compared to Time of the CC without an error (0.43). The main cause of the delay is that the PF requires a mental judgment to determine whether the post interaction of flick is needed or not. However, Time of the PF with an error (0.87 sec) was 1.7 sec shorter than Time of the CC with an error (2.57 sec). The main reason is that the PF can rapidly correct a click error through the post interaction of flick.

4 Conclusion

The PF developed in this study can be help of enhancing usability and user experience of website navigation in a smartphone when the size of target hyperlink is small.

References

1. Korea Internet and Security Agency (KISA). Survey of Smartphone Use in the First Half of 2011. Korea Internet and Security Agency
2. Korea Communications Commission, Wireless communication service statistics. (2013), `http://www.kcc.go.kr/user.do` (retrieved January 28, 2013)
3. Wikepedia, Smartphone (2013), `http://en.wikipedia.org/wiki/Smartphone#Market_share` (retrieved January 28, 2013)
4. Card, S.K., Moran, T.P., Newell, A.: The psychology of Human-computer Interaction. Lawrence Erlbaum Associates, Hillsdale (1983)
5. Chi, C., Chung, K.: Task analysis for computer-aided design (CAD) at a keystroke level. Applied Ergonomics 27(4), 255–265 (1996)
6. Holleis, P., Otto, F., Hubmann, H., Schmidt, A.: Keystroke-level model for advanced mobile phone interaction. In: Proceedings of CHI 2007 (2007)
7. Oyewole, S.A., Haight, J.M.: Determination of optimal paths to task goals using expert system based on GOMS model. Computers in Human Behavior 27, 923–933 (2011)
8. Kieras, D.E.: A Guide to GOMS Model Usability Evaluation using GOMSL and GLEAN3. University of Michigan, Ann Arbor (1999)
9. Dunlop, M.D., Crossan, A.: Predictive Text Entry Methods for Mobile Phones. Personal Technologies 4(2-3) (2000)
10. Mori, R., Matsunobe, T., Yamaoka, T.: A task operation prediction time computation based on GOMS-KLM improved for the cellular phone and the verification of that validity. In: Proceedings of ADC 2003 (2003)
11. Myung, R.: Keystroke-Level analysis of Korean text entry methods on mobile phones. International Journal of Human-Computer Studies 60, 545–563 (2004)

How Do Users Solve Software Problems?

Helmut Lang[1], Tanja Dolpp[2], and Florian Nothdurft[1]

[1] Ulm University, Institute of Communications Engineering, 89081 Ulm, Germany
[2] Ulm University, Institute of Psychology and Education, 89081 Ulm, Germany
{helmut.lang,tanja.dolpp,florian.nothdurft}@uni-ulm.de

Abstract. Problems with software programs can have negative consequences on a user's mood and efficiency. While the focus in research was on identifying the causes and the severity of frustration in the context of computer problems the present survey examines the strategies users employ in case of problems with software programs. Specifically, we were interested in what kind of assistance is used, in which order, and what kind of help would be preferred.

Our results show that the preferred and chosen approaches depend on factors like age, gender and perceived expertise. Furthermore the results indicate that there is a need for improvement concerning help systems integrated into software products.

1 Introduction

The interaction between computer users and software programs is not always straightforward and problems in dealing with computer systems can have negative consequences like frustration, personal dissatisfaction, a reduction in perceived self-efficacy [1] and even somatic discomfort [2]. In addition to these effects on the overall well-being, problems with computer software can also have economic consequences, like a loss of time from 30 % up to 50 % [3] caused for example by tinkering or searching for help in manuals [4].

While Ceaparu et al. [3] examined the causes and severity of frustration users experience using software systems, up to now there was only little research on the approaches chosen by users dealing with software related problems and the resources they consult in those cases. Hence the objective of the present survey was to investigate these approaches and to find out which kind of assistance users would actually prefer.

2 Method

2.1 Participants

The idea behind the setup of the survey was to get an overall impression by randomly recruiting a variety of people in a coffee shop. The survey involved 45 participants (17 female, 28 male) aged 17 to 65 years (M=28,91; SD=11,8). Completing the questionnaire took about 45 minutes and participants could either fill the form at the coffee shop or at home.

C. Stephanidis (Ed.): Posters, Part I, HCII 2013, CCIS 373, pp. 134–138, 2013.

2.2 Questionnaire

The questionnaire consisted of several parts. The first part assessed demographic data like age and gender. The second part consisted of three straightforward questions (e. g. "How competent do you feel using computers") evaluating participants' perceived expertise in a computing context. Those three items combined constituted an expertise scale (Cronbach's α=.94). The third part contained questions characterizing participants' typical behaviour in case of software problems. The kind of questions asked in this context will be elucidated along with the results in the next section.

3 Results

The data was analysed using descriptive statistics. To check for possible group differences one-factor ANOVAS have been computed. The following groups were considered for analysis:

Sex male (28) and female (17)
Age younger ($\leq$30 years, 33) and older (>30 years, 12)
Expertise competent (24) and less competent (20) (split at the median)

3.1 Scenario

In order to assess users' typical behaviour in case of encountering problems with software new to them, we asked them to note their usual steps in a given scenario. Participants were told to imagine that they have just installed a tax return software and after starting the program, they would not know how to proceed.

The categorized answers are depicted in Fig. 1 and show that, the first step for most of the participants (11) was to ask a third person (e.g. a co-worker, family member or friend) for help. Unexpectedly using Internet resources to get help was only the second most common answer along with a try and error approach that were both noted by 9 participants. 6 participants noted they would try to find help at the internal help system of the software and 4 mentioned to use some kind of manual. Since software usually does not ship with printed manuals anymore it is unclear if those answers also refer to the internal help system or if participants meant some kind of electronic document.

3.2 Where Users Search for Help

The next group of questions assessed users preferences when searching for help with software problems. It listed different resources for assistance and users had to decide on a 7-point Likert scale how often they use each one in case of problems. The endpoints of the scale were indicated with "never" and "always". Means and standard deviations of the results are summarized in Table 1. Here similar to the scenario case, searching the Internet (Mod=7) and asking a third

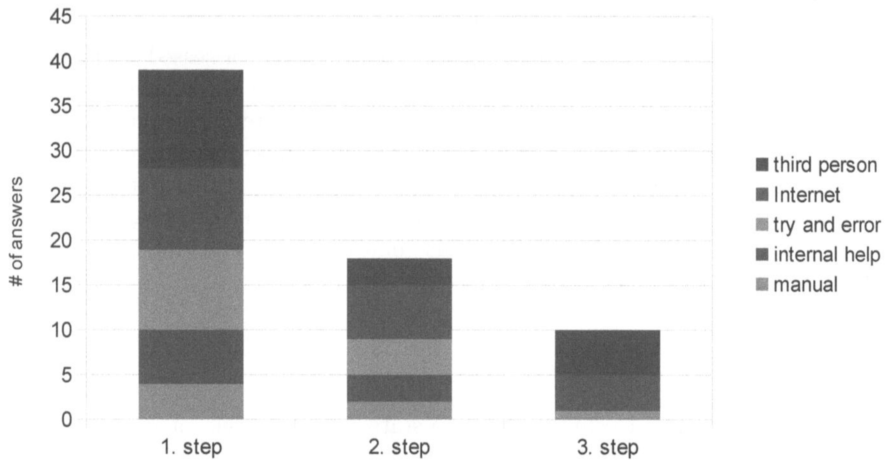

Fig. 1. Summarized steps undertaken in case of software problems

person (Mod=7) were the answers with the highest ratings. In this context female subjects and subjects with lower perceived competence values stated to ask a third person more often for help than male subjects and subjects with higher perceived competency (F(1,43)=4.09, p=.049; F(1,42) = 9.07, p=.004).

Subjects of lower competency also use the Internet significantly less to get help than more competent participants (F(1,42) = 20.62, p<.001). This is also true for subjects older than 30 years (F(1,43)=3.1, p=.008). Accordingly, participants from the senior group (M=4.25, SD=1.6) expressed that they would need significantly (F(1,43)=5.24, p=.027) more time finding relevant help on the Internet than younger participants (M=3.06, SD=1.52). Thus it is of no surprise that even though the overall rating for manuals is rather low, older subjects are more likely to consult a manual in case of problems than younger subjects (F(1,43)=7.26, p=.01). In addition to this subjects with lower perceived competence (M=4, SD=1.34) stated – similar to older subjects – to need more time to find relevant help on the Internet than subjects with higher competence values (M=2.75, SD=1.57; F(1,42)=7.91, p=.007).

The internal help of software is used significantly more often by participants from the expert group than by subjects with lower competence (F(1,42)=8.1, p=.007). Since usually this kind of systems is supposed to assist non-expert users, this clearly shows a deficiency in help system design and suggests that there is a need for improvement in this area.

As the Microsoft Office Assistant (Clippy the paperclip) was by far one of the most well-known attempts to improve this situation, we also asked participants, if they remembered Clippy. Additionally, we also assessed if subjects perceived him to be rather useful, likeable, annoying and if they miss him on a 7-point Likert scale. Only two subjects did not remember Clippy and concerning his usefulness (M=3.45, SD=1.61) and likeability (M=3.71, SD=1.98) participants were rather indifferent. However, the majority of subjects rated him to have been quite annoying (M=5.12, SD=1.8) and accordingly does not miss him (M=2.57, SD 2.99). The feeling of annoyance was marginal significantly smaller (F(1,40)=5.36, SD=1.8) for older (M=4.22, SD=1.56) than for younger subjects (M=5.36, SD=1.8).

Following a "try and error" approach (Mod=6) as well as internal help systems were also perceived to be useful in case of problems. Getting help from journals or magazines was perceived to be less useful and female participants stated to rely even less on this kind of help (F(1,43)=4.09, p=.049).

Overall it can be stated that especially non-expert and older users rely less on obtaining help on the Internet and prefer asking somebody. Additionally, older subjects also prefer to use a manual over searching help on the Internet.

Table 1. Means and standard deviations of help usage

	overall		sex				age				expertise			
			f		m		≤30		>30		⇓		⇑	
	M	SD	M	SD	M	SD	M	SD	M	SD	M	SD	M	SD
Internet	5.71	1.89	6.06	1.29	5.50	2.16	6.15	1.37	4.50	2.57	4.50	2.25	6.67	.56
third person	5.24	1.69	6.00	.86	4.79	1.91	5.21	1.61	5.33	1.96	6.05	1.14	4.63	1.83
internal help	4.67	2.02	4.18	2.21	4.96	1.87	4.73	1.87	4.50	2.46	3.75	2.19	5.38	1.58
try and error	4.27	1.92	4.41	1.90	4.18	1.96	4.52	1.90	3.58	1.88	3.90	1.86	4.50	1.97
manual	3.91	1.88	3.94	1.78	3.89	1.96	3.48	1.78	5.08	1.67	3.65	1.75	4.17	2.01
technical literature	2.31	1.49	2.35	1.41	2.29	1.56	2.36	1.51	2.17	1.46	2.45	1.60	2.17	1.43
journals/magazines	2.18	1.42	1.65	.86	2.50	1.59	2.12	1.29	2.33	1.77	1.70	.86	2.46	1.61

3.3 What Kind of Help Users Would Wish for

We also asked for the kind of help users would like to get in case of problems. The questions in this group were focused on assessing what kind of help software companies are supposed to provide. Participants were given different options that had to be rated on 7-point Likert scales. Means and standard deviations of the results are summarized in Table 2. The results are quite similar to the results of Section 3.2. While the Internet is overall again the preferred resource for assistance subjects with lower values in expertise significantly are less into obtaining information from the Internet than participants with high values in expertise (F(1,42)=16.11, p<.001). The same is true for participants from the senior group (F(1,43)=10.66, p=.002).

Again users with lower competence values significantly less appreciate internal help systems than users with higher expertise (F(1,42)=4.1, p=.049). This is especially interesting since for non-expert users the absolute value for internal help systems is higher than that for the Internet help. Indicating that less competent users would nevertheless prefer to use the internal help over searching the Internet. This also seems to be true for subjects from the senior group. Furthermore, subjects from the non-expert group as well as older participants expressed a rather strong wish for manuals.

Table 2. Means and standard deviations of preferred help

	overall		sex				age				expertise			
			f		m		≤30		>30		⇓		⇑	
	M	SD	M	SD	M	SD	M	SD	M	SD	M	SD	M	SD
Internet	5.40	1.80	5.76	1.48	5.18	1.96	5.88	1.31	4.08	2.31	4.40	2.13	6.29	.80
internal help	5.24	1.61	5.12	1.49	5.32	1.70	5.12	1.72	5.58	1.24	4.75	1.77	5.71	1.36
manual	4.64	1.88	4.76	1.85	4.57	1.93	4.39	1.83	5.33	1.92	5.25	1.91	4.12	1.77
training course	4.20	1.70	4.82	1.42	3.82	1.76	3.97	1.72	4.83	1.52	4.75	1.65	3.79	1.66
e-mail/call-center	3.62	2.15	4.29	2.20	3.21	2.06	3.73	2.22	3.33	2.01	3.25	1.94	3.83	2.31

4 Conclusion

The results attained with the present study show that the choice of help can depend on gender, age and perceived expertise of users. While searching the Internet and asking somebody are currently the dominant ways to get assistance, especially older subjects and subjects not feeling very tech-savvy seem to prefer to get help from the software itself or have a manual provided with the software.

It also seems like there are two groups of computer users. Young expert users that rely on the Internet to get help and a second group that prefers to ask one of these experts facing trouble with computers.

Since non-expert users hardly seem to use the help systems integrated into software and these help systems are usually developed to assist primarily this kind of users, there is definitely a need for improvement in this area.

References

1. Lazar, J., Jones, A., Hackley, M., Shneiderman, B.: Severity and impact of computer user frustration: A comparison of student and workplace users. Interacting with Computers 18(2), 187–207 (2006)
2. Schleifer, L.M., Amick III, B.C.: System response time and method of pay: Stress effects in computer-based tasks. International Journal of Human-Computer Interaction 1(1), 23–39 (1989)
3. Ceaparu, I., Lazar, J., Bessiere, K., Robinson, J., Shneiderman, B.: Determining causes and severity of end-user frustration. International Journal of Human-Computer Interaction 17(3), 333–356 (2004)
4. Wahlster, W., Bauer, M., Biundo, S., Dengler, D., Köhler, J., Paul, G., Thies, M.A.: Kooperative Hilfesysteme für Anwendungssoftware Entwicklungsstand und Forschungstrends. Innovative Softwaretechnologien, 401–426 (1994)

A Study on the Usability Testing of Gesture Tracking-Based Natural User Interface

C.J. Lim[1] and Y.G. Jung[2]

[1] Korea Polytechnic University, Dept. of Game and Multimedia Engineering, Korea
[2] Media Interactive Inc.
{scjlim,sadmyth7}@gmail.com

1 Research Significance

This paper compares the difference between the commercialized gesture tracking-based interface and the traditional computer mouse through a usability testing. It is then examined the possibility of applying this technological difference to a variety of content. To achieve this, Kinect sensor device, which is one of the commercialized gesture tracking-based interface, has been used and evaluated its performance through Fitts' law. Fitts' law is mainly used in human-computer interaction, which is an authorized tool to evaluate a cursor click and movement on the computer screen. In this paper, three factors – distance, width, and angle – between cursor and target are used to define the index of difficulty into 96 steps. The response time between two randomly selected cursor positions is then measured for each step. By comparing the measured time values, the possibility of using gesture tracking as an alternative interface to the computer mouse is verified.

2 Experiment Environment (Usability Testing)

2.1 Experimental Subject

50 users who are familiar to computer usage are involved in the experiment. In this way, a total number of 4800 data are collected from the experiments of 50 users. The left-handed or right-handed users are randomly selected, where all experimental subjects have been used computer for more than eight years and composed of either undergraduate or graduate students with the average age of 28. Note that subjects having trembling hands and low visions are excluded for an accurate calibration of gesture tracking-based interface. Among 50 users, 40 users have been classified as an expert group, whereas the rest of 10 users as a non-expert group.

2.2 Experimental Setup

Fitts' law is used to evaluate the usability of gesture tracking-based interface technology presented in this paper. Fitts' law provides an indicator that can quantitatively evaluate the operation time according to the index of difficulty. Thus, it can be used as a qualified tool to evaluate the performance of cursor click and movement on the computer screen. [1-3]

C. Stephanidis (Ed.): Posters, Part I, HCII 2013, CCIS 373, pp. 139–143, 2013.

At each step, the proposed experiment considers as a successful task if the user is able to move its cursor to click on the target. To achieve this, the usability testing program has been developed as shown in Fig. 1(b). As shown in Fig. 1(a), the index of difficulty is determined by three parameters: the distance between the current cursor position and the target position (D), the width of target (W), and the approach angle between the cursor and the target (A). Thus, the index of difficulty is judged to be difficult if the value of distance (D) increases whereas the value of width (W) decreases. The advantage of using Fitts' law is that it provides a linear relationship between the index of difficulty and movement time. Thus, the index of difficulty can be defined in a variety of ways depending on its purposes of using Fitts' law. [4-6]

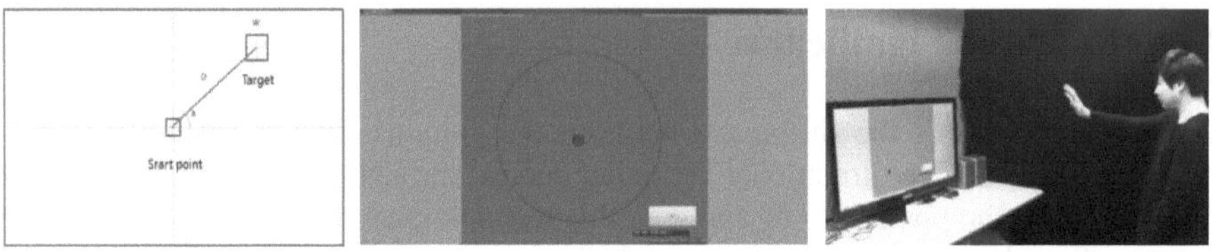

(a) (b) (c)

Fig. 1. (a) Three parameters (distance (D), width (W), and approach angle (A)) that define the index of difficulty, (b) Snapshot of the proposed usability testing program, (c) Snapshot of usability testing

The index of difficulty is consists of 96 steps, where the distance parameter (D) is divided into 3 levels ({125 pixel, 250 pixel, 375 pixel}), the width parameter (W) is divided into 4 levels ({50 pixel, 75 pixel, 100 pixel, 125 pixel}), and the approach angle parameter (A) is divided into 8 levels ({0°, 45°, 90°, 135°, 180°, 225°, 270°, 315°}) as shown in Table 1. Since the cursor position is randomly generated at each step, the experimental subject is not able to predict the cursor location of next step. Note that the position and size of the target are appropriately determined in a left and right direction with respect to the cursor location according to the difficulty at each step.

Table 1. The number of experiment parameters and their level values

Parameters	Parameter Level Values	Level Number
Distance to the target (D)	125, 250, 375 [pixel]	3
Width of the target (W)	50, 75, 100, 125 [pixel]	4
Approach angle to the target (A)	0, 45, 90, 135, 180, 225, 270, 315 [°]	8

2.3 Experimental Procedure

Prior to each experiment, the experiment procedure and correct posture are informed to each subject for an accurate calibration. Experiment environment is organized so that each subject can focus on the experiment. In addition, the lighting condition of environment is adjusted to increase the recognition rate by reducing the maximum amount of reflected light.

Prior to each experiment, five minutes of practice period is given to each subject. The actual experiment starts when the subject presses 'Start' button in 'Experiment' toolbar. Before generating the target point, the subject waits after moving its pointer on the top of 'Start Point' button. When the experiment is started, each target is randomly generated according to the condition of three parameters: position, width, and approach angle (a total of 96 steps).

The subject presses 'Start Point' button when he/she recognizes the position of target point. The response (movement) time is recorded when the subject immediately moves and presses its pointer to the target. In order to maintain the consistency of experiment results, five minutes of break period is given to each subject between each session to avoid additional factors such as concentration and fatigue. In this way, the experiment is progressed to a total of 50 users in accordance with four conditions in each session.

3 Experiment Results and Analysis

3.1 Average Response (Movement) Time

To examine the impact of response time for each parameter, the response time with respect to each parameter is presented as graphs. Fig. 2(a) shows the average response (movement) time for each width value when the distance between cursor and target is set as 125 pixels. As shown in Fig. 2(a), the average response time was decreased as the value of width pixel increases.

Fig. 2(b) shows the average response (movement) time for each distance value when the width of cursor and target are set as 100 pixels. As shown in Fig. 2(b), the average response time was increased as the value of distance between cursor and target increases.

Fig. 2(c) shows the average response (movement) time for each approach angle value. A short average response time was observed when the target was located relatively above the horizontal center of display. Particularly, the minimum average response (movement) time was observed when the approach angle to the target was

Table 2. Experiment results of each parameter

Distance [pixel]	Width [pixel]	Approach Angle [°]	Movement Time [msec]
125	50	0	2965
125	75	45	2837
125	100	90	2752
125	125	135	2654
250	50	180	3625
250	75	225	3561
250	100	270	3327
250	125	315	3412
375	50	0	4021
375	75	45	3829
375	100	90	3551
375	125	135	3315

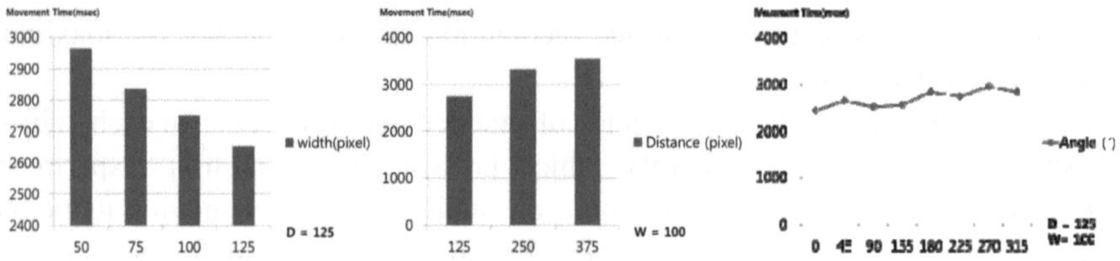

(a) (b) (c)

Fig. 2. (a) Average response (movement) time for each width value, (b) Average response (movement) time for each distance value, (c) Average response (movement) time for each approach angle value

Table 3. Comparison between mouse and gesture tracking-based interface

Distance [pixel]	Width [pixel]	Index of Difficulty [bits]	Mouse Movement Time [msec]	Gesture Tracking Movement Time [msec]
125	75	1.4150	1263	2837
125	100	1	1316	2752
250	75	2.1154	1349	3561
250	100	1.5849	1451	3327
375	75	2.5849	1451	3829
375	100	2	1578	3451

0°. Note that the response time was slightly increased when the approach angles were 45°, 90°, and 135°. As shown in Fig. 2(c), the average response time was increased as the value of approach angle to the target increases.

Table 2 shows the usability evaluation results between computer mouse and gesture tracking-based interface. Based on the measurements in both cases, it was confirmed that the index of difficulty and the movement time were linearly distributed as shown in Fig. 3. Fig. 3(a) shows the results when the computer mouse was used, where the measured index of difficulty was 1.2680 bits/sec. In contrast, the measured index of difficulty was 0.5312 bits/sec when the gesture tracking-based interface was used as shown in Fig. 3(b). Thus, if the numerical results of the index of difficult from the proposed experiment were only considered, we could conclude that the performance of gesture tracking-based interface is less efficient compared to the performance of computer mouse.

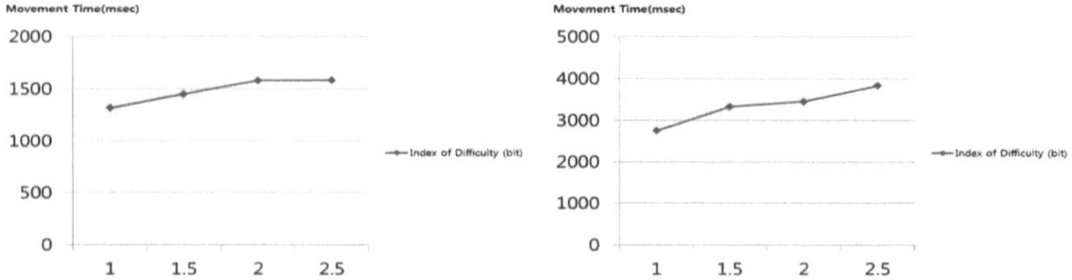

(a) (b)

Fig. 3. The relationship between movement time and index of difficulty (a) mouse, (b) gesture tracking-based interface

4 Conclusion

While it is important to know the capabilities and limitations of computer in an interface design, it is even more important to understand the capabilities and limitations of user first. This applies for both gesture tracking-based interface and regular computer mouse.

This paper examined the impact of response (movement) time for a recently commercialized gesture tracking-based interface by varying the distance to target, the width of target, and the approach angle between cursor and target.

The experiment results of the proposed interface showed that there is no problem with the usability of gesture tracking-based interface in contents such as games that have relatively large menu size and the accuracy is not critical. However, the computer mouse showed the outstanding performance for the tasks that require sophisticated user interface.

In the previous studies, several factors were not able to consider at the same time and there was a drawback that the index of difficulty in Fitts' law was not able to combine with other factors. Thus, more research is needed to provide a natural user interface to user while maintaining the performance. In addition, the detailed verification is further required by using the modified Fitts' law. [7-8]

These experiment results may help us to predict the performance degree of Kinect as well as to provide the guidelines for the development and evaluation of all interfaces that use gesture tracking-based interface.

Acknowledgement. This research was supported by the Culture Technology Research & Development Program funded by Ministry of culture, Sports and Tourism(MCST) and Korea Creative Content Agency (KOCCA), and the Technological innovation R&D program of SMBA [SA112908].

References

1. Andres, R.O., Hartung, K.J.: Prediction of head movement time using Fitts' law human factors 31, 703–713 (1989)
2. U.S NRC. Human-system interface design review guideline, NUREG-0700, REV. 1. U.S. Nuclear Regulatory Commission, Washington, D.C. (1996)
3. Parasurman, R.: Human-computer monitoring, the human factors society 29(6), 695–706 (1987)
4. Fitts, P.M.: The information capacity of the human motor system in controlling the amplitude of movement. Journal of Experimental Psychology 47(6), 381–391 (1954)
5. MacKenzie, S.: Fitts' law as a performance model in human-computer interaction, Doctoral Dissertation, University of Toronto (1991)
6. Pino, A., Kalogeros, E., Salemis, E., Kouroupetroglou, G.: Brain computer interface cursor measures for motion-impaired and able-bodied users. In: Proceedings of HCI International 2003: The 10th International conference on Human-Computer Interaction, Crete, Greece, pp. 1462–1466 (2003)
7. Hoffmann, E.R., Sheikh, I.H.: Effect of varying target height in a Fitts' movement task. Ergonomics 36(7), 1071–1088 (1994)
8. Casiez, G.: The impact of control-display gain on user performance in pointing tasks. Human-Computer Interaction 23, 215–250 (2008)

Development of a Usability Evaluation Method Based on Finger Movement

Nobuyuki Nishiuchi, Yutaka Takahashi, and Ayako Hashizume

Department of Management Systems Engineering, Tokyo Metropolitan University, 6-6 Asahigaoka, Hino, Tokyo, 191-0065, Japan
{nnishiuc,yataka-takahashi,hashiaya}@sd.tmu.ac.jp

Abstract. Current techniques for usability evaluation are costly, time-consuming, subjective, and often require operation logs, which are difficult to obtain from electrical products. To overcome these limitations, we developed a usability evaluation method that is applicable for various types of interfaces and involves extracting the video-recorded fingertip movements of a user during operation through image processing, and then evaluating usability based on several measurable parameters. Specifically, users' hand movements are first video recorded during the operation of either an actual product or a reproduced interface on a touch screen, and then operation time, and the distance and patterns of the moving locus, including stationary time and frequency of directional changes, are then extracted using image processing. To evaluate the usability of the interface, the ratio between novice and expert users for the parameters of operation time and distance traveled by the moving locus is used. Here, we conducted a comparative usability experiment using facsimile interfaces of two different manufacturers to evaluate the performance our method.

Keywords: evaluation method, image processing, interface, usability.

1 Introduction

Current techniques for usability evaluation encompass several approaches [1],[2], such as video capture and eye-tracking during user operation, conducting interviews and questionnaires, and recording user operation logs. However, these evaluation approaches are costly, time-consuming, subjective, and are often not feasible, as it is difficult to acquire the operation logs of many electrical products.

To overcome these limitations, we developed a novel usability evaluation method that involves extracting the video-recorded fingertip movements of a user during operation through image processing, and then evaluating the usability of the interface based on several measurable parameters. In particular, operation time and distance traveled by the moving locus were used to evaluate usability based on the ratio of each parameter between novice and expert users (NE ratio).

The present study is organized as follows. In Section 2, the methodology of our proposed usability evaluation is described in detail. Section 3 presents the results of an evaluative experiment. Finally, conclusions are discussed in Section 4.

C. Stephanidis (Ed.): Posters, Part I, HCII 2013, CCIS 373, pp. 144–148, 2013.

2 Methodology for Usability Evaluation

2.1 Extraction of Finger Movement and Action

Users operated the target interface wearing a rubber sleeve with a green-colored fingertip on the index finger of the right hand to aid in image extraction and processing. During operation, the users' index fingertip movements were recorded from above with a video camera (Fig. 1) and were then extracted by image processing (Fig. 2).

To detect button depression, an electric bulb that is activated whenever a button on the target interface is pushed was attached on the fingertip of the rubber sleeve. Thus, in addition to tracking fingertip movement, our system can be used to detect when buttons are pushed during the operation of an interface, a capability that is particularly useful for commercial products that do not record operational logs.

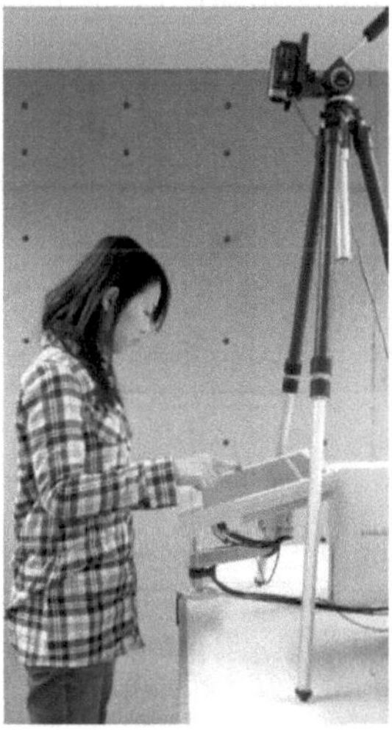

Fig. 1. Experimental setup

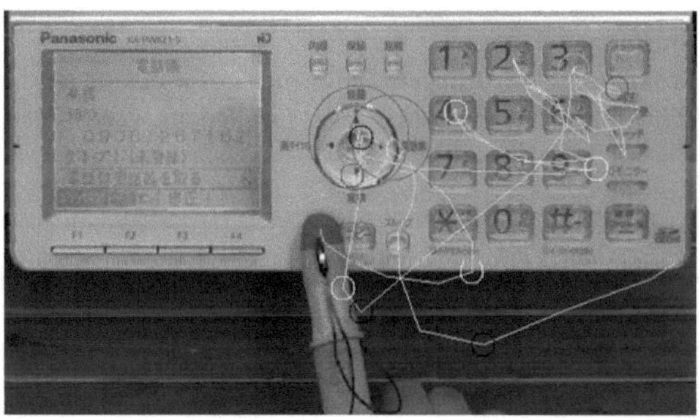

Fig. 2. Image processing for extracting hand movement (yellow lines) and stationary time (circle size)

2.2 Parameters for Usability Evaluation

Operation time, distance traveled by the user's fingertip, stationary time, and frequency of directional changes were used as usability evaluation parameters. All of the parameters were extracted from recorded videos using image processing algorithms.

Operation Time

We proposed a new parameter for usability evaluation termed the iNE ratio (improved Novice Expert ratio), which is derived from the previously described NE ratio [3]. To estimate the iNE ratio, ideal operation time, *Tm*, was modeled using Fitts' law (Section 2.3) and is considered to represent the indispensable time for finger movement and button operation. In addition, the ratio is a measure of the operation time of an expert user, *Te*, which includes the parameter *Tm*, and the delay time, *Td*, which is the response delay of the interface and can be calculated from equation (1).

$$\text{iNE} = (Tn - Td) / (Te - Td) = (Tn - Td) / Tm$$

$$Td = Te - Tm \tag{1}$$

Tn: Operation time of novice user, *Te*: Operation time of expert user, *Tm*: Ideal operation time, *Td*: Delay time

Distance

In addition to iNE, a second new evaluation parameter, the NE_d ratio (Novice Expert ratio of distance), was used. NE_d is the ratio between *Ln*, which is the total distance traveled by the movement locus (fingertip) during interface operation by a novice user, and *Le*, which is the sum of the shortest distance between the buttons depressed during operation of an expert user.

$$NE_d = Ln / Le \tag{2}$$

Stationary Time

From the recorded fingertip movements, the stationary time of the hand was determined. If the following equation (3) was fulfilled, the user's hand was judged to be stationary.

$$\sum_{i=1}^{T} L_i \leq L \times T \tag{3}$$

where L_i represents the distance between the positions of the finger in the current and preceding (i) video frame, and T indicates the number of previous frames in which the user's hand is considered to be stationary for at least $T\times(1/30)$ seconds. L represents the average distance that a user's finger moves between each frame for $T\times(1/30)$ seconds. Constants T and L were determined by a preliminary experiment. Fig. 2 shows an image of the locus of finger movement (yellow lines) and stationary time, which is represented by circles that are proportional in size to the duration of non-movement.

Frequency of Directional Changes

If the distance before and after the change of the moving direction exceeded a threshold value, the user's hand was judged to be in a state of directional change. The ratio of the frequency of directional changes between novice and expert users was also used as a parameter for usability evaluation. In Section 3, however, this parameter is not presented.

2.3 Model of Ideal Operation

Fitts' law was used for modeling ideal operation time. *MT*, which is the average time taken to acquire the target, was estimated using equation (4). In the model, Fitts' law was applied to estimate the operation time from the time required to depress two buttons based on the distance between the buttons. The sum of these operation times from a series of button-pressing operations represented the ideal operation time, *Tm*.

$$MT = a + b\,log_2(0.5 + \frac{D}{W}) \tag{4}$$

Where *W* is the width of the target, *D* is the distance from the starting point to the center of the target, and *a* and *b* are empirical constants determined through linear regression analysis. An exploratory experiment was conducted to estimate the two empirical constants (*a*, *b*) for eight directions.

3 Evaluative Experiment

3.1 Experiment Description

We conducted an evaluative experiment involving five users operating two different manufacturer's facsimile interfaces composed of buttons and a display (facsimile P), or buttons and a touch screen (facsimile S). Although users performed several defined tasks here, one task involving the transmission of a fax using the redialing function of the facsimile interface is focused and discussed.

3.2 Experimental Results and Discussion

The average values for the usability evaluation parameters of iNE, NE_d, and stationary time for the facsimiles P and S interfaces are shown in Tables 1 and 2, respectively.

Table 1. Evaluation parameters (facsimile P)

Operation step	iNE	NE_d	Stationary time [s]
Push redialing button	1.94	1.10	0
Select call recipient	7.93	9.26	1.5

Table 2. Evaluation parameters (facsimile S)

Operation step	iNE	NE_d	Stationary time [s]
Push phone call button	12.89	2.42	2.9
Push redialing button	5.75	2.57	0.4
Select call recipient	3.93	7.14	0.6

For the operation step "Select call recipient" on the facsimile P interface, both iNE and NE_d were large, and an average stationary time of 1.5 s was observed. As iNE and NE_d showed the same tendency, this operation step on the P interface appeared to have a problem with usability. The length of the observed stationary time also shows that the user's finger had stopped during the "Select call recipient" operation step. This finding was confirmed during post-task interviews with users, who reported that this operation step was difficult to perform on the P interface.

For the facsimile S interface, a long stationary time (2.9 s) and high iNE were detected for the operation step "Push phone call button", likely because there was no re-dialing button in the initial display of this interface, resulting in user confusion and operational errors. For the operation step of "Select call recipient", iNE was not notably large. However, NE_d was large because it was necessary that users remove a hand from the operation panel to check the operation. This result indicates that this operation step could use further improvement.

4 Conclusions

We have proposed a new method for usability evaluation that involves video recording the user's operation, extracting fingertip movements by image processing, and then evaluating usability based on operation time, distance, stationary time, and frequency of directional changes. From the results of an evaluative experiment involving two interfaces, our proposed usability evaluation method appears to be potentially suited for quantitative analysis and has applicability that is comparable to classical methods.

References

1. Bojko, A.: Using Eye Tracking to Compare Web Page Design: A Case Study. Journal of Usability Studies 1(3), 112–120 (2006)
2. Siegenthaler, E., Wurtz, P., Groner, R.: Improving the Usability of E-Book Readers. Journal of Usability Studies 6(1), 25–38 (2010)
3. Urokohara, et al.: A usability evaluation method that compares task performance between expert and novice. In: Proceedings of Human Interface Symposium, pp. 537–542 (1999)

Examining the Quality in Use of Web 2.0 Applications: A Three-Dimensional Framework

Tihomir Orehovački[1], Dragutin Kermek[1], and Andrina Granić[2]

[1] University of Zagreb, Faculty of Organization and Informatics
Pavlinska 2, 42000 Varaždin, Croatia
{tihomir.orehovacki,dragutin.kermek}@foi.hr
[2] University of Split, Faculty of Science
Nikole Tesle 12, 21000 Split, Croatia
andrina.granic@pmfst.hr

Abstract. Quality in use plays an essential role in a wide acceptance of software applications. It includes two complementary concepts: usability and user experience. With an aim to assure the quality in use of websites, researchers have proposed various metrics, but without guidelines for their use. Additionally, research on this topic in the context of Web 2.0 applications is fairly modest. In this paper, we introduce a framework composed of three dimensions related to categories of the quality in use, functions of Web 2.0 applications, and agile software development methods. The proposed framework can be used for the classification of metrics as well as for a sound and systematic evaluation of the quality in use of Web 2.0 applications.

Keywords: Web 2.0, Quality in Use, Evaluation Framework.

1 Introduction

More recently, quality in use has been recognized as an essential property of successful websites. Development of a methodology for ensuring the quality in use is therefore one of current research objectives of the HCI community. Although literature on evaluation of websites offers a number of diverse metrics, guidelines for their use are fairly scarce. With an aim to address this problem, Ramler et al. [9] suggested a generic cube scheme in which they considered quality aspects, website features, and lifecycle phases as three basic dimensions for evaluating website quality. Following their idea, Ruiz et al. [10] developed a three dimensional web quality model (WQM) meant for the classification of web metrics [2].

There are two main reasons why the aforementioned models, although useful for the assessment of websites, are not suitable for the evaluation of Web 2.0 applications. Firstly, dimensions on web features and quality aspects are exclusively intended for the product-centered usability evaluation while the hedonic-based assessment of user experience is neglected. Namely, the evaluation of Web 2.0 applications should take into account both pragmatic and hedonic facets of the quality in use [5]. Secondly, the lifecycle dimension encompasses diverse phases in a website

C. Stephanidis (Ed.): Posters, Part I, HCII 2013, CCIS 373, pp. 149–153, 2013.

monolithic release which is specific for the waterfall approach to software development. Conversely, the perpetual beta as a core design pattern [3] of Web 2.0 applications enables user driven release of new features during iterative lifecycle and is supported by agile development philosophy.

With an objective to facilitate the assessment of Web 2.0 applications, we introduce a framework that distinguishes three dimensions concerning categories of the quality in use, functions of Web 2.0 applications, and agile software development methods. The proposed framework is illustrated in Figure 1, while each of its dimensions is explained in the following section.

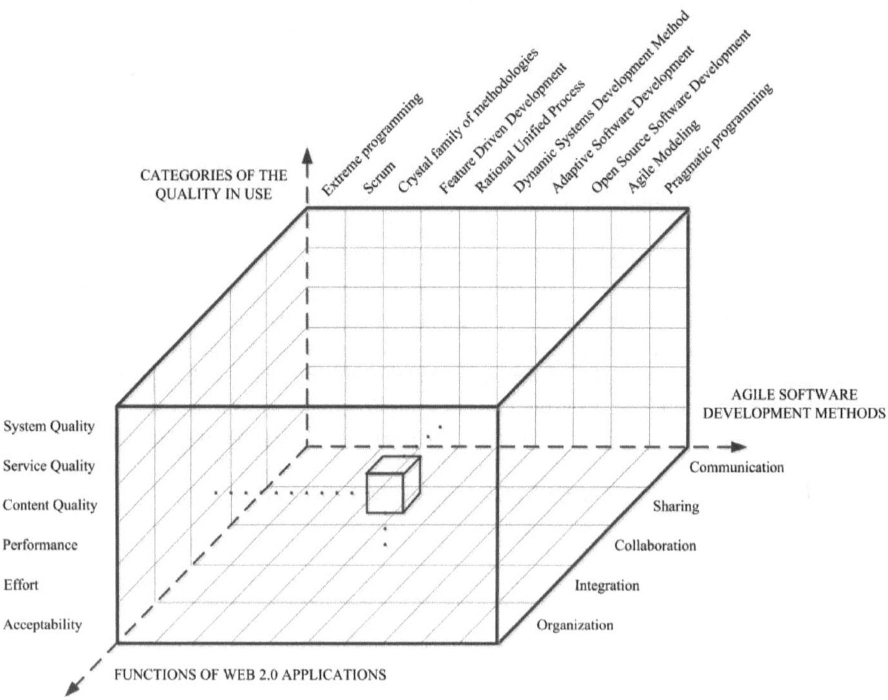

Fig. 1. Graphic representation of the framework

2 Dimensions in the Framework

2.1 Categories of the Quality in Use

As a foundation for the description of the dimension which addresses categories of the quality in use, we use six crucial categories aimed for evaluating the quality in use of Web 2.0 applications: System Quality, Service Quality, Content Quality, Performance, Effort, and Acceptability [4]. Both reliability and validity of the set forth categories were empirically validated in the context of Web 2.0 applications for collaborative writing [6] and mind mapping [8]. To enable fine-grained assessment of various facets of the quality in use, each category is further refined into measurable attributes.

System Quality refers to the attributes that measure the quality of a web application as a system and is comprised of six attributes: *navigability* (extent to which web interface features are well organized and various navigation mechanisms are provided), *consistency* (degree to which the same structure, design, and terminology are used throughout the web application), *aesthetic* (degree of visual attractiveness of a web interface design), *familiarity* (extent to which interaction with the web application is similar to previously used applications), *customizability* (degree to which a web application can be customized to meet users' needs and suit the characteristics of the task), and *security* (degree to which a web application contains functionalities and mechanisms that protect data from unauthorized use).

Service Quality refers to the attributes that measure the quality of interaction between the web application and users. This category is further decomposed into eight attributes: *helpfulness* (extent to which various forms of help are available and useful), *availability* (degree to which a web application and interface features are continuously available), *interactivity* (extent to which a web application creates the feeling of use of a desktop application and contains functionalities that facilitate different types of interaction among users), *error prevention* (degree to which a web application prevents the occurrence of errors and provides the features for their correction), *reliability* (extent to which a web application is dependable, stable, and bug-free), *recoverability* (extent to which a web application can recover from errors and operational interruptions), *responsiveness* (extent of the speed of a web application's response to users' requests and actions), and *feedback* (extent to which a web application appropriately displays messages and notifies the user about its status or progress of the task at hand).

Content Quality can be viewed from two different aspects. The first one is the quality of information that is located or displayed on a website, while the second one encompasses the quality of the content that is the result of using a web application. Content Quality is measured with five attributes: *correctness* (degree to which the content is correct, accurate, and valid), *coverage* (degree to which the content is complete, displayed clearly, and appropriately represented), *credibility* (degree to which the content is unbiased, trustworthy, and verifiable), *timeliness* (degree to which the content can be supplemented, modified, and updated), and *value-added* (degree to which the content is advantageous and contributes to making new decisions).

Performance refers to the attributes that measure the quality of tasks execution using the web application, including *effectiveness* (extent to which tasks can be executed accurately and completely by using the web application), *usefulness* (extent to which using the web application improves the user performance in task execution), and *efficiency* (extent to which the task execution using the web application saves resources).

Effort refers to the attributes that measure the effortlessness of the web application use. It is comprised of eight attributes: *minimal action* (the perceived amount of keyboard- and mouse-assisted motor activity required to complete a task), *minimal memory load* (the perceived amount of mental and perceptive activity required to complete a task), *accessibility* (extent to which the web application can be used by people with the widest range of characteristics and capabilities), *controllability* (extent of ease to make the web application do what the user wants), *ease of use* (extent to which interaction with the web application is free of effort), *learnability* (degree to which it is easy to learn to use the web application), *memorability* (degree to which it is easy to remember how the web application is used and where particular interface features are located), and *understandability* (extent to which interface functionalities are clear and unambiguous to the user).

Acceptability refers to the attributes that measure likeability and behavioral intentions related to the web application usage, including *playfulness* (extent to which the use of web application holds the users' attention and stimulates their imagination), *satisfaction* (extent to which the web application use meets user's expectations) and *loyalty* (extent to which the user is willing to continue to use the web application or recommend it to others).

2.2 Functions of Web 2.0 Applications

By introducing the dimension which deals with the functions of Web 2.0 applications, we are considering the fundamental functions of Web 2.0 applications: Communication, Sharing, Collaboration, Integration, and Organization [7]. Each Web 2.0 application can be assigned to the function that best describes its purpose. However, we must emphasize that Web 2.0 applications are not necessarily restricted to a single function. For instance, cloud based office suites can be employed for collaboration on document authoring, communication during document creation, and dissemination of created document. On the other hand, wikis enable users to collaborate on joint projects and integrate shared artifacts.

Communication refers to (i) web applications meant for synchronous or asynchronous interaction (e.g. audio and video forums, microblogs, or instant messengers), and (ii) web applications that provide a feature for communication between users (e.g. chat in a social network or virtual world). *Sharing* encompasses web applications (e.g. social networks and social bookmarking sites) that enable users to disseminate diverse types of artifacts, including photos, podcasts, documents, social bookmarks, etc. *Collaboration* includes web applications such as wikis and cloud based office suites where users work jointly with the aim to reach a common goal. *Integration* refers to web applications (e.g. wikis, blogs, e-portfolios, and mashups) that allow users to generate a repository of created artifacts. *Organization* includes web applications intended for visual representation of information (e.g. mind mapping and diagramming services) as well as web applications (e.g. podcasting services) that allow users to edit or combine previously created artifacts.

2.3 Agile Software Development Methods

The dimension which addresses agile software development methods encompasses diverse agile methods that can be used for the development of Web 2.0 applications such as Extreme programming, Rational Unified Process, Dynamic System Development

Method, Open Source Software Development or Agile Modeling [1]. The main reasons why agile methods are more appropriate for developing Web 2.0 applications than traditional methods are small releases with rapid cycles, adaptability, and collaboration among stakeholders. Adoption of the particular method depends on the size of development team, support for certain lifecycle phases, and type of Web 2.0 application.

3 Conclusion

The contribution of the proposed framework is twofold. Firstly, it can be used for the classification of both subjective and objective metrics thus providing guidance for their effective employment during the evaluation. Secondly, it can be applied for a sound and systematic assessment of the quality in use of Web 2.0 applications. In order to ensure that all important aspects of the introduced dimensions are appropriately considered, our future work will be focused on the refinement, revision, and validation of the introduced framework.

References

1. Abrahamsson, P., Salo, O., Ronkainen, J., Warsta, J.: Agile software development methods - Review and analysis. VTT Publications, Espoo (2002)
2. Calero, C., Ruiz, J., Piattini, M.: Classifying web metrics using the web quality model. Online Information Review 29(3), 227–248 (2005)
3. O'Reilly, T.: What is Web 2.0: design patterns and business models for the next generation of software (2005), `http://oreilly.com/web2/archive/what-is-web-20.html`
4. Orehovački, T.: Proposal for a Set of Quality Attributes Relevant for Web 2.0 Application Success. In: 32nd International Conference on Information Technology Interfaces, pp. 319–326. IEEE Press, Cavtat (2010)
5. Orehovački, T.: Development of a Methodology for Evaluating the Quality in Use of Web 2.0 Applications. In: Campos, P., Graham, N., Jorge, J., Nunes, N., Palanque, P., Winckler, M. (eds.) INTERACT 2011, Part IV. LNCS, vol. 6949, pp. 382–385. Springer, Heidelberg (2011)
6. Orehovački, T.: Perceived Quality of Cloud Based Applications for Collaborative Writing. In: Pokorny, J., et al. (eds.) Information Systems Development – Business Systems and Services: Modeling and Development, pp. 575–586. Springer, Heidelberg (2011)
7. Orehovački, T., Bubaš, G., Kovačić, A.: Taxonomy of Web 2.0 Applications with Educational Potential. In: Cheal, C., Coughlin, J., Moore, S. (eds.) Transformation in Teaching: Social Media Strategies in Higher Education, pp. 43–72. Informing Science Press, Santa Rosa (2012)
8. Orehovački, T., Granić, A., Kermek, D.: Exploring the Quality in Use of Web 2.0 Applications: The Case of Mind Mapping Services. In: Harth, A., Koch, N. (eds.) ICWE 2011 Workshops. LNCS, vol. 7059, pp. 266–277. Springer, Heidelberg (2012)
9. Ramler, R., Weippl, E., Winterer, M., Schwinger, W., Altmann, J.: A Quality-Driven Approach to Web Testing. In: Ibero-american Conference on Web Engineering, ICWE 2002, Santa Fe, vol. 1, pp. 81–95 (2002)
10. Ruiz, J., Calero, C., Piattini, M.: A three-dimensional web quality model. In: Cueva Lovelle, J.M., Rodríguez, B.M.G., Gayo, J.E.L., del Pueto Paule Ruiz, M., Aguilar, L.J. (eds.) ICWE 2003. LNCS, vol. 2722, pp. 384–385. Springer, Heidelberg (2003)

Desirability Methods for Evaluating Visual Design

Julie Schiller and Edward De Guzman

Autodesk, Inc., One Market St., Suite 500, San Francisco, CA 94105 USA
{julie.schiller,edward.deguzman}@autodesk.com

Abstract. Previous studies show that traditional usability evaluation methods can be problematic for collecting feedback on visual design [1]. Desirability studies have been used by usability practitioners to collect feedback on the affective response to interactive systems, but none allow end users to contribute feedback in the language of visual design experts. We describe how we adapted two traditional user research techniques (card sort, directed storytelling) to collect feedback on visual design. We then compare and contrast the kinds of data gathered from these methods with data gathered in a think-aloud exercise. A mixed-methods research strategy that includes methods adapted for visual design offers a path to engaging end users in a conversation that results in concise and actionable feedback for visual designers.

1 Introduction and Related Work

Traditional usability evaluation methods can be difficult to adapt for accurately assessing visual design in later design iterations because feedback for visual design is less about the user's ability to accomplish tasks and more about the affective response to a design. Desirability research methods can collect attitudinal reactions to a design rather than behavioral reactions. The data collected helps designers understand why different design directions alter the emotion of a user experience.

While several groups have reported case studies of desirability studies [1,2,4,5], it is unclear how desirability methods can be adapted to focus on visual design. End-users of software are not usually expert visual designers and do not have the appropriate vocabulary to provide concise actionable feedback to visual designers as part of a user-centered design process. There is a need for projection techniques that give end users a framework to express deeper feedback on visual design and to start discussions with end users that typically couldn't happen using traditional usability research methods.

In [3] De Guzman and Schiller described the Visual Design Card Sort (VDCS) as a technique to assess visual design and presented several explorations of visualizations for presenting data from this method. The work in this paper builds upon this previous research in two ways. First, it proposes another method for assessing visual design -- the Visual Design Mad Libs (VDML). Second, in order to better understand the benefits of VDCS and VDML as rapid user research methods, we compare the data collected from VDCS and VDML with the data collected from a think-aloud protocol study. Finally, we propose future directions for user research to partner and support visual design.

C. Stephanidis (Ed.): Posters, Part I, HCII 2013, CCIS 373, pp. 154–158, 2013.

2 Visual Design Card Sort

The Visual Design Reaction cards use a set of 75 Visual Design Reaction cards. 71 of the cards are a subset of the 118 Microsoft Product Reaction Cards from the Desirability Toolkit. Two researchers performed a card filtering exercise to inform and validate the set of cards, only keeping those that are relevant for providing feedback on the visual treatment of a design. Up to four additional cards can be used to add words that may be specific to the project or content being studied and/or to allow the participant to use their own word. Participants are then shown a set of images, one at a time. Once the image appears on the monitor, the participant has three to five minutes to select between three to five visual design reaction cards that best answers the question, "How does this look?" After the participant has selected a set of reaction cards, he/she is asked to explain why the card was chosen before moving on to the next image.

3 Visual Design Mad Libs

Visual Design Mad Libs is a hybrid of two research methods: directed storytelling and sentence completion tests, a semi-structured projective technique. To conduct a VDML, participants are shown a set of alternative visual designs along with control images. Once the image appears the participant has one minute to complete a one- to two-sentence statement where parts of the sentence(s) is left blank. For example, to assess the visual design of a product logo, the sentence to complete might be: "This is a logo for [company name]. The logo is a ______________ because ___________". The design alternatives are placed in a randomized order among the control imagery such as popular competitor products. After the participant has completed the sentence, the researcher may ask follow-up questions to better understand the participant's response.

4 Case Study: Evaluating Early Designs for an Autodesk Web Service

During the development of three Autodesk web products, the Visual Design Card Sort and the Visual Design Mad Libs were used to collect feedback on a proposed visual redesign. The purpose of this research was to collect feedback from Autodesk users about a new look-and-feel and report on trends observed across the participants. The visual design team identified several design goals such as: "simple", "easy to use", "focused", "efficient", and "humanized" also identified a target emotional response -- a "sense of wonder".

4.1 Materials

Participants were shown a set of high-fidelity static images that reflected a redesign of the Autodesk brand. They were also shown a set of images for a visual redesign of a Web application for collaboration. The materials included an image of the applications landing page, an image of a list of documents stored in the Web service, and screenshots of how the application would be redesigned for a mobile device.

4.2 Methodology

Three different methods were used to collect feedback on these materials: the Visual Design Card Sort, Visual Design Mad Libs, and a think aloud protocol. These methods were used over three rounds of user research focused on visual design. Table 1 summarizes the methodologies used in each of the three rounds of research. The research strategy builds on [3] which focused solely on the VDCS and lacked a comparison of the data from VDCS with any other technique (row 1). In the second round of research (row 2) we compared VDCS with data from a think aloud protocol. Having data from both methods gave us a stronger picture of the reactions from the participants but left us unsure if it was the complete picture. In the third round of research (row 3) we used all three methods. We found the data collected from each method to be complementary: VDCS gave deep actionable specific feedback on design while VDML provided good direction on choosing between several alternative designs.

Table 1. Research methods used in each round of research

	VDCS	Think Aloud	VDML
Study 1	✔		
Study 2	✔	✔	
Study 3	✔	✔	✔

The Visual Design Mad Libs were used to collect feedback on three company logos. Participants were asked to describe what they saw and give a reason why the logo represents Autodesk in the following sentence:

"It is a ______________ because ________________"

Finally, the think aloud protocol was used as part of a semi-structured follow-up interview about the three variations of the redesigned Autodesk logo.

4.3 Results

Visual Design Card Sort: The VDCS is displayed as a word cloud reflecting the most popular cards chosen by participants in the study. Cards that were chosen more often appear in a larger font and bolder type.

*Visual Design Mad Libs:*One participant's responses comparing three Autodesk logos:

- [Logo1] "It is a Folded 'A' because 'A' is for Autodesk. Kinda vague."
- [Logo 2] "It is a Bowtie or 3D glasses because you're making 3D TVs! Not good. Don't like the font"
- [Logo 3] "It is a perspective pyramid because you make software to build 3D designs"

Think aloud: Of the three logos presented to the participants, the strongest preference was for Logo 3:

- "More represents what Autodesk is known for. [It's] more recognizable as Autodesk."
- "…very precise, has gridlines."
- "Explains what we do. 3D design has volume."

5 Discussion

The past distance between visual design and HCI practices made it hard to get end-users engaged in the visual design development of an interactive product. Visual designers' complex vocabulary to discuss their work clashed with small sample user experience research feedback. However, in this case study, data was gathered both early and later in the development process. Accordingly, visual design was evaluated both holistically and in depth on specific pieces of the user interface.

HCI practitioners advocate including end-user feedback in the creation of user interfaces. Visual design for UIs has long the domain of experts due to the intricate, nuanced effect it has on user experience. In this paper, we advocate for more methods to express user experience along with brand or visual design needs. The techniques described contribute to deeper refinement, engagement, and a path to integrate these two fields.

6 Conclusion and Future Work

The use of desirability study methods has been documented in case studies but there has been little research and innovation in desirability research methods focused exclusively on assessing visual design. This is an opportunity for end-users to contribute to visual design goals. Techniques to make this feedback meaningful, actionable, and quick are needed.

Future directions include validation of some of the assumptions made which guided the design of this research method. We suspect that novice users are more subject to the acquiescence bias and would provide a significantly higher proportion of positive feedback than expert users.

Another direction for future work is the compare the VDCS and VDML methods to expert review of visual designers, rather comparing it to the think-aloud method. Finally, these techniques offer projective surfaces for end-users. The VDCS and VDML methods are given to demonstrate that a shared vocabulary and evaluation framework can generate strong results for the visual design of UI development. Additionally, these findings engage in a discussion with visual design professionals on the opportunities for direct user feedback. Hopefully, these techniques will do justice to the intricate and nuanced work of visual design while providing a strong UCD focus.

References

1. Barnum, C.M., Palmer, L.A.: More than a feeling: understanding the desirability factor in user experience. Ext. Abstracts CHI 2010. ACM Press (2010)
2. Benedek, J., Miner, T.: Measuring Desirability: New Methods for Evaluating Desirability in a Usability Lab Setting. In: Proc. Usability Professionals Association Conference (2002)
3. De Guzman, E.S., Schiller, J.: How does this Look? Desirability Methods for Evaluating Visual Design. Ext. Abstracts of HCII 2011 (2011)
4. Petrie, H., Precious, J.: Measuring user experience of websites: think aloud protocols and an emotion word prompt list. Ext. Abstracts CHI 2010. ACM Press (2010)
5. Williams, D., Kelly, G., Anderson, L.: MSN 9: new user-centered desirability methods produce compelling visual design. In: Proc. CHI 2004. ACM Press (2004)

Scale Development to Measure Usability of Text-Based CAPTCHA

Samar Swaid

Philander Smith College, 900 Daisy Bates Dr., Little Rock, AR
sswaid@philander.edu

Abstract. Completely Automated Public Turing Tests to Tell Computers and Humans Apart (CAPTCHA) is one of the important security mechanisms to avoid spamming and hacking on websites. This study focuses on identifying the usability dimensions of text-based CAPTCHA based on multi-method approach. Research methods of Think-Aloud protocol, factor analysis and equation modeling are applied. Analytical work shows that usability of CAPTCHA is formed of (i) content; (ii) format; (iii) distortion and (iv) services. The scale is used to evaluate the usability of ReCAPTCHA, JCAPTCHA and GIMBY. The main contribution of the study is constructing a scale, systematically, to quantitatively evaluate the usability of text-based CAPTCHA.

Keywords: Usability, Security, CAPTCHA, Usable Security, Users Perceptions, Design, Factor Analysis.

1 Introduction

Today, CAPTCHA is a widely used security tool to differentiate humans from automated agents by requesting a solution to a problem. Because text-based CAPTCHA is the most widely applied one [12], designers of text-based CAPTCHAs should give more attention not just to create robust ones, but also usable CAPTCHAs [7]. Recent studies underpins the necessity to focus on usability challenges in CAPTCHA [18,12] mainly for three reasons: (i) text-based CAPTCHA are the most common ones utilized by websites and the most ones preferred by web users [12] (ii) users do not necessarily share common cognitive backgrounds in which might affect their perception of the CAPTCHA and its usability [2]; and (iii) CAPTCHA generation is derived by an economic reasons to stop any abuse can be caused by automated agents [14], which make it an essential security tool. To my knowledge, no study has been dedicated to construct a scale to measure the usability of text-based CAPTCHA. This study is designed to cover this gap.

2 Literature Review

It is common knowledge that CAPTCHA should be secure and usable. Unlike the large number of studies on how to develop robust CAPTCHA, it is surprising to find

C. Stephanidis (Ed.): Posters, Part I, HCII 2013, CCIS 373, pp. 159–163, 2013.

that there has been little number of attempts to understand CAPTCHA usability. For example,W3C Working Group listed some concerns to problems posed by CAPTCHA for users with disability and suggested some alternatives to text-based CAPTCHA[15]. Another study recognized the impact of different distortion techniques on the usability of CAPTCHA designed by Microsoft [3]. Others applied usability criteria of accuracy, response time and perceived difficulty to measure usability (e.g., [8]), but no criteria were proposed. Another study examined usability aspects of CAPTCHA in a form of proposed framework of three dimensions of distortion, content and presentation[16]. Although this study forms a serious attempt to understand CAPTCHA usability, its framework cannot be used to quantify usability. Similarly, the study of [14] analyzed different properties of text-based CAPTCHAs that might explain usability.

3 Study and Findings

In this study a multi-method approach is applied. First, think-aloud protocol is used to understand usability measures and dimensions. Second, a scale is constructed to measure text-based CAPTCHAs implementing factor analysis. Finally, equation modeling is implemented to confirm reliability and validity of scale [9].

3.1 Think-Aloud Protocol

Think-aloud protocol is a well documented method in usability studies to understand cognitive processes. This method has been a proven way to highlight features and usability issues that can be improved [7].Six college students, participated in think-aloud study. Their ages ranged from 21 to 29 years old with 50% females and one male student with English as a second language. Participants were provided with six different text-based CAPTCHAs to solve. Input from participants was matched with identified usability criteria found in literature (see Table 1). It is interesting to note 66% of participants proposed issues related the “service” dimension.

3.2 Scale Construction

Several psychometric researchers have proposed different procedural models to develop better instruments. In general, scale construction follow the following pattern: (i) conceptualization; ii) operationalization; and (iii) purification; and (iv)testing psychometric properties of the scale. Dimensions conceptualization was made based on literature [14,16], and think-aloud study. The dimensions then, were opertionalized [6], and pilot tested generating 25 measures. The variable ease of use was adopted from literature [4]. CAPTCHA usability dimensions were treated as formative indicators of the second-order latent construct [5,6,9].

Table 1. Proposed Dimensions of Text-based CAPTCHA

Dimension	Definition	Source
Content	The extent the content embedded in CAPTCHA is understandable to users(e.g., character set, meaningfulness of words, combination of lowercase and uppercase, friendliness of words to non-English speakers, words are inoffensive, number of words)	[14],[16], think-aloud study
Format	The extent CAPTCHA content is formatted and presented to users (e.g., string length, font shape, font color, background color, background pattern, integration with website, uniformity of presentation, text box size)	[14],[16], think-aloud study
Distortion	The extent CAPTCHA content is distorted (e.g., stray lines, collapsing, and level of distortion)	[14], [16], think-aloud
Services	The solvers are provided with a number of services that make it easy to solve CAPTCHA (e.g., number of trials to solve, options to use other forms of CAPTCHA other than text, using appropriate symbols to indicate services	Think-aloud study

All items were measured using seven-point Likert-type scale ranging from (1) strongly disagree to (7) strongly agree. Data was collected from 135 participants with 76% of them females, their ages range from 19-43 years old. Factor analysis was conducted following Hair et al.'s recommendations [9], to identify the number of factors that adequately represent the underlying dimensions of CAPTCHA usability. Factor analysis resulted in identifying four-factor solution of: (i) content; (ii) format; (iii) distortion and (iv) services (see Table 2). Following the recommendation of [5,6,9], equation modeling is performed to understand the links among the dimensions of CAPTCHA usability and the "ease of use" variable. Conducting equation modeling reveals that identified factors relate significantly to overall ease of use. The developed scale demonstrated acceptable psychometric properties based on variety of reliability and validity indices drawn from exploratory factor analysis, and equation modeling, based on recommendations of [5],[6], and [13].

4 CAPTCHA Evaluation

Three of the commonly used CAPTCHAs were evaluated using the developed scale. Total of 26 participants, more than 70% of them are females with ages range from 21-30 years old, evaluated the text-based CAPTCHAs of ReCAPTCHA, JCAPTCHA and GIMBY. ReCAPTCHA scored the highest in terms of usability, then comes JCAPTCHA, to place GIMBY in the third place. Data Show that users find CAPTCHA with appropriate type of distortion that does not confuse them, supported with text of reasonable length and services that enable them to try again or switch to audio-based CAPTCHA make CAPTCHA easy to use by humans.

Table 2. Factor Solution for Usability of Text-based CAPTCHA

	Construct/ Measure	Factor Loading	VIF
	Content:		
1.	Text is clear and easy to solve	0.851	1.20
2.	Text is understandable	0.834	1.23
3.	Text is from dictionary	0.822	1.18
4.	Text is not offensive	0.820	1.33
5.	Text is appropriate for native language speakers	0.811	1.54
6.	Text is of appropriate number of words	0.811	1.70
7.	Text is of appropriate character set	0.809	1.61
	Format:		
1.	Text is presented in an appropriate way	0.901	1.21
2.	Text is of appropriate length	0.883	1.65
3.	Text is of predictable length	0.667	1.44
4.	Text is of appropriate font shapes	0.854	1.271.
5.	Text is of appropriate font sizes	0.848	71
6.	Text is of appropriate color	0.830	1.34
7.	Background is of appropriate color	0.829	1.51
8.	Background is of appropriate level of complexity	0.828	1.89
9.	Text is always presented in standard way	0.822	1.67
	Distortion:		
1.	Distortion applied does not make it hard to solve CAPTCHA	0.877	1.38
2.	Distortion is of appropriate level and do not stop me from solving CAPTCHA	0.856	1.41
3.	Noise added to text is of appropriate level and do not stop me from solving CAPTCHA	0.833	1.34
4.	Distortion type applied is appropriate and do not stop me from solving CAPTCHA	0.803	1.91
	Services:		
1.	CAPTCHA provides me with extra services and features that help me solve CAPTCHA	0.846	1.71
2.	CAPTCHA services improves my ability to solve	0.821	1.93
3.	CAPTCHA services enables me to choose other forms of CAPTCHA such as audio CAPTCHA	0.799	1.89
4.	CAPTCHA is provided with appropriate symbols such as symbol 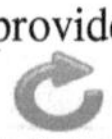 as an icon to try again	0.767	1.75

5 Conclusion

It has become a standard practice to employ CAPTCHA to differentiate between human users and automated agents. The purpose of this study is to present results of an in-progress study, with the aim to construct a scale to measure text-based CAPTCHA. The next phase of the study aims into collecting another dataset and confirm the dimensionality of the scale and its properties. This study contributes to efforts related to usable security on the World Wide.

References

1. Baecher, P., Fischlin, F., Gordon, L., Langenberg, R., Lutzow, M., Schroder, D.: CAPTCHAs: The Good, the Bad, and the Ugly, http://www.dominique-schroeder.de/resources/captchas.pdf
2. Belk, M., Fidas, C., Germankos, P., Samaras, G.: Do Cognitive Styles of Users Affect Preference and Performance Related to CAPTCHA Challenges? In: CHI 2012, Austin, Texas, pp. 1487–1492 (2012)
3. Chellapilla, K., Larson, K., Simard, P.Y., Czerwinski, M.: Building Segmentation Based Human-Friendly Human Interaction Proofs (HIPs). In: Baird, H.S., Lopresti, D.P. (eds.) HIP 2005. LNCS, vol. 3517, pp. 1–26. Springer, Heidelberg (2005)
4. Davis, F.: Perceived Usefulness, Perceived Ease of Use, and User Acceptance of Information Technology. MIS Quarterly 13(3), 319–340 (1989)
5. Diamantopoulos, A., Siguaw, J.: Formative Versus Reflective Indicators in Organizational Measure Development. JMR 17, 263 (2006)
6. Diamantopoulos, A., Winklhofer, H.: Index Construction with Formative Indicators: An Alternative to Scale Development. JMR 38, 369 (2001)
7. Erricsson, K., Simon, H.: Verbal Reports as Data. Psychol. Rev. 87(3), 215–251 (1980)
8. Fidas, C., Voyiatzis, A., Avouris, N.: On the Necessity of User-Friendly CAPTCHA. In: CHI 2012, pp. 2623–2626 (2012)
9. Hair, J., Anderson, R., Tatham, R., Black, W.: Multivariate Data Analysis, 5th edn. Prentice – Hall, Englewood Cliffs (1998)
10. Hwang, K., Haung, C., You, G.: A Spelling CAPTCHA Systems By Using Click. In: International Symposium on Biometrics and Security Technologies, pp. 1–8 (2012)
11. Nunnally, J.C.: Psychometric theory, 2nd edn. McGraw-Hill, New York (1978)
12. Sauer, G.H.: Towards a Universally Usable CAPTCHA. In: 4th Symposium on Usable Privacy and Security, SOUPS 2008, Pittsburgh, pp. 8–12 (2008)
13. Straub, D., Boudreau, M.-C., Gefen, D.: Validation Guidelines for is Positivist Research. Communications of the Association of IS 13, 380–427 (2004)
14. Sutherland, C.: Usability and Security of Text-Based CAPTCHAs. In: UMM CSci Senior Seminar Conference, Morris, MN (2012)
15. W3C Working Group.: Inaccessibility of CAPTCHA-Alternatives to Visual Turing Test on the Web, http://www.w3.org/TR/turingtest
16. Yan, J., El-Ahmad, A.: Usability of CAPTCHA or Usability Issues in CAPTCHA Design. In: Proceedings of the 4th Symposium on Usable Privacy and Security, pp. 44–52. ACM, New York (2008)

Optimizing Usability on Video Streaming Devices and Smart TV's

Sahar Tanabian[1] and Moe Tanabian[2]

[1]San Jose State University
[2]Intuigence Group, Irvine CA
sahar.tanabian@sjsu.edu,
moe.tanabian@intuigencegroup.com

Abstract. This presentation will provide a study of usability aspects for four Video Streaming Devices (VSD's) including Apple TV, Vizio Co-Star Google TV, Hisense Pulse Google TV, and Roku 3devices. The objective is to show the evaluation of user experience on these devices across multiple usability dimensions; and compile a list of what works best and what needs to improve in each device to compile a list of guidelines for designing better-optimized UX.

We employ Cognitive Walkthrough techniques to evaluate the usability aspects of each device. We selected a group of common tasks to make our evaluation more objective, and comparison more precise. We hope that these results can be used as a checklist for UX designers when designing Video Streaming Devices.

Keywords: Usability, User Experience, Cognitive Walkthrough, Smart TV, Testing.

1 Introduction

There has been rapid growth in consumer adoption of devices such as Roku, Apple TV and Google TV boxes from several OEM's over the last few years. This is indicative that Video Streaming Devices (VSD) are positioned to become one of the main components of the connected home concept as it is emerging.

Yet, studying the user experience (UX) of many of these VSD's, even the popular and successful ones, shows that the user interface (UI) and other user impacting aspects of these devices are not yet fully matured. We performed usability study on four of the available VSD's in the market to evaluate their UI and UX design. In this study we aimed to evaluate each device's UX and identify areas that the UX is well designed, and also the areas that the UX is poorly designed. The devices in our study included Apple TV generation3, Vizio Co-Stare Google TV, Hisense Pulse Google TV, and Roku 3 which are illustrated in Fig.1. We later summarized our findings in a series of suggested guidelines for other UX designer to use.

C. Stephanidis (Ed.): Posters, Part I, HCII 2013, CCIS 373, pp. 164–168, 2013.

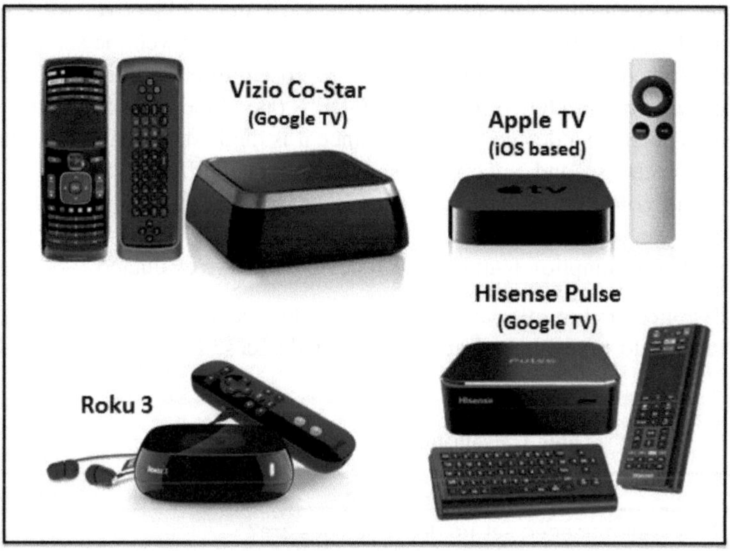

Fig. 1. Devices used for evaluation

2 Methodology

Our methodology begins with building a framework to objectively compare usability issues from a novice user's perspective, based on cognitive walkthrough technique. We first performed task analysis to identify tasks that are common across all devices. For example, "Find the latest episode of The Daily Show", constitutes a task. We then decomposed each task into its atomic subtask. In the next step, we evaluated each subtask across five usability dimensions: Visibility, Accessibility, Feedback, Responsiveness and Efficiency, and quantized the results. We then analyzed the data to identify where each device excels, and where it falls short to compile a list of best practices in user experience design. At the end we distilled this into a set of guidelines on optimizing usability on VSD's. Fig. 1 illustrates our approach.

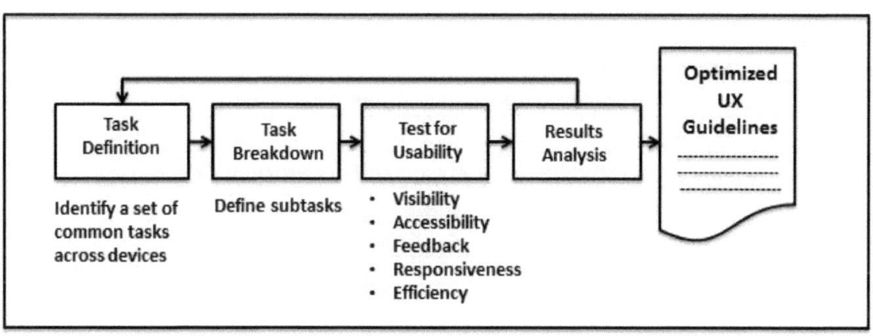

Fig. 2. Usability Evaluation and Analysis methodology

In order to streamline our analysis and make it more objective, we limited our scope of evaluation to two areas. First we wanted to see how well the set up procedure has been designed on each device. The set up procedure is often referred to as "Out Of Box Experience" or OOBE for short. OOBE is one of the main determinant factors in how users perceive a device's usability since it is the first encounter they have with a device. For the second area we opted to evaluate different aspects of content discovery and consumption tasks. Netflix is an application that is available on all devices that we studied, and hence Netflix was chosen as the proxy for content discovery and consumption features for all devices that we evaluated.

OOBE Evaluation: For evaluating OOBE, we defined six distinct criteria for set up process that could be evaluated across all four devices. These criteria are shown in Table-1.

Table 1. Evaluation criteria for OOBE procedure

	OOBE Use Case	Score range
1	How well managed set up dependencies are?	1-5
2	How easy it is to locate the Setup procedure?	1-5
3	How logical and sequential are the series of steps in the Setup procedure?	1-5
4	Can Setup be completed in less than 20min?	1, 5
5	Does Setup process provide enough feedback and control to the user?	1-5
6	Is end of Setup well communicated?	1-5

Video Content Discovery and Consumption Evaluation: For evaluating content consumption, we defined nine distinct tasks in a way that we could perform and evaluate across all different implementations of Netflix in these four devices.

Table 2. Common Use Cases

	Video Discovery & Consumption Common Use Cases
UC1	Launching Netflix
UC2	Search for content
UC3	Accessing recently watched content - Top 5
UC4	Accessing recently watched content - All
UC5	Browse recommended
UC6	Play a title (movie or TV episode), Forward/Rewind/ Pause
UC7	Play a TV show from Episode 1 in sequence
UC8	Play a title/ Forward/ Rewind/ Pause
UC9	Browse categories

Additionally, we evaluated each use case outlined in Table 2 across five different Usability dimensions to rate each device for these common use cases. We used the following Usability dimensions:

Table 3. Usability Dimensions for evaluating each Use Case

	Usability Dimensions	Description
1	Visibility	How visually easy it is to identify the right UI element
2	Accessibility	How easy it is to start the use case from the Gateway page?
3	Feedback	How much feedback and control is provided to the user
4	Responsiveness	How responsive and snappy the device is when performing the use case?
5	Efficiency	How fast the use case can be completed, i.e. how many steps needed to complete the use case?

3 Summary of Analysis and Results

The result of our analysis revealed interesting facts on how product, UX and UI design decisions could impact usability of the device. In general, we found that the design of the remote control has significant impact on the usability of the device, across variety of use cases. Our analysis shows that even though minimalist design for remote control may be aesthetically superior, it hinders several usability dimensions. Again, we found due to various needs of connected devices for alphanumeric data entry during the setup procedure, having a remote with full keyboard enhanced the usability of the setup procedure. The summary of our analysis is illustrated in Fig. 3. Fig. 3-a illustrates the usability scores for each device, across each of the nine use cases outlined in Table 2. Fig. 3-b illustrates the overall average score for each of the usability dimensions outlined in Table 3, and finally Fig. 3-c shows the average scores for overall OOBE software setup procedure across the usability criteria outlined in Table 1. In short, based on our findings we found that the following guidelines can be useful when designing UI/UX for VSD's:

- A remote control with full keyboard on one side and navigation, playback and quick lunch buttons on the other side enhances overall usability. GoogleTV based devices all ship with a remote with this design.
- Optimal navigation UI for TV episodes is multi-pane set of left to right panels. The first panel allows for selecting the desired season, the next one to the right the episode and next panel displays the detail information on the series and the episode.
- Google TV based devices provide this type of TV episode navigation UX.
- On the detail page of a movie, providing a list of similar items – or "More-Like-This" –increases Efficiency and Accessibility of discovery -as in Apple TV.

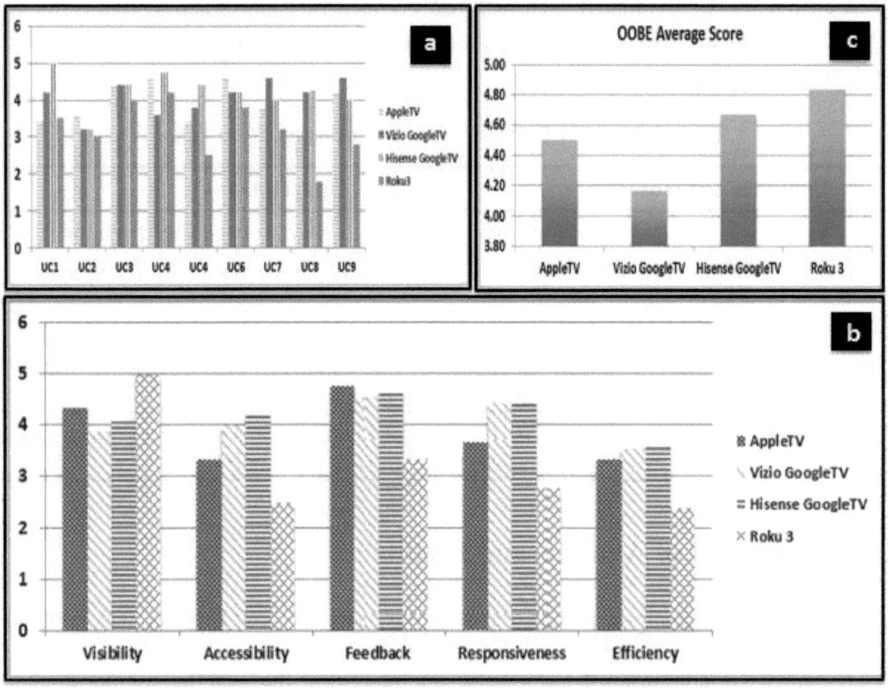

Fig. 3. a) Usability evaluation of each Use Case, b) Usability Dimensions and c) OOBE scores

- While larger icons increase Visibility, they severely limit screen's real-estate utilization and navigation speed, and lower Accessibility and Efficiency of content search and discovery. Roku 3 suffers from large icons, and in contrast, Apple TV and both Google TV devices have cut a good balance between Visibility and optimizing screen area utilization. 3-4 rows of content can be optimally placed on each screen for a typical TV screen size and watching distance.
- Explicitly outlining the stages of OOBE at the beginning is very confidence building, while the user is going through the setup procedure. We found that Roku exceled here, and provided the best OOBE setup experience.
- Including touch based UI, and touchpad on the remote decreases the usability scores of the experience. We found that touch based UI is not a good input method for TV based interactions.

Optimum UX/UI Design for DSV: As a result of our analysis, we combined best practices from each device we evaluated, to design an optimum device:

1. Hisense remote control – minus the touchpad
2. TV episode control of Google TV – either of the Vizio or Hisense devices
3. Movie detail page of Apple TV
4. Physical design and aesthetics of Apple TV box
5. OOBE setup procedure of Roku 3

Bonus Feature: Roku 3's on-remote headphone jack.

Insights from Eye Movement into Dynamic Decision-Making Research and Usability Testing

Benoit R. Vallières, Cindy Chamberland, François Vachon, and Sébastien Tremblay

Co-DOT Laboratory, School of Psychology, Université Laval, Québec, Canada
benoit.roberge-vallieres.1@ulaval.ca,
{cindy.chamberland,francois.vachon,
sebastien.tremblay}@psy.ulaval.ca

Abstract. This study shows how the use of various measures of eye movement can serve to portray dynamic decision-making (DDM) in a coherent fashion. We extracted eye movement metrics relative to 1) scanpath, 2) eye fixations, and 3) pupillary response, to characterize DDM during the process of risk assessment. Results from Experiment 1 revealed that incorrect classifications were associated with 1) less efficient information search, 2) difficulties in making sense of critical information, and 3) a low level of cognitive load. In Experiment 2, we used eye tracking to assess the impact on DDM of introducing a decision support system. The addition of a temporal-overview display seems to affect processing time in DDM as indexed by shorter scanpaths and fixations during classifications. These findings illustrate how event-based eye movement measures can reveal characteristics and limitations of the ongoing cognitive processing involved in DDM and also contribute to usability testing.

Keywords: Eye movements, dynamic decision-making, usability testing, decision support system.

1 Introduction

Dynamic decision making (DDM) involves a series of interdependent real-time decisions and actions made in an environment that continuously changes, and evolves according or not to operators' actions [1]. Air traffic control and military operations are examples of complex dynamic situations in which DDM is difficult to the point that it often taxes operators' cognitive capabilities [2]. In such situations, decision makers have to process and categorize information coming from multiple sources within a limited time frame [3].

The demands to support DDM are growing rapidly, but providing such support requires a good understanding of the underlying cognitive processes involved in DDM. One avenue that we wish to explore is to reveal these cognitive processes through the use of eye tracking in a manner that is closely linked to the dynamics of the situation [4-5]. Indeed, eye movements can provide non-obtrusive, online indices

C. Stephanidis (Ed.): Posters, Part I, HCII 2013, CCIS 373, pp. 169–174, 2013.

of cognitive functioning [6]. There are various ways in which eye movements can be measured to study a wide range of cognitive processes. Poole and Ball [5] highlighted different categories of eye movement metrics, each reflecting the action of specific cognitive processes. *Scanpath metrics* relate to saccade-fixation-saccade sequences of eye movements and can be used to index the efficacy in information seeking [5]. *Fixation metrics* measure how long the gaze is relatively stationary and can serve as estimates of processing (or encoding) time during DDM [6-7]. *Pupilometry* measures variations in the pupil diameter during DDM and can index the level of cognitive load [8].

In DDM studies, such metrics are usually exploited in isolation and are rarely used to investigate how a decision support system can affect information intake during DDM. The purpose of the present study was twofold. The first experiment aimed at demonstrating how the combination of different types of eye movement measures during the information intake can contribute to pinpoint the sources of errors in the context of a simulation of radar-based risk assessment. The goal of the second experiment was to test the potential of such an event-based eye-tracking approach to usability testing by assessing the impact of introducing a decision support system (DSS) on cognitive processes engaged in DDM.

2 Experiment 1

2.1 Method

Twenty-one adults reporting normal or corrected-to-normal vision and normal hearing took part in the experiment. We employed the S-CCS microworld (Figure 1), a low-level computer-controlled simulation of a naval anti-warfare [see 8-9] in which participants play the role of a tactical coordinator onboard of a frigate by conducting threat evaluation and weapon assignment. The simulation dynamically evolves according to a pre-determined scenario and takes into account participants' actions.

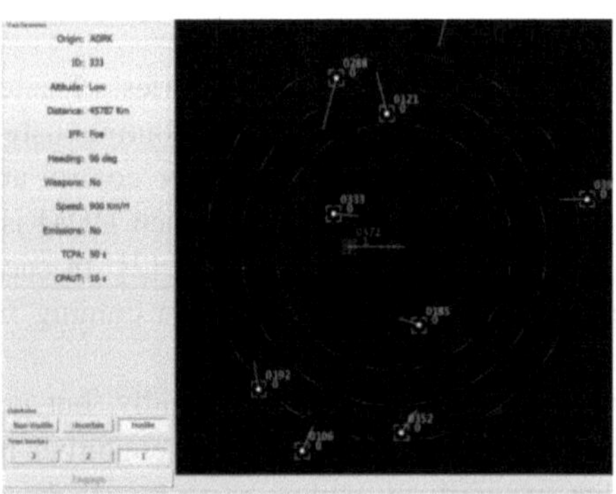

Fig. 1. The S-CCS display in Experiment 1

Participants performed three subtasks: threat-level and -immediacy evaluation and neutralization of hostile aircraft. Our analyses focused on the threat-level assessment subtask. In this task, participants had to categorize all aircraft moving on the radar according to a classification rule. This rule took into account 5 out of 11 parameters appearing in the list. Aircraft could be non-hostile, uncertain or hostile, and participants clicked on the classification buttons to record their decision. For hostile aircraft, participants must also judge threat immediacy and engage weapons.

The experimental session started with a tutorial explaining the context of the simulation, the mission and the task to perform, followed by a practice phase with static screenshots. Then, participants familiarized themselves with the S-CCS dynamic environment through eight training scenarios. The session ended with 16 4-min test scenarios, each including a set of 27 aircraft varying in speed and trajectory on the radar.

2.2 Results and Discussion

Eye movement measures were extracted from over 10,000 classifications (mean accuracy: 85.9%) and were classify as correct or incorrect decisions. Table 1 describes the eye-tracking metrics used in the present study with their meaning.

Table 1. Description of the eye movement metrics extracted during each classification

Type of metric	Metric	Description	Meaning
Scanpath	Scanpath duration	Mean duration (in ms) of the scanpath	Longer-lasting scanpath = Less efficient searching
	Scanpath length	Mean number of fixations in the scanpath	Longer scanpath = Less efficient searching
	Spatial density	Mean % of areas looked at to perform a classification	Higher density = Less efficient searching
Fixation	Mean fixation duration	Mean duration of a single fixation on relevant areas	Longer duration = Difficulty in extracting information
	Total fixation duration	Time spent fixating relevant areas	
Pupil response	% of change in pupil size	Pupil dilation when looking at relevant areas compared to a "baseline" dilation level	Larger pupil dilation = Increased cognitive load

Table 2. Eye movement metrics' mean obtained for correct and incorrect classifications

Metrics	Control (Exp. 1)		With TOD (Exp. 2)	
	Incorrect	Correct	Incorrect	Correct
Scanpath	•	•	•	•
Length	8.78	8.27	8.11	7.55
Duration (ms)	3077.41	2879.29	3282.35	3042.12
Spatial density	48.1	46.7	38.5	37.1
Fixation	•	•	•	•
Mean duration (ms)	246.72	233.38	187.91	183.5
Total duration (ms)	967.47	855.85	680.74	617.84
Pupillometry	•	•	•	•
% of change	-1.12	-0.27	-0.66	-0.62

Table 2 presents the results obtained for all metrics according to classification accuracy. Dependent-samples *t* tests performed on participants' means revealed a significant difference between correct and incorrect classifications for each metric. These results suggest that in the context of radar-based risk assessment, DDM errors were associated with impoverished efficacy to search for relevant information, difficulties in making sense of critical information, and transient slackening in the overall level of cognitive effort. This study illustrates how eye movements can be used to discriminate between correct and incorrect decisions in dynamic environments and, hence, provide insights into potential solutions (e.g., DSS, training) to improve the various aspects of cognitive functioning involved in DDM.

3 Experiment 2

The objective of Experiment 2 was to show how eye movement analyses can serve usability testing by examining the impact on threat evaluation of adding a DSS designed to support priorization and scheduling activities. A temporal overview display (TOD) was integrated to the original S-CCS interface (Figure 2) to support threat-immediacy assessment and defensive-measures management. While this tool was shown to promote temporal awareness for executing these subtasks [9], the holistic evaluation of its impact on other subtasks using eye-tracking is recommended.

3.1 Method

Twenty-two new adults participated to the experiment. Added to the right of the radar, the TOD represents temporal components such as time-to-decide and time to hit a target by presenting each aircraft (represented by a rectangle) across a timeline. An aircraft hits the ship when the right end of its rectangle crosses the red line.

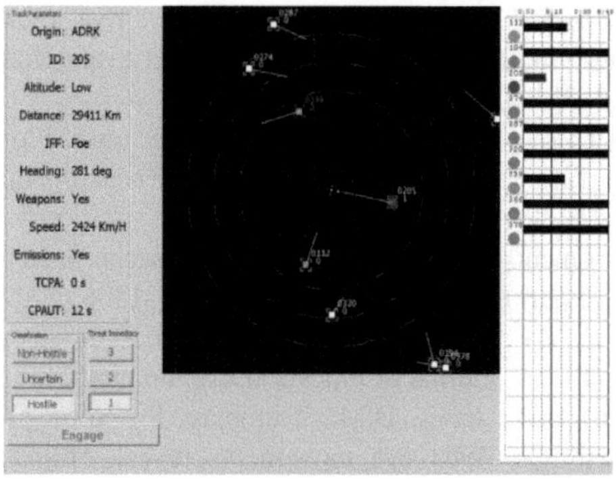

Fig. 2. The S-CCS display with the TOD located to the right of the radar screen

3.2 Results and Discussion

As shown in Table 2, the comparison of correct and incorrect classifications yielded the same results as in Experiment 1. When contrasting eye movement metrics between the two studies, independent-samples t tests revealed significantly lower spatial density and shorter fixations in the presence of the TOD. Such results suggest that promoting temporal awareness through the TOD influenced temporal aspects of the classification subtask as participants took less time to gather relevant information necessary to assess threat level. This experiment illustrates the potential of eye movements in uncovering the consequences of adding DSSs on cognitive functioning.

4 Conclusion

The present study was successful in showing that eye movements can be used not only to discriminate between correct and incorrect decisions in dynamic environments, but also to assess the impact of adding a DSS on different aspects of cognitive functioning, such as search efficiency. Taken together, our findings testified that dynamic, event-based measures of eye movement provide a window onto the ongoing cognitive processing in complex dynamic situations. The use of eye-tracking metrics in a convergent manner constitutes a powerful tool to portray DDM and can contribute to DSS usability testing.

References

1. Edwards, W.: Dynamic decision theory and probabilistic information processing. Human Factors 4, 59–74 (1962)
2. Gonzalez, C.: Decision support for real-time, dynamic decision-making tasks. Organizational Behavior and Human Decision Processes 96, 142–154 (2005)
3. Brehmer, B.: Micro-worlds and the circular relation between people and their environment. Theoretical Issues in Ergonomics Science 6, 73–94 (2005)

4. Morrison, J., Marshall, S.P., Kelly, R.T., Moore, R.A.: Eye tracking in tactical decision making Environments: Implications for decision support evaluation. In: Proceedings of the 3rd ICCRTS, pp. 355–364 (1997)
5. Poole, A., Linden, B.J.: Eye tracking in human-computer interaction and usability research: Current status and future. In: Ghaoui, C. (ed.) Encyclopedia of Human-computer Interaction, pp. 211–219. Idea Group, Hershey (2006)
6. Rayner, K.: Eye movements and attention in reading, scene perception, and visual search. Quarterly Journal of Experimental Psychology 62, 1457–1506 (2009)
7. Goldberg, H.J., Kotval, X.P.: Compute interface evaluation using eye movements: Methods and constructs. International Journal of Industrial Ergonomics 24, 631–645 (1999)
8. Vachon, F., Vallières, B.R., Jones, D.M., Tremblay, S.: Nonexplicit change detection in complex dynamic settings: What eye movements reveal. Human Factors 54, 996–1007 (2012)
9. Tremblay, S., Vachon, F., Rousseau, R., Breton, R.: Promoting temporal awareness for dynamic decision making in command and control. In: Stanney, K., Hale, K.S. (eds.) Advances in Cognitive Engineering and Neuroergonomics, pp. 3422–3431. CRC Press (2012)

A Usability Study of Dynamic Geometry Software's Interfaces

Serap Yağmur and Kürşat Çağıltay

Middle East Technical University, 06800 Çankaya Ankara, Turkey
{Yagmur,kursat}@metu.edu.tr

Abstract. The use of information technology such as dynamic geometry software in mathematics teaching has become more popular and essential. There are several benefits of using this software. In spite of the benefits, they have some difficulties in terms of usability, so users have some problems while using them in learning mathematics. The purpose of this study is to investigate the usefulness of these software interfaces. For this purpose, firstly, we selected two dynamic geometry software. One of them is GeoGebra and the other one is Geometer' Sketchpad. After selecting, 6 tasks designated using this software. In usability test, the participants tried to do task. While doing the tasks, in order to analyze the process, the participants were observed and their eye movements were recorded with eye tracker system. Then their opinions about software asked. Finally all data were analyzed, and discussed.

Keywords: GeoGebra, Geometer's Sketchpad, Usability, Eye Tracking.

1 Introduction

The computer is a powerful and helpful tool in teaching and learning mathematics [10]. With multimedia capabilities, students are able to visualize mathematical concepts which are difficult using traditional methods [5]. There are a lot of powerful software which can be used in classroom teaching such as Logo, Geometer's Sketchpad, Cabri, Derive, Mathemetica and GeoGebra. In the recent years, a number of studies in which dynamic mathematics software GeoGebra and Geometer's Sketchpad are used are seen in the literature. One of this software, GeoGebra can be defined as a software program that was e designed to combine geometry, algebra, and calculus in a single, dynamic geometry [10]. The other software; Geometer's Sketchpad uses exploratory in mathematics. This software allows teachers and students to use the construction and the animation of an interactive mathematics model [7]. There are several benefits of using this software. Previous studies show that the teaching materials, which prepared with GeoGebra, are more successful than traditional method [11]. Other study indicates that teaching the subject of symmetry with GeoGebra is enabling students to teach the subject better [1]. The other study about Geometer's Sketchpad shows that the use of interactive multimedia increases student attention and understanding of mathematics [7].

C. Stephanidis (Ed.): Posters, Part I, HCII 2013, CCIS 373, pp. 175–179, 2013.

2 Research Questions

There are a few studies on usefulness of this software. Dynamic geometry software has some difficulties in terms of usability, so users have some problems while using them in learning mathematics. The purpose of this study is to investigate the usefulness of these software interfaces. For this purpose, we selected two popular dynamic geometry software. One of them is Geogebra which of most features are free and it is open source and written in Java and thus available for multiple platforms [4]. The Geometer's Sketchpad is a popular commercial interactive geometry software program for exploring Euclidean geometry, algebra, calculus, and other areas of mathematics [9].In this study; we will try to find answers of questions: (i) What are the major problems when using these software interfaces? (ii) How much time the user spent for doing a basic task? (iii) Is there any difference doing basic or complex task? (iv) Is there any difference doing same task while using different software?

3 Methodology

The model of this survey is an end-user based research model. At this research, the steps were followed according to this model.

Apparatus. Our study was carried out at the HCI Research and Application Laboratory at the Middle East Technical University. In this laboratory, the devices enable to monitor screen shots on the computers. To record eye movements a Tobii 1750 Eye Tracker System was used. The Tobii 1750 Eye Tracker software provides a video of screen records, watching and analyzing these videos, participants behaviors' observed. Moreover, the records of Eye movements' data analyzed.

The Participants. Our population in this study was six end-users who are research assistant in Middle East Technical University. All of them were female and were at 23, 23, 27, 28, 29, 32 ages (M=27). Two of them were at PhD and the others were at master degree (M=1, 33). The degree of computer usage of this participation was advance (M=6, 83). Half of the participations have experience of using GeoGebra (M=2). However, the others have not any experience. On the other hand, two of them have no experience of using Geometer's Sketchpad, the others have (M=1, 83).

The Tasks. In usability test, 6 specific tasks were done by using GeoGebra and Geometer's Sketchpad. Two of them were easy, two of them had medium degree of difficulty and two of them were difficult. First two of them were basic task. After doing these basic tasks, the difficulties of other tasks increased. (Table 1).

The Application. In application step, we collected data while users do the tasks, the participants were observed and their eye movements were recorded with eye tracker system and they were asked to their opinion about software, giving a questionnaire which consists of 40 questions about each software. It asks users' opinion about the appearance of the interface and the terms which used in the program, and the learning of the system usage. Also this questionnaire was in the users' native language (Turkish). In addition to this questionnaire, we applied John Brooke's System Usability Scale (SUS).

"SUS can be used on very small sample sizes (as few as two users) and still generate reliable results." [8]. We asked 10 item questionnaire which were in Turkish with 5 response options. For each item users gave one response. These two questionnaires were translated from English to Turkish by Kürşat Çağıltay [3].

The Criteria. The other step was that we determined criteria for analyzing the results. Although there were a lot of criteria which used to evaluate systems' usability, we took into consideration Nielsen ten user interface design criteria [6].

Table 1. Tasks

Task 1:	Draw any triangle, show its angle and edge length and add any edge length of this triangle.
Task 2:	Draw any irregular polygon, show its angle and calculate its circumference and area.
Task 3:	Draw a straight line passing through the A (5, 0) and B (0, 2) points and indicate the equation of the line.
Task 4:	Draw a graph of the equation $y = 3x^2+5$.
Task 5:	$f(x) = 2x^3-x^2 +6x +4$ Take the derivative of the function. Draw a graph of a derivative.
Task 6:	Draw any circle; calculate its circumference, the radius and area. Create a table of values found by changing the radius of the circle. Draw a graph from the data in this table.

4 Results and Discussion

Qualitative Results. We observed participants and noticed some problems about this dynamic geometry software. The main problem with GeoGebra was not finding and opening "Input Help". The other problem was finding any function under menu options. The icon of "Input Help" menu was not visible and easy to click. Half of the participants opened and used this menu incidentally or they had experience for click and opened it. The other problem was data transferring between windows. Two of the participants tried to transfer input data to from "Algebra" to "CAS" but she did not. And another participant tried to transfer data from "Graphics" to "Spreadsheets", after lots of mouse click she did. The other problem was about error messages which only show errors but not give the correct type or any hints. The other problem was no instruction for using tools. Another problem was that about right click menu options. Some of participants tried to use right click for calculating area and circumference but GeoGebra did not allowed this. Last problem with GeoGebra which we observed was that "CAS" tools were not enough for using easily. One of the participants indicated that learning usage of this software takes long time and its menu was complex and remember the steps were not easy. The main problem with Geometer's Sketchpad was about instructions place on interface. The participants could not recognized instructions while doing the tasks. Instructions are bottom of the page and not recognizable. The other problem was about selecting the objects. The participants had difficulties while calculating and showing the angle. Another problem was menu's classifications of properties and functions. For example; one of the participants looked "Construct" menu for creating table. But she could not find it under "Construct" menu, she find it under "Number" menu. One participant indicated that there were not enough error messages.

Quantitative Results. Firstly, we compared fulfillment of the tasks in this dynamic geometry software. All tasks were completed by all participants using Geometer's Sketchpad. However, Task 6 was not completed by the half of participants using Geogebra. Secondly, we got time to first fixation, total visit duration, mouse click count, and time to first mouse click records of the participants by Tobii software. We calculated the time to first fixation for each task for each software and analyzed the average time to first fixation. We attended to total visit duration time for each task completion. And we calculated mouse click count for each task comparing the software. This gives information about the amount of steps. Lastly, we calculated time to first mouse click for each task. To compare the results we used Paired-Samples t-test for a task which was completed by using this software. We implemented 24 paired samples t-test for the results of Tobii records. We analyzed that there was no big differences for this data. Time to first fixation and time to first mouse click was similar for this software. The results were $p>0.05$ so this results were not meaningful. On the other hand, total visit duration and mouse click count for each task showed differences. Total visit duration for Task 1 in GeoGebra (M= 115, 6283, SD=72, 58297), for Geometers' Sketchpad (M=187, 1700, SD=75, 72062). Paired Samples t-test $p<0.01$. Total visit duration for Task 3 in GeoGebra (M= 25, 7617, SD=6, 92604), for Geometers' Sketchpad (M=54, 7717 SD=54, 7717). Paired Samples Test p<, 029. Total visit duration for Task 6 in GeoGebra (M= 679, 9283, SD=468, 29070), for Geometers' Sketchpad (M=159, 1317SD=32, 80426). Paired Samples t-test p<, 040. This results shows that Total visit duration in the task for Geometer's Sketchpad was longer than GeoGebra except from task 6. The reason of the task 6 was longer than the other was the participants had some problems while using the spreadsheets. And Task 6 was not completed by some participants because of this reason. Mouse Click Count for Task 1 in GeoGebra (M=41, 0000, SD=29, 09983), for Geometer's Sketchpad (M=106, 5000, SD=42, 49588) and $p<0.00$. Mouse Click Count for Task 3 for GeoGebra (M=7, 5000, SD=1, 87083), for Geometer's Sketchpad (M=20, 5000, SD=11, 29159) and $p<0.020$. This result shows that Mouse Click Count while doing a task using Geometer's Sketchpad was bigger than using GeoGebra. This means that users do much steps while using Geometer's Sketchpad. The other quantitative analyzed was done according to the questionnaire. The Paired-Sample t-test was used. The results of this test were that GeoGebra Average (M=6, 1917, SD=1, 80705), Sketchpad Average (M=7, 2208, SD=, 93640). Paired-Sample t-test p>, 05. So the differences are not meaningful as statistics. The last analyzed was done according the SUS. SUS is a reliable, low-cost usability scale that can be used for global assessments of systems usability [2]. The results of Sketchpad's SUS score (71, 66) was higher than GeoGebra's SUS score (58, 33). We investigated this difference and implemented Paired-Samples T-test for this SUS. We found that SUS Score for GeoGebra (M=58,333, SD=19, 5363) and SUS Score for Geometer's Sketchpad (71,667, SD=12, 2134) $p>0.05$. We concluded that this difference has no meaning as statics. Moreover, we decided to compare the questionnaire and SUS results. We analyzed the correlation between these results. First correlation was between SUS Score for GeoGebra and GeoGebra Average (data from questionnaire).The results were; r = 0,930 shows that there was a strong relation between our questionnaire and SUS Score for GeoGebra. r =0, 723 shows that there was middle level of relation between SUS Score for Geometer's Sketchpad and Geometer's Sketchpad Average (data from questionnaire). The relation between Geogebra's data was stronger than Geometer's Sketchpad's data. The reason was the difference that limitations of participants size.

5 Conclusion

In this study, we aimed to evaluate dynamic geometry software interfaces. According to the results there are no big differences between GeoGebra and Geometer's Sketchpad in terms of usability. We cannot say that this software have major usability problem. Some of participants were familiar the usage of these software. This provides the adaptability of learning usage new functions. We answered the question was about how much time a user spent while doing a basic task. We observed that there were differences between basic and complex task. Complex task took long time and required much steps. In this study, we cannot make definitive judgments because of some limitations. The participants' size of the study was at the lowest limit of eye tracking studies. Our participants were specific group so reaching more participants was impossible. Future Studies should increase the number of participants to obtain reliable and definitive results. The other limitation was Tobii Eye Tracker Software blocked some functions of Geometer's Sketchpad. So, Task 3 was done again by the user. Finally, in a further study, the task should designed specifically and try to test all functions of the dynamic geometry software.

References

1. Adnan Akkaya, E.T.: Using Dynamic Software in Teaching of the Symmetry in Analytic Geometry: The Case of GeoGebra. Procedia Social and Behavioral Sciences, 2540–2544 (2011)
2. Brooke, J. (n.d.): System Usability Scale, AHRQ Agency for Healthcare and Research and Quality, http://healthhit.ahrq.gov (retrieved January 19, 2013)
3. Çağıltay, K.: İnsan Bilgisayar Etkileşimi ve Kullanılabilirlik Mühendisliği: Teoriden Pratiğe. Odtü Yayıncılık, Ankara (2011)
4. GeoGebra-Wikipedia (n.d.): Wikipedia, http://en.wikipedia.org/wiki/GeoGebra (retrieved November 30, 2012)
5. Kamariah Abu Bakar, A.F.: Exploring secondary school student's motivation using technologies in teaching and learning mathematics. Procedia Social and Behavioral Sciences, 4650–4654 (2010)
6. Nielsen, J. (n.d.): Ten Heuristic User Interface, http://www.useit.com/papers/heuristic/heuristic_list.html (retrieved January 12, 2012)
7. Norazah Nordin, E.Z.: Pedagogical Usability of the Geometer's Sketchpad (GSP) Digital Module in the Mathematics Teaching. In: 7th WSEAS International Conference on Education and Educational Technology (EDU 2008) (2008)
8. Sauro, J.: Measuring Usability with the System Usability Scale (SUS), Measuring Usability, http://www.measuringusability.com/sus.php (retrieved January 19, 2013)
9. The Geometer's Sketchpad-Wikipedia (n.d.): Wikipedia, http://en.wikipedia.org/wiki/The_Geometer%27s_Sketchpad (retrieved November 30, 2012)
10. Yılmaz Zengin, H.F.: The effect of dynamic mathematics software GeoGebra on student achievement in teaching of trigonometry. Procedia Social and Behavioral Sciences, 183–187 (2012)
11. Zerrin Ayvaz Reis, S.O.: Using GeoGebra as an information technology tool: parabola teaching. Procedia Social and Behavioral Sciences, 565–572 (2010)

Conclusion

Part III
Universal Access and eInclusion

The E-training Caravans: An e-Inclusion Initiative in Saudi Arabia

Hend S. Al-Khalifa

Information Technology Department
College of Computer and Information Sciences
King Saud University, Riyadh, Saudi Arabia
hendk@ksu.edu.sa

Abstract. Today's technological world requires that individuals are capable of using Information and Communications Technology (ICT) effectively. In fact, more and more services are offered using technology, e.g. communication with family and friends, carrying out business, and interacting with governments.

To close the gap between "the technology-empowered communities and the technology-excluded communities" an initiative called the e-training caravan is presented in this paper. This initiative aims to enable the segments of society from dealing with telecommunications and information technology effectively, bridging the digital divide and raising awareness of the importance of ICT for all individuals. This initiative focuses on population of rural areas and low-income areas. In this paper we discuss the e-training caravan initiative proposed by the Ministry of Communication and Information Technology (MCIT) in Saudi Arabia, and highlight its objectives and training program. We also discuss the results obtained after running the caravan for one year along with the encountered barriers.

Keywords: e-Inclusion, Digital Divide, ICT Literacy, Rural Communities, Empowerment, Saudi Arabia.

1 Introduction

European Commission defines e-inclusion as "structural investment" for innovation and economic growth. It is both the inclusion and the use of Information and Communications Technology (ICT) to achieve wider inclusion and focus on participation of all individuals and communities in all aspects of the information society [1]. E-inclusion is concerned with "the goal of ensuring that everyone is included in and gains from developments enabled by ICT" [2].

The concept of e-Inclusion drives us to the term "Digital Divide" which refers to "the difference in access to, and usage of, information and communications technologies between people within the same country" [10]. This means that the lack of internet and computer access is one aspect of digital divide; yet, the other aspect includes people skills and capacities in using ICT.

C. Stephanidis (Ed.): Posters, Part I, HCII 2013, CCIS 373, pp. 183–187, 2013.

Many governments' worldwide [2] started e-inclusion policies, programs and activities aimed at ensuring the participation of individuals and communities in all dimensions of the knowledge-based society and economy through their access to ICT. These governments have made many initiatives to remove access and accessibility barriers to ICT resources. Examples of worldwide initiatives include: the eInclusion European project [1], the eInclusion Foundation initiative, appointed by the Government of the Hong Kong Special Administration Region [3], and the Chile project aimed at bringing hope to people excluded by disability and poverty [4], to name a few.

Turning briefly our attention to Saudi Arabia, the current situation indicates the spread of computer illiteracy and Internet in rural and poor areas more than others [9]. To start bridging the digital divide and raising awareness of the importance of ICT for all individuals, as well as focusing on people living in rural areas and low-income, the provision of basic training and free use of ICT became a government necessity [5].

This paper reports on the e-Training caravans' initiative, proposed by the Ministry of Communication and Information Technology (MCIT) in Saudi Arabia, along with its objectives and training program. Furthermore, we will discuss in details the initiative obtained results and barriers pertaining to the features of the initiative.

2 Case Study: E-Training Caravans Initiative

In January 2012, MCIT launched the e-training caravans' initiative (http://www.eqwafil.gov.sa) which aims to provide computer and Internet literacy courses for both young and old citizens in rural areas and low-income people in Saudi Arabia. The objectives of this initiative are [6]:

- Introducing the importance of ICT to the targeted groups.
- Conducting training of the basic skills of using computers and the internet by the targeted groups.
- Providing the appropriate training environment to teach the basic skills of using computers to people in areas that large institutes and training centers are not available in.
- Encouraging people in rural areas, villages and hamlets to learn how to use computers and the internet, and
- Facilitating the access to government and commercial services easily to ensure equal access and inclusion for all citizens.

The trainers and the driver traveled between cities and villages within planned route specified by the ministry [6]. For the first year of the initiative, the e-training caravans routes were planned to visit ten provinces (Saudi Arabia is divided into 13 provinces) and 61 governorates (Saudi Arabia's provinces are further divided into 118 governorates).

The e-training caravan stays for one week (5 working days) in each place. During the week, the caravan provides four training sessions daily in the use of computers and the Internet, for ten training hours for each session in a total of 40 hours of training per week.

The e-training caravan target audience was selected based on their age and literacy criteria: students of the upper grades of elementary and middle school students in public schools; adults who do not have experience in the use of computers; and low-income families from urban and rural areas and villages.

The training is conducted in mobile classrooms in specially adapted five big buses. The maximum number of trainees for each class is sixteen. The classrooms are equipped with equipments and training materials such as LCD Screens, PCs, Printers and Wi-Fi connection (as shown in Figure 1).

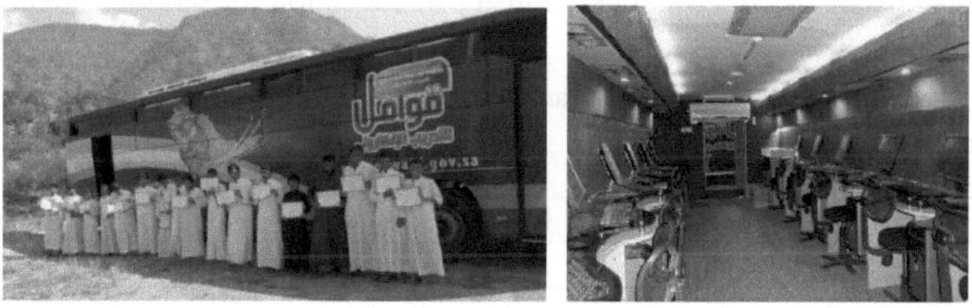

Fig. 1. Standard E-Training shuttle bus: Outside and inside view [9]

The training materials consist of a stripped down version of International Computer Driving License (ICDL), and tackles the following topics: (1) Introduction to ICT, (2) Computer and its components, (3) Using the computer and managing files (4) Word processing and presentations, (5) Introduction to Internet, and (6) Using E-Mail. The training materials also cover a topic about introduction to Government e-services with examples on how to deal with the main e-services that benefit the citizens.

The training materials are provided in printed format for both the trainer book and the trainee book and in an electronic format as a CD, which contains the training materials. The training materials were designed by a board of experts in MCIT.

The trainers were selected based on a number of criteria to help ensure their success in the training. The criteria include: the trainer qualifications, ICT competencies and experience in conducting training.

The training is given in two versions: one targeting students, where the content covers how to search for information, use communication and presentation tools and benefit from government e-services; the other targeting adult users, where the content covered includes the basics of using computers and the internet and benefiting from government e-services.

During the caravans' trips, each trainee has a chance to enroll in the offered sessions, practice their content and have a certificate after completing the required hours.

3 Results and Discussions

The results (Table 1) inform the first year (2011/2012) of the caravans that travelled to ten provinces and 61 governorates, covering a total of 70,672 Km.

Table 1. E-Training caravan overall results for the first year [7]

Provinces	Governorates	Caravans	Courses	Total no. of trainees
10	61	120	443	9254

Table 2 shows the breakdown of registered and attended students and adults. We can see that the uptake of students was around 97% compared to 94.5% for non-students. This may be attributed to the previous arrangement and collaboration between the ministry of education and MCIT. The trainees were enrolled by a prior arrangement between MCIT and the ministry of education for school students.

Table 2. E-Training caravan enrolled trainees for the first year [7]

Students Courses		Adult Courses		Total no. of trainees
Registered	Attended	Registered	Attended	
5609	5431	4044	3823	9254

Based on qualitative data collection using both semi-structured interviews and observations among students and adults, the results of the first year of the e-training caravans were promising.

Observations showed that the caravan have helped elderly people get over their fears of using computers and helped curious young people who wanted to learn how to use the Internet. The elderly had the opportunity to use the Internet and benefit from the government and commercial services available online. They have also been trained on how "to sign up for emails, how to use chat and video programs to contact and see their children studying abroad, how to set up accounts for business purposes and how to access cultural, social and marketing sites" [8].

On the other hand, students were curious and excited about how to "use social networking sites, play games on the Internet and download different smart phone programs" [8]. Besides, high school graduates learned how "to register on various sites, including universities, Ministry of Higher Education, language learning centers, and how to chat with their friends and exchange photos and video files" [8]. Also students profited from the wealth of content in science, culture and entertainment provided by the caravan.

Switching to the encountered barriers, the semi-structured interviews showed that the most common barrier by adults was not knowing how to use computers and the Internet. This barrier is complemented by fear of using the technology and lack of self-confidence.

Also the cost of having decent internet access is another barrier, knowing that most people living in rural areas have low-income. Another barrier was the culture, since Saudi society is largely conservative and religious, therefore any actions against Islamic norms and values is inappropriate. The final noticed barrier was ICT infrastructure. In fact, the existing ICT infrastructure in most rural areas in Saudi Arabia is not that well-established.

4 Conclusion

The goal of this case study was to showcase the experience of conducting the e-training caravan and highlight the barriers encountered during running this initiative. The experience of the first year can be put to practice in improving the training for the next years and help in bridging the digital divide in Saudi Arabia.

Given the results of the first year of this initiative, it has shown success in achieving its main objectives and contributed to educating rural areas' residents about computer and the Internet.

This project was divided into three main phases, for the first phase lasting for one year, the second phase for two years, and the third phase for two years, in total the life span of this initiative will last for five years. This division was planned so as to benefit from the results of each stage in the implementation of the next phase. Also MCIT long term goal is to target 36 thousand students from primary and middle schools through 2400 training courses within 600 caravan trips [9].

Finally, MCIT continues to work on plans, policies, programs, projects and initiatives that assist in developing ICT awareness among Saudi citizens as well as stimulating the growth and spreading the use of ICT at all life aspects.

References

1. eInclusion | Europa - Information Society, http://ec.europa.eu/information_society/activities/einclusion/index_en.htm (accessed: February 15, 2013)
2. Cunningham, M.: Exploiting the Knowledge Economy: Issues, Applications and Case Studies. IOS Press (2006)
3. eInclusion Foundation, http://www.e-i.hk/ (accessed: February 21, 2013)
4. Molina, A.: The Digital Divide: The Need for a Global e-Inclusion Movement. Technology Analysis & Strategic Management 15(1), 137–152 (2003)
5. Badger, M., Khan, M., Lanvin, B.: Growing Talent for the Knowledge Economy: The experience of Saudi Arabia. Best Practices in Networked Readiness: Selected Case Studies. World Economic Forum – 2011 Global Information Technology Report (GITR). Efficient Governance Global Information Technology Report (GITR) (2010-2011)
6. E-training Caravans - MCIT ePortal, http://www.mcit.gov.sa/english/initiatives/E-trainingCaravans/ (accessed: February 15, 2013)
7. E-Training Caravan Statistics, http://www.eqwafil.gov.sa/statistics.html (accessed: February 21, 2013)
8. Saudi Gazette - E-training caravans spread Internet literacy in villages, http://www.saudigazette.com.sa/index.cfm?method=home.regcon&contentid=20110723105836 (accessed: February 21, 2013)
9. MCIT National IT Plan 2011/2012 Annual Report – MCIT ePortal, http://www.mcit.gov.sa/arabic/NICTP/Report/(accessed: February 28, 2013)
10. Norris, P.: Digital divide?: Civic engagement, information poverty, and the Internet worldwide. Cambridge University Press, Cambridge (2001)

Interactive Serious Gaming for Children with Auditory Processing Difficulties in the Arabic Language

Arwa Alamoudi, Modhi Almozaini, Rawan Alabdulrahman, Sara Alkoblan, and Sarah Drine, Areej Al-Wabil

Department of Software Engineering, King Saud University, Saudi Arabia
{aalamoudi,ralabdulrahman,salkoblan,aalwabil}@ksu.edu.sa

Abstract. Sada is an interactive multimedia program for auditory discrimination therapy in the Arabic Language. Sada was designed to extend speech therapy beyond clinical settings and provide patients with a computer-based therapy system which can be used between sessions with speech therapists; at school or at home on an 'on-demand' basis. The program provides local Arabic dialects and a configurable knowledge-base which allows for extending the therapy and customizing the pronunciation of words for different Arabic-speaking populations. The Sada architecture and its interaction design are described and the advantages of computer-based therapy for auditory perceptual problems are discussed.

Keywords: Speech Therapy, Auditory Processing Disorders, APD, SpLD, Dyslexia.

1 Introduction

In recent years, there has been proliferation of technology solutions available for users with special needs. However, there remains a scarcity in assistive technologies for native Arabic speakers, especially people with disabilities. In the field of speech therapy, aural rehabilitation often involves complex programs to rehabilitate disorders of the auditory system [1]. Examples of disorders that involve auditory discrimination difficulties include cochlear implants; attention deficit disorders with and without hyperactivity (ADHD and ADD); Auditory Processing Disorders (APD); Specific Learning Difficulties (SpLDs) such as dyslexia; and autism spectrum disorders.

The rehabilitation process of auditory perceptual difficulties often involves a medical specialist and continuous training, which are often hard to find in large geographic regions such as the context of Saudi Arabia. In this context, families face the challenge of providing essential training for their children. In addition, there are several software programs for speech therapy activities that have been shown to be effective in improving auditory skills [e.g. 3-5]; however these programs inadequately support speech therapy in the Arabic language. Technology solutions for this user populations include auditory rehabilitation programs in English such as AUDIX [3], Hearing your Life [4], Sound and Way Beyond [5]. The most comprehensive program

C. Stephanidis (Ed.): Posters, Part I, HCII 2013, CCIS 373, pp. 188–191, 2013.

designed for Arabic-speaking users is Rannan which is based on Modern Standard Arabic (MSA) [6]. Moreover, exploratory studies and field studies that we have conducted in our local context have suggested that some bespoke software is actually used in clinics; however, these are not available as products accessible to a wide range of specialists or for the general population.

In this paper, we describe the background, motivation, and nature of the problem that this interactive multimedia program, called Sada, addresses. Sada was designed to address the need for accessible auditory discrimination therapy programs for auditory perceptual problems (i.e. inability to perceive differences between phonemes) by providing training techniques in MSA and local dialects through interactive exercises that aim to improve auditory perceptual skills of children with auditory-related problems and learning difficulties, and assist them in effective communication. This design can be extendable for other dialects in a configurable interface. The novelty of this system is the contribution towards Arabized technology for our local context as well as the approach adopted in the design cycle. In this project, we followed the User Centered Design ISO 13407 standard in the analysis and design of the system [2]. The goal was to develop a system that provides effective solutions through interactive games to improve the auditory skills of children with auditory discrimination difficulties beyond clinics and in home environments.

2 Sada's Interactive Therapy Programs

The system is comprised of three types of activities which include auditory discrimination, articulation, and auditory attention as depicted in the interface screenshots of Figures 1 and 2. From within categories, the child can select the type of game to launch an activity.

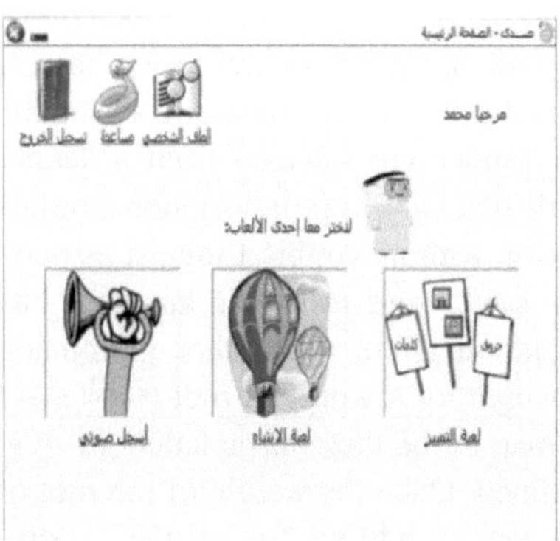

Fig. 1. Configurable Visual Design of Sada's Interface

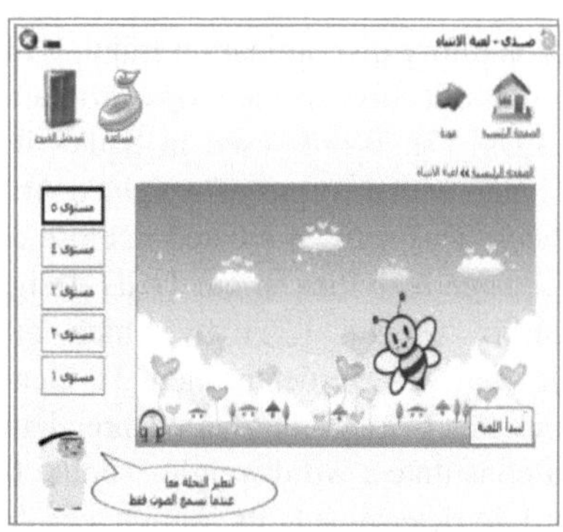

Fig. 2. Auditory Attention Training

Sada was designed to be configurable by an administrator to adapt the program flow and the interface, to fit the needs and personal preferences of the target user populations. Accessibility standards have been adhered to by allowing key aspects of the interface to be configurable by users including font type, size, color as well as background color. Algorithms were developed in collaboration with Arabic Linguists to include a gradual increase in complexity to ensure motivation and engagement in the user experience in the therapy program. Advancing levels in the game involves accomplishing at least 60% of the active level. Furthermore, presentation of Arabic words in activities is based on randomization of selection from a pool of words which were pre-categorized based on the weight of the Arabic word as depicted in Figure 3.

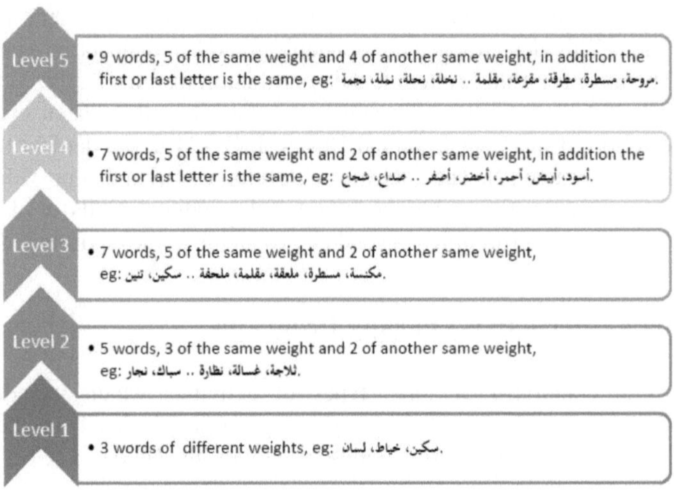

Fig. 3. Algorithm for word-based auditory discrimination

For auditory discrimination training of Arabic letters, categories were used based on the classification in the Cops program developed for Specific Learning Difficulties (SpLDs) [7]. Words used in Sada's interactive games are selected from a database designed with a corpus of weighted Arabic words that vary in pronunciation similarity indices. This set was created in close collaboration with an Arabic Linguist as part of the design activities in our UCD design cycles. Each word in Arabic language has a specific "weight" (وزن) by which its pronunciation along with other grammatical characteristics are determined. To identify the weight of a word, its root (أصل الكلمة) – which is a word composed of three letters that map to the three basic letters (ف، ع، ل) that constitute a word weight– should be determined. Once the weight of the root of a word is determined, its weight can be concluded by adding any of the "addition letters" (حروف الزيادة) –which are these ten letters (س، أ، ل، ت، م، و، ن، ي، ه، ا) – the word may have in addition to the weight of its root. Table1 shows some examples of words and its roots and weights.

Table 1. Examples of weights of Arabic words used in Sada

The word	The word root	The root weight	The word weight
أحَر	حَر	فَعَل	أفْعَل
يَذْهَب	ذَهَب	فَعَل	يَفْعَل
كَوْثَر	كَثَر	فَعَل	فَوْعَل
مُكْرِم	كَرَمَ	فَعَل	مُفْعِل

3 Conclusion

This paper describes the conceptual design of Sada, an interactive game suite designed to support practitioners in speech therapy with computerized-training for auditory discrimination. There is a dire need for technology support for speech and language therapy in Arabic-speaking regions, and in Saudi Arabia in particular. The prohibitive costs and the limited availability of specialists have led to limited availability of rehabilitation programs for children who need auditory discrimination training beyond clinical settings. This system aims to bridge this gap with an innovative bespoke solution for Arabic speaking populations.

Acknowledgment. The authors extend their appreciation to the Deanship of Scientific Research at King Saud University for funding the work through the research group project number RGP-VPP-157. The authors would like to express their appreciation for the assistance provided by speech therapists in the PFMAC Autism Center and Learning Difficulties' specialists in Manarat Schools in Riyadh and for all the children who have participated in the evaluation sessions of this program.

References

1. Martin, M.: Software-based auditory training program found to reduce hearing aid return rate. Hearing Journal 60(8), 32, 34, 35 (2007)
2. International organization for standardization, ISO 9241-210: 2010–Ergonomics of human-system interaction: Human-centred design for interactive systems (2011)
3. Grawemeyer, B., Cox, R., Lum, C.: AUDIX: A Knowledge-based System for speech-therapeutic auditory discrimination exercises. In: Studies in Health Technology and Informatics. Medical Infobahn for Europe, vol. 77, pp. 568–572 (2010)
4. `http://www.advancedbionics.com/hearingyourlife/HYLDemo.htm` (accessed in 2011)
5. `http://professionals.cochlearamericas.com/cochlear-academy/sound-and-way-beyond` (accessed in 2011)
6. Al-Ghamdi, N., Al-Ohali, Y.: The design and development of an interactive aural rehabilitation therapy program. In: Proceedings of the 12th International ACM SIGACCESS Conference on Computers and Accessibility (ASSETS 2010), pp. 285–286. ACM, New York (2010)
7. Kuwait Dyslexia Association, Arabic Cops version 1.0 User Manual: Computerised Screening and Assessment for Dyslexia for Schools and Individuals (2007)

Issues with Designing Dementia-Friendly Interfaces

Claire Ancient and Alice Good

University of Portsmouth, School of Computing, Portsmouth, United Kingdom
{claire.ancient,alice.good}@port.ac.uk

Abstract. People with dementia are a rapidly growing demographic. In a world which is increasingly dependent on computing, this large group of people is becoming technologically isolated, due to the ill-suited design of interfaces. This paper looks at the possible 'roadblocks' which need to be considered when designing interfaces in order to ensure they are dementia-friendly. By considering the unique needs of a person with dementia, designers can ensure that their software is accessible to this demographic, hence potentially reducing the feelings of technological exclusion.

Keywords: Dementia, Interface Design, Accessibility.

1 Introduction

Dementia is a degenerative brain condition which is not a natural part of the aging process. Generally, the symptoms of dementia include memory loss, communication problems and mood changes. However, each person will experience the condition differently depending on the type of dementia and their individual circumstances [1].

In the next 8 years, the number of people with dementia in the UK is expected to reach 1 million [2]. In a world were computing is increasingly ubiquitous, it is important that all users are catered for when designing interfaces. Research suggests that elderly people are keen to utilise the latest technology [3, 4] in spite of the fact that their understanding of the products is minimal. When this limited knowledge is combined with inappropriately designed interfaces, it could enhance the person with dementia's feelings of technological isolation. The result being an entire demographic which is being alienated by interface designers, possibly leading to a greater divide between the digital native and digital immigrants [5].

Designing interfaces for people with dementia is difficult. It involves a delicate balance of accessibility features, usability features and elements which are designed to improve the user experience. In addition to this, the people with dementia will not only suffer from condition related decline, but also problems linked to the natural aging process. Despite the rapidly increasing number of computer users with dementia, the W3C WAI currently has no specific guidelines designed to make interfaces dementia-friendly [6]. There are existing guidelines which inform the development of interfaces allowing access to people with age-related decline. However, these do not take into account the special needs of a person who is living with a diagnosis of dementia.

C. Stephanidis (Ed.): Posters, Part I, HCII 2013, CCIS 373, pp. 192–196, 2013.

Table 1. (*Continued.*)

Motor Impairments	• Movements are slower	• Slower movements can be accentuated by symptoms of dementia with Lewy bodies (which are similar to Parkinson's disease) [11]
	• Elderly people struggle with complex movements - particularly if they are novel [7].	• May not be able to learn new complex motor skills.
	• Find manipulating scroll-bars challenging, leading to disorientation [4, 7]	
	• Reduced ability for typing [7]. • Comments made during a pilot study [9] suggest typing on a tablet or smartphone is not natural for older people.	
Visual Impairments	• As people age, their eyesight ability declines [7, 12]	• Damage to occipital lobe can cause problems with perception due to problems with interpretation in the brain [13]
	• Larger text is easier to read for older people [10] – Should avoid text becoming too big, so there is no requirement for scrolling windows	
		• Maximise readability in order to provide the occipital lobe with enough information to provide an accurate reading [13]

3 Conclusion

Given the range of requirements for this user group, designing dementia-friendly interfaces will not be easy. However, with the number of people with dementia increasing, it will become a necessity of the interface design process, if we are to strive towards inclusiveness. By accounting for the additional needs of this important demographic, interface designers may be able to reduce feelings of technological isolation and improve interaction with modern technologies, by enabling a positive user experience.

The aim of future research will be to devise a set of guidelines to aid interface designers with the development of dementia-friendly interfaces. The diverse nature of dementia symptoms together with the increased variability of individual needs as people get older certainly make this a difficult challenge.

Research has shown that older people are not averse to adopting new technologies [3, 4], if designers can ensure that their interfaces are accessible to people with dementia, a new realm of possible treatments aimed at mitigating the symptoms could be developed.

References

1. Alzheimer's Society, What is Dementia? http://www.alzheimers.org.uk/site/scripts/documents_info.php?documentID=106
2. Alzheimer's Society, Demography, http://www.alzheimers.org.uk/site/scripts/documents_info.php?documentID=412
3. Chou, J., Hsiao, S.: A Usability Study on Human-Computer Interface for Middle-aged Learners. Computers in Human Behavior 23, 2040–2063 (2007)
4. Ziefle, M.: Information Presentation in Small Screen Devices: The Trade-Off between Visual Density and Menu Foresight. Applied Ergonomics 41, 719–730 (2010)
5. Holsapple, C., Pakath, R., Sasidharan, S.: A Website Interface Design Framework for the Cognitively Impaired: A Study in the Context of Alzheimer's Disease. Journal of Electronic Commerce Research 6, 291–303 (2005)
6. Web Accessibility Initiative, Web Content Accessibility Guidelines, http://www.w3.org/WAI/intro/wcag.php
7. Hawthorn, D.: Possible Implications of Aging for Interface Designers. Interacting with Computers 12, 507–528 (2000)
8. Gregor, P., Newell, A.F., Zajicek, M.: Designing for Dynamic Diversity - Interfaces for Older People. In: Proceedings of the Fifth International ACM Conference on Assistive Technologies, pp. 151–156. ACM Press, New York (2002)
9. Ancient, C., Good, A., Wilson, C., Fitch, T.: Can Ubiquitous Devices Utilising Reminiscence Therapy be Used to Promote Well-being in Dementia Patients? An Exploratory Study. In: Ambient Assisted Living, Part of HCI International 2013, Las Vegas, July 21-25 (2013)
10. Dickinson, A., Newell, A.F., Smith, M.J., Hill, R.L.: Introducing to the over-60s: Developing an Email System for Older Novice Computer Users. Interacting with Computers 17, 621–642 (2005)
11. Alzheimer's Society, What is Dementia with Lewy Bodies? http://alzheimers.org.uk/site/scripts/documents_info.php?documentID=113
12. Lorenz, A., Oppermann, R.: Mobile Health Monitoring for the Elderly: Designing for Diversity. Pervasive and Mobile Computing 5, 478–495 (2009)
13. Alzheimer's Society, The Brain and Behaviour, http://alzheimers.org.uk/site/scripts/documents_info.php?documentID=114

Gesture Recognition Using Commodity RGB-D Sensor for Imitation Learning Platform for Children with Autism

Esubalew Bekele, Jake Bumpus, Shuvajit Das, Julie Crittendon, Zachary Warren, and Nilanjan Sarkar

Vanderbilt University, 518 Olin Hall 2400 Highland Ave Nashville / TN 37212, USA,
University of Michigan · Ann Arbor, MI 48109 USA
{esubalew.bekele,jacob.m.bumpus,julie.a.crittendon,
zachary.warren,nilanjan.sarkar}@vanderbilt.edu, shudas@umich.edu

Abstract. Autism Spectrum Disorders (ASD) is characterized by profound impairments in social interaction and communication. Children with ASD have deficits in core areas of social interactions such as gesture imitation. Gesture imitation is one of the early developed social communication skills and is thought to be linked with concurrent as well as later complex social skills such as language development, play and joint attention skills. Thus early identification of such a deficit and providing appropriate intervention regarding gestural imitation skills are quite important. This work, which is a part of a larger study that aims at building a gesture imitation intervention platform for children with ASD, leverages the intrinsic interest of the children with ASD in robotic technology. In this paper, we discuss the part of the robot-mediated intervention system that deals with gesture recognition and present preliminary recognition results.

Keywords: Gesture recognition, hidden Markov models, autism intervention, adaptive interaction, RGB-D sensor, assistive robotics.

1 Introduction

Young children with autism spectrum disorders (ASD) display profound impairments in social communication and atypical patterns of behaviors [1] such as delayed language development, pretend play, joint attention and imitation [2]. Imitation impairments were associated to co-occur with other impairments concurrently or affect later developmental outcomes [3,4] including language development, pretend play, and joint attention for children with ASD [3,5]. Children with autism lack the use of gestures, which are related to joint attention and expression of affective states, than typically developing children [6]. Therefore improvement in gesture imitation may translate into improvement in complex social and communication skills. Ingersoll et al. [6] argued that very few research has been done in teaching imitation of meaningful gestures to children with autism and most research focuses on directly commanding the children to do a particular isolated gesture or sequence of gestures

C. Stephanidis (Ed.): Posters, Part I, HCII 2013, CCIS 373, pp. 197–201, 2013.

which limits the children from learning novel gestures and hinders generalization. They suggest a more naturalistic intervention called reciprocal imitation training (RIT) that was aimed at teaching imitation skills to young children with autism within an ongoing play interaction. It was reported that RIT not only improved the gesture imitation capability but also helped with increase in pretend play skills. However, intensive behavioral interventions such as RIT require trained behavioral therapists and entail repetitive intervention over an extended period of time and hence, are not available to the wider ASD population. Due to the repetitive nature of the intensive behavioral therapy, robotic technology is suited for such service delivery. It is documented that children with ASD are interested in robots and technology and may prefer to play with a robot than humans [7,8]. Robot-mediated joint attention therapy was piloted in earlier study and found that it created increased engagement while performing as well as a human therapist [9]. Imitation learning and robot programming by demonstration have been an active research area in the past decades [10,11]. Also, traditional gestural imitation learning intervention for children with autism have been an active area of research separately [6]. In recent years, applications of robot-based imitation learning for therapy have also been investigated [12,13].

The overall objective of our project is to develop an innovative robot-mediated imitation learning intervention environment for children with autism based on RIT. The overall system will have two main subsystems: gesture recognition of the participants by the robot, and demonstration of correct gestures and providing feedback by the robot. The contribution of this paper is in the development and evaluation of the gesture recognition part of the system. The recognized gestural data has been mapped to the robot workspace for validation.

2 General System Overview

The robot-mediated imitation learning platform in its current state is composed of the Microsoft Kinect, NAO - a humanoid Robot, and a gesture recognition module. The current system that recognizes a gesture demonstrated by the child and maps it to the robot is shown in Fig. 1 (left). The gesture recognition module consists of data pre-processing, gesture training, gesture recognition, and workspace mapping components.

2.1 The Humanoid Robot, NAO

The robot used in this project is the humanoid robot NAO (www.aldebaran-robotics.com). Its software was built around a programming architecture with a network broker called NAOqi. Task specific modules can be written and attached to the broker either inside the robot's operating system locally or remotely. This broker process, which is based on the Simple Object Access Protocol (SOAP) specification, allows extending NAO's capabilities via distributed system architecture. We leveraged this ability and run most of the computationally intensive tasks of the system such as the gesture recognition component on separate machines.

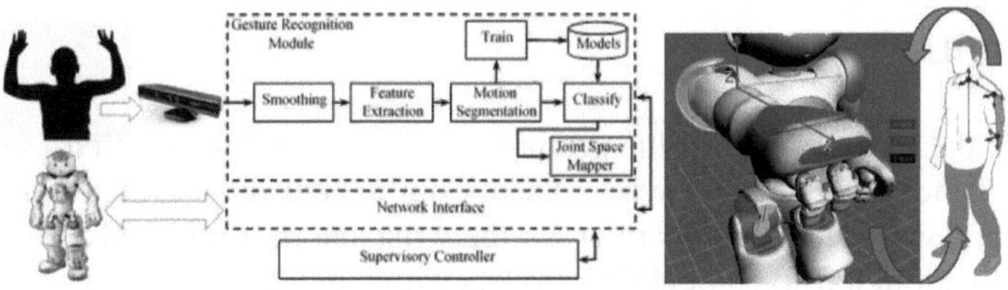

Fig. 1. Overall system diagram (left), and joint mapping (right)

2.2 Gesture Monitoring with Kinect

The Microsoft Kinect skeletal tracker can track up to two humans in its field-of-view and provides the ability to fit a 20-joint skeletal model to each user that is being currently tracked. The raw skeletal joints data were first filtered to eliminate spurious data outside of the workspace limits, data that produces jerky motion as well as noise. The data were filtered both in time and space and a time median filter was used to smooth the trajectories of a particular gesture demonstration. We have extracted various features from the raw data such as relative distance of the joint from a shoulder center reference for each joint involved in a particular gesture and then applied a forward feature selection procedure called sequential forward selection (SFS). A direct joint to joint mapping between the robot and the human space was used as shown in Fig. 1 (right) to demonstrate the recognized gestures.

2.3 Gesture Recognition with HMM

A gesture is inherently composed of sequence of primitive action sequences that can be modeled efficiently by the Hidden Markov Model (HMM) [14]. Given: *N*, the number of states in a model, *M*, the number of distinct observable output symbols per state, $A = \{a_{ij}\}$ (the transition from state i to j), the state transition probabilities, $B = \{b_j(k)\}$ (symbol V_k given state j), the observation symbol probability distribution, and the initial state $\Pi = \{\pi_i\}$, a discrete HMM can be defined as $\lambda = (A, B, \Pi)$. HMM models are generated from a sequence of training dataset. The recognition phase evaluates the observation likelihood of the observation sequence given the model, $P(O/\lambda)$. The solution to the training problem is in the form of locally maximizing the $P(O/\lambda)$. The feature vector stream was first clustered and labeled into M number of output symbols before the sequence is fed to training. In this work, we used the k-means clustering. We have selected two sets of five gestures. The first gesture set is composed of symbolic gestures including moving the arm in a circle, 'come here', move the arm in a rectangle, swipe, and wave. The second set includes gestures which are part of the unstructured imitation assessment (UIA) imitation action gestures from Ingersoll et al. [2]. We have recorded 30 instances of each gesture (with two different people at different poses) and used 20 examples as the training set and the remaining 10 as the testing set.

3 Results

To evaluate the performance of the gesture recognition system we first used the 3-D trajectory of the end effector (wrist). Then from a high dimensional feature vector (105 features), we selected the features for the wrist and performed SFS. We used two degrees of freedom left-to-right HMM models with 8 hidden states and 12 output with 3 dimensional feature vectors taken at a time. There were two sets of gestures. Fig. 3 shows segmented two dimensional three gesture trajectories from each set. Different colors indicate different segments of each gesture that are grouped for a particular output symbol in the vector quantization stage.

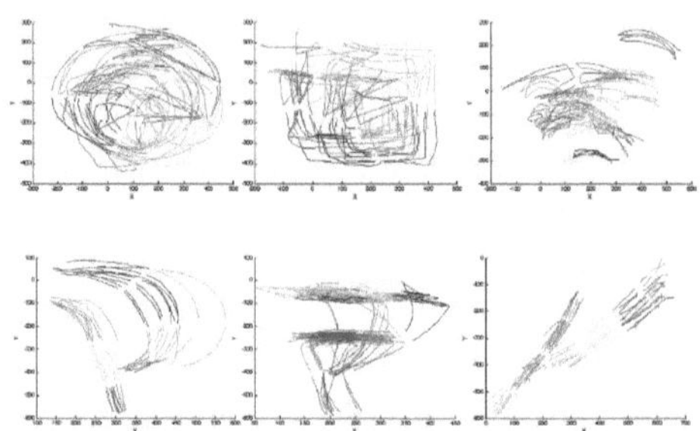

Fig. 2. Top: Set 1 (Circle, Rectangle, and Wave). Bottom: Set 2 (hands on head, move fingers in circle and point)

The average recognition rate for gesture set 1 was 68% using raw trajectory while gesture set 2 resulted in average recognition rate of 96%. So, gesture set 2 was selected for further SFS analysis. The recognition results using the individual feature categories in the first level of the SFS process was more than 95% for all the 5 gestures and that of final winner feature combination was 100%. The best feature set was found to be combination of Euler angles, polar, Cartesian and spherical velocities, and relative distance of the wrist relative to the shoulder.

4 Discussion and Conclusion

The recognition system was validated for known gesture sets and was able to recognize them accurately. However, there were several limitations of the current system including inability to handle novel gestures. In the future, the system will be expanded to include an intelligent supervisory controller that is able to perform in a bi-directional manner to make the robot-mediated therapy resemble closely to that of the human therapist by demonstrating a gesture to the child. In the case of partial or complete success, the robot should be able to give reinforcement contingent upon success and imitate back the child in the case of contingent imitation. Isolating gesture from a movement stream, transferring summery information about the gesture using continuous HMM, mapping it to the robot workspace in a generalized manner and completing incomplete attempt of a gesture by the child are also part of future extensions of the system. Gesture sequence matching algorithm in time domain such as dynamic time warping could also be employed to make the sequences equal length before clustering.

References

1. Diagnostic and Statistical Manual of Mental Disorders: Quick reference to the diagnostic criteria from DSM-IV-TR, American Psychiatric Association, Amer. Psychiatric Pub. Incorporated, Washington, DC (2000)
2. Ingersoll, B., Meyer, K.: Examination of correlates of different imitative functions in young children with autism spectrum disorders. Research in Autism Spectrum Disorders 5(3), 1078–1085 (2011)
3. Stone, W.L., Yoder, P.J.: Predicting spoken language level in children with autism spectrum disorders. Autism 5(4), 341–361 (2001)
4. Stone, W.L., Ousley, O.Y., Littleford, C.D.: Motor imitation in young children with autism: what's the object? Journal of Abnormal Child Psychology 25(6), 475–485 (1997)
5. Rogers, S.J., Hepburn, S.L., Stackhouse, T., Wehner, E.: Imitation performance in toddlers with autism and those with other developmental disorders. Journal of Child Psychology and Psychiatry 44(5), 763–781 (2003)
6. Ingersoll, B., Lewis, E., Kroman, E.: Teaching the imitation and spontaneous use of descriptive gestures in young children with autism using a naturalistic behavioral intervention. Journal of Autism and Developmental Disorders 37(8), 1446–1456 (2007)
7. Diehl, J.J., Schmitt, L.M., Villano, M., Crowell, C.R.: The clinical use of robots for individuals with Autism Spectrum Disorders: A critical review. Research in Autism Spectrum Disorders 6(1), 249–262 (2011), doi:10.1016/j.rasd.2011.05.006
8. Scassellati, B., Admoni, H., Matarić, M.: Humanoid Robots for Use in Autism Diagnosis/Research. Annual Review of Biomedical Engineering 14(1), 275–294 (2012)
9. Bekele, E., Lahiri, U., Swanson, A., Crittendon, J., Warren, Z., Sarkar, N.: A Step Towards Developing Adaptive Robot-Mediated Intervention Architecture (ARIA) for Children With Autism. IEEE Transactions on Neural Systems and Rehabilitation Engineering 21(2), 289–299 (2012)
10. Schaal, S.: Is imitation learning the route to humanoid robots? Trends in Cognitive Sciences 3(6), 233–242 (1999)
11. Calinon, S., D'halluin, F., Sauser, E.L., Caldwell, D.G., Billard, A.G.: Learning and reproduction of gestures by imitation. IEEE Robotics & Automation Magazine 17(2), 44–54 (2010)
12. Duquette, A., Michaud, F., Mercier, H.: Exploring the use of a mobile robot as an imitation agent with children with low-functioning autism. Autonomous Robots 24(2), 147–157 (2008)
13. Fujimoto, I., Matsumoto, T., De Silva, P.R.S., Kobayashi, M., Higashi, M.: Mimicking and Evaluating Human Motion to Improve the Imitation Skill of Children with Autism Through a Robot. International Journal of Social Robotics, 1–9 (2011)
14. Rabiner, L.R.: A tutorial on hidden Markov models and selected applications in speech recognition. Proceedings of the IEEE 77(2), 257–286 (1989)

Pee-democracy: Opening Data to the Great British Public Toilet Map

Jo-Anne Bichard and Gail Ramster

Helen Hamlyn Centre for Design, Royal College of Art,
Kensington Gore, SW7 2EU London
United Kingdom
Jo-anne.bichard@rca.ac.uk, Gail.ramster@network.rca.ac.uk

Abstract. This paper and the accompanying poster will present a case study of the development of The Great British Public Toilet Map http://greatbritishpublictoiletmap.rca.ac.uk/ through the use of UK open data. The map acts as an information resource but also as an access point for members of the public to campaign for open data to be released concerning publicly available toilet provision in their local area. In addition, the map also provides members of the public, who may be unfamiliar with the concept of open data and the possibilities for greater e-democracy it may hold, an entry point for engagement through the seemingly mundane, yet essential issue of public toilet provision.

Keywords: Open data, e-democracy, participatory design, public toilets.

1 Introduction

The Great British Public Toilet Map was developed through a participatory design methodology conducted by the authors at the Helen Hamlyn Centre for Design; Royal College of Art. It formed a key deliverable for the TACT3 (Tackling Ageing Continence through Theory Tools & Technology) research project. Incorporating an inclusive design philosophy and participatory design methods, the researchers worked with two stakeholder groups to identify how toilet provision could be made more accessible, especially regarding the needs of an ageing population.

This paper will describe how through interviews and participatory design games, the research was able to identify a singular issue for both stakeholder groups and design an intervention to meet their needs. Identifying a shared concern between users and providers was paramount, as previous research (Greed, 2003) [1] had noted that within the design and management of public toilet provision there is often conflict between what users require and desire for toileting in comfort and dignity, and what providers can deliver within wider management concerns.

Often the resulting design solution has met the needs of the providers over the users and focused on the anti-social behaviour of a minority opposed to the access requirements of the majority. Such a design lead creates an 'access versus fortress' agenda which finds many users withstanding uncomfortable and sometimes unusable provision, which in moments of urgency can be unpleasant.

C. Stephanidis (Ed.): Posters, Part I, HCII 2013, CCIS 373, pp. 202–205, 2013.

2 Methodology

Working under the title 'Challenging Environmental Barriers to Continence' the authors undertook 101 interviews with members of the public as users of publicly accessible toilets, and members of professional bodies involved with the delivery of publicly accessible toilet provision. This second group included architects who specialise in the siting, design and planning of provision, managers of provision from local authorities, department stores and transport terminals, and community groups interested in promoting local provision.

The interviews focused on the contexts of use and provision and were directed towards both users and providers. Initially the research focused on the physical design and management aspects of the environment such as the need of a larger toilet cubicle and assurance from cleaning regimes. However, following the interviews the project developed a participatory design game in which participants worked together in teams to design their own toilets.

Whilst these games highlighted design and management needs they also directed the research to consider the effective technological solutions concerning provision both from a users and providers perspective (See Bichard et al, 2013) [2].

3 The Great British Public Toilet Map

To address the need for providers to distribute accurate information about toilet provision, and for users to be able to access such information, the research team developed The Great British Public Toilet Map http://greatbritishpublictoiletmap.rca.ac.uk/ as a key deliverable for TACT3 a multidisciplinary collaboration between:

- Brunel University
- the Universities of Sheffield
- the West of England and Manchester
- the Dalarna Research Institute and
- the Bristol Urological Institute and the Royal College of Art.

TACT3 ran between 2008-2011 and was funded by the New Dynamics of Ageing (NDA) Research programme http://www.newdynamics.group.shef.ac.uk/ 'a seven year multidisciplinary research initiative with the ultimate aim of improving quality of life for older people'.

The NDA, which was funded by all of the UK's research councils, has been considered 'the most ambitious research programme on ageing ever mounted in the UK'.

The projects user driven refocus moved away from critiquing physical space to exploring the opportunities of digital space to deliver a framework for improved service delivery. Initially, the research explored an inclusive philosophical perspective through consideration of crowd sourcing as a data capture method on current toilet provision. However an analysis of a series of smartphone applications that had incorporated crowd-sourced data revealed a number of inaccuracies and highlighted how crowd-sourced information alone is insufficient as it can be inaccurate and quickly become obsolete [3].

Within the UK there is currently no centrally collated information, database or inventory of UK publicly accessible toilets. The research saw an opportunity to address this with the UK government's call for more open data to be released especially in relation to public services, by requesting local authorities to collect collate and release their data regarding their public toilet provision. The open data on provision would then be used to populate The Great British Public Toilet Map.

However, the Great British Public Toilet Map also incorporates public participation features in which it not only retrieves released open data on public toilet provision but also provides a platform for members of the public to request that such data is made available by their local authorities to populate the map.

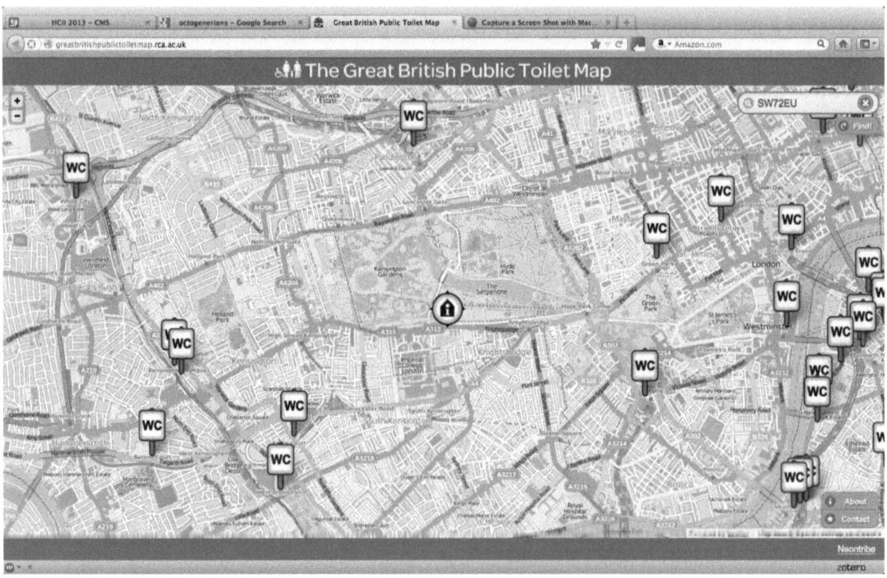

Fig. 1. The Great British Public Toilet Map

4 Conclusion

The development of the Great British Public Toilet Map through a participatory methodology would incorporated a participatory function for members of the public to request that open data be released on local toilet provision. This information not only populates the map but helps raise awareness that open data on local authority services and expenditure exists and where released can be accessed and used by members of the public.

References

1. Greed, C.: Inclusive Urban Design: Public Toilets. Architectural Press, Elsevier, Oxford (2003)
2. Bichard, J., Greene, C., Ramster, G., Staples, T.: Designing Ethnographic Encounters for Enriched HCI. In: Proceedings HCI 2013, Las Vegas, Nevada (July 2013)
3. Knight, G., Bichard, J.: Publicly Accessible Toilets: An inclusive design guide. Helen Hamlyn Centre for Design. Royal College of Art, London (2011)

Applying an Approach to Develop Web Applications Considering Accessibility Practices Using Design Rationale

Thiago Jabur Bittar[1,2], Leandro Agostini do Amaral[2], Luanna Lopes Lobato[1], and Renata Pontin de Mattos Fortes[2]

[1]Universidade Federal de Goiás – UFG, Brazil
{thiago.bittar,lll}@catalao.ufg.br
[2]Universidade de São Paulo – USP, Brazil
{jabur,ordnael,renata}@icmc.usp.br

Abstract. Regardless of the techniques and methods that have been developed to improve web applications, there are still gaps that need to be solved in order to reduce the accessibility barriers. Aiming to contribute to this area, this study presents an controlled experiment to validate an approach which uses Design Rationale. The participants attended an initial training and, after being classified according to their experience and divided into different groups, they were asked to develop a web application. Such process gave rise to useful concerns that were shared among the work teams. This paper reports this experiment and presents relevant contributions to approach accessibility issues.

Keywords: Web, Accessibility, Design Rationale.

1 Introduction

The lack of accessibility has become a prevalent issue that challenges developers of web applications. Through the implementation of good accessibility practices it is possible to remove the barriers that prevent certain groups of people from accessing information.

Accessibility is very important to software applications and several studies have been dedicated to it. In spite of this, the current scenario presents a mismatch between the requirements imposed to apply accessibility during system development and what is really performed and presented to the market. Thus, there is a gap related to accessibility in web applications development due to the lack of guidelines and recommendations which, once adopted, would provide access for many users.

For this reason, our study is focused on the use of good accessibility practices, since there is an increased awareness about the topic and a growing demand for applications that take into consideration the needs of all potential users.

To ensure the development of accessible web applications, it is important to train developers. In view of this, this study proposes and presents an approach to guide developers during system's development. In this way, they will learn what must be done in several cases to ensure accessibility to web content.

C. Stephanidis (Ed.): Posters, Part I, HCII 2013, CCIS 373, pp. 206–210, 2013.

In order to test the proposed approach, a controlled experiment was undertaken in an academic environment, involving undergraduate students from the Computer Science Department of Federal University of Goiás - Brazil. First of all, the students were trained and after they were divided in groups to perform a task. A questionnaire had been previously applied to identify the participants' profiles so that they could be distributed in similar groups. The groups were asked to develop a web application for scheduling scientific evaluation committees. The experiment resulted in several considerations and useful findings that contributed to improve the approach. Such results were shared among the development teams.

As a result of this study we identified an increasing awareness of the participants relating to accessibility issues. This is relevant since the academy and the industry can take profit of the insights presented in this study and incorporate the lessons learned to new web projects.

The remainder of this paper is organized as follows: Section 2 presents the concepts of accessibility which may be used as guidelines to achieve it. Section 3 addresses the Design Rationale concept. Section 4 presents the methodology used in this study and the findings. Section 5 presents final remarks and envisages future work.

2 Web Accessibility: Concepts, Tool Support and Guidelines

Accessibility can be interpreted as the possibility of using a resource universally, without barriers or through alternative access means. In the web context, the resource to be accessed is constituted by the pages content. The idea of this concept is that the users, using every agent, can understand and interact with the offered content [10].

In web projects, it is a common practice to consider accessibility only at the advanced stages of development or when the applications are entirely coded. At this point, making applications accessible is a real challenge that involves redesign and reprogramming. Moreover, developers almost always do not know details about accessibility practices or, if know, they do not use such knowledge during the application development. Thus, most programmers have no essential knowledge or experience to ensure that their code meet accessibility requirements.

A solution for this problem is the use of lessons learned from other projects, since the same mistakes may be avoided and the accessibility practices already tried with success may be reused. This solution reduces costs related to the process of choosing the practices that should be applied during the application's development. For this reason, in general, the use of patterns and templates is recommended.

According to Bigham et al. [1] very few developers have been explicitly trained for accessible pages creation. Evaluating pages using assistive technology may reveal problems related to the complexity of defining systems.

Aiming to explain how to produce accessible web contents, World Wide Web Consortium (W3C), through its Web Accessibility Initiative (WAI), released a collection of accessibility guidelines in a document named Web Content Accessibility Guidelines (WCAG). These guidelines present recommendations to produce web content (texts, images, forms, sounds) accessible for people with disabilities including blindness and low vision, deafness and poor hearing, learning difficulties, dyslexia, cognitive limitations, movement limitations, speaking inability, photosensitivity and combinations of them.

The WCAG guidelines are in their 2.0 version since December 2008 [10]. Their objective is to support developers and to be a reference for tests undertaken by automated tools and by humans.

3 Design Rationale

Design Rationale (DR) can be defined as a reference for the reasoning that justifies a project as well as for discussions that justify the choice of structure on other alternatives [5][8][9]. MacLean, Young & Moran [8] and Lee [7] consider that DR not only includes a description of the potential artifact, but also defines reasons for decisions, experiences, alternatives and arguments that lead to the decisions that best fit to the system development.

The interest in DR has grown, since the approach presents relevant tools that consider not only the reasons behind a design decision but also the justification for it. DR presents, as well, other alternatives, as the tradeoffs evaluated and the argumentation that led to the decision.

The DR concept was selected to assist the use and register of decisions and techniques concerning web accessibility, since we aim to build a useful basis for knowledge management and reuse by the work team. This approach is based on previous studies with intensive domain research [2][3].

According to Lee [7] as the use of DR's systems increases, new tools have been developed to capture and to make DR easily accessible. Such tools improve dependency management, collaboration, reuse, maintenance, learning, and documentation.

However, storing DR can take a significant time and be expensive, since the most current DR system can fail to consider practical concerns, such as cost-effective use and smooth integration. In order to solve these problems, it is possible to automate the capture process and associate it with the work object, i.e. the development itself.

4 Methodology and Results

This section presents a controlled experiment performed with the aim of assessing the benefits and drawbacks of the reported approach. The experiment was carefully designed and validated by two main researchers: i) a Ph.D. expert in empirical Software Engineering, who helped to define the processes to be followed; and ii) a Ph.D. student that has worked with web development and accessibility in the last five years, who is the main author of this paper and who proposed the approach.

In this study we developed an academic experiment since experiments in a real scenario demand several external interventions, take more time to be performed and require additional investments. Moreover, it is difficult, sometimes, to find companies that agree to undertake academic experiments in their development process.

The methodology used in this study consists in executing a sequence of stages, like the general planning, the analysis of developers experience and their division into groups aiming to have a technical balance on each team. To define the stages and to set other methodological details, we used the recommendations, concepts and techniques for experiments described in [6].

In order to perform a systematic experiment, we followed the recommendations defined in Wohlin *et al.* [11], which describe the plan, or protocol, used to perform the experiment and also to analyze its results.

To verify the quality of the insights from each group we performed a quantitative evaluation. This evaluation was based on the criteria defined in this research. A value 1 was assigned for each fulfilled criterion and a value 0 was assigned when the development was not in accordance with the criterion. These scores are presented in the Figure 1.

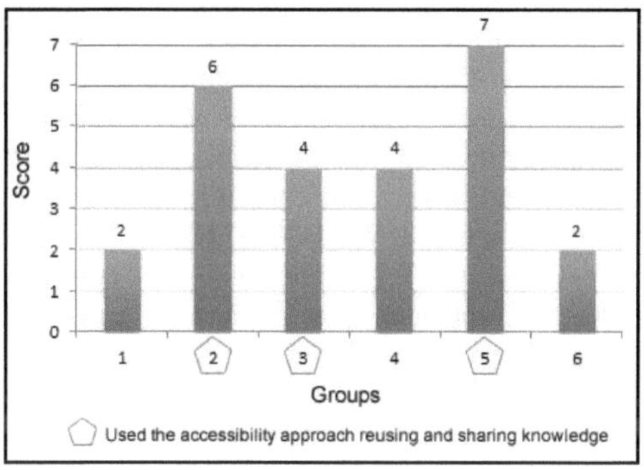

Fig. 1. Graph showing the score obtained by each group in the assessment

Figure 1 demonstrates that groups using the approach presented higher scores than those not using the approach. However, Groups 3 and 4 obtained the same score in spite of the first one having used the approach and the second having not used it. This is justified because using the approach constitutes an aid and not a guarantee. In other words, not using the approach does not imply necessarily a bad development.

Additionally, the Figure 2 displays the corresponding box-plot graph for the data distribution of the obtained results.

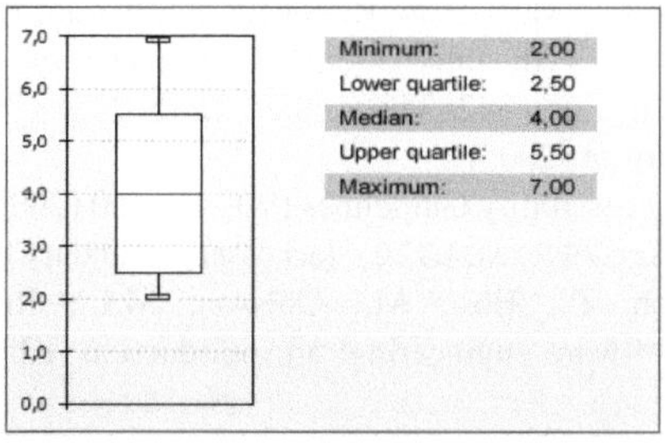

Fig. 2. Data distribution in a box-plot graph

As observed in Figure 2, none of the groups obtained a zero score, indicating the importance of the initial training, regardless the approach used.

5 Conclusions

As a result of this study we identified an increasing awareness of the participants relating to accessibility issues. This is relevant since the academy and the industry can take profit of the insights presented in this study and incorporate the lessons learned to new web projects.

References

1. Bigham, J.P., Brudvik, J.T., Zhang, B.: Accessibility by demonstration: enabling end users to guide developers to web accessibility solutions. In: Proceedings of the 12th ACM SIGACCESS Conference on Computers and Accessibility (ASSETS 2010), pp. 35–42. ACM, New York (2010)
2. Bittar, T.J., Lobato, L.L., Fortes, R.P.M.: Guidelines2Model2Code: uma Abordagem para incorporação de diretrizes no desenvolvimento Web orientado a modelos. In: Actas da Conferencia IADIS Ibero Americana, WWW/INTERNET 2010, Lagoa – Algarve (2010)
3. Bittar, T.J., Neto, D., Lobato, L.L., Lucredio, D., Fortes, R.P.M.: Definição de metamodelos para Web incorporando boas práticas de acessibilidade e usabilidade. In: Anais da XXXVI Conferência Latino-Americana de Informática, CLEI 2010, Assunção (2010)
4. Freire, A.P., Russo, C.M., Fortes, R.P.M.: A survey on the accessibility awareness of people involved in web development projects in Brazil. In: Proceedings of the 2008 International Cross-disciplinary Conference on Web Accessibility (W4A 2008), pp. 87–96. ACM, New York (2008)
5. Grubber, T.R., Russel, D.M.: Design Knowledge and Design Rationale: A Framework for Representation, Capture, and Use. Technical Report KSL 90-45, Knowledge Systems Laboratory, Stanford, California, 40 p. (1991)
6. Lazar, J., Feng, J.H., Hochheiser, H.: Research Methods in Human-Computer Interaction, 448 p. Wiley (2010) ISBN 978-0-470-72337-1
7. Lee, J.: Design Rationale Systems: Understanding the Issues. IEEE Expert/Intelligent Systems and Their Applications 12(3), 78–85 (1997)
8. Maclean, A., Young, R.M., Moran, T.: Design rationale: the argument behind the artifact. SIGCHI Bull. 20, 247–252 (1989)
9. Paiva, D.M.B., Fortes, R.P.M.: Design Rationale in Software Engineering: A Case Study. In: Proceedings of the 17th International Conference on Software Engineering & Knowledge Engineering, pp. 342–348. United Daily News Digital Co. and Tung Tai University, Taipei, Taiwan (2005)
10. W3C. Web Content Accessibility Guidelines (WCAG) 2.0 (2008), `http://www.w3.org/TR/WCAG20/` (accessed at January 2013)
11. Wohlin, C., Runeson, P., Höst, M., Ohlsson, M.C., Regnell, B., Wesslén, A.: Experimentation in software engineering: an introduction. Kluwer Academic Publishers, Norwell (2000)

iPad 2013: A Leaning Tool for Students with Special Needs

Khalid Buragga[1], Amandeep Dhir[2], and Abeer A. Boreqqah[3]

[1] Department of Information Systems, CCSIT, King Faisal University, Saudi Arabia
[2] Department of Computer Science and Engineering, Aalto University, Finland
[3] College of Education, King Faisal University, Saudi Arabia
{Kburagga,aboregeh}@kfu.edu.sa, amandeep.dhir@aalto.fi

Abstract. Interactive technologies such as iPad are considered as perfect learning tool for students with special needs. Lately, educational researchers and technology specialists have coined the idea of using iPad as a learning tool for students with Autism spectrum disorder (ASD). However, our literature review on the subject matter shows that scientific investigations on using iPad with ASD students are scarce. Therefore, academic researchers should organize longitudinal studies examining this subject. In this work in progress submission, we have provided broad overview of our ongoing research focused on investigating as if and how iPad and similar interactive devices could be used for the betterment of students with ASD in Saudi Arabia i.e. supporting students with ASD in learning and play. This work in progress paper pinpoints recent work on this subject covering some of major challenges faced by the iPad for Autism research.

Keywords: Autism spectrum disorder (ASD), educational technology, information technology, information systems, iPad, learning.

1 Introduction

Interactive forms of technologies are considered to have a special place in the lives of young students. Various interactive technologies including iPad, surface table and other touch based interactive learning devices are known for contributed towards education, learning and play among young students. However, not all students are same when compared against learning, social and cognitive abilities. Few students possess cognitive disabilities since their biological birth and we refer them as students with special needs due to their inherited biological learning related disabilities (Vera et. al., 2005). Students with special needs face significant problems in learning and gaining instruction and even score below average marks in academic exams (Falcão and price, 2010). Other prominent characteristics of special needs students are week concentration; poor recall and memorization skills, cognitive disabilities, reduced social, practical and academic development (Falcão and price, 2010). Due to all of the aforementioned differences in the cognitive abilities of students, their potential needs, expectations and requirements in context to interactive technologies, are also different

C. Stephanidis (Ed.): Posters, Part I, HCII 2013, CCIS 373, pp. 211–215, 2013.

in contract to ordinary students without any learning disabilities (Falcão and price, 2010). This has resulted in the need for adapting the interactive technologies as per the needs of the students with special needs.

Lately, developing appropriate interactive educational technologies for students with special needs has attracted the attention of multidisciplinary researchers from various disciplines including education, educational psychology, human-computer interaction and information systems (Alper et. al., 2012; Duncan and Tan, 2012). This reflects a popular sentiment among research community towards supporting educational needs of the developmental disorders e.g. learning disabilities.

The aim of our ongoing research is to understand various needs, expectations and requirements of students with special needs from interactive devices such as iPad for educational purposes. Our research philosophy is influenced from the user-experience research. This current research involves development of various processes and procedures within the framework of interactive technologies, so as to support students with special needs in variety of ways. Interactive technologies might help them in grasping difficult concepts in easy fashion, directly aide their learning in classroom as well as non-classroom environment, relives them from any sort of academic stress and/or embarrassment. The focus of this research is mainly on the Arabic-speaking students with special needs in Saudi Arabia. Based on our review of existing literature on the subject, it was found that design considerations and theoretical framework for designing interactive technologies for students with special needs in Saudi Arabia are missing (Al-Wabil et. al., 2012). Therefore, in order to bridge this gap in the existing literature, our ongoing research is focused on addressing "Can iPad be used as a learning tool for Students with Special needs". This open research question involves examination of different aspects namely determining the impact of iPad use on the learning, academic performance, social, communication and concentration skills of students with special needs.

At present, cognitive disorders or learning disabilities among students can be classified into several different types e.g. Autism spectrum disorder (ASD), Dyslexia, etc. Due to the presence of several different types of cognitive disorders, we decided to focus on single type of cognitive disorder, which is ASD among students. There were two main reasons behind choosing only one type of cognitive disorder namely: 1) Recent statistics have shown that ASD is on rise among students and it is found to be the most common learning disability among young students these days. 2) By focusing on single type of cognitive disorder, we can examine different perspectives of this disorder in better way and investigate if and how iPad could support ASD students. ASD is recognized as a qualitative impairment in social interaction and communication, restricted repetitive and stereotyped patterns in terms of habits, activities and interests (Autistic Disorder, 2012). Autistic students have problems in understanding and processing the verbal instructions and even performing basic cognition based generalizations and abstractions. Some of the specific cognitive problems with ASD students are difficulty in filtering extraneous sensory information and motor control (Autism Spectrum Disorder, 2011; Autism, 2011). According to (CDCP, 2012), 1 our of every 88 students in the US in 2012 were diagnosed with ASD and this rate has increased by 23% compared to 2009 statistics. These statistics clearly reveal that tomorrow's classrooms will witness sharp increase in the number of students with ASD.

2 Research Methodology

Innovative interactive technologies can support students with ASD by enabling them to express and communication in educational settings (Alper et. al., 2012). Recently researchers and practitioners have made various efforts at exploring how the existing interactive technologies such as iPad could be made better fit for the student with special needs in addition to designing newer technologies aimed at student with special needs (Alper et. al., 2012).

Lately, iPad has received immense response from people suffering from autism spectrum disorders (ASD) (Herbert, 2010). Some of the notable affordances of iPad that makes it ideal tool education for student with ASD includes lightweight, portability, affordability offered by touch screen as compared to single-use special education devices, screen size, low cost as compared to other special education devices, graphical scheduling aspects, support different applications and abundance of iPad applications available on Apple iTunes (Herbert, 2010). All these aforementioned reasons make iPad an appropriate candidate for integration into the educational for student with ASD and also for application developers so that they can develop applications that suit the needs of student with ASD.

iPad act as a reinforce agent due to its inbuilt support for various highly preferred reinforces for-example, iPad provide access to various reinforces such as game applications, viewing pictures, videos with friends and family (King, 2011). (King, 2011) argued that iPad is socially acceptable and socially appropriate and it provides engagement to individuals with autism who obviously suffer from challenging behaviours. (Mozaffar et. al., 2012) pointed out several design considerations that govern the potential use of iPad for student with ASD. These design considerations are: 1) students must be supervised when using iPad so as to ensure that full educational exposure and device safety. 2) iPad acts as an incentive and self-reinforcement agent for students with ASD. 3) iPad enables ASD student to self-regulate their activities within educational settings, verbally and physically communicate with their peers, perform turn taking and mentoring own peers. 4) Teachers particularly appreciated iPad's accessibility features, media and portability support and finally ease of using it.

3 Challenges in iPad for Autism Research

During the review of existing literature on the given subject, we found some of the prominent challenges faced by research dealing with developing interactive technology for students with ASD. These challenges are:

1. Although, large numbers of mobile applications are available for teaching and aiding students with ASD but there is a shortage of software applications specifically for adults i.e. ASD adults (Duncan & Tan, 2012).
2. Recent research has shown that iPad is not equally suitable for all students with ASD (Mozaffar et. al., 2012). Therefore, teachers need to adapt the usage of iPad based on the needs of students with ASD so as to attain maximum benefit from iPad technology.

3. There is a pressing need for a strong collaboration between academic researchers, technology designers and educational technology practitioners for the task of innovating interactive technologies aimed at students with ASD (Alper et al. 2012).
4. Since the research involving the development of interactive technologies such as iPad-based applications for ASD is still young so future research should consider practicing of longitudinal methods on examining the impact of iPad on learning and academic performance of students with ASD.
5. Recent research on the subject has shown that academic research currently lacks the design and development of iPad based applications for students with ASD however, private sectors has undertaken several initiatives in this regard such as: Apple iPad apps for students with ASD (Alper et al. 2012).

4 Conclusion

Educational technologies researched have seen a potential in iPad that it can be used as a learning tool for students with Autism spectrum disorder (ASD). Our literature review on the subject matter shows that scientific investigations on using iPad with ASD students are scarce and this research field is still in its young phase. Therefore, considering the importance of this subject, our ongoing research is focused on investigating as if and how iPad or similar interactive devices could with used as a learning tool for the students with ASD. This research further investigates into other aspects of this subject namely determining the impact of iPad use on the learning, academic performance, social, communication and concentration skills of students with special needs. We argue that through this scientific examination and research will result in the betterment of students with ASD in Saudi Arabia, a community which otherwise is often ignored or less studied.

Acknowledgements. The Deanship of Scientific Research (DSR), King Faisal University (KFU), Saudi Arabia, funds this ongoing research.

References

1. Vera, L., Herrera, G., Vived, E.: Virtual reality school for children with learning difficulties. In: Proceedings of the 2005 ACM SIGCHI International Conference on Advances in Computer Entertainment Technology (ACE 2005), pp. 338–341. ACM, New York (2005)
2. Falcão, T.P., Price, S.: Informing design for tangible interaction: a case for children with learning difficulties. In: Proceedings of the 9th International Conference on Interaction Design and Children (IDC 2010), pp. 190–193. ACM, New York (2010)
3. Al-Wabil, A., Dhir, A., Al-Musaaed, H., Al-Sheaha, A.: Screening Program for Learning Difficulties in Arabic Speaking Students: Design Considerations for Educational Interfaces. In: Workshop on Interaction Design in Educational Environments (IDEE), 15th International Conference on Enterprise Information Systems (ICEIS) (June 28, 2012)
4. CDCP: Center for Disease Control and Prevention, New Data on Autism Spectrum Disorders (2012), http://www.cdc.gov/Features/CountingAutism/ (retrieved)

5. Autism, PubMed Health, http://www.ncbi.nlm.nih.gov/pubmedhealth/PMH0002494/ (retrieved November 2011)
6. Autistic Disorder Definition, Autism Spectrum Disorder, ASD (2012), http://education.qld.gov.au/students/disabilities/adjustment/verification/asd.htm
7. Autism Spectrum Disorder (ASD) – Sign and Symptoms, Centre for Disease Control and Prevention (CDC), http://www.cdc.gov/ncbddd/autism/signs.html (retrieved November 2011)
8. Alper, M., Hourcade, J.P., Gilutz, S.: Interactive Technologies for Children with Special Needs. In: Workshop on Special Needs, IDC 2012, Bremen, Germany, June 12-15 (2012)
9. Duncan, H., Tan, J.: A visual task manager application for individuals with autism. J. Comput. Sci. Coll. 27(6), 49–57 (2012)
10. Herbert, M.: The iPad—Breaking New Ground in Special Education (November 2010), http://techworkshops.pottsgrove.wikispaces.net/file/view/The+iPad%E2%80%94Breaking+New+Ground+in+Special+Education.pdf/248317743/The%20iPad%E2%80%94Breaking%20New%20Ground%20in%20Special%20Education.pdf
11. King, M.L.: Effectiveness of the iPad in enhancing the mand repertoire for children with autism. Southern Illinois University at Carbondale. ProQuest Dissertations and Theses, 144 (2011)
12. Mozaffar, S.S.: iPad for Autism: How can the iPad serve as a teaching tool for students on the Autism Spectrum? In: Proceedings of the Fourth Annual Teachers College Educational Technology Conference, May 19-20 (2012)

An Accessible Chat Prototype for Screen Reader Users in Mobile Devices

Rocío Calvo, Ana Iglesias, and Lourdes Moreno

Computer Department, Universidad Carlos III, Leganés, Spain
{mrcalvo,aiglesia,lmoreno}@inf.uc3m.es

Abstract. Chats present accessibility problems for screen reader users. This work presents a prototype of an accessible chat for Mobile Devices (MD). The main aim of this research is to remove the accessibility barriers that screen reader users face when they use a chat in a MD. Thus, this prototype is based on the requirements which have been elicited considering background research and with the use of Software Engineering (SE) and Human Computer Interaction (HCI) methods as well as accessibility standards and guidelines.

Keywords: Accessibility, chat, interaction, screen reader, mobile device.

1 Introduction

The use of chats in Mobile Devices (MDs) is being increased in the last years. However, chats are not accessible for everybody [1]. For instance, screen reader users face accessibility barriers related to updated content without advising [2] and keyboard traps [3]. Furthermore, chats in MDs present additional accessibility barriers [4]. Related works, which include accessibility improvements, have been found; nevertheless, most of them do not follow a Use Centered Design (UCD) approach and do not include accessibility requirements to improve the interaction. Considering it, this research aims to create an accessible chat prototype which solves the barriers that screen reader users face when they use chats in MDs. To achieve it, some new or improved requirements have been added to progress the accessibility of chats in MDs.

2 Background

This section introduces the accessibility barriers that screen reader users face when use chats in MDs. Moreover, some previous accessible chats are studied.

2.1 Accessibility Barriers of Chats

Chats are synchronous communication tools and most of them present problems of accessibility for a huge variety of people. However, this kind of tools in MDs could present additional problems than other information technology (IT) systems like

C. Stephanidis (Ed.): Posters, Part I, HCII 2013, CCIS 373, pp. 216–220, 2013.

interaction problems or auto-refresh content [5]. Furthermore, some people cannot follow the conversation [6]. For instance, if one of the emitters is not able to write quickly and if there are not ways to establish the turn to write, he could have problems to follow the rhythm of the conversation [7][8]. Besides, screen reader users face other specific problems related to the web page's auto-refresh or updated content because it causes the restart of the screen reader [3]; the use of keyboard traps [4]; or the lack of support for text-to-speech or text-to-braille functions [5].

With regard to the accessibility problems of chats in MDs, these problems are similar to the chat's barriers of desktop computers. However, there are some additional specific problems that users could experience due to the technology of MDs and nevertheless of their functional limitations [2].

2.2 Previous Proposals of Accessible Chats.

Some researchers have tried to solve the accessibility problems of chats. For instance, the Reef Chat [9] follows the specifications of WCAG 2.0 [10] and WAI-ARIA [11]. Moreover, the mobile chat, AssistiveChat[1], provides features for people with speech disabilities like the suggestion of words.

Furthermore, some learning software like Moodle or Atutor, which include chats, has improved their chats. For instance, Moodle avoids the use of frames or Javascript technology and the auto-refreshing time can be configured [12]. Also, Atutor's Chat solves some technological aspects to guarantee access to users who use assistive technology because they can configure the refresh rate of the application. These approximations try to improve the user experience. However, none of them follow the UCD approach and most of them do not accomplish with accessibility guidelines. Moreover, they do not solve accessibility problems related to the interaction and the flow and rhythm of the conversation. Thus, the presented research aims to solve the interaction problems following a UCD approach and basing on standards and guidelines.

3 Accessible Chat Approach for Mobile Devices

This works is part of a Ph.D which main goal is to create a model-driven design and a strategy development process of an accessible chat [13]. Currently, the Ph.D is in the requirement engineering phase. The requirements have been elicited and now they must be validated. To achieve it, the prototype has been created. This section details the elicited requirements and the chat prototype.

3.1 Elicited Requirements

The requirements elicitation phase combines SE and HCI methods as a complement of each other to include the user in this phase and follow a UCD approach. Some of these techniques are: brainstorming, user interviews, analysis of existing system/competitors,

---

[1] `http://www.assistiveapps.com`

scenarios and personas and standards and guidelines related to accessibility [14]. The obtained functional requirements which improve the user experience and accessibility in MDs are showed in the Table 1. It is important to emphasize, that some of these requirements are new functionalities and other requirements are improved classical functionalities of chats.

Table 1. Functional Requirements to Improve the User Experience and Accessibility in MDs

Requirement	Description of the Improvement
Add an interlocutor	Users could stop the new interlocutor addition to the conversation.
Predefined Sentences	Users can select predefined sentences provided by the system.
Add File	The user should specify a description for the uploaded file and the system informs the users about the size's file.
Add URL	The user should specify a summary of the URL and its language.
Refresh Conversation	Allow users to pause and refresh the conversation.
Convert Conversation	Transform the conversation to other formats like audio or braille.
Messages Preferences	Include preferences related to the way in which messages are showed such as: time refresh interval or chronological order.
Clean Messages	Allow users to clean the messages which are showed in the screen.
Reception Messages	Inform users when the message has been delivered.
Writing	Inform users when other users are writing.
Check Spelling	Inform users about grammatical errors.
Translate	Translate messages if the sentence language is different to the predefined language.

3.2 Chat Prototype

Basing on the obtained requirements the chat prototype is created to improve the accessibility and user experience in MDs. Next sections explain the chat development.

Responsive Web Design

The prototype has been created to be adapted to different viewports. It has been developed in a web environment because it can be executed in more MDs than native applications and a responsive web design with the use of standards like HTML5 and CSS3 is followed to guarantee the layout adaptation to a huge variety of MDs [15].

Chat Functional Requirements to Improve Accessibility and Interaction

The prototype includes some of the functional requirements which improve the accessibility and the interaction of the chat in MDs. The selected requirements for the prototype are: the *Refresh Conversation* and the *Add File.* It is important to remark that these requirements are improved using the WAI-ARIA specification because it adds semantic information to HTML code to specify screen readers how to align keyboard navigation to landmarks, the page structure, updated content and expanded information[11]. Next, these requirements are explained in detail.

With regard to the *Refresh Conversation,* the user is able to control the flow and the rhythm of the conversation. If the user feels overwhelmed, he could pause the conversation by pressing the button *Pause.* The system informs the other users about it, they could write more sentences but the user who has stopped the conversation does not receive any sentence until he refreshes the conversation again. Then, these messages will be showed together. The Fig. 1 includes screenshots of the chat related with the "pause/refresh" functionality. The first figure shows the perspective of the user who stops the chat and the second one the perspective of the other user.

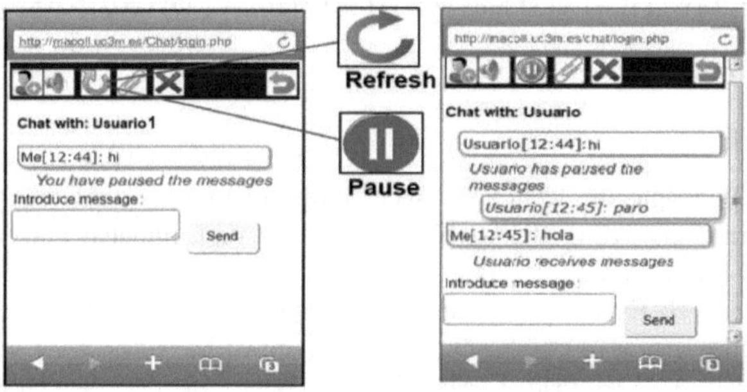

Fig. 1. Refresh/Pause Functionality

Moreover, the *Add File* requirement is improved too, Fig. 2. Users exchange files between them but sometimes the user cannot access to them. Thus, if the user sends a file, he should specify a description of the file and the system should inform the other users about the size and the description of the file. Then, the user who receives the file decides if he downloads it or not depending on his network circumstances and his necessities.

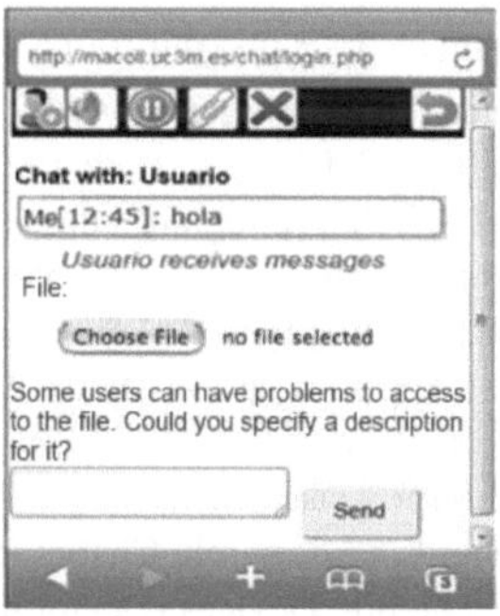
Chat with: Usuario
Me[12:45]: hola
Usuario receives messages
File:
Choose File
no file selected
Some users can have problems to access to the file. Could you specify a description for it?
Send

Fig. 2. Add File Functionality

4 Conclusion

This paper reveals accessibility barriers that screen-reader users face when they interact with chats. Previous works include accessibility improvements in this kind of tools. However, most of them do not include accessibility improvements in the user-interaction. The chat prototype presented in this paper has been designed following a UCD approach including specific features for improving the screen-reader users experience like the *Refresh Conversation* or *Add File* which have been created using WAI-ARIA specification.

Currently, a user evaluation of the prototype is being carried out to check the accessibility of the tool and the effectiveness of the new proposed features.

Acknowledgements. This research work has been partially supported by MA2VICMR (S2009/TIC-1542) and MULTIMEDICA (TIN2010-20644-C03-01).

References

1. Hackett, S., Parmanto, B., Zeng, X.: Accessibility of Internet websites through time. In: The 6th International ACM SIGACCESS Conference on Computers and Accessibility, pp. 32–39. ACM Press, New York (2004)
2. W3C. Shared Web Experiences: Barriers Common to Mobile Device Users and People with Disabilities, http://www.w3.org/WAI/mobile/experiences
3. Lazar, J., Allen, A., Kleinman, J., Malarkey, C.: What Frustrates Screen Reader Users on the Web: A Study of 100 Blind Users. International Journal of Human-Computer Interaction 22(3), 247–269 (2007)
4. Resta, P., Laferrière, T.: Technology in Support of Collaborative Learning. Education Psychology Review 19(1), 65–83 (2007)
5. Schoeberlein, J.G., Wang, Y(K.): Evaluating Groupware Accessibility. In: Stephanidis, C. (ed.) UAHCI 2009, Part III. LNCS, vol. 5616, pp. 414–423. Springer, Heidelberg (2009)
6. IMS Access for All v 2.0, http://www.imsglobal.org/accessibility/
7. National Center on Accessible Information Technology in Education. Accessibility of Electronic Tools & Features Used in Distance Learning, http://adasoutheast.org/ed/edpublications/itseries/8_etools.pdf
8. Guenaga, M.L., Burger, D., Oliver, J.: Accessibility for e-learning environments. In: Miesenberger, K., Klaus, J., Zagler, W.L., Burger, D. (eds.) ICCHP 2004. LNCS, vol. 3118, pp. 157–163. Springer, Heidelberg (2004)
9. Thiessen, P., Russell, E.: WAI-ARIA live regions and channels: ReefChat as a case example. In: Disability and Rehabilitation. Assistive Technology, vol. 4(4), pp. 276–287 (2009)
10. W3C. Web Content Accessibility Guidelines, http://www.w3.org/TR/WCAG/
11. W3C. Accessible Rich Internet Applications (WAI-ARIA) 1.0, http://www.w3.org/TR/wai-aria/
12. Moodle. Using chat, http://docs.moodle.org/23/en/Chat
13. Calvo, R., Iglesias, A., Moreno, L.: Accessible Chats for Computer Supported Collaborative Learning Environments in Mobile Devices (Doctoral Consortium). In: 7th IEEE International Conference on Research Challenges in Information Science (in press, 2013)
14. Calvo, R., Moreno, L., Iglesias, A.: Requirements elicitation for designing an accessible chat. In: Fernández, L. (ed.) REICIS Spanish Journal on Software Engineering, Quality and Innovation, vol. 8(1), pp. 7–21 (2012)
15. Gardner, B.: Responsive Web Design: Enriching the User Experience. In: Gilbert, H. (ed.) Sigma Journal: Inside the Digital Ecosystem, vol. 11(1), pp. 13–20 (2011)

An Approach to Design with People Who Have Special Needs

Selene Chew[1,2]

[1] School of Design & Environment, National University of Singapore,
4 Architecture Drive, Singapore 117566
[2] The Ohio State University
chew.40@osu.edu

Abstract. The main challenges when designing for people with disabilities are that 1) designers have difficulties empathizing with them; 2) designers tend to focus too much on the disability rather than the individual; and 3) people with disabilities have difficulties articulating their desires outside of their disabilities. A new approach is proposed to help designers overcome these problems. This involves getting insights from people without disabilities to understand the underlying desires of people with disabilities. Disabled people are then engaged as experts of their situations and invited to collaborate closely with the designers. This helps designers to focus on what people with disabilities want, instead of what they cannot do, and create solutions that have the greatest relevance and positive impact while maintaining minimal disruption to their everyday lives. The new approach is presented through the design process of "Blindspot", a white cane that uses smart technology to improve the lives of blind people.

Keywords: people with disabilities, blind people, white cane, Blindspot.

1 Introduction

Imagine a blind person walking along a busy street with a white cane. Along the same street, a friend is texting on the phone. Without the friend taking the initiative to spot the blind person, they miss each other along the same street. A little further down the street, a long stick is carelessly protruding from a trashcan. Unable to detect the stick with the white cane, the blind person walks right into the stick, leaving a bruise on his face.

Now imagine the blind person walking along the busy street with a smart white cane. The friend has checked-in his location through a social network on his phone. A notification informs the blind person of the check-in through a Bluetooth earpiece. Among the choices of calling, finding or ignoring, he chooses to give his friend a surprise by finding him. The blind person is guided to the location of his friend with the help of the smart white cane. On the way, the long stick protruding from the trashcan is avoided with the help of a sensor on the white cane. The blind person finds his friend and said "hi".

C. Stephanidis (Ed.): Posters, Part I, HCII 2013, CCIS 373, pp. 221–225, 2013.

"Blindspot" is the smart white cane. It empowers blind people to locate friends who are nearby and can direct visually disabled people to their friends and/or any destinations. It can also detect overhanging objects not contactable by the cane. A new approach was used in designing "Blindspot" that expanded design opportunities and developed a solution that has impact. This paper aims to explain the new approach through the design process of "Blindspot".

2 Challenges When Designing for People with Special Needs

"Blindspot" began with the traditional design approach of literature research, brainstorming and ideation, and user interviews. However, there were several difficulties in this process. Blind people have articulating their desires outside of their disabilities. The designer, on the other hand, finds it challenging to look beyond the disabilities of blind people and identify their real desires. Several assumptions about blind people were made because the designer couldn't empathize with them.

Through research on existing products or conceptual design for blind people, some product problems were identified. Some of the products either made blind people look more handicapped than they already look, or try to hide all of the handicapped signs of the blind person. The products also do not consider what will happen if the technology breaks down.

3 New Approach

A new approach was developed to overcome these barriers and is described below.

3.1 Expanded Literature Research

There are a number of books and articles about the physical conditions of blind people and how to cope with blindness [1], [2]. However, most methods and approaches to designing for visually disabled people discuss technologies, interface design, etc. This research was sufficient for a start on the technicalities surrounding blindness; however it was limiting in helping the designer to empathize with the blind people.

Fictional novels or non-fictional bibliographies of blind people are better sources of literature to understand and empathize with them. These books [3]–[5] have more descriptive narrative about the emotional and mental state of the people, which are not typically articulated by the participant or observable through their actions. The books also give a better understanding of their capabilities and issues of daily living.

3.2 Comparison to People without Disabilities

The fictional and non-fictional literature research revealed a pattern that blind people want the same things as everyone else; such as social connections, convenience, information access, etc. Based on this assumption, people without disabilities can be a reference to understand the underlying desires of disabled people. In designing "Blindspot", the emotional needs of sighted people were used as a source of insight to identify deeper emotional needs of blind people that are hard to articulate.

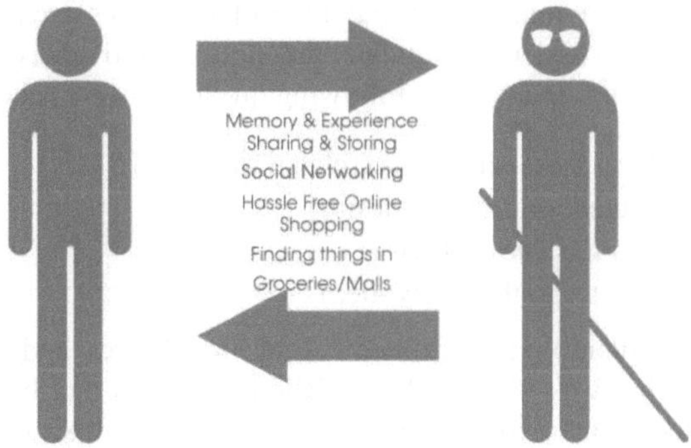

Fig. 1. People with and without disabilities share the same desires

Insights were derived by asking the following questions:

- What would people without disabilities do in this situation?
- What would people without disabilities want in the same situation?
- What about disabled people in the same situation?
- How would disabled people achieve what they want in that situation now?
- If it's not possible now, how can they achieve it through design?

By concurrently comparing what sighted people want and what blind people can do now, several insights about the opportunities surrounding the unmet desires of blind people were identified. When comparing people with and without disabilities, it is important to compare between culturally and demographically similar people. That is, a European 60 year old blind person is very unlikely to have the same desires as an Asian teenager.

3.3 Interviews with Experts

Ideas and assumptions about blind people were verified through a professional expert on the "Blindspot" project. There are several benefits of approaching experts prior to the meeting with the blind participants. First, learning about how to communicate with blind people is important to avoid unnecessary misunderstandings. Second, experts have vast knowledge about the legal and administrative constraints with regards to blindness in the country. Third, experts can arrange suitable participants based on the project scope.

3.4 Validating Desires and Ideas with Participants through Interviews

The expert may not have an accurate account for issues regarding the emotional needs and desires of blind people. For instance, during an interview with a therapist for blindness, he mentioned that knowing the identity of people is not important for blind people. This contradicted what the blind participants said later in an interview.

Desires and ideas were generated through the literature research, and comparisons with sighted people. In order to validate the desires and ideas, interviews were conducted with blind participants. The following questions were asked:

- What would you do in these situations (related to desire)?
- Why would you do that? (validating desire)
- What if you could do this (new idea)?
- Why would you want to do this (new idea)?

Through repeated validation and refinement of the desires and ideas with blind people, the insight that was identified for "Blindspot" was that blind users want to initiate everyday social interactions but are unable to due to their inability to identify people around them.

3.5 Co-creating with the Disabled Participants Using Interactive Models

Blind people are then involved as experts of their situation in the creation of the design concept. When trying to present a concept to blind people, they often have difficulties imagining an idea. In addition, their suggestions are often limited to their knowledge of technology. Therefore physical and interactive models helped blind people imagine concepts better, and break through their limitation of technology knowledge. In a co-creating session, blind people were able to propose better features for the designs with responsive and interactive models rather than stagnant models.

3.6 Continued Collaboration with Disabled Participants and Experts

As experts of their own situation, people with disabilities can collaborate closely with designers to develop an effective solution. Blind people provided inputs from the

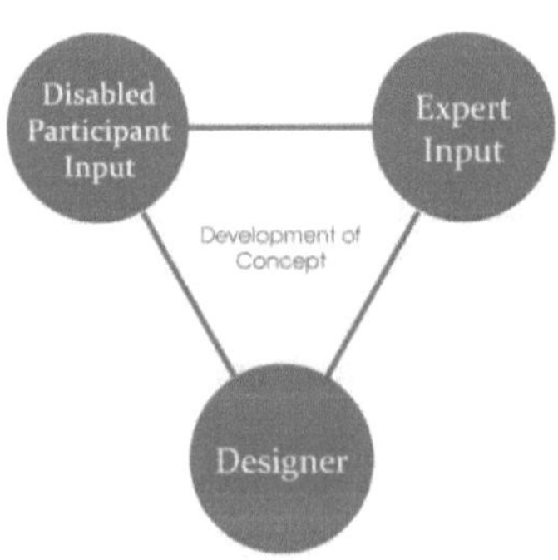

Fig. 2. Input from Experts, Disabled Participants and the Designer to develop the concept

user's desire standpoint, while the professional experts informed about legal and administrative constraints. This triangulated collaboration ensured that the problem to solve or the solution to propose was of significant impact to blind people's lives.

4 Conclusion

"Blindspot" broke through conventional norms of targeting solely on disabilities when designing for people with disabilities. Instead, it focused on designing with people who have disabilities in order to provide for their desires. It won James Dyson's Finalist Award 2011 and was the Netexplo 2011 Grand Winner. The approach helped identify deeper desires of blind people and created a holistic solution that can change lives.

In the future, the approach is likely to be applied not only to designing with blind people, but also people with other disabilities.

5 Limitations

This approach is developed based on one case study, "Blindspot". The case is also only focused on designing with blind people. The approach has yet to be applied to other projects, nor other cases of disabilities.

"Blindspot" is also a conceptual product that is not yet available for sale in the market.

"If you manage to design something that has a positive impact for one blind person, your design is likely to also have positive impact for most blind people."

– Quote from an interview with a blind participant.

References

1. Roberts, A.: Coping with blindness: personal tales of blindness rehabilitation. Southern Illinois University Press, Carbondale (1998)
2. Lende, H.: American Foundation for the Blind. In: Federal Legislation Concerning Blind Persons in the United States and Insular Possessions. American Foundation for the Blind, New York (1952)
3. Green, H.: Blindness. Viking Press, New York (1978)
4. Saramago, J., Pontiero, G.: Blindness: a novel. Harcourt, New York (1998)
5. Monbeck, M.E.: The meaning of blindness: attitudes toward blindness and blind people. Indiana University Press, Bloomington (1973)

Inclusive Websites for the Elderly: User Friendly Guidelines for Designers and Managers of Websites and Applications

Alireza Darvishy[1] and Alice Good[2]

[1] School of Engineering, Steinberggasse 13, 8400. Winterthur
[2] University of Portsmouth, PO1 3AE UK
alireza.darvishy@zhaw.ch, alice.good@port.ac.uk

Abstract. This research aims to define the most significant criteria for guidance on accessible design. It highlights 9 significant areas of guidance which we consider to be very important for the design of accessible, elderly friendly websites and web-applications. These areas look at specific elements of web design, including: structure; navigation; language; multimedia; links; search as well as others. Each of these areas has defined checkpoints which can be used to test the accessibility of a website. The criteria and checkpoints are presented in the form of a user friendly brochure. This brochure is aimed at two target groups: an instrument for website managers and secondly a checklist for web designers.

Keywords: Accessibility, Elderly, Disability, Web design.

1 Introduction

There is a definite need to 'bridge the gap' between elderly users and the Internet and with almost a fifth of the population aged over 65, it is a significant market to exclude. The concern at the growing 'digital has led to a number of initiatives being employed to encourage web usage for the older generations and to ensure they are not excluded from the digital world. Many elderly people now make use of the Internet in controlling their finances, keeping up to date with current affairs and staying in contact with family and friends (DRC, 2004, Good, 200,). In considering that the elderly are very likely to develop age related impairments such as visual and/or mobility related disabilities, web accessibility then becomes an important consideration. However if web designers do not understand the guidelines that are put in place, then the problem of poor accessibility will inevitably continue.

The focus of this paper is to present recommendations for the design and development of age appropriate websites. These recommendations form the basis of a brochure which presents are nine areas for web design tailored to senior citizens, each of which is dealt with on a double page. For each area, principles are formulated which are important for the design of websites tailored to senior citizens. The principles are primarily geared to clients, i.e. people who commission websites while

C. Stephanidis (Ed.): Posters, Part I, HCII 2013, CCIS 373, pp. 226–230, 2013.

web design and development specialists will also find specific instructions in the check lists regarding the implementation of the recommendations. The purpose of this booklet is to increasingly reduce the restrictions senior citizens face on a day-to-day basis when viewing not only residential and external areas on the web but also virtual areas.

2 Methodology

To be able to investigate the needs and requirements of the 65+ generation with regard to user-friendly web design in greater detail, four focus groups with a total of 24 older participants, (average age 73 years), who use the Internet on a regular basis, were created in our project. The aim of the focus groups was to record the point of view of older web users as well as any obstacles that may arise which have been caused by the web design. An important result of the study revealed that the participating parties placed a great deal of importance on how well the web pages were designed. A few people reported that they were not able to use the websites in the way they wanted due to poor design and navigation.

Following the group interviews, the statements were compared with the latest specialist literature and discussed and extended by two circles of experts (specialists from the worlds of research, further education and senior citizens' organizations). Based on this multi-layered survey involving literature-based research, user focus groups and circles of experts, it was possible to formulate the recommendations outlined for "age-appropriate website design".

3 Recommendations

Nine areas for web design tailored to senior citizens are examined in greater detail below. Recommendations for implementation are also assigned to each area. The sequence of the areas is not relevant in itself, however, the discussions in the focus groups have shown that the first three of the following aspects were regarded in all groups as being very important:

Clarity and Structure: The clarity and good structure of a website are important, if not in fact the most important prerequisites for achieving user-friendly web design. Senior citizens prefer information on a website to be ordered in as self-explanatory a way as possible, for the information to be restricted to what is absolutely essential and like having clear user guidance.

- The purpose of a website and its logical structure should be obvious the second a user looks at it. This means the various content, search and navigation areas must be well structured and their benefits or function must be self-explanatory. The selected layout must be applied as consistently as possible across all the web pages.

- If the content of the pages is arranged well, this makes the website easier to read and understand. Longer texts should be divided up in a sensible way. Related content areas can be linked together by navigational elements.

User Guidance and Navigation: User guidance which provides simple step sequences enables users to use the Internet on their own. Constructive and consistent navigation means older users feel they have adequate support

- Navigation elements must be self-explanatory and identifiable as such and must have the same design throughout the website.
- If icons or symbols are used for navigation purposes, their functions must be readily recognizable.
- Information about the user's current location on the website and the path the user took to get there help with orientation and contribute to effective user guidance.

Text and Language: The text is designed in such a way that it comprises a content component and a design component. The combination of both elements makes the site easier to read and understand. The design component also includes taking contrasts into account.

- Visitors to the website must be able to follow the information and understand it.
- With regard to the text design (line length, line spacing, spacing, contrasts), it is important to bear legibility and compatibility with different terminal devices in mind.
- Tools such as text enlargement are a good idea but should not impair the layout.
- Complementary (opposite each other in the chromatic circle) color combinations should be avoided.

Graphics, Animated Features and Multimedia: Graphics and multi-media content are not only design elements, but are also used to display information and operate the web application. If they are reduced exclusively to their creative benefits, they can have a diverting influence or be very off-putting. The proportion of text to images should be balanced.

- As already discussed for text and language, there must be sufficient contrast with the images as well. From the point of view of readability and detectability, the size in which the images are displayed is important and it should be possible to adjust this size individually without any loss of quality.
- In the case of downloads, additional information regarding the content, the size as well as the loading times to be expected is helpful.
- Decorative elements such as animated images and background music often have a more jarring effect.

Links: Links allow you to navigate within a website and to tap into additional as well as external information. If you are going to use links, make sure that they are clearly identifiable and self-explanatory.

- Links on a website should be clearly identifiable as such, also for visitors with restrictions such as color blindness and should be presented in a uniform manner throughout the entire website.
- Mouse-over effects (texts that are displayed as soon as the mouse pointer hovers over the link) have become an additional source of information for many users. However, these effects do not work with touchscreens (tablet PCs and smartphones) and for this reason you must provide alternatives.

Search: The search engine makes it easier to locate web content. Older people appreciate this function. They do, however, say that the manner of the search process is frequently not transparent and the order of the search results presented to them does not appear to be very logical. They have trouble, however, influencing this order.

- That the search fields are positioned well is just as important as the transparency of the search process. An option for refining the search through further criteria is welcomed.
- When the search results are displayed, the range of sorting options, for example, by date, place or other criteria can improve the overview.

Currentness, Consistency and Robustness: Older people appreciate it if the websites they use regularly as far as possible do not change their appearance (design) at all or only a little. They do, however, expect that the content is always up-to-date. Websites which are kept up-to-date usually provide a range of information of a very high standard. The structure and presentation of the entire website should therefore be as stable as possible. For users, finding their way on a newly designed page always involves a degree of learning. If the layout of web sites changes constantly, this reduces users' motivation to use the website.

- When it comes to layout, it is a balancing act between currentness and consistency. This, of coursc, docs not apply to thc contcnt or thc functionalitics which must bc kept up to date.
- The important thing is that the user quickly gets to grips with the website.
- It is important to note that the community of users is visiting the website from all kinds of terminal devices and the website should therefore be accessible on all such dcviccs.

Contact Information and Support: In order to be able to support users of a website in the event of questions or problems, they must have some contact options. Ilere, in addition to web forms and e-mail, traditional contact options are also important for older people, namely the telephone or face-to-face contact at a counter. Older people also like to know who they are dealing with. For this reason, it is important to provide information about the provider of the website in the masthead. This helps to promote transparency.

- The contact information and the masthead should not just be available but should also be displayed in a prominent position on the site.
- This also applies to other tools such as text enlargement, read-out function, glossary, FAQs, etc.

Registration and Forms: Registrations and online forms require a self-explanatory design. The purpose and benefits of the data entry should make sense to the users immediately. With regard to data protection, data use, archiving and access by third parties must be able to be detected by users or explained on an additional page. For the design of online forms tailored to senior citizens, impaired sight and slower reaction times must also be taken into account.

- When personal data is entered, the meaning and purpose of the data and the necessary steps must be visible to the users before the data is input.
- As far as possible, incorrect entries should be eliminated when the data is first entered. In the event of errors, you should provide meaningful advice and a targeted correction function.
- What are known as captchas are often used to provide protection against spam. These, however, are difficult to read for older users and also for many people with "normal" vision. We recommend that you offer alternative security methods.

4 Summary and Conclusions

The recommendations presented in this document do not claim to be complete as the ever-changing Internet is constantly creating new challenges for older people in terms of accessibility. The recommendations and the checklist in this brochure can be used by clients and web developers alike. They provide clues for creating websites tailored to senior citizens. After a new website has been created, it should, however, also be checked and optimized using usability tests. Involving older users early on in the process can help identify and rectify specific problem areas in a website.

The premise of this paper is to present the principles for age appropriate design. The main brochure however proves full recommendations and guidance for the implementation of these guidelines. It is anticipated that providing a user friendly brochure on the most prominent areas of accessible design guidance will inform designers better and subsequently lead to improved web accessibility.

References

1. Disability Rights Commission, The Web: Access and Inclusion for Disabled People, London (2004)
2. Good, A., Stokes, S.: Elderly, Novice Users and Health Information Web Sites: Issues of Usability and Accessibility. Journal of Healthcare & Information Management 21(1) (2007)

Relationship between Weight of Our Developed White Cane and Muscle Load on the Upper Limbs during Swinging Action of the Cane

Kouki Doi[1], Atsushi Sugama[2], Takahiro Nishimura[3], Akihiko Seo[4], Shuichi Ino[5], Kiyohiko Nunokawa[6], Kazuhiko Kosuge[7], Akito Miyazaki[8], Masaaki Sugiyama[9], Yoshihiro Tanaka[1], Mayumi Sawada[1], Ken Kaneko[1], Susumu Ouchi[1], and Katsuhiro Kanamori[1]

[1] National Institute of Special Needs Education, Yokosuka, Kanagawa, Japan
[2] Graduate School of System Design, Tokyo Metropolitan University, Hino, Tokyo, Japan
[3] Graduate School of Human Sciences, Waseda University, Tokorozawa, Saitama, Japan
[4] Faculty of System Design, Tokyo Metropolitan University, Hino, Tokyo, Japan
[5] Human Technology Research Institute, National Institute of Advanced Industrial Science and Technology, Tsukuba, Ibaraki, Japan
[6] School of Human and Social Sciences, Tokyo International University, Kawagoe, Saitama, Japan
[7] KOSUGE Co., Ltd, Itabashi, Tokyo, Japan
[8] A-tech Co., Ltd, Kakogawa, Hyougo, Japan
[9] Japan Braille Library, Shinjyuku, Tokyo, Japan

{doi,yoshihiro,sawada,kaneko,oouchi,kanamori}@nise.go.jp, {sugama-atsushi,aseo}@sd.tmu.ac.jp, t.nishimura@akane.waseda.jp, s-ino@aist.go.jp, kazu-kosuge@adagio.ocn.ne.jp, miyazaki@a-tech.org, sugiyamam@nittento.or.jp

Abstract. The present study aimed to investigate the influence of the weight of white canes on upper limb load. Concretely, we conducted quantitative evaluations of the load on upper limb muscles during swinging action of the cane. The white canes used were a new type of white cane newly fabricated using aramid fibers, as well as a conventional type of white cane fabricated using carbon fibers. The results indicated that the newly developed cane reduced the load on the muscles by about 50% in comparison with the conventional type of cane. It became clear that it was possible to sustain the same posture even when used continuously over a long period of time.

Keywords: White cane, Aramid fibers, Electromyogram, Upper limb load.

1 Introduction

White canes are not only a symbol for the visually impaired, but they are tools for acquiring information from road surfaces and surroundings. However, it had been pointed out that users tend to suffer from excessive load on the upper limbs, due to the swinging action of the cane over a long period of time when the user walks alone.

C. Stephanidis (Ed.): Posters, Part I, HCII 2013, CCIS 373, pp. 231–235, 2013.

The operating methods of the white cane vary, but what is called the touch technique, often used by those walking alone, requires a single manipulation of the cane for each step, which results in an enormous number of repeated movements. Furthermore, users swing the cane in a steady rhythm with the movement of the wrist alone. This can lead to the continuous use of certain muscles on the wrist, resulting in the accumulation of load and triggering tendovaginitis.

Accordingly, we fabricated a white cane using aramid fibers instead of carbon fibers, which has been the main material used in the past [1]. This newly developed white cane made of aramid fibers, is more lightweight than the ordinary white cane. However, evaluations of the influence on upper limb load of the user had not been sufficient. Therefore, in this research, we investigate the influence from the weight of white canes, for the new white cane made of aramid fiber and the conventional white cane made of carbon fiber.

2 Method

2.1 Participant and the Canes Used in the Experiment

A male adult participated in the experiment. His age, height and weight was 23 years, 186 cm and 71 kg respectively. The upper limb was 80.5 cm and the lower limb was 106 cm. This participant wore a sleeping mask during the experiment.

Table 1 shows the properties of the canes used in the experiment. Two types of canes were used in this experiment. One was the new white cane made of aramid fiber, the other was conventional white cane made of carbon fiber. In order to restrict the white cane positions, two plastic plates were placed at a position in front of the participant and the participant was instructed to thrust the tip of the cane onto these plates. This regulated the participant to ensure that he did not swing the cane in an excessively wide range.

Table 1. The properties of the cane used in the experiment

Cane	Type		Material		Total	Total
	Cane	Tip	Cane	Tip	Length	Weight
New	Folding	Standard	Aramid Fiber	Aramid Fiber	121.9 cm	113 g
Conventional	Folding	Standard	Carbon Fiber	Nylon	122.5 cm	252 g

2.2 Manipulation of White Canes

In this experiment, it was decided to evaluate the movement, "manipulation while in a stationary position [2]". The participant was instructed to grip the white cane by placing the index finger on the grip and extending it along the shaft, so that the grip was held at the center of the palm. The touch technique, the way often used when users walking alone, was adopted as the method for thrusting the white cane.

Furthermore, the participant was instructed to swing the white cane in such a way that the position of the wrist, positioned at the center of the body trunk, remained the same while the cane was swung to draw an arc with the wrist as the fulcrum. The participant was instructed to swing the cane about 5 - 10 cm beyond his shoulder width on both left and right sides. The participant was asked to swing the cane in an even manner in both left and right directions and to consciously manipulate the cane with the wrist.

A summary of the experiment was explained to the participant before the experiment. The participant was then instructed to practice and master the movement of swinging the white cane using the touch technique. The participant was then asked to start manipulating the cane once the signal was given. The measurement time was 10 minutes.

2.3 Electromyogram

For the purpose of evaluating upper limb load during swinging action of the cane, the muscular activities were measured by the electromyogram (EMG). EMG measurements were taken at 5 locations. The manipulation of the cane was considered a motion realized by isokinetic contraction of the wrist joint in this research and it was determined that the evaluation [3] ought to be conducted based on the integral value of the electric potential of the electromyogram (iEMG). Concretely, once a full-wave rectification was performed on the raw waveform, the average electric potential for the initial one second was deducted from the overall figure to offset the baseline. The electric potential for every minute since the start of the operation was then integrated to observe the transition over 10 minutes.

3 Results

Figure 1 shows the results of the integrated EMG. Each graph depicts a comparison for the transition of the EMG integratedvalues per minute for 10 minutes between the new type cane and conventional type cane.

A comparison in the time transition for the variable integration of the EMG indicated that based on the results of (a), (b) and (c), with the electric potential rose after about 7 minutes for the conventional type cane but minthen took the course of a declining trend thereafter. However, the new type cane showed hardly any change over a 10 minute period. On the other hand, with (d) and (e), the conventional type cane indicated a gradual rise from approximately 5 minutes and the trend of a monotone increase was indicated. However, with the new type cane it was revealed that hardly any changes occurred in the 10 minute period. From this it is clear that although the load on muscles acting on the flexion of the wrist increased once and then decreased, the muscles acting on extending the wrist were in a monotone increasing trend.

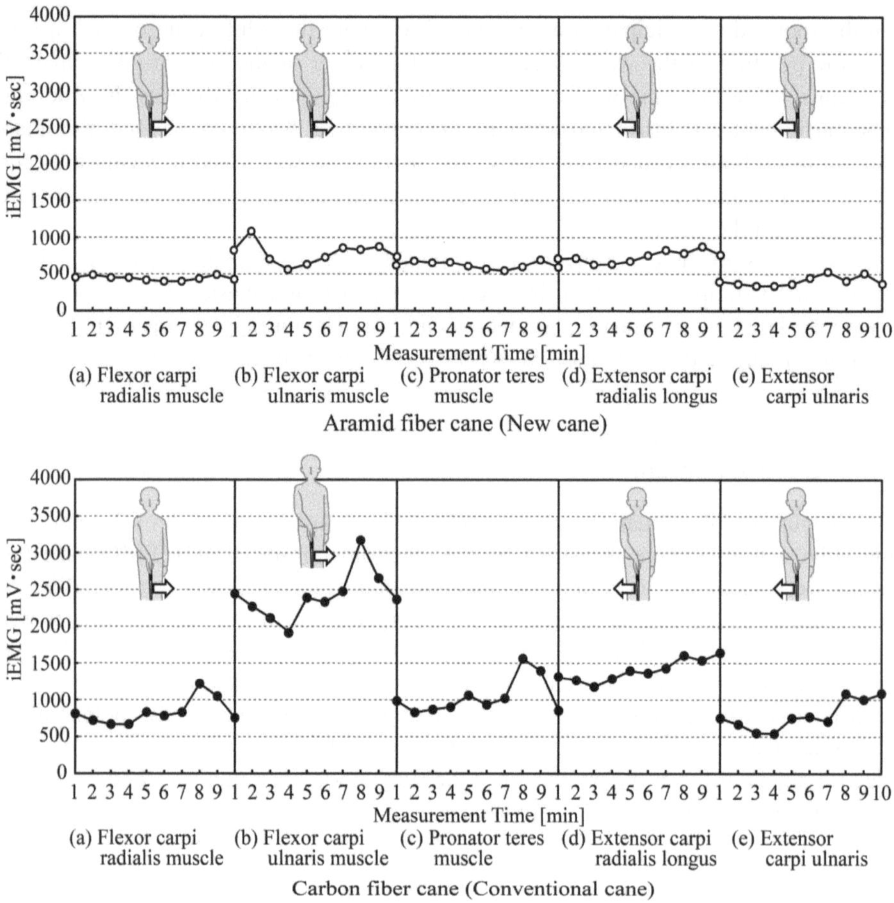

Fig. 1. Results of iEMG

4 Discussion

First of all, with regard to the difference muscle load tendencies, it is believed that for the touch technique, the inward rotation motion of the forearm by the pronator teres muscle occurred simultaneously during the flexing movements of the wrist, since the pronator teres muscle that acts on the inward rotation of the wrist indicated similar variations in load to the flexor muscles of the wrist. This transition of iEMG for the flexor muscle and the pronator muscle of the wrist revealed that there was a similar trend in the change for the value of the iEMG over time, showing a tendency of increased muscle load after approximately 7 minutes and then decreasing. This is believed to have been due to the avoidance of load concentration arising from the use of specific muscles only by the participant, who substituted the movement of swinging the cane towards the left from the perspective of the test subject with the inward swing and the inner rotation of the shoulder, as the load on the flexor muscle of the wrist and the pronator muscle of the forearm increased, due to continued movements of the touch technique conducted over a relatively long period of time. On the other hand, a monotone increasing trend of the load was seen with the passing of time for the extensor muscle of the wrist. This is considered to be due to the necessity of more extensive extensions of the wrist in order to secure the breadth of swinging for the tip of the cane, as the position of the wrist approached the trunk with the passing of time. Furthermore, it is considered that unlike the flexion of the wrist, the extension of the wrist was not substituted by the movement of the upper arm or forearm. For this reason, it is considered that when the cane is manipulated primarily by the wrist, the load tends to accumulate particularly on the extensor muscle of the wrist.

5 Conclusion

In order to investigate the influence of the weight of white canes on upper limbs loads, a quantitative evaluation of upper limb muscle loads for the manipulation of a white cane over a long period of time with the test subject remaining in a stationary standing position was conducted in this research, between a newly fabricated type of white cane made of aramid fibers and a conventional type of white cane made of carbon fibers. The results indicated that the newly developed cane reduced the loads on muscles by approximately 50% compared to the conventional type of cane.

References

1. Doi K.: The Development of a White Cane Made of Aramid Fiber reinforced resin for People with Visual Impairment. J. Text Mach. Soc. Japan 63, 196–197 (2010) (Proceedings, in Japanese)
2. Shibata, Y.: Orientation and Mobility Training for People with Visual Impairment in Japan: A Comparison of Training in 1965 and in 2005. Jpn. J. Spec. Educ. 43(2), 93–100 (2005)
3. Horita, T.: Relationships between Muscle Lactate Accumulation and Surface EMG Activities during Isokinetic Contractions in Man. Eur. J. Appl. Physiol. 56, 18–23 (1987)

Developing a Mobile Application for Language Disabled Children with User Centered Design

Lizeth Islas, Víctor M. González, and Marcelo Mejía

Department of Computer Science, Instituto Tecnológico Autónomo de México, Mexico City, Mexico
{ana.islas,victor.gonzalez,marcelo.mejia}@itam.mx

Abstract. This paper describes the design and implementation of an alternative communication device implemented as a mobile application for tablets. The application was developed applying user-centered design techniques and allows children between 3 and 12 years old with severe language impairments improve their communication skills with others. Several prototypes have been developed and evaluated with users. This paper summarizes the results and the advantages versus other apps.

Keywords: Alternative communication, language disorders, tablets, user centered design.

1 Introduction

In Mexico is estimated that over 5 million people with any kind of handicap exist, and 8.3% of this people have a handicap related with language disabilities [1]. A lot of children with language disabilities do not count with special education in the schools. Sometimes they are supported by special education teachers in Service Units and Regular Education Support. The tools that they have for the inclusion of language-disable children are, most of the time, made by the own teacher. We can find paper cards with drawings and pictures that allow expressing the children needs and wants. There are enormous opportunities to provide solutions through technologies that support them in solving their challenges of communication anytime and anywhere. The goal of this study is design and develop a mobile application oriented to language disabled children between 3 and 12 years old using techniques of user centered design and usability providing a tool for communication with the people. The inspiration of the app is based on the communication boards. Today many technologies are available on the Internet for use by people with different disabilities. However several barriers inhibit the commercialization and widespread use of this devices and applications, specially the training of the parents and teachers [2] and the elevate cost. Augmentative and Alternative Communication applications and devices are usually made for each person need and are quite expensive [3]. There are many apps that use different default pictograms and allow doing the basic communication avoiding high

C. Stephanidis (Ed.): Posters, Part I, HCII 2013, CCIS 373, pp. 236–240, 2013.

costs. The apps that allow the use of your own pictures or pictograms are scarce. The most popular in the market and the most similar to our application is "TapToTalk". They have a free version of their app but, in order to customize it you need to pay a license. The license is expensive thinking in the Mexican market. The cost is about 99 dollars which suppose a cost of over 1200 pesos per year [4]. "TapToTalk" is an entire system that provides to the user the possibility of having it in several mobile platforms and in your PC [4]. The process to load a photo or an audio recorder is pretty complicated. Consequently, what do we offer like an added value? First of all we intend to reduce the cost of the application orienting it to just one mobile platform. On the other hand, the difference between the other apps and our app is the way of loading and configuring it. For example, with "TapToTalk" you need another app that allows to take the pictures and load them. Then you need to download the picture to your app. Also, the upload of the sounds is via Internet with a PC or in the case of the application for the iPad you need to synchronize it with your iTunes library in which the sounds you want to load must be located. The user is totally unable to edit or load anything of the app in real time. Also, the parents need to read a lot of manuals to do this. Our application is designed to avoid all of these issues. In the same app you can take the photos and edit the names. Similarly, you can record with the microphone of the device your sound and be able to use it almost instantly. We offered an added value based on simplicity by making our app totally centered in user and 100% usable. That will provide the kid the feeling of owning the application because he is going to be able to manage it almost by himself and making it usable will grant that people will be more interested in use it. Another advantage of our app is that we can use it also as a reading tool. It shows us the spelling of the word we are listening to and you can easily change it for a better fits to each user and their needs. We pretended to not only do another app for people with language disabilities; we pretended to create an app totally usable and centered in kids with language disabilities at low cost.

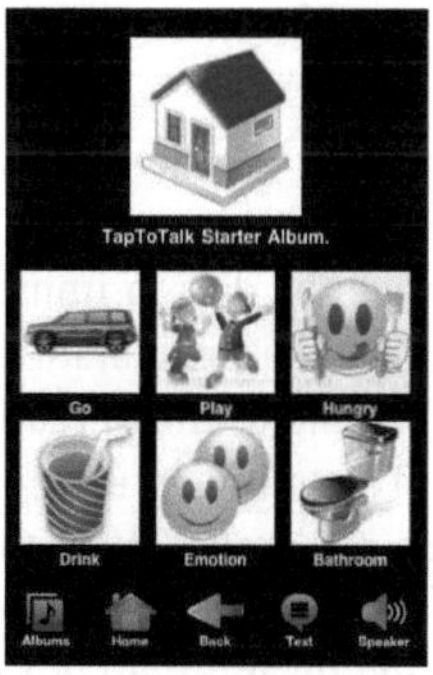

Fig. 1. TapToTalk Screen Shot (Source:"AAC|speech n stuff' http://speechie.littlelioness.net/tag/aac/)

2 Methodology

At the first part of the work we made the design of the application. For this part we used a low and a high fidelity prototype. A specialist in language therapy helped us to select the profile of the kids that could help us with the evaluation during the work. We selected kids that don't have language disabilities and in a range of 4 and 5 years old. The reason why this was done was that they can give us a feedback of the evaluation; they can tell us what thing like or dislike about the application but they can't read yet, so they basically made the tasks using only the guide of what they see. This is a really important subject if we are trying to make a design and an application with red routes well defined and a very intuitive use for our little users. The design tests were made with 3 children. We used tools like the creation of persons and storyboard for supporting the tests and ensure that the kids understood the idea. We evaluated first the low fidelity prototype with the design that we thought was more appropriate for the kids and then a second test with the changes made to the prototype but in high fidelity, all of this based on the feedback that each child provided us. We were looking for a design that could be easy to use and understand and for that reason we made two tests with each kid. On the second part of the work we made new tests with 8 kids to find patterns of usage, difficulties of usage and how they envision the application in some situations of their lives. The tests were made using the app on the iPad. We used techniques of thinking aloud and cognitive walkthrough questions, that allowed us to find out why our users were making the choices they were making while interacting with the interface of the application. We recorded in audio the tests to analyze the behavior of the users. After that, we summarized the data collected and analyzed it to identify what we could do next to improve even more the interface of the application. Finally we report the results of the whole work and the next steps for the application.

3 Design Evaluations and Results

We used two different prototypes for the design evaluation. The first one is a low fidelity prototype. We made it with post-its, scissors, glue, colored sheets and stickers. This prototype allowed us to change the design immediately almost without expenses. In this way we could find the best data presentation for the user. We evaluated two simple tasks that the users must be able to finish really easily. In addition, we used the techniques of thinking out loud. This allowed us to know what the users are thinking when they are trying to complete the tasks. With these evaluations we were able to notice that the abstraction of an adult is pretty different from the abstraction of a kid. The kids (with or without language disabilities) are not able to differentiate semantic information that they have on words or letters, although they can read, but the kids with language disabilities also have less valid and more invalid phonological information [5]. We used storyboards to tell the story to the children. The tasks were: 1) Find and point a part of the body to communicate that it's hurting, and 2) find and point some food to communicate what you want to eat. What did we find with this evaluation? Usually the kids got distracted very easily. We must put only the necessary things on the interface to avoid distraction. The letters in the principal screen are not too important, the image is the one that catches the attention and it must be clear. All the images must be consistent, maintain same patterns and format. At the beginning the application had to may buttons and options that are useless for the user. They need to have only the essential options in the screen, they must be easy to understand and easy to find or locate. Once, a kid couldn't end the task because he never found the "body" option.

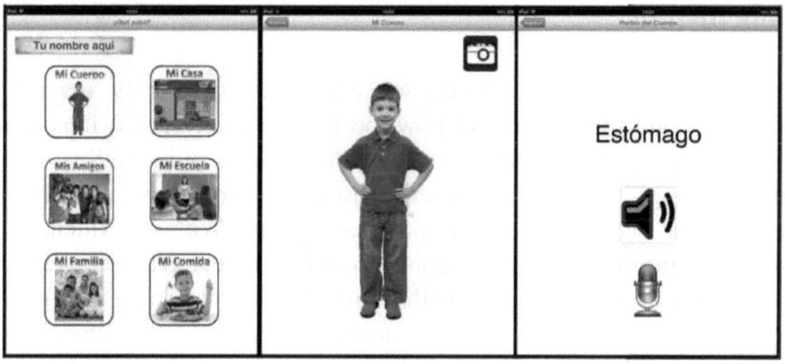

Fig. 2. Screenshots of the flow for the category "My body" (Source: Screen shots from the app)

The second prototype was a high level one. This was made using a program called "Axure". This prototype allowed us to know if the flow of the application was correct, prove if the interface based on big icons distributed in columns was more intuitive than having too many options in the principal screen. The users did the same tasks than above but with the changes in the new prototype. The images were consistent, the letters were not too big, and the options were presented with big icons. The tasks that we evaluated were the same that the ones above. What did we find with this evaluation? The high level prototype caught the children attention very easily. The flow of the interface was pretty simple to follow, so they could manage it by themselves with no additional help. They could end all the tasks with no big problem. The distribution of the interface in big icons helped the kids to understand the options that were showing.

4 Usability Evaluations and Results

After the design evaluations we did a prototype design for the iPad. This prototype was programed in iOS. It has the basics categories of communication and has pre-recorded the sounds of the pronunciations. It doesn't have the option for loading the photos, just the icon that will allow this. First we asked the children look and navigate through the entire application, pointing and testing all the options and icons they wanted. After that we asked to the kids in this evaluation to do three simple tasks: 1) Find and point the option "Escuela" (School) in the app and point an object that you use regularly, 2) find and point a part of the body, and find and point a meal or food.

What did we find with this evaluation? We needed to implement more gestures in the interface; the kids are really familiarized with them. They could end the task without issues once they get a look to the entire app. In the case of practicing with the pronunciation, the kids only repeated the words they wanted to. We needed to do it in a more encouraging manner if we wanted that our tool help in pronunciation too. They were able to find quickly the option that let them reproduce the sound of the vocabulary.

5 Conclusions

With the test of design and usability we were able to identify several areas of improvement for our app. We found how the images must be distributed, how kids identify patterns really easy and how intuitive the gestures of the iOS system are. We noticed the challenges for children to understand the application with the low level prototype when we had big letters and no clear options. We saw evidence that often the ornaments in the images are not good because the kids get distracted. Although our system is small comparing it with "TapToTalk", we have a big chance of improving the way of presenting the information. Our system allows a direct and easy use by the kids from the first time. They don't need so much time to get to know it. It doesn't count with a menu with options to avoid distracters and to make it easier. The form of upload and customization of the sounds and vocabulary is as simple as taking a photo or recording with the own device. The parents or teachers don't need to have an Internet connection to get the photos uploaded. We have consistency in the pictograms that we used; we don't mix drawings and photos, we use only pictures to make sure the user don't get confuse. We are making a tool designed and developed for children. Each child has a unique temperament. Unlike many other aspects of children, temperament is unlikely to change over time, we need to understand it and make the app adaptable to avoid frustration problems and make their lives simple and easier.

Acknowledgements. This work has been supported by Asociación Mexicana de Cultura A.C.

References

1. INEGI, Censo de población y vivienda de México, México (2011)
2. Hasselbring, T., Williams, C.: The Use of Computer Technology to Help Students with Special Needs. The Future of Children 10(2), 102–122 (2000)
3. Braddcock, D., Rizzolo, M., Thompson, M., Bell, R.: Emerging Technologies and Cognitive Disability. Journal of Special Education Technology 19(4), 49–56 (2004)
4. Tap to Talk ACC Information (2013), http://www.taptotalk.com/
5. Miriam, F., Lilly, D.: Naming difficulties in language-disabled children: preliminary findings with the application of the tip-of-the-tongue paradigm. Journal of Speech, Language & Hearing Research 40(5), 1026 (1997)

R&D Strategy of HCI Technology for Aging

Sangil Kim

Korea Institute of S&T Evaluation and Planning, Korea
cappy@kistep.re.kr

Abstract. The prevention or elimination of causes of death in early life has resulted in a population consisting of an increasing proportion of elderly people. With this increasing proportion of elderly people, we will encounter many problems like a degenerative disease, the depletion of welfare money like public medical insurance and the lowering growth rate of nation, and so on. In this research, at first every possible expected issue related to aging population was drawn through literature review and expert interview. Then products and service need to tackle aging population issues was drawn. The last step is to draw key technologies to realize these products and services. Among such technologies, we studied which technology belongs to the HCI technology, and carried out survey of the impact of each technology economically or socially. Based on these results, we presented a R&D strategy of the Korean government for the HCI technology development in response to the future aging society.

1 Introduction

Death rate reduction due to the advancement of modern medicine and improvement of daily healthcare and low birth rate, the Korean society is becoming aging population rapidly. Also, as a low birth rate is evident throughout the world, aging society rapidly proliferate as well all over the world. In particular, China, which has the largest population in the world, is predicted to have more than 400M aging population by 2033. Japan has already entered into an aging society in 1970 when population over 65 year's old exceeded 7% out of total population, and has become a super aging society in 2006 when aging population exceeded 20%. For Korea, proportion of aging population in 2000 exceeded 7.2% and has become the world's fastest aging society since then. The working population in Korea will start to decrease from 2016, and its decreasing rate will be expected to be faster than Europe and Japan. The average age of the population in Korea, currently 37.9 year's old, is already more than that in the USA, and is expected to exceed Europe by 2020. Thus, this study analyzed aging population-related issues, which are expected to be the most significant impact on the Korean society and require urgent action, and studied how the HCI technology can contribute to this issue response. To achieve these objectives, first, problems due to aging society were identified. Then, products and services for solving these problems were identified followed by selecting core technologies required for implementing the identified products and services. Among the selected core technologies, we identified which technology belongs to the HCI, and via the evaluation of each technology, future direction of technology development was presented.

C. Stephanidis (Ed.): Posters, Part I, HCII 2013, CCIS 373, pp. 241–245, 2013.

2 Identification of the HCI Technologies in Response to Aging Society

2.1 Analysis of the Aging Society Related Major Issues

The web search query data of DAUM was utilized for analysis of issues with regard to aging society of population structure. Through this process, major keywords were identified and structured, and then detailed contents per issue were identified via literature reviews and examination of experts on aging society. The detailed issues regarding the identified population structure aging were categorized in terms of health, economy, living, and society.

Table 1. Detailed issues regarding the population structure aging

Category	Main issues
Healthy life	Degenerative brain disease increase (Alzheimer, Parkinson's disease) Increase in chronic disease prevalence (Hypertension, Diabetes, and Arthritis) Mental stress increase Physical/Cognitive impairment Increased need for anti-aging and health care
Economic stability	Economic difficulties due to stable income loss Financial insecurity of social welfare due to the increase in the burden of health expenditures Decrease of economic vitality due to reduction of production and consumption population
Safe and convenient living life	Increase in demand on age-friendly information devices Difficulties in voluntary motion (Physical and cognitive ability degraded) Lacking in voluntary daily living ability
Continuous social relationship	Difficulties in voluntary motion (Physical and cognitive ability degraded) Conflict between members of family or intergenerational conflict around the elderly Conflict between the elderlies (polarization within the elderly society) Elderly alienation deepened Information gap deepening

2.2 Products and Services in Response to the Aging Society Issues

Products and services in response to the previously identified major issues of population structure aging were identified. During the identification process, candidates were limited to products and services which were only implementable by utilizing science and technology. That is, services simply given through policy support were excluded.

Table 2. Products and services in response to the aging society issues

Issue	Products and services that can be implementable via science and technology
Degenerative brain disease increase	Early diagnosis system for degenerative brain diseases Medication for degenerative brain diseases Life-care service robot
Increase in chronic disease prevalence	U-health remote healthcare system Life-care service robot
Mental stress increase	Artificial intelligence chat robot
Physical/Cognitive impairment	Rehabilitation robot Artificial intelligence robot
Increased need for anti-aging and health care	U-health remote healthcare system
Economic difficulties due to stable income loss	Providing work-at-home jobs for the aged/ Remote work support system Lifelong learning infrastructure (u-learning)
Financial insecurity of social welfare due to the increase in the burden of health expenditures	Drugs for curing chronic diseases Inexpensive drugs for chronic diseases Custom-tailored exercise healthcare system
Increase in demand on age-friendly information devices	User-friendly interface
Difficulties in voluntary motion	Muscle assistance equipment Self-driving vehicles A vehicle system which is easy to control by the aged
Lacking in voluntary daily living ability	Muscle assistance equipment Daily living assistance robot
Information gap deepening	User-friendly interface

2.3 HCI Technologies in Response to the Aging Society Issues

Technologies required to implement the products and services in response to the aging society identified previously were identified. For this identification, a group of seven experts per each technological area was configured and total three workshops have been carried out. As a result, 75 candidate technologies were selected. With regard to these 75 candidate technologies, a survey was conducted to prioritize the technologies based on criteria of likelihood of success of implementation within 10 years, responsiveness to the aging society issues, and impact (economically and technologically) by the technology experts. The survey used a 5-point scale for each question. As a result, top 20 technologies in total were chosen as the core technologies. The table below shows some of them that can be categorized into the HCI technology among the top 20 technologies.

Table 3. Result of evaluation on the HCI technology

	Technology	Likelihood of success of technology implementation	responsiveness to the aging society issues	Impact	
				Economically	technologically
1	Brain-computer interface	2.83	3.14	3.78	3.95
2	Life-care service robot	3.17	3.48	3.50	3.58
3	Wearable power assisting suit	3.63	3.77	3.47	3.53
4	Natural language process	3.89	3.20	3.48	3.53
5	Autonomous vehicle	3.84	3.16	3.70	3.58
6	Automated manufacturing	4.22	2.44	3.61	3.16
7	Smart-work technology	3.98	3.55	3.41	3.27
8	Bio-signal based Human-computer interface	3.77	3.53	3.41	3.41
9	Artificial neural network	2.89	2.84	3.08	3.53
10	Life log data mining	3.61	2.64	2.95	3.02

3 Direction of the HCI Technology Development for Aging Society

By the categorization of the HCI technologies based on the evaluation results, future direction of the technology development was derived. First, in the cases of Brain-computer interface, life-care service robot, and Artificial neural network , which have low likelihood of success of technology implementation compared to their impact, it is required to invest in education for the skilled workforce in basic technology and related technology areas, taking the future impact into consideration. Second, technologies, which have higher likelihood of success of technology development but low economic impact, can be considered. These technologies have achieved their commercialization already but lacked their social penetration due to administrative limitation or market creation. Therefore, in order to accept the technology penetration by the society, the government should provide policies to create related markets. The technologies requiring the government institutional support are Wearable power assisting suit, Natural language process, Smart-work technology, and Bio-signal based Human-computer interface . Third, technologies, which have low likelihood of success of technology development but have high economic and social impact as well as having low responsiveness to the aging society, can be considered. That is, Life log data mining is not really difficult to implement currently but it is expected to have a low possibility of market creation and low demand in future. Hence, such technologies require re-review with regard to continual investment needs. Finally, technologies, which require technology development led by a private sector, can be classified. These technologies include Autonomous vehicle and Automated manufacturing, which have high likelihood of success of technology development and high economic impact. These areas are considered as being matured for commercialization and expected to create a sufficient market in future, which is preferred to be led by a private sector rather than being led by the government.

References

1. Demiris, G., Hensel, B.K.: Technologies for an Aging Society: A Systematic Review of "Smart Home" Applications (2008)
2. Bouma, H.: Gerontechnology: emerging technologies and their impact on aging in society. Stud., Health Technol. Inform. 48, 93–104 (1998)
3. Charness, N., Scaie, K.W. (eds.): Impact of Technology on Successful Aging. Springer Publishing Company (2003)
4. Cash, M.: Assistive technology and people with dementia. Reviews in Clinical Gerontology 13(4), 313–319 (2003)
5. Rialle, V., Rumeau, P., Ollivet, C., Herve, C.: Smart Homes. In: Wootton, R., Dimmick, S.L., Kvedar, J.C. (eds.) Home Telehealth: Connecting Care Within the Community. RSM Press (2006)

A Study for Web Site Color Guideline for Universal Access for Color Vision Deficiencies: Focusing on the Best General Hospitals in Korea and in the United States

MiGyung Lee, YoungEun Kim, and Jin Wan Park

Department of Advanced Image Graduate School of Advanced Imaging Science, Multimedia and Film, Chung-Ang University, Korea
miklee755@naver.com, naankim@gmail.com, jinpark@cau.ac.kr

Abstract. In the modern society, the access and use of the internet for the individual is a crucial factor. However, the color vision deficiencies experience many difficulties in accessing the web because of their visual defects or when they are using the websites, experience many inconveniences because of the color issues. This study has realized the internet appointment screen colors in 4 general hospitals that have been selected as the best general hospitals in Korea and in the United States in 2012 for the color vision deficiencies perspective. In the websites that have been voted as the best general hospitals, the convenience of approachability was analyzed for the color vision deficiencies and improvements were suggested for an equal access to the web for the color vision deficiencies by considering the certain color guidelines.

Keywords: universal design, color deficiency, web accessibility, websites color, color schemes.

1 Introduction

The government in Korea has started a policy that mandates the web approachability since 2008 and currently the web approachability for the disabled in the main administrative organizations has improved significantly, but the financial, portal, education areas as well as the truly needed general hospital websites have not guaranteed the approachability in their websites.

Currently, the medical welfare market shows an acceleration of globalization with WTO, DDA, and FTA along with the deepened competition between countries to gain an advantage in the global medical market and the individual can choose the desired medical services in any countries in the world through the internet.

2 Color Analysis for Korean and American General Hospital Websites

The targets for analysis were selected as the 4 general hospital websites that have been voted as the best in 2012 for Korea and the United States through the Medipana Internet News in Korea and U.S. News & World Report (USNW) in the United States.

C. Stephanidis (Ed.): Posters, Part I, HCII 2013, CCIS 373, pp. 246–250, 2013.

Table 1. Analysis Targets list

Country	General Hospital list
Korea	1. Seoul National University Hospital
	2. Samsung Medical Center
America	1. Massachusetts General Hospital
	2. Johns Hopkins Hospital

The internet appointment screen colors that are often used by the users were realized and analyzed by the color vision deficiencies perspective. The analytical tool used was the color Doctor 2.1 program by Fujitsu company as a web approachability evaluation tool as recommended by the international standardization organization, WAI. The screens was used to select the text and background colors to show the RGB and Munsell values and were used for substitution to comparatively analyze the hue, brightness, saturations and the color contrast relationship.

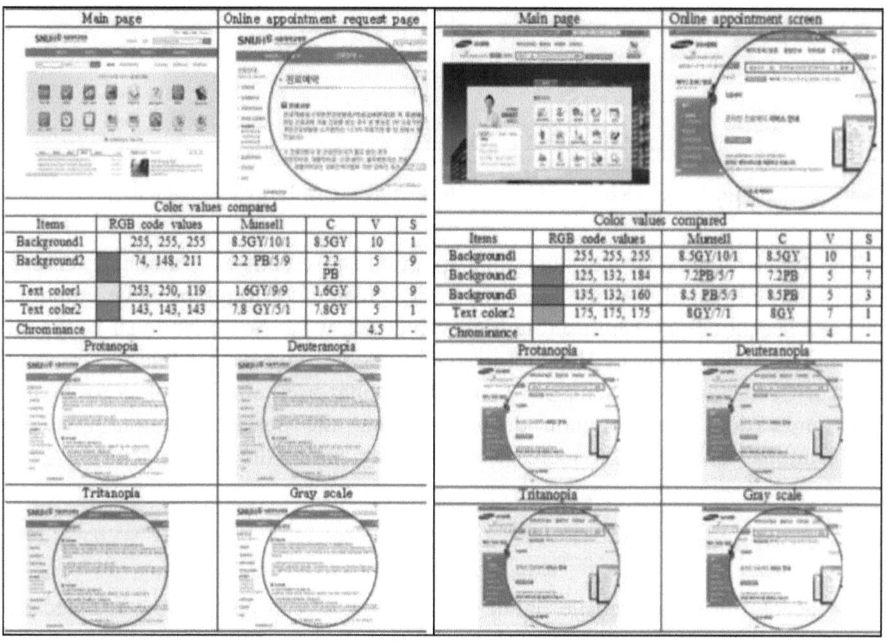

Fig. 1. Seoul National University Hospital & Samsung Medical Center

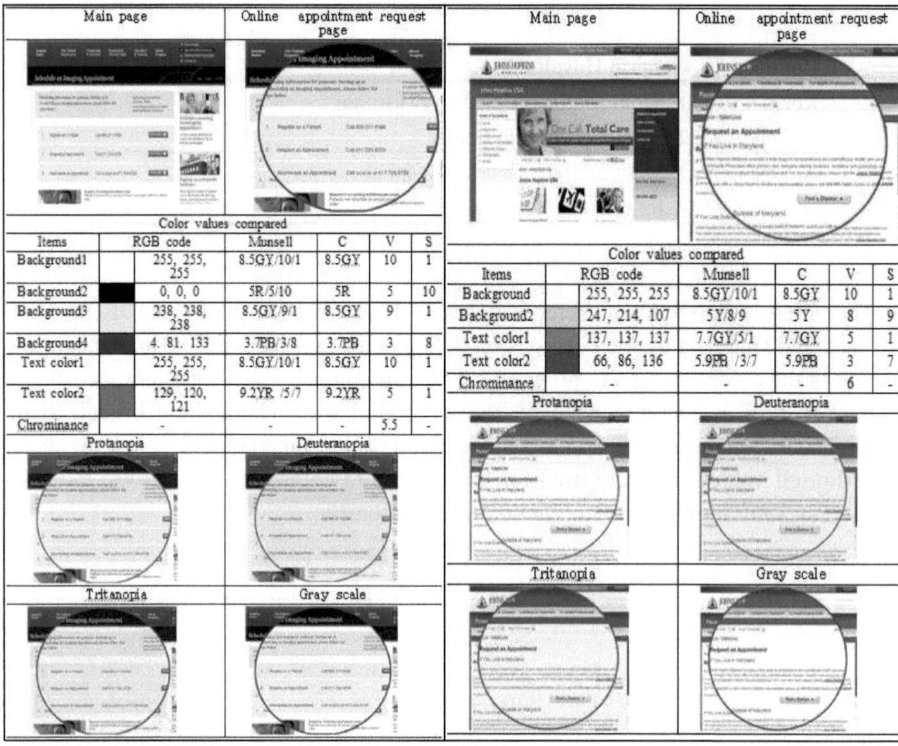

Color values compared

Items		RGB code	Munsell	C	V	S
Background1		255, 255, 255	8.5GY/10/1	8.5GY	10	1
Background2		0, 0, 0	5R/5/10	5R	5	10
Background3		238, 238, 238	8.5GY/9/1	8.5GY	9	1
Background4		4. 81. 133	3.7PB/3/8	3.7PB	3	8
Text color1		255, 255, 255	8.5GY/10/1	8.5GY	10	1
Text color2		129, 120, 121	9.2YR /5/7	9.2YR	5	1
Chrominance		-	-	-	5.5	-

Color values compared

Items		RGB code	Munsell	C	V	S
Background		255, 255, 255	8.5GY/10/1	8.5GY	10	1
Background2		247, 214, 107	5Y/8/9	5Y	8	9
Text color1		137, 137, 137	7.7GY/5/1	7.7GY	5	1
Text color2		66, 86, 136	5.9PB /3/7	5.9PB	3	7
Chrominance		-	-	-	6	-

Fig. 1. Massachusetts General Hospital & Johns Hopkins Hospital

The 4 general hospital website online appointment screens were simulated and the results showed that all 4 places used the basic screen color usage of white, gray, and blue and accent colors were used in high value yellows in Seoul National University Hospital an Johns Hopkins Hospital to give a strong impression while the Samsung Medical Center and Massachusetts General Hospital used similar colors to create a clear impression. The common theme was that the purple blue and non-color combinations were applied to increase the visibility among the color schemes.

3 Conclusion

The 4 general hospital website online appointment screen colors were realized and analyzed to show that the Samsung Medical Center had the lowest visibility even with non color vision deficiencies, which prompted the color improvement suggestions.

The improvement suggestions were simulated to prove to the color vision deficiencies perspective.

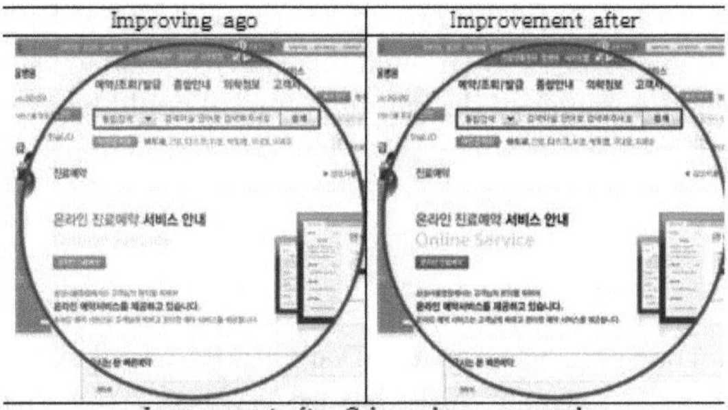

Improvement after Color values compared

Items	RGB code values		Munsell	C	V	S
Background1		255, 255, 255	8.5GY/10/1	8.5GY	10	1
Background2		86, 92, 150	7.5PB/3/7	7.5PB	3	7
Background3		106, 109, 146	7.2PB/4/5	7.2PB	4	5
Text color1		255, 255, 255	8.5GY/10/1	8.5GY	10	1
Text color2		97, 97, 97	7.2GY/3/1	7.5GY	3	1
Chrominance		-	-	-	7	-

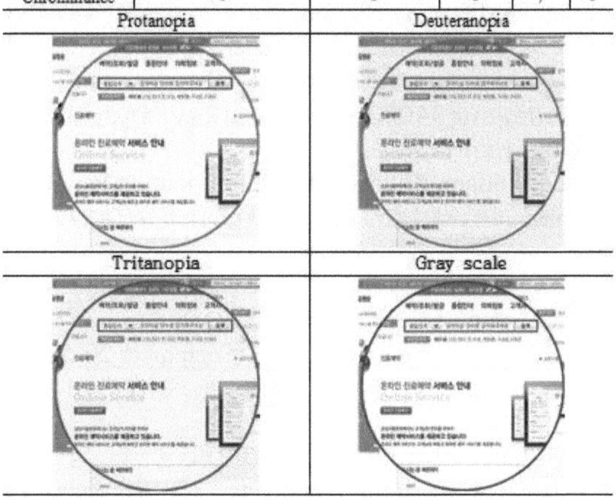

Fig. 2. Improvement

Before the Improvement, Samsung Medical Center screen had small differences in brightness between the background colors and text colors, which made the overall screen, look blurry as it presented the information. Therefore, the improvement increased the brightness differences to 7 between the background colors and text colors and the headline background colors did not change but the brightness and hues were adjusted to increase the color contrast. After the improvement, each information section became clearer even from the non color-blind person's perspective and even in black and white screens without any colors showed higher visibility.

Therefore, the following color guidelines can be suggested to be used in website color planning to be used.

A simple and direct screen should be organized with the minimum brightness difference between the background and text colors to be 5 and as high as possible to increase visibility. In addition, when using the similar color combinations, the brightness contrast should be increased or an outline should be used to distinguish them.

This study aims to be useful by providing a model for websites to consider the needs of color vision deficiencies. Through this study, I wish to establish a foundation to realize the concept of universal design; therefore, it could be used in many ways in the design field.

References

1. Rigden, C.: Now You See it, Now 954 You Don't. IEEE Computer 35(7), 104–105 (2002)
2. Dr. Dobbs, Chuck Newman (Web Techniques, August 2000) (September 20, 2012), `http://www.drdobbs.com/sitesearch?sort=publishDate+desc&queryText=Considering+the+Color-Blind&type=site`
3. Japanese Color Universal Design Organization (CUDO) (September 30, 2012), `http://www.cudo.jp/rrqcuw/bjuiss/c4727r`
4. Mace, R.L.: Universal design: Barrier free environments for everyone. Designers West 33(1), 147–152 (1985)
5. Medipana Internet News (August 2012) (September 20, 2012), `http://www.medipana.com/news/news_viewer.asp?MainKind=A&NewsKind=100&Newsu=84052&vCount=12&vKind=1Num=84052&vCount=12&vKind=16`
6. Ministry of Health and Welfare, National Health Information Portal (March 2010) (October 1, 2012), `http://health.mw.go.kr/HealthInfoArea/HealthInfo/View.do?idx=4`
7. NIA, Korean Web Contents Accessibility Guidelines 1.0 (March 2009) (September 20, 2012), `http://www.iabf.or.kr/`
8. U.S. News & World Report (USNW) (July 2012) (September 20, 2012), `http://health.usnews.com/health-news/best-hospitals/articles/2012/07/16/best-hospitals-2012-13-the-honor-roll`
9. W3C WAI, Web Content Accessibility Guidelines 2.0 (December 2008) (September 20, 2012), `http://www.w3.org/TR/WCAG/`

Older Adults' Experiences with Technology: Learning from Their Voices

Chaiwoo Lee, Richard Myrick, Lisa A. D'Ambrosio, Joseph F. Coughlin, and Olivier L. de Weck

AgeLab, Engineering Systems Division, Massachusetts Institute of Technology, Cambridge, MA 02139, United States
{chaiwoo,dmyrick,dambrosi,coughlin,deweck}@mit.edu

Abstract. When developing technologies for older adults, it is important to have them involved in the design process to identify needs, expectations and requirements correctly and comprehensively. However, communication gaps often exist, which call for the need to have continuous relationships with the target segment. In this study, older adults who have previously participated in a home technology study are interviewed to comfortably talk about their thoughts and experiences. User comments on various technologies are analyzed in relation to various stages of technology use. This paper discusses design implications, as well as topics for future research. The study can be expected to contribute to setting strategic design goals.

Keywords: User-centered design, user experience, gerontechnology, assistive technology, technology adoption.

1 Introduction

When the target users of a technology are older adults, it is more difficult to identify needs and translate them into design than when products are targeted toward younger people. For example, it is hard to simply ask what they need due to communication barriers, as well as experiential, cultural and knowledge gaps between designers and older users [1-2]. Due to such difficulties, many technologies have been designed based on incomplete understanding that focus only on the physical and cognitive limitations. Also, many have relied on stereotypes for the design of features [3-4].

It has been claimed that building a strong, continuous relationship with older adults is essential to minimize possible communication gaps [2]. In this exploratory study, we use an in-depth interview method to investigate older adults' perceptions, experiences and behaviors around various technologies. To minimize potential gaps and to have a common context in which the older respondents can comfortably talk about their thoughts, participants of a previous long-term field study were interviewed.

This paper describes the study design, including the original study and the interview, and detailed results with voices from older adults. The results are discussed as general design properties that can be applied to a broad range of technologies.

C. Stephanidis (Ed.): Posters, Part I, HCII 2013, CCIS 373, pp. 251–255, 2013.

2 Study Design

2.1 Original Field Study

In the original study, an integrated system was developed for medication management and remote communication. The system integrated a medication management component with an RFID reader and a precision scale, and a communication module with notes and video chat function, along with a PC for user interaction.

The system was evaluated in an eight-week field trial with potential users in their homes. More detailed descriptions can be found in [5] and [6]. Older adults taking at least one medication without any management services and living at least 25 miles apart from family were eligible for participation. Based on a questionnaire and an interview, four older adult and adult child pairs were selected. The age range of the older adults selected for the field study was from 65 to 76. The systems were kept on all day during the study, and were used as needed. Researchers visited each participant four times to collect data and to get feedback. The PCs used for the study were given to the participants after the study ended, with the software removed.

2.2 Follow-up Interview

The participants were contacted ten months after the original study for a follow-up interview. Out of the four older adults, three took part in the interview. At the time of the interview, they had aged a year since the original study. Each session lasted between 30 to 60 minutes. Interviews were done in participants' homes to have a comfortable setting, and to enable observation of the types of technologies being used.

The interview was designed to discuss their experiences with the original system, thoughts around various technologies, and behaviors around purchase and use of new technologies. Questions were prepared to investigate their perceptions about the original study and the study system, interactions with technologies they have experienced in the past, and thoughts around new technologies. In the semi-structured, open-ended interviews, questions with broader coverage, listed below, were asked first, and questions for probing details were asked later as necessary.

- In general, what were the impacts of having the system in your home?
- You were provided with the PC after study. How are you using it now?
- What suggestions do you have for improvement or extension of the system?
- Did your study experience have an impact on the way you think about technology?
- Have you bought or started using any new technologies recently? What and why?

3 Interview Results

3.1 Reflection on Field Study Experience

Retrospective comments were given around the system design. Since the system for the original study was a prototype, it was found to be sometimes "a little bit frustrating" and "kind of aggravating" to operate the system. One older adult said that he had to "slow down" when using it. In terms of detailed physical design, they found the interface to be "real easy," but thought "it would be better if the printing was bigger."

Respondents agreed that they benefited the most from the communication features, as in the comment "it was good because I could get to see my grandkids a little bit more." They also talked about how the system gave them a sense of presence, as they liked "having the little thing beep at me" and thought it was "good to come home and see that light." It was found that communication was made more frequent and richer by sharing medication information, as in "more of a connection and a conversation… a little bit more about me." Medication information seemed to have triggered conversation, as in "that started interaction, which branched off and blossomed."

When they were asked about the PC they were given after the original study, their answers varied. One said that she "got rid of the computer," because "it was too much money" to "have an Internet thing." The other two said that they "installed Windows 7" instead of the XP that the PCs originally had. One of the two was planning to move it to a different room because "it will be a lot more useful in there."

Suggestions for the system were also collected. A concern was raised on the involvement of family as "if you don't have the right person on the other end, it's kind of a waste," and suggested "a company or service that would do it, so if you don't have family, you can pay somebody to do it." Ideas for additional features were included tools for managing nutrition, fitness, and medical appointments.

3.2 Thoughts on Various Technologies

The effect of the field study experience on their perceptions toward technology in general was discussed. Positive effects were found, as one person said "it just opened up my eyes to different things that might be helpful," while another respondent said "I feel more confident (about using technology) now." One mentioned that she "would love to have the whole house computerized," and explained it as, "maybe that had come about from the study, because that's something that had not been in my life to have something beeping at you and helping you manage your medication and stuff."

Similar to their thoughts on the system used for the original study, emotional values seemed to be important for technology in general. For example, while they had different opinions about using Facebook, they all based their thoughts on emotional gains and losses. One who liked Facebook said "I'm more on Facebook just to know what my kids are doing… I just look at their page and I know what's going on. I don't have to worry," but another older adult who didn't like using Facebook said "I'd rather talk to your face here like this. I think it's taking away from a lot of things."

As they talked about getting new technologies and choosing what to buy, several factors were found to be important. When they were first introduced to the existence and key functions of a new technology, social connections played a big role. For example, one respondent said that her grand-sons put her on Facebook, and another older adult started using computer tutorials after her boss told her about it.

When choosing what to get after they become aware of a new technology, they based their decisions on the fit with their lifestyle. For example, one recently replaced his old air conditioner with a new one because "the management (of his residence) gave me a hard time". Another said that she recently bought a coffee machine and chose the particular model because "it was small… I have a small kitchen." Another key criterion was the related costs. High cost was described as "the stopping factor," because "when you're retired, you look at cutting costs not adding costs." They, however, said that they evaluate costs in relation to potential benefits, as in "(it's) a matter of the service you get as to whether it makes sense financially." Also at this stage of use, accessibility, visibility and past experiences were important as they just "went to the store" to see what's available and wanted to "stick with" brands they have used.

Technical support was found to be important through long-term use, as well as at the initial learning stage. For example, one older adult "bought an extended warranty" and was happy about the "help line." On the other hand, one older adult wasn't using her Kindle because she "hasn't figured it out yet." One expressed frustration with computer training programs because "they really don't tell me what I want to know."

During continued use, older adults said they often decided if they liked or disliked a technology based on its usability. For example, one complained about his mobile phone because "I get arthritis in the thumbs. The buttons are way too small. You can't see enough on the screen. I have to wear glasses for reading and stuff. When you go to a website, it's like next to impossible to read it."

Older adults complained about the lack of interoperability in the technologies that they are using. For example, one described his data back-up process as "every-thing goes into this machine, and then I duplicate it onto this computer and I put it onto my netbook, and I have external hard drives… time-consuming and not automatic."

Problems were also discussed on conceptual compatibility. For example, they were confused with the use of the word "friend" on Facebook. One older adult didn't get that her daughter-in-law's friend could add her as a "friend" on Facebook, and another said "I posted it (a picture) on Facebook and so my grandson got it, because he happens to be listed as a friend, not family. Why, I don't know." Frustrations related to service structures were also expressed. For example, they had problems with communication services because they "get a lot of dropped calls," experienced "the services has all gone down," and "don't trust when you do it out in the cloud or online."

4 Discussion and Conclusion

In this study, results from a set of interviews with older adults, who participated in a previous study, are described. Because they were familiar with the research setting, they comfortably shared perceptions and experiences in detail. In the interviews, they shared retrospective thoughts about the system they used during the original study, experiences with technologies in general, and perceptions toward new technologies.

User comments collected from the interview can be interpreted as design properties that address broader issues. Particularly, past experiences, practical value, emotional benefits, ease of use, social support and technical assistance, are consistent with findings from existing studies on older adults' technology adoption factors [7-8, 9].

However, results also suggested that there may be important factors that were not identified by previous studies. These factors include making systems reliable and trustable, and designing for compatibility with other systems, life-styles, and conceptual models. While these have rarely been discussed for older adults, other areas of study, including ergonomics and engineering systems, have already described them as important system properties [10-11]. Such gaps in research address the need for a more comprehensive understanding of older adults' thoughts, behaviors and values.

While the interviews were conducted in depth with probing questions, the study is limited in that it is based on a small sample. For a better representation, the process can be replicated to see how results converge. While this study took a more exploratory approach, future studies can also make use of quantitative methods for description or explanation of related topics, such as the effect of the design factors identified on user satisfaction. In addition, the mapping between the design properties and product lifecycle can be discussed in future studies, as respondents talked about various design properties at various stages of use.

Acknowledgements. The original study with system design and field trial was funded by NTT Japan. C. Lee is supported in part by Samsung Scholarship.

References

1. Sixsmith, A., Sixsmith, J.: Smart Care Technologies: Meeting Whose Needs? J. Telemed. Telecare 6(suppl. 1), 190–192 (2000)
2. Eisma, R., Dickinson, A., Goodman, J., Syme, A., Tiwari, L., Newell, A.F.: Early User Involvement in the Development of Information Technology-Related Products for Older People. Univers. Access Inf. Soc. 3(2), 131–140 (2004)
3. Niemelä-Nyrhinen, J.: Baby Boom Consumers and Technology: Shooting Down Stereotypes. J. Consum. Mark. 24(5), 305–312 (2007)
4. Turner, P., Turner, S.: Is Stereotyping Inevitable When Designing with Personas? Des. Stud. 32(1), 30–44 (2010)
5. Asai, D., Orszulak, J., Myrick, D., Lee, C., D'Ambrosio, L., Godfrey, K., Coughlin, J.F., de Weck, O.L.: Enhance Communication between Parents and Mature Children by Sharing Medication Information. J. Inf. Process. 20(3), 738–748 (2012)
6. Lee, C., Orszulak, J., Asai, D., Myrick, R., Coughlin, J.F., de Weck, O.L.: Integration of Medication Monitoring and Communication Technologies in Designing a Usability-Enhanced Home Solution for Older Adults. In: Proc. ICTC 2011, pp. 390–395. IEEE (2011)
7. Conci, M., Pianesi, F., Zancanaro, M.: Useful, Social and Enjoyable: Mobile Phone Adoption by Older People. In: Gross, T., Gulliksen, J., Kotzé, P., Oestreicher, L., Palanque, P., Prates, R.O., Winckler, M. (eds.) INTERACT 2009. LNCS, vol. 5726, pp. 63–76. Springer, Heidelberg (2009)
8. Coughlin, J.F.: Understanding the Janus Face of Technology and Ageing: Implications for Older Consumers, Business Innovation and Society. Int. J. Emerg. Technol. Soc. 8(2) (2010)
9. Demiris, G., Rantz, M., Aud, M., Marek, K., Tyrer, H., Skubic, M., Hussam, A.: Older Adults' Attitudes Towards and Perceptions of "Smart Home" Technologies: A Pilot Study. Med. Inf. Internet Med. 29(2), 87–94 (2004)
10. de Weck, O.L., Roos, D., Magee, C.L.: Engineering Systems: Meeting Human Needs in a Complex Technological World. MIT Press, Cambridge (2011)
11. Scott, K., Bakker, C., Quist, J.: Designing Change by Living Change. Des. Stud. 33(3), 279–297 (2011)

Providing Access to Social Networking Services for Elderly People

Andrea Nutsi, Martin Burkhard, and Michael Koch

CSCM Cooperation Systems Center Munich, Bundeswehr University Munich, Germany
{andrea.nutsi,martin.burkhard,michael.koch}@unibw.de

Abstract. The aim of the Ambient Assisted Living Project Social Interaction Screen is to support social interaction of elderly people by easing access to existing Social Networking Services. In this paper, we present the solution that was developed in the project, the elderly interaction and service assistant (elisa). We discuss the design of the prototype and present first results of its evaluation in Germany and Spain. In general, the results showed that elderly participants with different social activeness and technical affinity enjoyed the social interaction with family and friends through a user-oriented tablet interface. Nevertheless, we were unable to convince members of social networks to share their activity streams due to privacy concerns.

Keywords: Ambient Assisted Living, Social Networking Services, Social Interaction Screen, elderly people.

1 Introduction

Research suggests that Social Networking Services on the Internet foster social interaction and awareness of individual activities resulting in a feeling of connectedness that could eventually lead to real life meetings and new relationships [1]. In Germany 88% of persons aged 14-19 already use private online communities, but only 10% of people 60 years and above [2]. Based on our findings in the Ambient Assisted Living (AAL) project Social Interaction Screen (SI-Screen), we propose that the reason for the low presence of older people in Social Networking Services (SNS) is that older people encounter existing user interfaces of computer hardware and Internet platforms as usage barriers [3]. Elderly people with low technical affinity seem to have more difficulty learning to use computers [4]. As an alternative to requiring computer training, we focused on developing a simpler user interface and interaction paradigm suiting their personal needs. In our holistic approach, we recombined existing hardware components, applied new graphical user interface concepts and created a new way of accessing different SNS. In this paper we will present the solution we developed to make access to SNS easier and discuss the results of the first evaluation of the elderly interaction and service assistant (elisa).

C. Stephanidis (Ed.): Posters, Part I, HCII 2013, CCIS 373, pp. 256–260, 2013.

2 Related Work

Several approaches exist to address user interface barriers and make SNS accessible for elderly users. Particular contributions can be found in projects on Ambient Displays and in the field of AAL.

The CareNet Display by Consolvo et al. [5] and the ePortrait by Tentori et al. [6] use digital displays to enable social interaction by connecting elderly people with SNS. With ePortrait Tentori et al. [6] developed a digital picture frame enabling elderly people to stay aware of the activities of their kin network. In their study elderly people tested ePortrait at home watching family photos of their relatives on the digital picture frame supplied by SNS. They found that elderly people in their tests began to integrate the ePortrait device in their daily life routine. In addition, family members started to upload photos and status messages more than usual. Even though the presented digital photo frames offer access to activity streams including awareness support, the devices' social interaction capabilities for the end users are rather limited. The Go-myLife AAL project[1] uses a web interface customized for elderly users to consume aggregated content from various SNS. However, computer skills are mandatory for using these advantages. Similar to our effort, InclusionSociety[2] develops a comprehensive solution supporting the elderly person with a tablet device. In contrast to our solution they require communication partners to use a dedicated web portal. A holistic approach comprising of dedicated hard- and software, relying on touchscreens was followed by Doyle et al. [7]. A commercial product focusing on fostering social interaction of elderly people is the Doro Experience[3] offering applications for desktop and tablets. Instead of integrating SNS they rely on email communication.

3 Social Interaction Screen

The core innovation of the SI-Screen project is the creation of an easy to use digital device supporting social interaction of elderly people via the Social Web motivating the participation in real-life activities. Elisa is a portable tablet computer with customized graphical user interface and a server-based social middleware. Essential part of the solution is an innovative middleware that simplifies access to different SNS.

3.1 Overview

The basis of the hardware design is a 10.1-inch Android tablet. It is surrounded by a leather-covered frame, has a softly shaped back part that improves the grip and a solid stand for a safe two-hand operation for touch interaction. Hardware shape, user interface colors and tablet materials were evaluated by elderly people.

---

[1] http://www.gomylife-project.eu/

[2] http://www.inclusionsociety.com/

[3] http://www.doro.com/

The graphical user interface of elisa (elisa UI) is a replacement for the classical Android home screen that hides apps and technical details. The front end is dedicated to visualize activity and content streams of SNS using a consistent card layout. The card layout is designed as simple and comprehensible metaphor for an information unit, abstracting from the appearance of underlying web platforms. For instance, a card resembles an article, a friend's status or an event summary.

The Social Software Integration Layer (SSIL) middleware enables elderly users on their portable elisa devices to individually access various SNS in a unified way while technical details remain opaque to them [3]. For this purpose the SSIL uses CommunityMashup [8] to unify profile data, activity streams (status updates) and content streams (comments, recommendations, photos) of existing social networks (e.g. Facebook, Google+), content sharing platforms (e.g. Flickr, Picasa), contact management (e.g. Google Contacts) as well as emails, website feeds, and personal blogs. The combination of the SSIL and the elisa UI enables the homogenous presentation of content from different sources in the front end. New information is frequently collected for each user from various SNS sources and synchronized for visualization.

3.2 User Interface Views

The elisa UI is divided into three main views offering information according to personal interests of the user: 1. Interests view presenting articles and news, 2. Friends view combining activity streams from different online communities, and 3. Activities view proposing daily events in the user's neighborhood.

The Interests view enables internal and external publishers to provide articles and news for elderly readers either through their proprietary web interfaces or using a content management system (CMS). We also introduced a photo of the day article taking high-quality photos from Flickr.

The Friends view promotes awareness of the family's and friend's activities. Users see one aggregated activity stream of emails and status messages from members of online social network services (Facebook and Google+). To achieve the homogenous presentation of the elisa UI we avoided to visually differentiate between direct messages (e.g. email) and status messages from different SNS. Instead we abstracted from the technical platform and ensured that every comment or reply from the elisa user is forwarded to the originating email server or SNS.

The Activities view is about the discovery of daily events to facility social activity within the near environment according to the interests of the elderly person. The elisa user is able to participate in any event and invite their acquaintances to join in the activity. In preparation for the field test we used predefined activities supplied by the SSIL. In Germany we were also able to integrate the web feed of a cultural center.

3.3 Limitations

The implementation of elisa and the integration of external SNS for the field test revealed several organizational and technical obstacles.

Articles view: Existing web content is semi-structured and cannot be easily extracted and presented in our layout. Due to copyright issues, reusing articles from publishers like newspapers would require a license agreement. As articles might be shared by elisa users publishers refrained from supporting the field test.

Interests view: The integration of members of family and friends was challenging due to privacy concerns. In order to protect the privacy of our elderly test persons, we tried to setup anonymous Facebook accounts, which were against the Facebook guidelines resulting in blocked accounts. Furthermore family and friends of test participants denied the integration of their personal Facebook accounts. Consequently, we were not able to integrate activity streams for the duration of the field test. Moreover it was difficult to convince family and friends to share their email addresses and Skype usernames for communication purposes.

Activities view: Integrating content on web feed basis had additional limitations. Most of the tested websites did not provide structured web feeds on RSS or Atom basis. For every remaining web feed we tested no images were available and the description text was cut off after a specific character length, requiring the user to visit the corresponding website. However, using a web browser broke with our card layout.

4 Evaluation

For verifying our concept we built and evaluated three evolutionary prototypes based on requirements gathered from end users. We followed a user-centered design process in order to assure a usable solution for our target group. Involvement of elderly people was archived by focus groups, interviews and user studies.

The first prototype was realized as clickable mockup application to evaluate the comprehensibility of our graphical layout designs. For the second prototype, we concentrated on testing the user's acceptance of the elisa UI with horizontal navigation and animated transitions. The evaluation revealed a high acceptance rate for applied usability concepts [9]. Finally, for the third prototype, we improved the usability of elisa and introduced the SSIL back end system to synchronize data from SNS.

The third prototype was tested during field studies in Spain and Germany over a period of 12 days. For every country we selected ten elderly participants differing in social activeness and technical affinity. The aim was to evaluate the effectiveness of elisa with different types of elderly people and if our solution achieves our goal to foster social interaction and activity. During the first week the test persons had to solve three tasks every day, for example to find and participate in an interesting event. In the second week, no specific tasks were assigned and the users had to use elisa on their own. Besides automatic logging in back end and front end, the user had to fill in a prepared diary every day, noting down difficulties, duration and location of use.

First results seem promising and qualitative data from the German field test [10] is provided in the following. The data was collected during a focus group at the end of the field test. All participants stated that the system is user-friendly and met their personal needs. Elisa was perceived suitable for people with low technical affinity. Test persons with prior no or little technical experience required guidance during the first week but they used the application confidently during the second week and finally enjoyed the advantages of elisa.

5 Conclusion

In this paper we presented the third prototype of the elderly interaction and service assistant with its three user interface views. We highlighted our limitations for integrating existing SNS during the field test and concluded with our initial findings. Although we were not able to test the integration of activity streams of members of social networks, elderly participants irrespective of their prior technical knowledge enjoyed the ability to communicate and stay aware about the activities of others using email. For a future product, we have to convince publishers to use elisa as platform for publishing articles or at least to make articles published elsewhere available for elisa with all the meta information. Apart from technical challenges, we still have to overcome social barriers in order to fully take advantage of online communities to foster social interaction for elderly people.

Acknowledgements. This contribution is funded by the European AAL Joint Programme (AAL-2009-2-088) and the German Ministry of Education and Research (BMBF–16SV3982).

References

1. Köbler, F., Riedl, C., Vetter, C., Leimeister, J., Krcmar, H.: Social Connectedness on Facebook–An Explorative Study on Status Message Usage, Citeseer
2. Busemann, K., Gscheidle, C.: Web 2.0: Habitualisierung der Social Communitys. Media Perspektiven 7-8, 380–390 (2012)
3. Burkhard, M., Koch, M.: Social Interaction Screen. Making Social Networking Services Accessible for Elderly People. i-com. 11, 3–7 (2012)
4. Kelley, C.L., Charness, N.: Issues in training older adults to use computers. Behavior and Information Technology 14, 107–120 (1995)
5. Consolvo, S., Roessler, P., Shelton, B.E.: The CareNet Display: Lessons Learned from an In Home Evaluation of an Ambient Display. In: Mynatt, E.D., Siio, I. (eds.) UbiComp 2004. LNCS, vol. 3205, pp. 1–17. Springer, Heidelberg (2004)
6. Tentori, M., Cornejo, R., Favela, J.: Sentient displays to connect elders with cognitive disabilities to the digital era of social interaction. In: Proceedings of Workshop on Interactive Systems in Healthcare (WISH) at CHI, Atlanta, Georgia, USA, pp. 1–4 (2010)
7. Doyle, J., Skrba, Z., McDonnell, R., Arent, B.: Designing a touch screen communication device to support social interaction amongst older adults. In: Proceedings of the 24th BCS Interaction Specialist Group Conference, pp. 177–185. British Computer Society, Swinton (2010)
8. Lachenmaier, P., Ott, F., Koch, M.: Model-driven development of a person-centric mashup for social software. Social Network Analysis and Mining, 1–15 (2012)
9. Barberà, R., Campos, N.: Results of the usability validation using SIMPLIT methodology. Update to Internal SI-Screen Deliverable 3.2, Valencia, Spain (2012)
10. Erdt, S., Vidal Cabello, U.: Deliverable 5.2: Validation in real context, Field test in Germany: March 08-22, 2013. Internal SI-Screen Deliverable, Munich, Germany (2013)

Design of User Manuals for Elderly People Focusing on Font Types: Refinement of Experimental Design

Tomokazu Shimada and Michiko Ohkura

Shibaura Institute of Technology, Japan
nb11104@shibaura-it.ac.jp, ohkura@sic.shibaura-it.ac.jp

Abstract. We focused on Japanese font types to design better user manuals for elderly people. We used four different Japanese fonts provided by Morisawa consisting of three universal design fonts and a font designed based on "kawaii". We created three user manual design elements and performed an experiment to reduce the number of candidates of combinations between font types and design elements and refine experimental design.

Keywords: Usability, User manual, Elderly, Universal design, Font type.

1 Introduction

According to the National Institute of Population and Social Security Research, by 2050 in Japan, one person in three is expected to be 65 years old or older. In such an aging society, products, services, and environments for the elderly and the handicapped must be designed using specialized design concepts, such as universal design, accessible design, inclusive design, design for all, and barrier free. Since Japanese society continues to age rapidly, it is necessary for us to consider methods beneficial to the elderly. Therefore, we must not only improve the design of such industrial products as IT devices, but also provide support for the elderly so that they can live safe, peaceful, and comfortable lives. To improve the usability of IT devices, we focused on the design of paper-based user manuals because few researches have addressed the use of IT-device user manuals by elderly people.

In a previous experiment, we ascertained that emphasis on target action is an effective design element for optimizing the ability of the elderly to understand user manuals [1].

In this paper, we focused on Japanese font types to propose a better user manual design for the elderly. We used four different types of Japanese fonts, provided by Morisawa, that consist of three universal design fonts and a font designed based on "kawaii" (the quality of cuteness). For our experiment, we defined three design elements: step title, target procedure, and details of operations. We created sixty-four combinations of user manuals that contain combinations of the four Japanese fonts under three design elements and performed a preliminary experiment to reduce the number of combination candidates for two of the design elements: target procedure and details of operations.

C. Stephanidis (Ed.): Posters, Part I, HCII 2013, CCIS 373, pp. 261–265, 2013.

We conducted a preliminary experiment and used the results to help us refine our experiment so that it is more effective for the elderly.

2 Candidates of Font Types

In this study, we focused on Japanese font types of user manuals and designed an experiment to investigate which font types affect the elderly's understanding of user manuals. We used a printer as a target device and the same user manual as in previous study. We selected Morisawa as our font vendor since Morisawa provided the fonts used in the prior user manual. Because our focus was on universal design, we selected UD Ryumin, UD Shin Go, and UD Shin Maru Go, recommended by Media Universal design[2] , as candidates for this experiment. As we also focused on a "kawaii" feeling for this study, we selected Kamoraimu, which was developed by Morisawa to represent "kawaii." Figure 1 shows the four font type candidates used in this study.

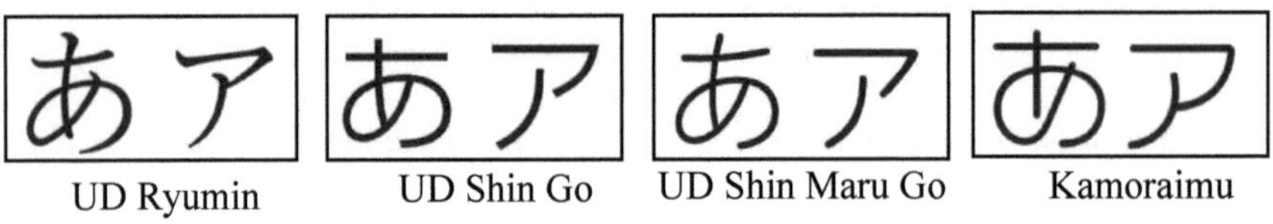

Fig. 1. Font type candidates

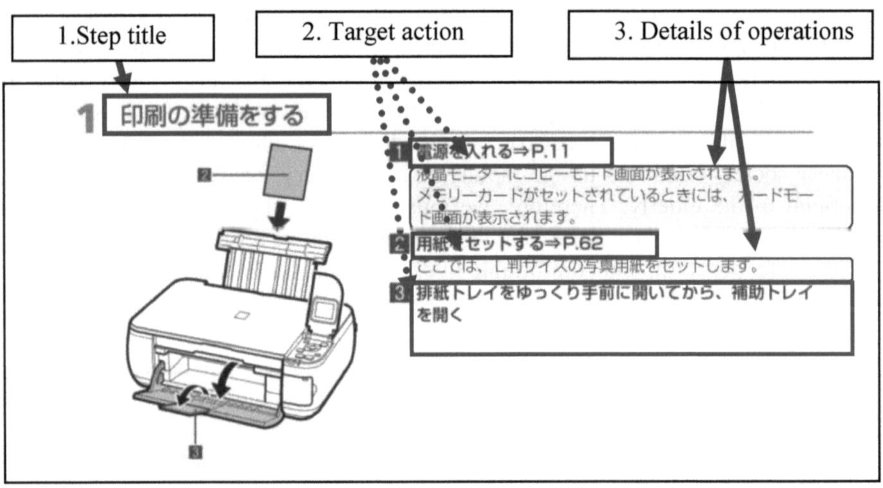

Fig. 2. Three design elements

3 Previous Experiment to Reduce Candidates

In our previous experiment, we defined the following three user manual design elements. Figure 2 shows examples of each design element.

1. Step title: The step title is the title of each procedure.
2. Target action: The target action indicates the operation location on the printer.
3. Details of operations: The details of operations describe the operation steps.

We performed a preliminary experiment to reduce the number candidates from the 64 combinations of the four font types and three design elements.

As a result, we obtained the font type combinations shown in Table 1. From this, we determined that UD Shin Go and UD Shin Maru Go are similar font types.

Table 1. Candidates for target action and details of operations

#	Target action	Details of operations
1	UD Ryumin	Kamoraimu
2	UD Shin Go (UD Shin Maru Go)	UD Ryumin
3	UD Shin Go (UD Shin Maru Go)	UD Shin Go (UD Shin Maru Go)

4 Experiment

4.1 Method

The purpose of this preliminary experiment is to refine the experimental design. The experimental method is the same as in our previous preliminary experiment.

The subjects read twelve variations of a section of the user manual containing a combination of the font types shown in Table 2 and answered a questionnaire. On the questionnaire, we used a three-point Likert scale to evaluate font type combinations: 1. Easy to read and high visibility; 2. Neither easy nor difficult to read nor high or low visibility; and 3. Difficult to read and low visibility. In addition, the subjects answered the following questions:

1. Why do you feel some manuals are easy to read or have low visibility?
2. Why do you feel some manuals are difficult to read or have high visibility?

4.2 Results

The subjects were sixteen male and female students in their twenties and thirties. Figure 3 shows the results of our questionnaire. The horizontal axis shows the ratio of the number of answers and the vertical axis shows the combinations of font types shown in Table 2.

Most subjects felt that the combination of UD Shin Go and UD Shin Maru Go on target action and details of operations was easy to read and had low visibility, followed by the combination of UD Shin Go or UD Shin Maru Go on target action and UD Ryumin on details of operations.

Table 2. Combinations of font types

#	Design elements		
	Step title	Target action	Details of operations
1	UD Ryumin	UD Ryumin	Kamoraimu
2		UD Shin Go (UD Shin Maru Go)	UD Ryumin
3		UD Shin Go (UD Shin Maru Go)	UD Shin Go (UD Shin Maru Go)
4	UD Shin Go (UD Shin Maru Go)	UD Ryumin	Kamoraimu
5		UD Shin Go (UD Shin Maru Go)	UD Ryumin
6		UD Shin Go (UD Shin Maru Go)	UD Shin Go (UD Shin Maru Go)
7	UD Shin Maru Go (UD Shin Go)	UD Ryumin	Kamoraimu
8		UD Shin Go (UD Shin Maru Go)	UD Ryumin
9		UD Shin Go (UD Shin Maru Go)	UD Shin Go (UD Shin Maru Go)
10	Kamoraimu	UD Ryumin	Kamoraimu
11		UD Shin Go (UD Shin Maru Go)	UD Ryumin
12		UD Shin Go (UD Shin Maru Go)	UD Shin Go (UD Shin Maru Go)

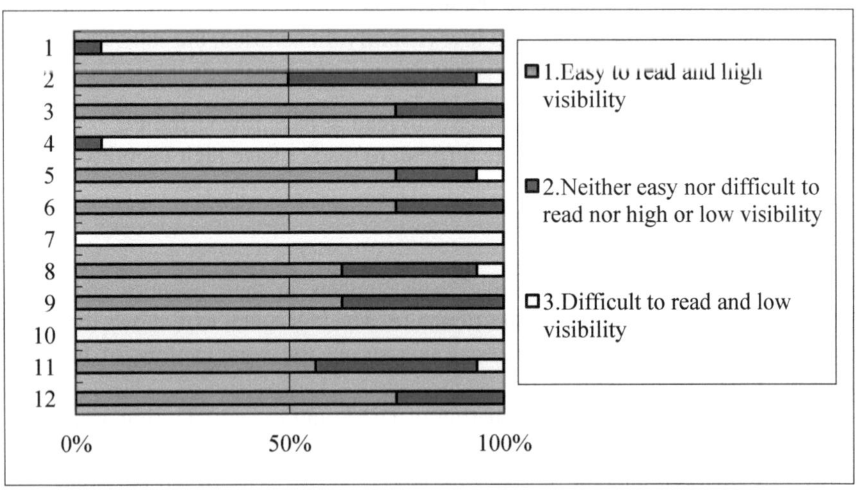

Fig. 3. Results of questionnaire

Table 3. Combinations of font types

#	Step title	Target action	Details of operations
1	UD Shin Go (UD Shin Maru Go)	UD Shin Go (UD Shin Maru Go)	UD Shin Go (UD Shin Maru Go)
2	UD Shin Go (UD Shin Maru Go)	UD Shin Go (UD Shin Maru Go)	UD Ryumin
3	Kamoraimu	UD Shin Go (UD Shin Maru Go)	UD Shin Go (UD Shin Maru Go)
4	UD Ryumin	UD Shin Go (UD Shin Maru Go)	UD Shin Go (UD Shin Maru Go)

5 Discussion and Conclusion

In this paper, we performed an experiment to refine our experimental design. Most subjects felt that the combination of UD Shin Go and UD Shin Maru Go was easy to read and had low visibility in target action and details of operations. From this, we obtained our candidates of the font type combinations shown in Table 3.

Based on this result, we will design an experiment on the usability of user manuals focusing on different font types and conduct the experiment with elderly people.

Reference

1. Shimada, T., Ikeda, S., Ohkura, M.: Designs of user manuals for elderly people. In: Proceedings of the 10th Asia Pacific Conference on Computer Human Interaction (2012)

Development of Support Applications for Elderly and Handicapped People with ICT Infrastructure

Ippei Torii, Kaoruko Ohtani, Takahito Niwa, and Naohiro Ishii

Faculty of Information Science, Aichi Institute of Technology, Aichi, Japan
{mac,x08062xx,ishii}@aitech.ac.jp, kohtani@comcast.net

Abstract. We work on studying and developing support applications for aged and handicapped people. First, we developed a new communication assistant application for autistic children, "Let's Talk!". We especially focused on an easy and simple manipulation. We also developed a to-do application for kids, "Hanamaru" and a scheduler application for elderly people, "Anshin". We used ICT infrastructure, especially computer network systems such as SNS (Twitter, Facebook), e-mail, Skype, Line, and a message board on the web site, to collect the requests and opinions of users, and tried to feed it back to improve the applications.

1 Purpose of the Study

Lately, an electrical device that support people who are unable to use natural speech to express their thoughts or needs has been developed. It is called a Voice Output Communication Aid (VOCA). And also, PDA (Personal Digital Assistant) is getting attention as assistant tools for communication with its advantages as a communication tool. Fist of all, it is easy to carry around. A user can create symbols by him/herself that are suitable his/her situation with easy steps. And also, a user can actually talk to others by the voice of the application. Some assistant applications for PDA, such as Drop Talks[1], Voice4u[2], Tap to Talk[3], aimed to help autistic children have already introduced. Although many studies about VOCA [4][5] had been made and school educational fields have adopted these applications, they are not come into general use because of the high price and complicated operations. Therefore, we tried to develop a new VOCA for PDA with simple and easy manipulation in low price, and named it "Let's Talk!"

2 Construction of the System

2.1 Usability of the Application

We focused on a simple manipulation without complicated explanation to develop this application. In most of the existing VOCA applications, a user needs to choose the suitable words from a large amount of symbols. (Figure. 1, Left) It is hard for the autistic children that have severe mental disturbance. On the other hand, in "Let's

C. Stephanidis (Ed.): Posters, Part I, HCII 2013, CCIS 373, pp. 266–270, 2013.

Talk!" a user needs to tap only one button and a sentence of two words comes out automatically. (Figure. 1, Right) The autistic children can learn this easy operation quickly. It gives them a feeling of satisfaction at having achieved to communicate with others by themselves.

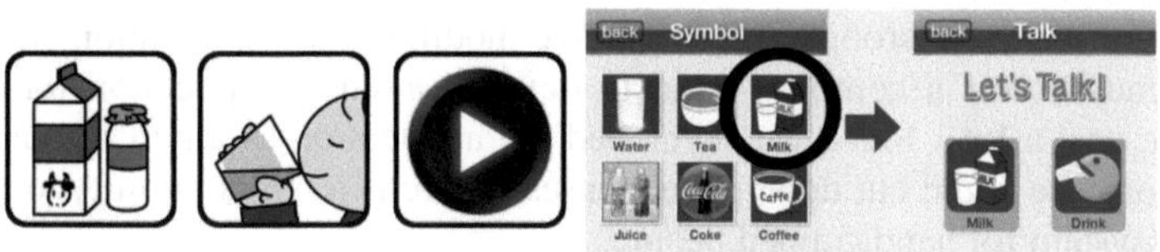

Fig. 1. Left: The example of screen of VOCA application Right: The example screen of "Let's Talk!"

2.2 Supportive Mode/Self-use Mode

On Supportive Mode of the application, a supporter starts to pick symbols fitting to the situation and the condition of an autistic child who needs assistant for communication. When an autistic child touches the symbol what he/she wants to tell, a sentence comes out by voice sound. It is difficult for autistic children to choose what they really need to say among too many choices. So we limited the numbers of symbols picked by a supporter from 1 to 4 and make it easy to choose.

If an autistic child understands how to manipulate this application, he/she can tell what he/she wants directly with categories or symbols in Self-use Mode.

2.3 Make / Original Page and Stamp Mode

This application has about 120 icons that fit our daily life, but more icons may be required depending on the situation. On Make Page, a user can make his/her original icons with a camera or a voice recorder the PDA has or using an illustration or sound founded on web sites. It is sure to broaden the communication if there are some original icons that suitable with an autistic child's dairy life, such as the places he/she goes frequently, familiar people or the dairy activities. Original Page is customizable to put icons that are created by a user or existing symbols freely.

On the newest version of "Let's Talk!"(iPhone / "Let's Talk!"AppVersionNumber:4.0 June 10, 2012), we added Stamp Mode. On this mode, a user can make a chart with a goal. Children get a stamp whenever they have done what they needs to do.

3 Updating the App with ICT Infrastructure

After we released "Let's Talk!", we have collected suggestions and requests from users through ICT infrastructure and the data from schools for handicapped children. We modified and updated the app 14 times till September 2012 referring to those opinions and the data.

We used ICT infrastructure, especially computer network systems such as SNS (Twitter, Face book), e-mail, Skype, Line, and a message board on the web site, to collect the requests and opinions of users, and tried to feed it back to improve the application. There were some inconveniences which beyond our expectations. For example, freezing when a child swipe the screen too fast, malfunctioning when the button is hit repeatedly, the icons were too small to see, the sound is not big enough to use outside or noisy classroom, and so on. We modified the application based on all of these requests. If a company tried to develop a same application for profit, it would have cost a lot. Since we developed the application as a part of our study in the laboratory, we could cut down on expenses. There is a big possibility to apply the supporting system for handicapped people.

4 Experiments at School for Handicapped Children

Introducing "Let's Talk!" on the experimental basis was carried out at Miai Yogo School, which is the school for handicapped children in Aichi, Japan.

4.1 Case Study 1

The subject of investigation was a 8 year-old autistic boy (T) with no ability to speak. T tried to tell his teacher he wanted to have another plate at lunchtime with the application. Figure 2 shows how his behavior had changed when he started to use this application.

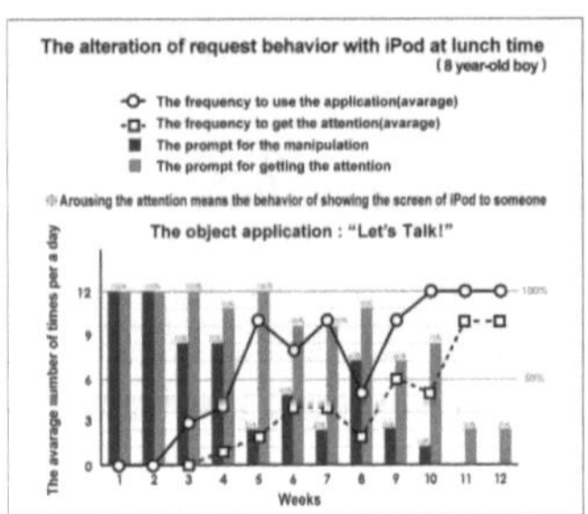

Fig. 2. The alteration of request behavior with iPod at lunchtime (8 year-old boy)

The dark bar graph shows how many times the teacher thought T the manipulation of this application. The manipulation is divided into 5 levels. 1) To get the iPod 2) To release the lock of the iPod 3) To start the application 4) To choose an icon 5) To show it to someone. Autistic children will learn 1) to 4) quite easily, but they will not understand 5), which means they need to show the screen to someone to communicate. The light bar graph shows how many times the teacher told him to get the attention of others. The teacher's support was needed more than 50% till 10th week for T. The Solid line graph shows how many times he actually used this application. The dashed line graph shows how many times he tried to get attention of his teacher. In this case study, it is clear that his motivation to communicate with the teacher had been increased by using iPod with this application..

4.2 Case Study 2

The subject of observation was a 11 year-old autistic boy (M) with severe mental disability. In April 2011, we gave iPad to M with "Let's Talk!" on the screen. He understood that the screen would change when he touched it immediately. In May, he became to show the words such as " Can I start?" "Can I have some more?" and so on with iPod at lunchtime. In late May, we took pictures of the lunch menu and saved them in "Let's Talk!" as original symbols. M showed what he did not like to eat when he saw the pictures. At this point, he did not try to arouse someone's attention. In June, M started to use "Let's Talk!" in different situations besides lunchtime. For example, he told his teacher that he had done with his test by tapping "I'm done" button. (Figure 3) He started to arouse someone's attention by tapping his/her shoulder or arm. In September, M became to be able to create original symbols by himself. And in November, he became to be able to use some other application besides "Let's Talk!". In February, M has been using "Let's Talk!" less often at this point. He used his gestures to tell us simple requirements such as "Can I start to eat?" or "Reduce some of this, please." If the person he tried to tell his request could not understand his gesture, he used pictures in iPod or typed words on memo function. He sometimes made voice sound to get someone's attention that he had never done before.

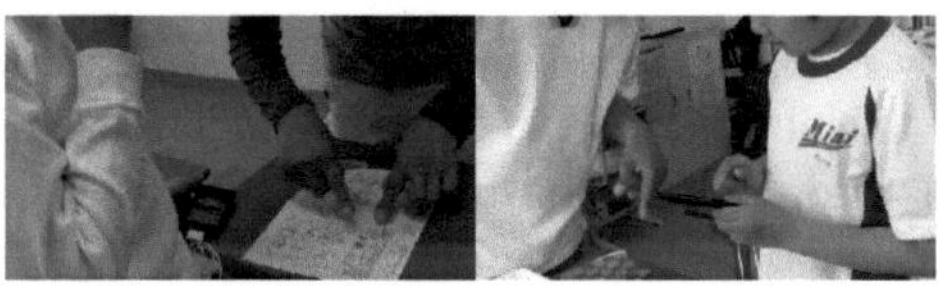

Fig. 3. M tells the teacher "I'm done" with iPod

M understood the function of communication quickly with this application and became to be able to communicate with others. We consider repeating the experiences to communicate with others stimulates the desire for communications and arouses initiative. It is obvious "Let's Talk!" is useful to raise the communication ability.

5 Another Support Application

5.1 Hanamaru

It is a To-do application for autistic children. It will show you a schedule by voice sound and text. A user can also show the processes of a behavior by symbols with this application. It is easy to understand for child what he/she needs to do next and he/she can get on the next step by him/herself. Figure 4 shows the situation of students in the school for handicapped children using "Hanamaru" to make a cake. The student confirms the process of "check the cake" on the screen of iPod. The students can figure out what they need to do next with this function by themselves without the instructions of the teachers.

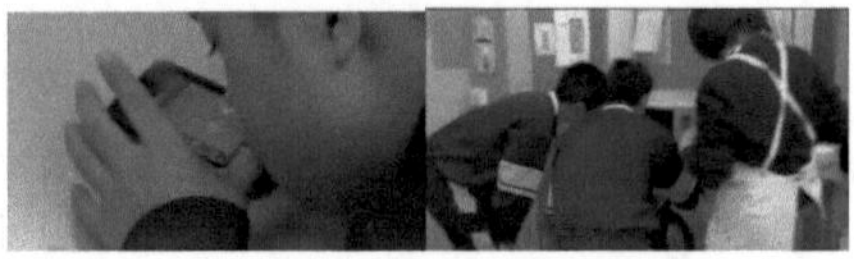

Fig. 4. Using "Hanamaru" to make a cake

5.2 Anshin

We also developed a scheduler application for elderly people, "Anshin". It is easy to understand "what to do next" at a glance by pictures, letters, and voice. We tried to make the manipulation as simple and easy as possible for the elderly people who are not familiar with portable equipments to be able to use it by own. In Japan, it has been a social problem that solitary death, which means someone who lives alone dies at home without anyone knowing. If a user doesn't use "Anshin" for 3 days, it will send e-mail to his/her family or friends (up to 2 people) automatically and let them know a user's situation.

6 Conclusion

We developed a new communication assistant tool with PDA, "Let's Talk!", for autistic children. If autistic children feel the joy of communication by using this application, they will be strongly motivated to try to understand others thoughts. This application may have much possibility to be used by not only autistic children but also people who have problems of communication because of some diseases, such as pharyngeal cancer, cerebral palsy from a stroke, or senile dementia. We think if people can communicate with each other regardless of disabilities, it will provide new human resources and encourage developing the society where people support each other. In future prospective, it is urgently necessary for us to develop supporting systems for children with Limb/Trunk Dysfunction or bedridden old people who even cannot touch the screen. We consider the core categories and symbols for basic communication is established through the development of "Let's Talk!" We will apply the method for future studies.

References

1. Drop Talk, `http://droplet.ddo.jp/droptalk/`
2. Voice4u, `http://voice4uaac.com/jp/`
3. Tap to Talk, `http://www.taptotalk.com/`
4. Nakamura, K.: Effects and limitations of communication aids. Journal of Communication Aids for People with Cognitive Disabilities, Higher Brain Function Research, 194–200 (2001)
5. Sakai, S.: VOCA application to Autistic Children. National Welfare Foundation for Disabled Children, 29–32 (1999), `http://voice4uaac.com/jp`

Interface Model for Accessible Forums for Blind, Deaf and Non-disabled People

Carla da Silva Flor, Ronnie Fagundes de Brito, Douglas Kaminski, Vania Ribas Ulbricht, and Tarcísio Vanzin

Federal University of State Santa Catarina, Florianópolis, Brasil
{carla.flor,ronniefbrito,kaminskidk,vrulbricht}@gmail.com, tvanzin@yahoo.com.br

Abstract. The objective of this article is to present an interface model that enables the integration of deaf, blind and non-disabled people on internet forums, considering their different linguistic features. Therefore we designed a theoretical model that uses Sign Language (LS) Sign Writing (SW), text and speech. The shortage of automatic SL translators makes it difficult to implement the interface and its evaluation, undermining researches in the area of digital accessibility.

Keywords: Interface, fóruns acessíveis, surdos, cegos.

1 Introduction

The integration between people on Internet forums depends on the Human-Computer-Human (HCH) interaction, considering not only the needs and goals of users, but also their characteristics and capabilities [1]. The implications increase as the user's sensing abilities become limited, making visual or auditory interaction impossible.

As blind, deaf and non-disabled people interact in an environment such as a forum, challenges rise. There is a need for a mediator capable of making a syntactic and semantic translation according to the different communication models being used. Language and comprehension problems arise, hampering the integration between users with different sensory capabilities.

This article aims to develop a model that supports communication between deaf, blind and non-disabled people, in order to minimize the difficulty of communication between these user profiles, facilitating learning and the exchange of experiences.

2 Method

2.1 User Profiles

Different groups of users participate in web forums. However, this study adhered to three specific groups of people: deaf, blind and non-disabled. The choice was not by

C. Stephanidis (Ed.): Posters, Part I, HCII 2013, CCIS 373, pp. 271–275, 2013.

chance, since deaf people make constant use of their vision to communicate [2], [3], while blind people basically use the oral-auditory canal and tact. Thus, there is a heterogeneous group with very different needs.

Deaf. Most deaf people use a language of their own that differs from their native country's spoken language. This language, known as Sign Language (SL), is based on the use of gestures, through movements of hands, face, eyes, lips and body, with different meanings as the position, orientation, movement and facial expression change. Moreover, the structure of sign language does not resemble the spoken language and it has its own grammar [3].

Even though SL is the natural language of the deaf, its use and acceptance is not unanimous among them, dividing opinions between those who advocate its use and those who advocate the use of spoken language. One of the main problems associated with SL is the difficulty of the written record. Recently, Valerie Sutton developed the Sign Writing (SW), a system that facilitates reading and can be applied to different communication platforms [4].

Blind. Blind people are distinguished from deaf people for having language as their primary communication channel. Unlike the deaf, all visual information that can not be played must be described in some way, either by a screen reader or a specialized browser. For multimedia content to be accessible to blind people, images, videos and other multimedia resources must contain an equivalent textual or audio description.

Non-disabled People. The non-disabled participate in those two user groups because they use both vision and hearing to communicate. However, most of these people do not know Sign Language.

2.2 Related Studies

Similar projects were studied by Campr et al [5], who developed a system capable of turning dactylology in speech and vice versa, assisting in communication between people with visual and hearing disabilities. Dactylology consists of a manual alphabet that corresponds to the alphabet of the spoken languages and not exactly to the SL, natural language of the deaf, as proposed by this work.

2.3 Theorical Model

Considering the standard language pattern used by deaf, blind and non-disabled, it was possible to establish a theoretical model that would enable communication between all users. It was found that as the deaf can be taught spoken language, they can make use of both Spoken Language or Sign Language. And the ones who use Sing Language may or may not be familiaar with Sign Writing. According to these parameters, we identified three profiles of deaf people: SL, SW and text. At the other end there are blind people who use text and speech. Non-disabled people most commonly use text, but can also make use of speech, SL and SW. The model that describes the transformation of the interface can be seen in Figure 1.

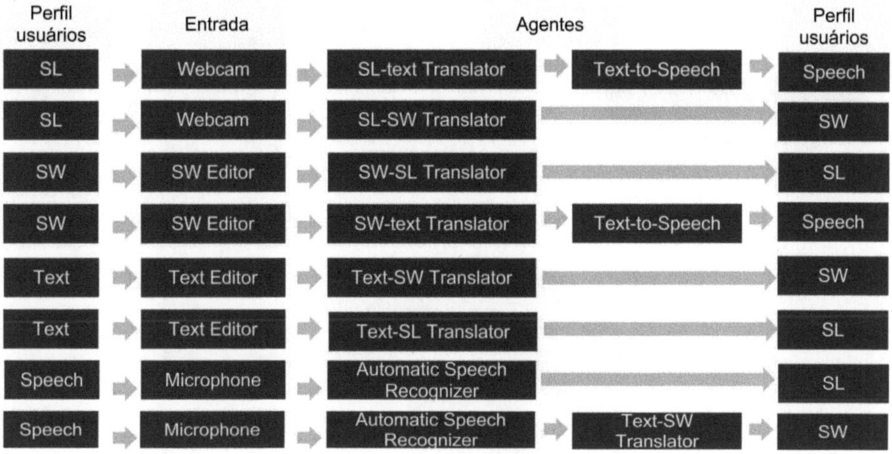

Fig. 1. Interface model for accessible forums to deaf, blind and non-disabled people. (Source: The authors)

For each user profile there is an input device that is required to interpret the type of communication used by them: webcam (SL), SW editor (SW), text editor (text) and microphone (speech). However, to be understood by people who are at the other end, these data must be interpreted and translated by technical agents, such as automatic translators SL-text/text-SL, SL-SW/SW-SL, text-SW/SW-text; speech recognition systems, and speech synthesizer system. This article does not focus on the development of these agents, but rather on the interface integration between users.

3 Graphical Interface Model

A graphical interface that integrates different user profiles is challenged to represent text, SW, LS and sound. Several studies [3], [6] show that the most common way to use SL video on a page, ie, which is at a specific location on the screen, is not the most appropriate way because it takes space from other elements such as images or multimedia. Furthermore, the use of a movable sign language video in a transparent background on the page is encouraged because it enables the visualization of elements on the lower part of the page. The use of semi-transparency in the video is suggested for the same reason [7], but in this case the level of transparency has to be adjustable by the user. In relation to the content in SW it is not advisable to use semi-transparency, nor the transparent background, because it impairs reading. A proposition of the interface can be visualized on Fig. 2.

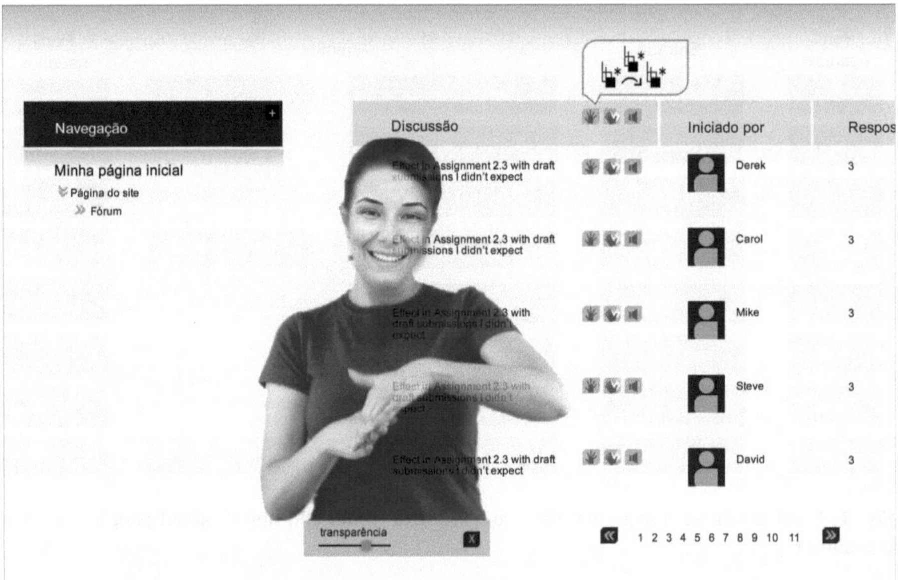

Fig. 2. Interface of the accessible forum to blind, deaf and non-disabled

In the proposed interface, each forum topic would have three icons next to it that correspond to the icons of SW, SL and speech synthesizer. As you click on the first icon a balloon with the SW translation would appear; clicking on the second icon would bring a SL video into view, and clicking on the last icon, would synthesize the text into speech. When editing messages, each user would use the most adequate mode for their needs: a deaf who uses SL would use a camera, a deaf who uses SW would use a SW editor (there are already a few options available in the market), a blind person would use a speech recognition software and a non-disabled person would use a text editor. All models would be arranged on the page in text form and converted to SW, SL or speech through the icons.

4 Research Limitations

There are many studies being held on SL automatic translators for LS, however, regarding the softwares in Portuguese, many are not yet ready for use and others are unstable [8], which hinders the implementation of the proposed interface. The lack of a working interface makes it impossible to test it with real users, based only on studies from the references submitted. Thus, validation of the interface is not part of this work and should be the focus of future researches.

5 Conclusion

Human-Computer Interface has provided, in addition to the human-machine communication, interpersonal communication, linking users with different characteristics and needs, as deaf, blind and non-disabled. Even if language barriers remain, advances in technology tend to allow these people to interact and to exchange ideas and experiences in accessible forums.

The proposed interface model considered linguistic differences, searching to present the most suitable language for each user profile. An evaluation will be needed in the future, when the proposal is implemented. In this course, other factors must be mastered by technology, such as providing a wide supply of eficient automatic translators.

References

1. Acuña, S.T., Castro, J.W., Juristo, N.: A HCI technique for improving requirements elicitation. Information and Software Tecnology 54, 1357–1375 (2012)
2. Bueno, J., Garcia, L.S., Junior, A.M.: Bilingual alphabetisation of deaf children: requirements for a communication tool. In: IADIS International Conference WWW/INTERNET, Anais...Texas (2010)
3. Debevc, M., Kosec, P., Holzinger, A.: E-Learning Accessibility for the Deaf and Hard of Hearing - Practical Examples and Experiences. In: Leitner, G., Hitz, M., Holzinger, A. (eds.) USAB 2010. LNCS, vol. 6389, pp. 203–213. Springer, Heidelberg (2010)
4. Rossi, D., Souza, V.C., Pinto, S.C.: Sign WebForum: um Fórum de Discussão que Utiliza a Troca de Mensagens em Libras na Web. SimpÓSio Brasileiro De InformÁTica Na Educaç ÃO, 15 (SBIE 2004), Anais...Amazonas, pp. 259–268 (2004)
5. Campr, et al.: Automatic Fingersign to Speech Translator. In: The 6th International Summer Workshop on Multimodal Interfaces (eNTERFACE 2010), Anais...Amsterdam (2010)
6. Debevc, M., Kosec, M., Holzinger, A.: Improving multimodal web accessibility for deaf people. Multimedia Tools and Applications 54, 181–199 (2011)
7. Miller, D., Gyllstrom, K., Stotts, D., Culp, J.: Semi-transparent Video Interfaces to Assist Deaf Persons in Meetings. In: Proceedings of the 45th Annual Southeast Regional Conference (ACM-SE 45), pp. 501–506. ACM, New York (2007)
8. Piveta, E.M., Ulbricht, V., Savi, R.: Mechanical translators of oral and written Portuguese. In: Congresso Nacional De Ambientes Hipermídia Para A Aprendizagem (CONAHPA), Pelotas (2011)

Evaluation of Accessibility with the Deaf User

Daniela Satomi Saito, Elisa Maria Pivetta, Vania Ribas Ulbricht, and Cláudia Mara Scudelari de Macedo

Post-graduate Program in Engineering and Management of Knowledge, Federal University of Santa Catarina, Florianópolis, SC, Brazil
{daniela.saito,vrulbricht,claudia.scudelari}@gmail.com, elisa@cafw.ufsm.br

Abstract. Learning mediated by teaching and learning virtual environments (AVEA in Portuguese) contributes to disseminating knowledge in a more pleasurable way to people who have disabilities. However, the technologies used for teaching should satisfy recommendations on usability and accessibility. This article sets out to present a case study regarding evaluating a virtual environment using the technique of interviews with deaf users. The case study enables issues relevant to accessibility as well as possibilities for development and innovation to be identified. Furthermore, the use of the tool of evaluation by interviews prompted reflections related to the specificities required for using the technique with deaf users.

Keywords: The Deaf, Web accessibility, AVEA.

1 Introduction

Distance Education (DE) in its design is a backdrop for making inclusion effective. However, this has been incipient. Therefore, discussions as to the accessibility of Teaching and Learning Virtual Environments (AVEA, in Portuguese) and the characteristics of their users are crucial to the inclusion of people with disabilities. With a view to assisting developers to produce accessible material, WAI (Web Accessibility Initiative) drew up Web Content Accessibility Guidelines (WCAG), for which there is currently a 2.0 version. [14]

This paper reports on the evaluation of the accessibility of an AVEA for deaf users, by means of a case study. The objective was to identify general aspects of accessibility from the point of view of the deaf. To do so, the Moodle environment [7], configured within the standards of an educational institution, was selected.

2 Evaluating Accessibility

There are different approaches to evaluating accessibility, some of which use automated tools, and are evaluated by experts and by the user. Although evaluation by the user is an onerous process, it gives the developer a better understanding of topics

C. Stephanidis (Ed.): Posters, Part I, HCII 2013, CCIS 373, pp. 276–280, 2013.

such as accessibility, namely, how these audiences use the web, the use of assistive technologies and the forms of interaction best suited to each of them [14]. Consequently, new perceptions of and insights into development can be obtained, thus generating more effective solutions in terms of accessibility.

2.1 Evaluation with the User

To work with users, use is often made of strategies for evaluating interfaces by: a focus group, testing interaction with participant observation and conducting evaluation interviews with the user [10]. Evaluation by interviews is a strategy of qualitative research. This approach seeks to analyze deeper aspects of the complexity of human beings, their habits, culture, and behavioral trends [6]. The authors identify two categories of interviews [6]:

- standardized or structured - script previously established and strictly followed;
- non-standardized or semi-structured - the interviewer has the freedom to explore and deepen the issues that he/she deems relevant.

3 Case Study

The study set out to obtain an overview of the elements of accessibility in a Teaching and Learning Virtual Environment for the deaf. The methodology for the study is given below:

- Selecting the AVEA to be studied;
- seeking information about the characteristics of the target audience by means of current readings on the topic;
- defining the profile of the audience that is to be evaluated;
- identifying partners or collaborators who may be members of the target audience;
- defining the structure and script of the evaluation instrument;
- selecting interviewees;
- implementing and recording the interviews (on video, audio or the most appropriate instrument);
- transcribing and analyzing the interviews;

The evaluation instrument was in the format of a semi-structured interview with a deaf user, with a view to the possibility of identifying barriers to and opportunities for innovation in the interface structure of the Moodle. This audience is characterized by communicating in a visual-spatial modality using Sign Language (SL). Because of the characteristics of communication and the history of different approaches in education, the deaf have difficulties with Portuguese in its written mode [3], [9], [11].

Within the group of deaf people, the profile defined for the data collection was that of deaf people who had had higher education, are teachers, and have a good command of Portuguese in its written form, and also of technology. This profile was determined while bearing in mind one of the dimensions of assessing the Moodle environment was to be evaluated. The choice aimed to identify how deaf people with a good knowledge of Portuguese evaluate the environment. In addition, the sample consisting of teachers set out to produce a vision of those who have daily contact with deaf students, and so are really involved in the processes of drawing up learning materials and content relevant to students.

The activity was applied in the context of an educational institution, the interviewees being three post-graduate deaf students, and teachers whose job it is to educate deaf people. Although the sample is small, the relevance of the respondents' profile of knowledge and activity was assessed as being extremely relevant. The interviews were conducted directly in Sign Language.

4 Results and Analysis

For discussion purposes, the results compiled from the analysis were summarized into five categories for discussion: the Portuguese language, viz., the relationship of the deaf with the Portuguese language in its written form; the need for value to be given to their own language, namely the Brazilian Sign Language (Libras); matters related to the visuality of the deaf, and the use of visual resources; and finally, the question of Distance Education and of the new tools and technologies as means to facilitate the education of the deaf. Each of the categories is described below.

4.1 The Portuguese Language

Despite their being deaf and yet having a high level of education and a good command of the Portuguese language, the respondents emphasized their difficulties with long texts as well as the difficulty of navigating a menu structure based on texts. The difficulty stems from their not knowing certain written words/ terms in Portuguese, as well as the cognitive effort they spend on the activity of reading. The turmoil that oral languages in the written form cause the deaf has been reported in the literature [3] [4] [9] [11] and derive from the approaches to educating deaf people that until recently they set in phonocentric logic.Another important question was with regard to the use of subtitles in videos, when the time set for reading is often not enough for deaf people to be able to follow the text properly. There is no denying the importance of this resource, but they are not always effective in their objective. However, respondents reported that the subtitles are sometimes very fast or have words that are unknown to the deaf. Similar arguments were identified when using interaction and communication tools, such as chat, which in practice has textual resources.

4.2 Giving Value to Sign Language, Called LIBRAS in Portuguese

All respondents were emphatic about the need to include resources in Libras or linked to it, such as SignWriting, to improve the accessibility of the AVEAs. SignWriting is the written form of sign language. [13]

4.3 Visual Resources

The importance of visuals also gained prominence in the search environment precisely because of the characteristics inherent in the mode of visual-spatial communication used by the deaf in SL. At various times in the interviews, the deaf reported the need for the presence of visual resources in the virtual environment and the materials and activities therein developed. Therefore, it is appropriate to reflect on the quality of the messages conveyed by visual elements. These should be used in order to inform, and to aid communication, besides meeting aesthetic ends.

4.4 Distance Learning and New Tools

The technological media combined with the Internet and its possibilities for communication, create opportunities to develop and evolve Distance Education. In Brazil, there are still few initiatives really targeted on the deaf. Starting in 2006, the Letters-Libras Distance Learning Program (BA and Licentiate in Brazilian Sign Language) of the Federal University of Santa Catarina (UFSC) in its face-to-face and distance modes is considered a pioneer and remains a reference centre for the deaf community. All respondents at some point cited the AVEA of that course, emphasizing that the interface and tools of the environment bring greater stimulus to its users. Reports give evidence of the need to develop a greater number of research studies and initiatives from the perspective of someone who is deaf.

5 Final Remarks

This article set out to present a case study on evaluating the accessibility evaluation of the Moodle environment for an audience of deaf users, who use the Brazilian Sign Language. By virtue of the specificities of the audience of this study, a set of reflections on the use of the interview technique could be raised. For effective results, it is important that barrier-free communication is carried out so that it is fluid.

The results, even though from a restricted sample, enabled reflections to be made on the deaf, who have a culture and a language of their own, but who are placed within a context where the vast majority do have hearing. Using indications from the deaf respondents' reports and by further reading, the need for in-depth studies became explicit as to the elements that lend greater accessibility to an AVEA. There is need to reflect on the current standards of design environments in order to exploit the visual-spatial communication characteristics of the deaf. The development of navigation features and support materials must not only be giving the logic of thought of oral languages, using transcripts and captions. Besides this, current technologies allow new features to be designed which bear the specificities of the deaf in mind. A proposal has been identified regarding the use of video in activities that normally take place in the form of preparation of written texts, quizzes and discussion forums. There is a need to propose new, more visual tools given that innovations which explore strategies for visual narratives and the visualization of knowledge lie in fertile ground for developing research in the field of teaching and learning in virtual environments.

For more effective results regarding the accessibility of the environment of this study, it is important that the same procedure be applied to deaf students with other educational profiles and that their profiles are identified using an AVEA. What is also recommended is the use of other participatory processes when evaluating and redesigning an AVEA interface so that drafting the concepts to be proposed is carried out by involving users to a greater extent.

References

1. Ceraulo, S.: Benefits of Upgrading to an LMS. Distance Education Report, 6–7 (2005)
2. Creswell, J.W.: Projeto de pesquisa: métodos qualitativo, quantitativo e misto. Artmed, Porto Alegre (2010)
3. El-Soud, M.A., et al.: A Proposed Web Based E-Learning and Dictionary Framework for Deaf Arab Students. IJECS/IJENS 10(1) (2010)
4. Huenerfauth, M.: American Sign Language Spatial Representations for an Accessible User-Interface. In: Proceedings of the 3rd International Conference on Universal Access in Human-Computer Interaction (2005)
5. IBGE, Instituto Brasileiro de Geografia e Estatística: Censo 2010 (2010)
6. Lakatos, E.M., de Marconi, M.A.: Metodologia Científica, 5th edn. Atlas, São Paulo (2011)
7. Moodle: Modular Object-Oriented Dynamic Learning Environment (2013), `http://www.moodle.org`
8. Neto, C.M., Ulbricht, V.R., Gutierrez, A.J.C.: Teoria da Atividade e suas Contribuições à Organização do Trabalho Docente em AVAA: o caso Polvo. In: Ulbricht, V.R., Pereira, A.T.C. (eds.) Hipermídia: Desafios da Atualidade, pp. 173–202. Pandiom, Florianópolis (2009)
9. Ottaviano, S., Merlo, G., Chifari, A., Chiazzese, G., Seta, L., Allegra, M., Samperi, V.: The Deaf and Online Comprehension Texts, How Can Technology Help? In: Miesenberger, K., Klaus, J., Zagler, W., Karshmer, A. (eds.) ICCHP 2010, Part II. LNCS, vol. 6180, pp. 144–151. Springer, Heidelberg (2010)
10. Preece, J., Rogers, Y., Sharp, H.: Design de Interação- Além da interação homem-computador. Bookman, Porto Alegre (2005)
11. de Quadros, R.M.: O ‘bi’ do bilingüismo na educação de surdos. In: Surdez e Bilingüismo, 1st edn., vol. 1, pp. 26–36. Editora Mediação, Porto Alegre (2005)
12. Santa Rosa, J.G., de Moraes, A.: Design Participativo. Rio Book’s, RJ (2012)
13. Stumpf, M.: Aprendizagem de Escrita de Língua de Sinais pelo Sistema SignWriting: Língua de Sinais no Papel e no Computador. [Tese]... Pós-graduação em Informática na Educação - Universidade Federal do Rio Grande do Sul, Porto Alegre (2005)
14. WCAG20: Web Content Accessibility Guidelines (WCAG) 2.0 (2008), `http://www.w3.org/TR/WCAG20/`

Design Touch Feedback for Blind Users

Shuang Xu and Kyle Bailey

Lexmark International, Inc.
740 West Circle Road, Lexington, KY 40550, USA
{shxu,kbailey}@lexmark.com

Abstract. Touch-screen interfaces do not offer tactile cues for the visually impaired users to distinguish interaction controls. As touch based interactions become more pervasive in our everyday lives, they present critical accessibility concerns. The recent advancement of touch screen technology makes design solutions possible. This research investigates the usability of accessible solutions on touch interfaces. Findings from our user study suggest that (1) proper voice feedback enables blind users to navigate touch-screen interface; and (2) different touch gestures have significantly different impacts on blind users' touch performances, such as efficiency and accuracy.

Keywords: Accessibility, touch interaction, gesture, auditory feedback.

1 Introduction

With the rapid advent of smart phones such as iPhone and Droid, touch screens are becoming pervasive across a wide range of technologies in our everyday lives. Touch based interactions are used in not only smart phones, but also personal computers (e.g., Windows 8), public kiosks, bank ATMs, printers, and various home appliances. This presents critical accessibility concerns for the 285 million world-wide visually impaired people [1].

Different from the physical controls on traditional interfaces, touch interfaces do not offer tactile cues to distinguish interaction controls and are extremely visual-demanding. In addition, the action controls and their positions vary from screen to screen, which makes it impossible for blind users to learn and remember the function and location of each control. As the physical keypad, knobs, buttons disappear from mobile phones, microwaves, and printers, it significantly reduces the degree of independence and equal opportunities for the visually impaired community.

A large body of research has been carried out in the last decade to improve the accessibility of touch interfaces [2-7]. These innovative techniques can be categorized in three areas: (1) gesture based interaction, (2) screen overlays with haptic or vibration for tactile feedback, and (3) earcons or readout as auditory feedback. These approaches alleviate the accessibility concern, but not without problems. Gesture interaction allows fast but less accurate input. It brings new challenges to the blind users as 82% of the blind people are 50 years and older [1] and many have cognitive or motor disabilities [8]. It is difficult for them to remember, distinguish, and accu-

C. Stephanidis (Ed.): Posters, Part I, HCII 2013, CCIS 373, pp. 281–285, 2013.

rately reproduce the required gestures like sighted users [9]. Tactile feedback helps because many visually impaired users are spatial and pressure sensitive [10]. However, the static physical overlays suffer from its inflexibility. Similarly, very limited information can be conveyed via the non-speech earcons or vibro-tactile feedback.

New solutions are made possible by the recent advancement in interaction technology. Tactus [11] provides a tactile solution by enabling application-controlled transparent physical buttons that dynamically rise up from the touch surface on demand. Neonode [12] introduces Z-force to allow accurate detection of different pressure on the touch screen. With such opportunities becoming available, this research investigates the usability and feasibility of accessible solutions on touch interfaces. We are particularly interested in understanding how to design touch gestures and feedback that are natural and effective, easy to use, and optimized for efficiency.

2 Experiment Design and Procedure

Our investigation comprised the following three phases:

Phase I. We carried out one-on-one interviews with 6 visually impaired participants (36 to 74 years old, 3 females and 3 males) to identify their needs and concerns with touch based interactions. All interviews focused on the discussion of how everyday activities were supported (or limited) by technologies. The outcome of the interviews has confirmed the increasing accessibility challenges introduced by touch screen interaction. For example, several participants mentioned that they had to add Braille tags on their home appliances to be able to identify the control buttons. Participants' top requests for accessibility improvement include:

- Equal opportunities to access information and technologies as sighted people.
- To use mainstream devices via effective yet inexpensive assistive technologies.
- Adjustable speed for screen read-out to optimize efficiency.
- Auditory feedback on the touch interface of home appliances and office devices.
- Simple and intuitive touch gesture that is easy to discover, remember, and use.

Phase II. We implemented the following five interaction methods (see Table 1) to investigate users' task performance (speed and accuracy) and satisfaction.

Table 1. Gestures examined in the users study

		Gesture to activate the selection			
		Press down	**Lift finger**	**Single tap**	**Double tap**
Gesture for speech feedback	**Touch**	Method 1	Method 2	Method 3	Method 4
	Single tap	(N/A)	(N/A)	(N/A)	Method 5

Eight (8) participants were recruited for this within-subject evaluation. Each participant completed 15 tasks, 3 tasks on each of the five prototypes. They were asked to start from a pre-defined screen position to locate a pre-defined target (on a 3x 3 grid-layout) as quickly and accurately as possible. Task assignments were randomized to reduce learning effect. We evaluated the five methods by examining participants' (1) task completion time, (2) error rate, and their perceived (3) ease of use, (4) learnability, (5) satisfaction. We also asked participant to indicate their preferred readout speed and overall ranking of the five interfaces. (Note: We will complete the data collection in Phase II with a total of twelve participants.)

Phase III. Based on the results from Phase II, we will adjust the proposed solution accordingly to develop a prototype that simulates the printer interaction experience. Participants in Phase II will be re-recruited in this follow-up study. The evaluation in Phase III includes more complex tasks such as making copies with changed settings, faxing a document to a given 10-digit number, and sending a scanned document to an email address. The complexity of these tasks allows us to further examine users' perceived effectiveness and efficiency of various (1) speech feedback and (2) audio confirmation of selection.

3 Preliminary Findings

As of the submission of this paper, we have completed the data collection of the first eight participants (4 totally blind, 4 legally blind.) in Phase II. One-way Analysis of Variance (ANOVA) was used to analyze the quantitative data collected in this study. Preliminary findings are discussed in the following sections.

3.1 Task Completion Time

Task completion time was defined as the time elapsed from starting to selecting the target item. Different gestures had a significant effect on completion time ($F_{4,115}$=5.04, p=.001), see Table 2. However, the difference was not significant ($F_{3,92}$=0.47, p=.704) amongst the first four gestures (touch-press, touch-lift, touch-tap, and touch-double tap). The main contributors to the difference in task completion time are (1) navigation gestures (touch vs. tap), where $Mean_{touch}$=25.88s, $Mean_{tap}$=60.14s ($F_{1,118}$=19.59, p<.001); and (2) selection gestures (non-double-tap vs. double-tap), where $Mean_{non\text{-}d\text{-}tap}$=26.06s, $Mean_{d\text{-}tap}$=42.73s ($F_{1,118}$=6.29, p=.014).

Table 2. Task Completion Time (in seconds)

	Touch-Press	Touch-Lift	Touch-Tap	Touch-Double Tap	Tap-Double Tap
All	23.41	31.50	23.27	25.33	60.14
Totally Blind	42.46	45.61	35.52	35.11	103.14
Legally Blind	11.98	23.03	15.92	19.46	34.33

Participants' vision status also affected their task efficiency. In general, legally blind participants (i.e., central visual acuity of 20/200 or less) were able to complete tasks faster than totally blind participants (i.e., no vision): $Mean_{LegalBlind}$=20.95s, $Mean_{TotalBlind}$=52.37s ($F_{1,118}$=25.11, p<.001). A significant interaction between Gesture and Vision was identified in this study ($F_{4,110}$=5.84, p<.001).

3.2 Error Rate

Error rate was measured as the total number of wrong selections divided by the total number of tasks. Results indicated that error rate was significantly impacted by different gestures ($F_{4,115}$=3.28, p=.014), see Table 4. Error rate with tapping-for-feedback was about 5 times higher than touching-for-feedback: $Mean_{Touch}$=10.42%, $Mean_{Tap}$=50.00% ($F_{1,118}$=10.15, p=.002). Double tapping for selection had much higher error rate than other selection gestures: $Mean_{non\text{-}d\text{-}tap}$=9.72%, $Mean_{d\text{-}tap}$=31.25% ($F_{1,118}$=4.30, p=.040). Error rate was also affected by participants' vision ($F_{1,118}$=5.26, p=.024) and age range ($F_{1,118}$=5.30, p=.023), but not gender ($F_{1,118}$=2.33, p=.128).

Table 3. Error Rate

	Touch-Press	Touch-Lift	Touch-Tap	Touch-Double Tap	Tap-Double Tap
All	0.00%	4.17%	25.00%	12.50%	50.00%
Totally Blind	0.00%	11.11%	55.56%	33.33%	66.67%
Legally Blind	0.00%	0.00%	6.67%	0.00%	40.00%

3.3 Subjective Ratings

Subjective ratings were collected on a Likert Scale (Perception: 1-lowest, 7-highest. Ranking: 1-lowest, 5-highest). No significant difference was found among the perception ratings (see Table 4), except Ease of Use ($F_{4,35}$=3.46, p=.017). Whether to touch or tap for speech feedback had a significant impact on perceived Ease of Use, where $Mean_{touch}$=6.3, $Mean_{tap}$=4.5 ($F_{1,38}$=13.91, p=.001). Perceived Learnability was rated higher by younger participants: $Mean_{35\text{-}44yr}$=7.0, $Mean_{55\text{-}74yr}$=6.4 ($F_{1,38}$=10.69, p=.002).

Table 4. Subjective Ratings and Overall Ranking

	Touch-Press	Touch-Lift	Touch-Tap	Touch-Double Tap	Tap-Double Tap
Ease of use (1~7)	6.375	5.938	6.375	6.375	4.500
Easy to learn (1~7)	6.500	6.875	6.875	6.750	6.500
Satisfaction (1~7)	5.750	6.188	6.500	6.313	5.125
Overall ranking (1~5)	2.875	3.000	3.625	3.250	2.250

4 Discussion and Future Work

Participants' comments explained why tapping-for-feedback was particularly difficult for blind users: (a) it had no point of reference – for totally blind users, tapping to find target was like "taking a stab in the dark"; (b) it was very easy to miss the target – sometimes they tapped on a target but moved away too quickly and missed the voice feedback; (c) continuous tapping on the same target was registered as a double-tap, which resulted in errors rather than voice feedback; and (d) several participants were able to find the target quickly, but they tapped slightly off the target, and had to spend much more time to re-find and select the target. In addition, the speed of double-tap varied individually, which made it difficult for the system to distinguish a slow double-tap from two quick single-taps. Other interesting findings are summarized below:

- Preferred speech rate for blind users is 256 words/minute (from 187 to 421wpm).
- Touching/sliding to navigate would have worked more effectively if the screen had different textures or haptic feedback for action area vs. non-action area.
- Lift-to-select was easy to use and to learn. But some concerned that they might make many mistakes if accidentally lifted finger off the wrong target.

We expect to finish data collection in Phase II and Phase III soon. Design guidelines will be proposed in the completed paper. We believe that results from this in-depth investigation will shed light on how to improve accessible design on touch interfaces universally. Applications of our design guidelines should provide blind users with easier access to information and technologies.

References

1. World Health Organization. New Global Estimates on Visual Impairment, `http://www.emro.who.int/control-and-preventions-of-blindness-and-deafness/announcements/global-estimates-on-visual-impairment.html` (cited October 10, 2012)
2. Kane, S.K., Bigham, J.P., Wobbrock, J.O.: Slide Rule: Making Mobile Touch Screens Accessible to Blind People Using Multi-Touch Interaction Techniques. In: Proceedings of ASSETS 2011, pp. 73–80. ACM Press, NewYork (2008)
3. Guerreiro, T., Nicolau, H., Jorge, J., Goncalves, D.: NavTap: A Long Term Study with Excluded Blind Users. In: Proceedings of ASSETS 2009, pp. 99–106. ACM Press, New York (2009)
4. Ferati, M., Mannheimer, S., Bolchini, B.: Acoustic Interaction Design through "Audemes": Experiences with the Blind. In: Proceedings of SIGDOC 2009, pp. 23–28. ACM Press, New York (2009)
5. Vidal, S., Lefebvre, G.: Gesture Based Interaction for Visually-Impaired People. In: Proceedings of NordiCHI 2010, pp. 809–812. ACM Press, New York (2010)
6. Parente, P., Bishop, G.: BATS: The Blind Audio Tactile Mapping System. In: Proceedings of ACM South Eastern Conference 2003 (2003)
7. Su, J., Rosenzweig, A., Goel, A., Lara, E., Truong, K.N.: Timbermap: Enabling the Visually-Impaired to Use Maps on Touch-Enabled Devices. In: Proceedings of MobileCHI 2010, pp. 17–26. ACM Press, New York (2010)
8. Kane, S.K., Jayant, C., Wobbrock, J.O., Ladner, R.E.: Freedom to Roam: A Study of Mobile Device Adoption and Accessibility for People with Visual and Motor Disabilities. In: Proceedings of ASSETS 2009, pp. 115–122. ACM Press, New York (2009)
9. Kane, S.K., Wobbrock, J.O., Ladner, R.E.: Usable Gestures for Blind People: Understanding Preference and Performance. In: Proceedings of CHI 2011, pp. 413–422. ACM Press, New York (2011)
10. Oliveira, J., Guerreiro, T., Nicolau, H., Jorge, J., Goncalves, D.: Blind People and Mobile Touch-based Text-Entry: Acknowledging the Need for Different Flavors. In: Proceedings of ASSETS 2011, pp. 179–186. ACM Press, New York (2011)
11. Tactus. White paper, `http://www.tactustechnology.com` (cited October 10, 2012)
12. Neonode Technology, `http://www.neonode.com` (cited October 10, 2012)

Development of Recognition System of Japanese Sign Language Using 3D Image Sensor

Yanhua Sun, Noriaki Kuwahara, and Kazunari Morimoto

Graduate School of Science and Technology Kyoto Institute of Technology Matsugasaki, Sakyo, Kyoto 606-85858, Japan
oo_alison@hotmail.com
{noriaki.kuwahara,morix119}@gmail.com

Abstract. The population of Japanese people with disabilities is growing day by day. And the population of sign language translator is too few to support them. In general life, people communicate with others through conversation but this is obviously impossible for deaf mute people who use sign language to communicate. So it is necessary to explore a recognition system of sign language which can help the deaf and mute to keep in touch with others. In order to solve that problem, a large amount of researches related to recognition system development and establishment have been reported by previous literatures. However, current paper introduced a novel method for system developing. In this paper, 3D sensors called Kinect were employed for hand gesture dataset's collection following by data dealing from transformation matrix based on specific formulas. Although the hand gesture can be captured, but there still are a lot of noises left, so PCL (Point Cloud Library) was applied to do the 3D data processing.

Keywords: Japanese Sign Language, Kinect, Recognition of JSL, 3D Sensor.

1 Introduction

In Japan, the population of people with disabilities who are deaf and mute or hard of hearing and speaking is about 2.7million. It is said that about 3 thousand people do a job as a sign language translator. There are so little people to support the deaf and mute. In general life, people take the communication with the others through talking, but it is impossible for the deaf mute people, who can take the communication with others just using sign language. So it is necessary to explore a recognition system of sign language, which can help the deaf and mute to keep touch with others.

So developing a recognition system of sign language is the purpose of this paper. About the system, Sign language recognition is such a system which translate the picture of the sign language to data, and then translate the data to words, sentences or sounds. This paper presents the front part of the recognition system. Several ways are used to research the sign language recognition, such as Facial movement analysis in ASL [5], human detection [3], 3D model tracking [4] and so on. But in most of the researches, even though they carry important grammatical and prosodic information, the rate of the recognition is still low.

C. Stephanidis (Ed.): Posters, Part I, HCII 2013, CCIS 373, pp. 286–290, 2013.

For increasing the rate of the recognition, we think that the most important step is taking a 3D data with the least noise. First we decided to use two Kinects to take the 3D data. Each kinect can take a part of hand, and if we can do a data combination, so that we can take more data of hand. The second step, we plan to do a 3D data processing with PCL. PCL is an abbreviation of Point Cloud Library. The Point Cloud Library (PCL) is a standalone, large scale, open project for 2D/3D image and point cloud processing. Use the advantage of the PCL, it not only can take the noise away, but also can reconstruct the surface of the hand, in some means, it can increase the rate of the recognition, however, the step of superimpose is introduced only in this paper.

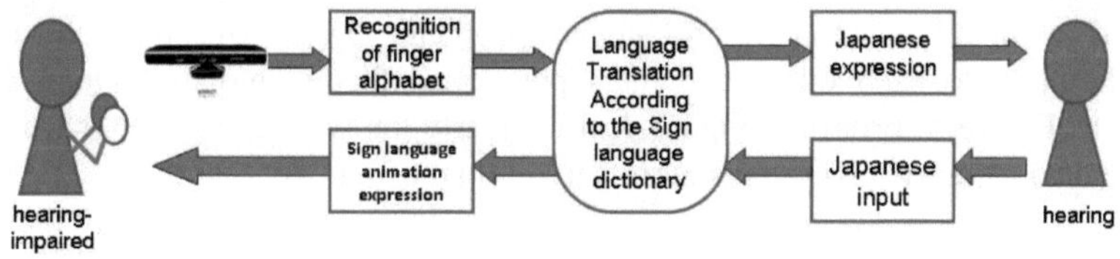

Fig. 1. Recognition system of finger gesture

2 Method and Condition

2.1 Research Condition

Launched in November 2010, Kinect is a motion sensing USB (Universal Serial Bus) input device by Microsoft that enables users to control and naturally interact with games and other programs without the need to physically touch a game controller or object of any kind. Kinect achieves this through a natural user interface by tracking the user's body movement and by using gestures and spoken commands [1, 2]. Kinect holds the Guinness World Record as the fastest selling consumer electronics device, with sales surpassing 10 million units as of 9 March 2011. Kinect works in all room

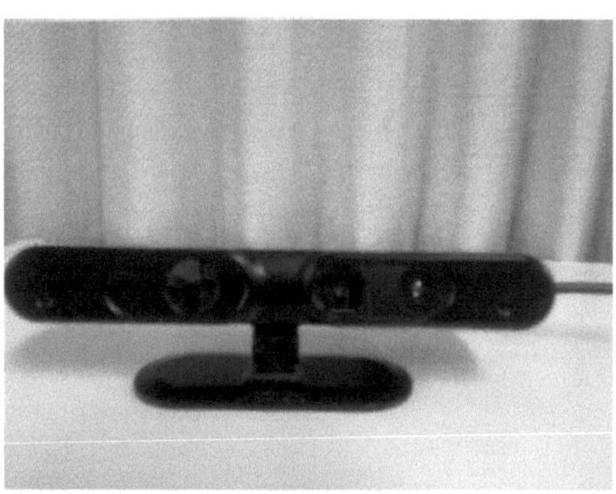

Fig. 2. Kinect Xtion

lighting conditions, whether in complete darkness or in a fully lit room, and does not require the user to wear or hold anything. Prime Sense also teamed up with ASUS to develop a PC-compatible device similar to Kinect, which they called ASUS Xtion and launched in the second quarter of 2011. Running proprietary firmware (internal device software), these components together can provide full-body 3-D option capture, gesture recognition, facial recognition, and voice recognition capabilities.

2.2 Research Methods

As it had been introduced, the Kinect is a strong powerful sensor, but it also has weakness. Certainly the front part of hand was easily captured and record by Kinect, however the data of side-part often be leaked without receiving. So in this part, we proposed a novel method to solve the problem. Two Kinects were located perpendicularly to each other, and hand positioned facing into the central of two Kinects as Figure 3. From the Figure 4, it is clearly known that no matter from each side, the data using two Kinects is more perfect than using one.

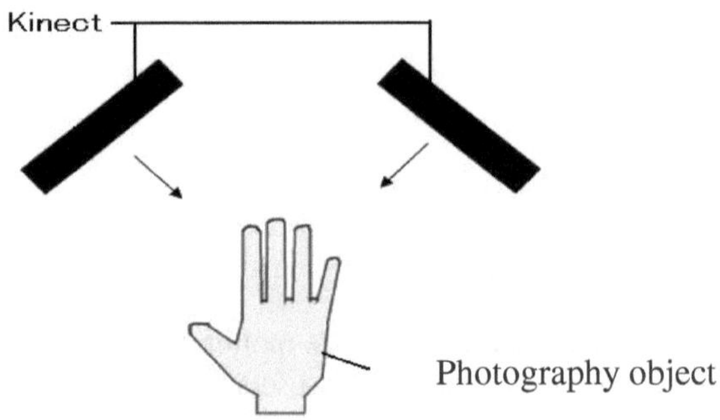

Fig. 3. Recognition system of finger gesture

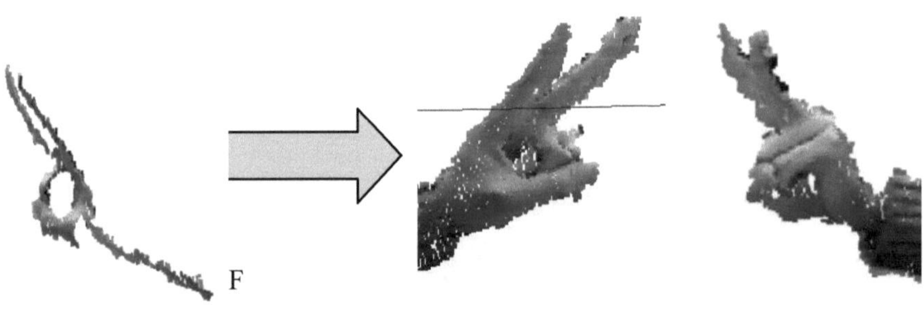

Fig. 4. Dataset combination

3 Experimental Results

3.1 Superimpose

For better analysis on two groups dataset's overlapping from two Kinects, datasets were illustrated in Figure.4 in the form of two-dimension plotting which were departed from original 3D dataset. In which, red circle expressed the measuring range, the blue one expressed all space and the green one expressed the range of parameter. Circles were smaller, more accurate the positions can be captured and recognized. Therefore, the points fell within parameters' scope were found smaller than outside of parameter range. However it also demonstrated that a lot of noises need to be removed, which can be done by the method introduced afterwards.

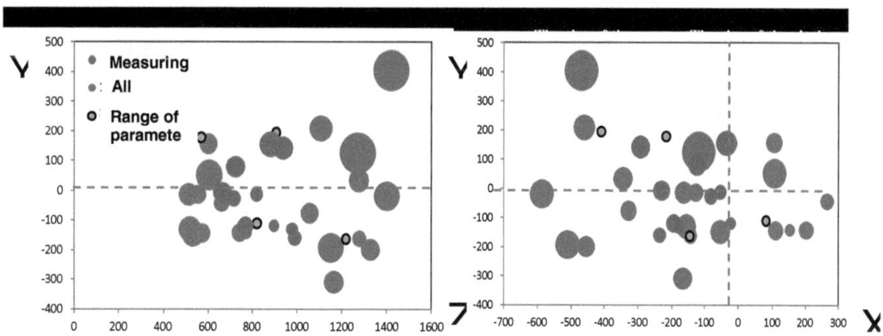

Fig. 5. Recognition system of finger gesture

4 Conclusions

We proposed to develop a recognition system of sign language with a 3D sensor in this research. To date, we had done the important first step, generating 3D data from the sensors. Until now, although Kinect had been used to research in all kinds of areas, this kind of method had not been reported. However the previous research still takes us very important messages and it is a very important part for us to research the recognition system of sign language.

3D camera was utilized in evaluating the sign language recognition system. 3D sensor is useful for developing sign-language recognition system because it is very easy to extract a hand shape. From the previous research it is said that the recognition rate of the finger alphabets was about 40%, and low recognition rate was the biggest problem. Through the method of using two Kinects, we found that we can get more datasets of hand than use one, from the section 2, it is fully proved that the data of superposition can construct hand gesture more consummately.

About the future research, the most main work is 3D processing and evaluation of the system of sign language. PCL had been introduced as a powerful filtering in this paper. Therefore 3D data processing will be implemented using PCL. Although the previous job had been finished as it was expected, it is not sure whether the method and condition match the JSL system until we get the data of rate of recognition. Evaluating the datasets which had not been processed and which had been can prove the significance of the proposed approach, so we will use some ways to evaluate the rate of the recognition. In future study it is the most important to perfect the JSL recognition system as much as possible.

References

1. Kinect Official Web Site, `http://www.xbox.com/kinect/`
2. Kinect, `http://en.wikipedia.org/w/index`
3. Xia, L., Chen, C.-C., Aggarwal, J.K.: Human Detection Using Depth Information by Kinect (2011)
4. Oikonomidis, I., Kyriazis, N., Argyros, A.: Efficient Model-based 3D tracking of Hand Articulations using Kinect (2011)
5. Vogler, C., Goldenstein, S.: Facial movement analysis in ASL (2007)

Part IV
Multimodal and Ambient Interaction

Smart Watches for Home Interaction Services

Gerald Bieber[1], Nicole Fernholz[2], and Mirko Gaerber[2]

[1] Fraunhofer IGD, Joachim-Jungius-Strasse 11, 18059 Rostock, Germany
gerald.bieber@igd-r.fraunhofer.de
[2] Basis Computer und Systemintegration GmbH, Luebsche Straße 187, Wismar, Germany
{nicole.fernholz,mirko.gaerber}@basis-wismar.de

Abstract. The demography of the Federal Republic of Germany predicts that the average age of the society rises in future. A generation ago, elderly people died only a couple of years after being retired. Nowadays elderly people enjoy their after work-life for approx. 20 additional years. These are very active and they enjoy traveling, meeting friends or find new purposes in life. The research project "Home Interaction Service" develops new mobile assistants by using Smart Watches for continuously monitoring of physical activities to identify life anomalies and to assist elderly people in their daily life. New algorithm also enables the Smart Watch also to be a new gesture interaction device to control home consumer products and to support new services that might become available in future.

Keywords: SmartWatch, Activity, Sleep, Pattern Recognition, Acceleration Sensor, Mobile Assistance.

1 Motivation

In future, the demographic change will affect the everyday life of elderly people. Years ago, each generation of a family lived together in one household and they did take care about each other. Nowadays the family is separated; elderly people often are living for their own or left alone in nursing homes. Furthermore, the low birth rate leads to the circumstance that fewer children can take care and communicate for a higher number of parents and grandparents. In the most European countries, the birth rate is very low. In Germany the total fertility rate has been rated around 1.4 in 2010 [1] but should be about 2 to ensure a constant population.

A century ago, elderly died in relatively young age (only a short period after their retirement), now people become much older. Even ill people who would die in the past are today obtaining a good medical care and enjoy additional years of living. This leads to the condition that the relation of available caregivers to elderly people is decreasing tremendously.

The elderly people in the age between 65+ and 85 are a new class of people in our society, the fit elderly. Some of the elderly people are using computer, mobile phones and touch pads, but the internet communication services are not well designed for them.

C. Stephanidis (Ed.): Posters, Part I, HCII 2013, CCIS 373, pp. 293–297, 2013.

Elderly people are used to wear wrist watches. Currently the technological progress provides a new kind of watches on the market: Smart Watches. Smart Watches with integrated sensor functionality and wireless connectivity are capable to provide new methods of user support. These devices are inexpensive and enabling a new usage of internet services for elderly people.

The aim of this work is to show that the integrated sensors of Smart Watch recognizes not only physical activity such as walking, doing homework or car driving but also provide important information about periods of being physically and socially inactive. Hereby a new algorithm enables a detection of the duration and performance of sleep, periods of recovery and number of received or sent messages and compares these parameters to activity pattern during the day.

2 Related Work

2.1 Hardware

Smart Watches are wrist watches with additional computer functionalities. Smart Watches provide a wireless connectivity to a phone or to the internet. An important component is the sensing feature of acceleration forces. The first Smart Watches were designed in the early 80s to be a permanent but small “window to internet news” [5]. Nowadays the main functionality of a Smart Watch is the displaying of short messages, e.g. SMS, facebook-, RSS messages, or incoming calls. One of the main advantages of smart watches is not to have to take the phone out of the pocket, to see who is calling.

Current models of Smart Watches provide a micro display in the dimension of approx. 100 x 100 pixel, an acceleration sensing with 32 Hz and Bluetooth connectivity. Some watches can´t compute data on board, they are event triggered. These watches have to transmit every event (display touch, button event, sensing data) via Bluetooth to a smart phone. Also the other way round, the action events (vibration, screen display) are also to transmit wirelessly which costs a lot of transmission energy on both devices.

The other type of watches are capable to process all data on board, a wireless connection is only needed for external data exchange. Depending on the hardware, internal design and application purposes, the battery stamina is about a week. For future watch models the prediction is a battery lifetime of up to a year.

Figure 1 shows a commercial Smart Watch (Meta Watch [6]), equipped with an activity recognition algorithm. The watch itself contains an integrated 3D acceleration sensor, light sensor, Bluetooth connectivity, 96x96 pixel monochrome display and 256kb ram/flash memory.

2.2 Application

The main purpose of Smart Watches is the usage of the micro displays to present various messages. For displaying social messages (by e.g. facebook) the watch need the access to the internet. Specialized hardware is designed to be applied in nursery or private homes to monitor elderly or handicapped people. The manufacture of Limmix watch, a device with integrated GSM module, Loudspeaker and microphone, is the world first watch which directly can call the emergency [4] by pressing an emergency button. Other watches [7] are using ISM connectivity to send button triggered messages to a connected external device or a phone. This phone is able to send emergency calls with phone generated GPS positioning information.

The usage of a constantly worn sensor enables new interaction possibilities as well as a monitoring of physical activity or vital life signals. Industrial applications are using Smart Watches as an interaction device to control maintenance video on tablet PCs, which is not possible in case of wearing gloves or having greasy fingers [2]. The constantly monitoring of physical activity might allow an automatic emergency call in case of detected anomalies. The idea of internet of the things could be shown by the eWatch [3], designed to be one of many connected devices of the wearer or intelligent environment.

The commercial Sophia Vivago watches are used for monitoring elderly people [8] and are sending alarms in case of a detected inactivity. Even these devices are excellent for elderly monitoring, they don´t cover social connectedness or social interaction.

The potential of using of physical activity, inactivity, and sleep pattern or communication behavior will be used in our approach to achieve new communication input for a social communication between the generations.

3 Basic Concept

The combination of Smart Watches, tablet PCs and smart phones can be used for a new approach of an unobtrusive, social connectedness. The basic concept is to support elderly people by providing an easy to use and inexpensive monitoring and interaction system that opens the internet world for them. Hereby a digital picture frame (realized by an android tablet or digital t.v.) is used as the main gateway to the internet. The metaphor of a digital picture frame is used because the user is not forced to react immediately to the displayed information. Some elderly people enjoy having more time to receive and work with information. The concept of asynchrony also occurs on SMS or Emails but unfortunately only a few elderly people are used to these new technologies.

Because a digital picture frame is just displaying information, a further back channel is needed. This back channel can be realized by touch interaction on the screen of the device, similar to a browser webpage. Another very promising approach is the constantly monitoring of the user by the integrated sensors of the Smart Watches. Beside the effect of retrieving activity data, the wearer can use the Smart Watch as a gesture interaction device and remote control for other devices e.g. t.v., light control or other purposes. The ensemble of all these devices is collecting data about the frequency of the received and outgoing messages.

This concept enables that for instance the adult son can check if grandma is doing fine, he can communicate by electronic messages and is able to post pictures or messages to the grandma´s display. The elderly still can use traditional information methods, e.g. to write a note on a piece of paper with a pen and hold it in front of a camera for sending these picture messages to their relatives.

4 Project Home Interaction Services

The research project "HIS – Home Interaction Service" combines the given basic concepts and intents to let elderly people live comfortable and safe in their own homes. Primarily, HIS is developed for seniors and people needing care. HIS is a central communication platform, which provide transparent, simple to configure and user-friendly intelligent services to connect seniors with their family members, careers or other peoples. Beside easy messages or picture posting, various services can be integrated by external service-providers.

Furthermore, the project supports the connection of seniors with the younger generation, the Facebook generation. The family members can check if the elderly person is doing fine (anomaly recognition, sleep and unconsciousness separation), communicate by electronic messages or pictures. Finally a senior gets useful information i.e. medical reminder, food plan or important dates.

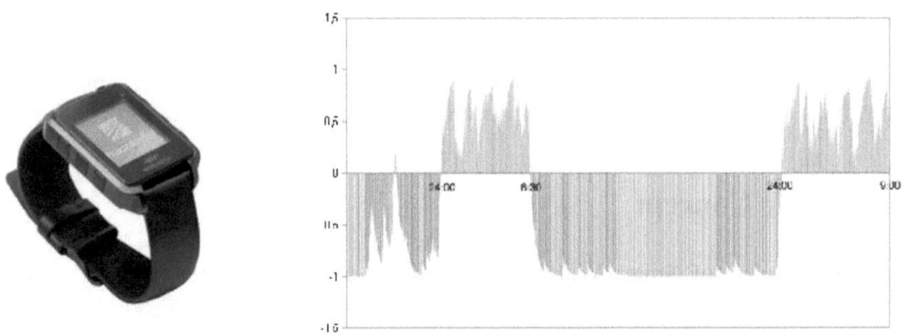

Fig. 1. Sleep (red) and Activity diagram (blue) of two days, recorded by a Smartwatch

HIS combines home automation and assistive technologies in the home environment for an ambient assisted living. The main features are security, health, comfort, information, activity, services, anomaly recognition supported by Smart Watches and social living. The frequency and quality of received or sent messages is checked and if someone seems to suffer of social communication, some auto-generated messages will transmit to the senior. Furthermore, coffee-meetings or other events between or with seniors will be automatically organized by electronically generated invitations (like senior flash-mob). The project HIS is funded by the Federal State of Mecklenburg-Vorpommern, Germany.

5 Conclusion and Future Work

Smart Watches are a new technology for the new generation of interaction, messaging (alarming) and micro displaying that is originally designed for the young internet generation. Smart Watches enable multiple application fields because of their free programming capabilities, the nice display and sensor functionality. Smart Watches will push especially elderly people into the world of internet. The research project "HIS – home interaction service" addresses new services and technologies to support healthy elderly people in their everyday life and enables their way into the internet. The first indicators show that Smart Watches and a specified backend technology are well suited for this purpose. The project HIS provides new services and possibilities, e.g. identification of anomalies, sleep recognition, gesture interaction.

The further work of this project is to improve activity monitoring with wrist worn sensors and to design a complete message pipe to the elderly people. This message pipe should provide the optimal tradeoff between too much information (information overflow) and only a few (seldom messages). This will raise the acceptance for the complete system.

References

1. Raftery, A., Alkema, L., Gerland, P., et al.: Probabilistic projections of the total fertility rate for all countries for the 2010 world population prospects. In: United Nations expert group meeting on recent and future trends in fertility (2009)
2. Bieber, G., Kirste, T., Urban, B.: Ambient Interaction by Smart Watches. In: International Conference on Pervasive Technologies Related to Assistive Environments, Petra 2012. ACM, Crete (2012)
3. Maurer, U., Rowe, A., Smailagic, A., Siewiorek, D.: eWatch: a wearable sensor and notification platform. In: International Workshop on Wearable and Implantable Body Sensor Networks. IEEE, Massachusetts (2006)
4. Limmex watch, Heinrichstrasse 267C, 8005 Zürich, Schweiz, Tel: +41 44 440 00 14, `https://www.limmex.com/de/de`
5. Krumm, J., Cermak, G., Horvitz, E.: RightSPOT: A novel sense of location for a smart personal object. In: Dey, A.K., Schmidt, A., McCarthy, J.F. (eds.) UbiComp 2003. LNCS, vol. 2864, pp. 36–43. Springer, Heidelberg (2003)
6. MetaWatch, Meta Watch, Ltd., Dallas, Texas | Espoo, Finland, phone: +1 469-278-META (6382), email: info@metawatch.org, `http://www.metawatch.org`
7. Emporia Telecom, Produktions- und Vertriebs-GmbH & Co. KG, Industriezeile 36, A-4020 Linz, Austria, `http://www.emporia.eu`
8. Mattila, E., Korhonen, I., Merilahti, J., Nummela, A., Myllymaki, M., Rusko, H.: A concept for personal wellness management based on activity monitoring. In: Second International Conference on Pervasive Computing Technologies for Healthcare, PervasiveHealth 2008, pp. 32–36. IEEE (2008)

My Music Mosaic

Jaylyn Dawson, Vesna Dragojlov, Ryan Meuth, Amanda McIntyre,
Molly Satterfield, and Joshua Vargas

University of Advancing Technology, Tempe, AZ, USA
{jaydawso,vdragojlov,rmeuth,amamcint,molsatte,josvarga}@uat.edu

Abstract. All Greater Good Foundation, in conjunction with students and faculty at the University of Advancing Technology, are using music as a tool to help children and teenagers in difficult circumstances communicate and express themselves visually. The program called, My Music Mosaic, will connect to a musical keyboard which will allow for real time visual/emotional input. My Music Mosaic gets children who have experienced trauma in their lives to share their feelings in a more innovative manner. The team will be making connections to abstract emotions with input like time, sound, and force. Input is then transferred into shapes, transparency, line, three dimensions, size, color and movement on the computer.

Keywords: new forms of communication, music as communication, music and emotions, high risk teenagers use music to express themselves, music mosaic, turning music into visual art, visualizing music.

1 Introduction

This paper will be used to describe the methodology and research behind the My Music Mosaic program. It will show research into the users, decisions behind color and design choices as well as how it was implemented. At the end there is brief section about the user testing that has been conducted since the first version of the program came out.

2 Defining the Users

2.1 Context of San Diego

San Diego is located in Southern California by the Pacific Ocean. The average temperature is 70 degrees Fahrenheit [1]. The San Diego area was approximately 4,206 sq miles with an overall population of about 3,095,313 in the 2010 census [2]. According to the same census, the San Diego area was composed of approximately 26.5% or 821,263 children and teens under the age of 19. The mean household income is $63, 857. About 2.6% of the population were victims of a crime in 2010; this number increased to 2.8% in 2012 [3].

C. Stephanidis (Ed.): Posters, Part I, HCII 2013, CCIS 373, pp. 298–302, 2013.

2.2 Children and Teenagers

Teenagers and children born around 1994 or beyond are considered part of both Generation Y and Generation Z. Cell phones become prevalent around 1995 along with computers, meaning most children and teens of the Y and Z Generation have always known about or owned cell phones and computers. A recent Pew survey indicates that nearly 25% of teens use their cell phone to access the internet [4].

2.3 Victims of Abuse

Abuse. According to the National Child Traumatic Stress Network (NCTSN) in 1997 nationally 64% of 12 to 17 year olds experienced a traumatic event like being sexual assaulted, physically assaulted or witnessing violence [5]. In 2011 3.4 million referrals were made to Child Protective Services and 19% were sustained [6]. These victims suffered neglect, physical, and sexual abuse. According to Administration for Children and Families 76,644 children and teens under the age of 18 were abused in California in 2010 [7].

Treatment Programs. There are treatment programs like the San Diego Center for Children that offer support to children and teens that have had traumatic experiences happen to them. Places like this offer counseling and learning. It is not just physical safety that is important after a child or teen is abused, but also emotional safety as he or she tries to get used to a new environment [8]. My Music Mosaic was specifically requested as a way for children and teens living at this group facility to express their emotions and reduce stress as they become familiar with their new surroundings. The artwork created can then be shared and put up in their rooms to help them feel a sense of accomplishment and to help with feelings of loneliness or stress.

3 Color

3.1 Basic Color Schemes

Color Palettes. My Music Mosaic allows the user to choose his or her own color palettes. Each note on the keyboard is assigned a color value based on the color palette chosen. The color palettes themselves have been designed to take various themes inspired by popular culture, different kinds of sight and everyday life. Some of the basic color palettes include a rainbow palette, a shades-of-blue palette, and a shades-of-purple palette.

Perception. While considering the users and the original intention of the project, a decision was made to research the effect color can have on the mind. Colors can represent certain ideas and feelings based on previously-cemented perceptions [9]. While choosing the color palettes, the team chose to create colors that stereotypically represented these perceptions. For example, rainbows are usually representative of things that inspire happiness and excitement, while grays paired with dark blues might represent depression.

3.2 Color Blindness

When developing this program, some careful consideration was put into the fact that the team did not have access to specifics about the intended users. One avenue that was explored was color blindness, because one of the main components of the program was the use of color. Using a triadic color scheme, a color palette was created representing a few different types of colorblindness [10]. These color palettes were designed specifically for color blindness so the series of colors may appeal to someone with color blindness, but may not be appealing to those who do not have color blindness. Since these colors are not commonly seen together in what is considered normal vision, these color palettes explore different areas of expression.

3.3 Borrowing from the World

Many of the remaining color palettes that were not considered basic or for color blindness were designed represent colors of objects in everyday life or experiences in everyday life. Some of these palettes include a fire palette (composed of reds, oranges and yellows), a traffic palette (composed of yellows, reds, greens, grays, whites, and blues), and an ocean water palette (composed of various shades of blues and greens).

4 Design

4.1 Overall Aesthetic

The My Music Mosaic interface was designed to be especially accessible for children and teens. The program was designed to incorporate the idea that the user should be able to interact with the keyboard and program as intuitively and easily as possible. The design limits complicated interactions by hiding the save menu and not cluttering the start menu with too many options. This allows for the users to focus on playing music and not having to go through the process of learning a complex program beforehand.

4.2 User Interface

The beginning start screen was designed to be minimalistic so users can explore the variety of color pallets and change the background color at their leisure. If the user did not want to choose anything, they can just hit start and go with the default options to begin playing. As users choose different palettes and backgrounds, their choices are reflected in the My Music Mosaic title and the on-screen background changes. After pressing the start button, a simple message appears on-screen that communicates to the user that they can start playing and that they can click for the menu. Once the user starts playing with the keyboard, the message disappears and brushstrokes start to appear on screen representing the colors chosen from the color palette and the instrument they are using. When the user has finished playing, they can click the mouse to access the pause menu where they can save, start over, quit, or get help. The pause menu is designed in a similar art style as the main menu, so that the user knows that he or she is still in the program.

4.3 Brushes and Paths

The brushes that are used in the main part of the program were made by the designers to represent different kinds of real world art supplies. The different types of brushes are roller brush, palette knife, dry brush, paint splat, paint drip, watercolor, calligraphy, spray paint and chalk. Most of the brushes were composed of three separate images combined in the code. The reason for this is that some brushes follow a different path than other brushes when they are being drawn. Each of the splats consist of only one image, as these images were intended to show up on screen very quickly to represent percussion instruments. All of the brushes start on a sine wave and a random angle is chosen in code for where they get drawn, but their path is either another sine wave or a straight line.

5 Implementation

Open Source Programs
Since the project was being completed on behalf of a non-profit organization, the choice was made to create the project using open source technology. My Music Mosaic was created in Processing [11] using a library called proMIDI [12]. One programmer completed all of the programming for the project for the sake of consistency.

Variables
The location of brushes, the effect of holding down a note on a brush, and the size of the brushes were modified throughout the process using code. The location of a note is dependent on when the key is pressed, and follows the path of a sine wave. If a user hits a note hard, it will appear larger than if he or she played it softly. When a user plays the notes quickly, the brush will appear short, whereas if they hold a note it will appear much longer. Otherwise, the colors of the notes and the background of the program are chosen by the user at the start screen.

Iterations
From the programming aspect of the project, the first step was to learn how to read input from the musical keyboard to draw a line on the screen. The line drawn was based on the timing of the note. The program uses a black and white brush image that is then colored in the specific manner created by the designers. Color palettes were added once the brushes were perfected.

6 User Testing

The first round of user testing provided meaningful feedback. It was a small sampling of college-aged students who volunteered to try the program. The students were given a small survey before they tried using the program to compare how similar these users were to the target audience. The students were observed by the team using the program with little to no direction, to test how intuitive and easy the program was for a first-time user. Afterwards, they were given another longer survey to see if their mood had changed, whether they felt the program represented the music they were playing, and to give them a chance to explain any problems they encountered. The user-testing yielded clues about some of our menus, how users exit a program or menu and whether they read instructions. Further user testing will continue in May in San Diego with the intended users being observed and surveyed.

References

1. San Dieg, CA (2013), http://www.sandiego.org (accessed April 11, 2013)
2. U.S. Census Bureau, State and County Quick Facts (2013), http://quickfacts.census.gov (accessed April 11, 2013)
3. San Diego Police Department, San Diego, CA (2013), http://www.sandiego.gov/police/pdf/2013/UCRRates1950to2012.pdf (accessed April 11, 2013)
4. Pew Research Center, Washington, DC (2013), http://www.pewresearch.org/daily-number/a-quarter-of-teens-mostly-access-the-internet-using-their-cell-phones/ (accessed April 11, 2013)
5. The National Child Traumatic Stress Network, Facts and Figures (2000), http://www.nctsn.org (accessed April 11, 2013)
6. United States Department of Veteran Affairs, PTSD in Children and Adolescents (2012), http://www.ptsd.va.gov (accessed April 11, 2013)
7. Children's Bureau, Children maltreatment (2010), http://www.acf.hhs.gov (accessed April 11, 2013)
8. Child Welfare Information Gateway, Treatment for Abused and Neglected Children: Infancy to Age 18 (1994), https://www.childwelfare.gov (accessed April 11, 1994)
9. Lamancusa, K.: Emotional Reactions to Color. Creative Latitude (2003), http://www.creativelatitude.com/articles/articles_lamacusa_color.html (accessed April 11, 2013)
10. Stanicek, P.: Color Scheme Designer (2002-2010), http://colorschemedesigner.com/ (accessed April 11, 2013)
11. Fry, B., Reas, C.: Processing (2003), http://processing.org/ (accessed April 11, 2013)
12. proMIDI (2013), http://creativecomputing.cc/p5libs/promidi/ (accessed April 11, 2013)

MAGIC: Developing a Multimedia Gallery Supporting mid-Air Gesture-Based Interaction and Control

Giannis Drossis[1], Dimitris Grammenos[1], Chryssi Birliraki[1], and Constantine Stephanidis[1,2]

[1] Institute of Computer Science (ICS), Foundation for Research and Technology – Hellas (FORTH) N. Plastira 100, Vassilika Vouton, GR-700 13 Heraklion, Crete, Greece
[2] University of Crete, Department of Computer Science, Heraklion, Crete, Greece
{drossis,gramenos,birlirak,cs}@ics.forth.gr

Abstract. Touchless remote interaction empowers users to interact with systems at a distance without the burden of actually coming to physical contact with any tangible object. The research presented in this paper focuses on motion-based interaction in public spaces through hand detection using Microsoft's Kinect, in order to allow natural interaction in mid-air. The paper presents the development of a system that allows browsing and exploring large collections of multimedia information (images and videos).

Keywords: Interaction Design, touchless interaction, interactive media gallery, Kinect, hand tracking, public display.

1 Introduction

Multimedia information browsing is a common task that may apply to a wide set of activities, ranging from medical information systems to public displays in museums and exhibition spaces. The ongoing decrease of hardware cost is leading to the incorporation of touchless interaction technologies in a variety of application domains, e.g., the manipulation of every-day objects such as household appliances [3], in operating rooms during surgery operations [7], etc. The majority of such systems in the past involved wearable components such as gloves or specially designed clothes. However, Microsoft's Kinect has been a breakthrough in terms of precision and responsiveness and is therefore widely adopted for supporting various natural interaction techniques such as 3D reconstruction, speech recognition and skeleton tracking [2]. Its primary advantages include a relatively low cost, the provision of both depth and RGB cameras and the lack of strict lightning requirements.

Touchless interaction is mostly accomplished through gestures, which are defined by Kendon [5] as "a label for actions that have the features of manifest deliberate expressiveness". Gestures are widely used supplementary to other interaction modes to accomplish specific tasks, providing a natural way of interaction similar to every-day human to human communication. For instance, a user may respond to a yes/no

C. Stephanidis (Ed.): Posters, Part I, HCII 2013, CCIS 373, pp. 303–307, 2013.

dialogue by raising or lowering his or her hand in order to communicate with a system. However, the inclusion of gestures in a system's interaction repertoire holds some important drawbacks, such as the necessity to memorize the rules defined by the interface in order to communicate with the system. Apart from task-specific gestures, another common procedure includes pointing with a hand in a specific direction so as to select an area or an object, usually using a cursor. In order to select items, many approaches exist in literature. For instance, Wilson et al. [9] embed a button in a physical wand in order to select items. Another approach suggests the application of a cursor dwell time threshold as a click event [4; 8]. Other solutions apply speech as a signal for making selections [1] but are limited by the addition of supplementary auditory constraints. Finally, another approach includes the combination of a small time threshold to focus on an item and successively a click in the air (by pushing and pulling) [6], in order to eliminate accidental selection.

2 MAGIC

2.1 System Design

The main goal of the MAGIC system is to provide a straightforward way for easily and efficiently browsing and exploring large collections of multimedia, i.e., images and videos, in public spaces. Some key requirements include that its users should be able to:

1. Have a quick overview of the entire collection.
2. Focus on a single item and obtain additional information (e.g., a short description) but also easily browse items in the vicinity of the selected one.
3. Zoom in the details of the selected item.

Based on the above, it was decided to support three distinct views/modes respectively:

1. A two-dimensional grid containing large thumbnails of the multimedia elements of the collection. Since the system is used from a certain distance, the thumbnails' size is fixed in order to ensure the visibility of their contents. Users can scroll the grid horizontally and vertically in order to view items which lie beyond the screen boundaries. To minimize the gesture distance between items located at opposite ends of the grid, the grid wraps around in both axes.
2. If users select to focus on a single item, it appears in full screen accompanied by a descriptive caption. This mode also allows scrolling to adjacent items on both axes, as well as changing the caption's language.
3. When in single view mode, users can utilize a magnified glass to zoom in on the details of the selected item.

In addition to the above, touchless interaction was deemed to be highly appropriate for public spaces for several reasons. First of all, it allows system manipulation from a distance, without the burden of physical contact, also avoiding hygiene-related issues and preserving the clearness of the visual display. Then, all the "fragile" technological components are situated far from the user's reach, thus minimizing potential vandalism acts. Last but not least, touchless interaction can support larger displays as well as interaction spaces, also allowing users to move around.

2.2 First Prototype

The first version of the system supported interaction through a small set of hand gestures. In order to initiate interaction, users had to wave their hand to "get the system's attention". To provide feedback about this fact, a waving hand appeared on the display when the system was inactive. Once interaction started, a virtual hand appeared over the grid of multimedia items, instantiating a cursor metaphor, i.e., the virtual hand moves in 1-1 correspondence to the user's one. Since the system is intended for use by a single person, any other hands are ignored until the current user's hand is no longer tracked. In order to select an image from the grid and view it at full size, the user had to perform a 'click' gesture over an item of interest. While viewing the item in detail, the user could perform swipe gestures (up, down, left or right) which resulted into scrolling to the adjacent item in the respective direction. The click gesture was used as a mechanism for toggling between different modes; i.e., clicking while viewing a single item resulted into entering zoom mode, where the hand worked as a virtual magnifying glass. A click in this mode would switch the system into the grid mode.

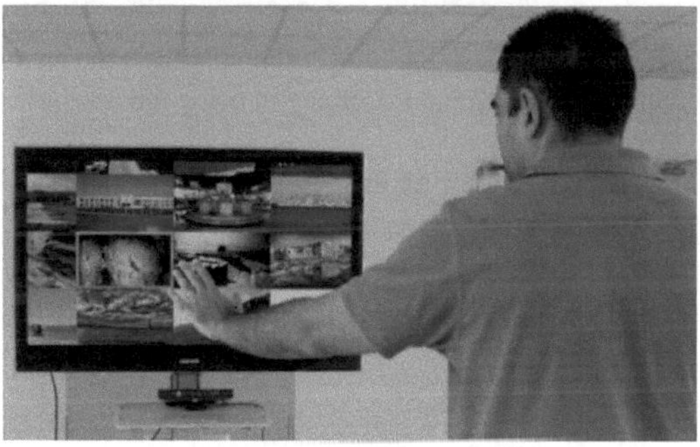

Fig. 1. MAGIC version A

This first prototype was meant to explore the potential of more "natural" interaction avoiding the use of typical computer-based metaphors such as buttons. The prototype was installed for one month in a public space inside the premises of ICS-FORTH and informally tested with visitors and staff members using observational methods and thinking aloud. As a result, a number of usability problems were identified. First of all, users not familiar with the system or other gesturing technologies could not figure out how to use it without a short introduction and some training. Furthermore, selecting an item from the grid view using a click gesture was not accurate, as jitter and minor instabilities often resulted in erroneous selections. Additionally, there was some unpredictable system behavior when a user tried to make a swipe gesture in one direction which was not successfully recognized, and subsequently, as the hand was moving towards the user's torso, a gesture in the opposite direction was recognized. Last but not least, the adoption of a single gesture to toggle between different views often puzzled the users, as the same action caused the system to respond in a different manner.

2.3 Second Prototype

In order to overcome the usability problems mentioned in the previous section, a radically different design approach was followed for creating a second prototype of the system, in which hand-gestures were replaced by virtual buttons. Additionally, the process for selecting an item was changed from clicking to time-based: the user should simply dwell the virtual hand over an item for some time period in order to select it. Upon hovering the hand cursor over an item, a virtual watch appears over it providing feedback about the time required for completing the selection.

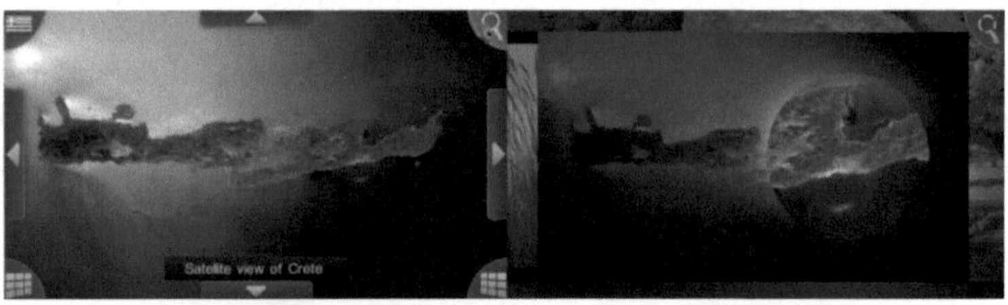

Fig. 2. The final view for exploring a single image, showing the hand enabling the magnifier by clicking the corresponding button (left) and zooming in using the magnifier (right)

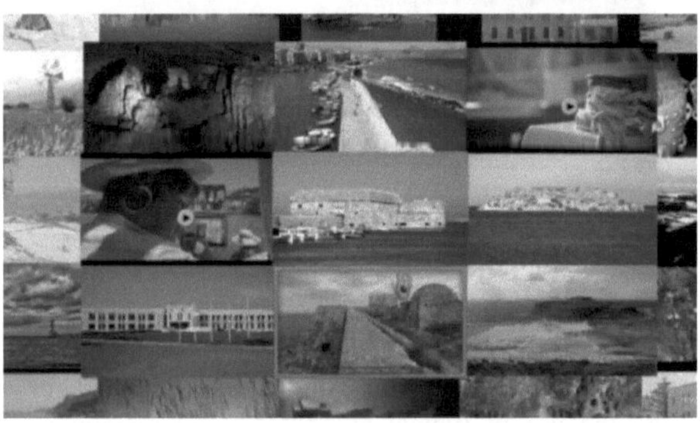

Fig. 2. The final view of the images grid

Apart from altering the selection metaphor, the notion of having a single gesture to toggle between different views was replaced by corresponding virtual buttons. Also, the magnifying glass functionality can be triggered through a toggle button on the top-right corner of the display. Moreover, the gestures to iterate through neighboring items were replaced by four buttons, one for each respective direction. Buttons are hidden when users hold their hand still, so as to make them as unobtrusive as possible. The grid view was also enhanced with an effect to favor the photos at the center of the display by enlarging them (Fig 3), while also shrinking the others. Finally, multilingual legends were added so as to enhance the multimedia elements with a short textual description. The active language may be changed at any time through a corresponding button on the top left corner of the display.

3 Conclusions

The usage of MAGIC led to the conclusion that although gestural interaction may be more natural, its employment is not so intuitive to the users, resulting in their inability to manipulate the system without guidance. Currently, the system's new version is in public display at the premises of ICS-FORTH and evaluated using both formal and informal methods. Preliminary results show that the usability and intuitiveness of the system has greatly improved. Future work involves supporting multiple users and also exploring the possibility of developing a hybrid approach which will include both virtual buttons and gestural interaction.

Acknowledgments. This work has been supported by the FORTH-ICS RTD Programme "Ambient Intelligence and Smart Environments".

References

1. Bolt, R.A.: "Put-that-there": Voice and gesture at the graphics interface 14(3), 262–270 (1980)
2. Cruz, L., Lucio, D., Velho, L.: Kinect and rgbd images: Challenges and applications. SIBGRAPI Tutorial (2012)
3. Garzotto, F., Valoriani, M.: Don't touch the oven: motion-based touchless interaction with household appliances. In: Proceedings of the International Working Conference on Advanced Visual Interfaces, pp. 721–724. ACM (2012)
4. Hansen, J.P., Johansen, A.S., Hansen, D.W., Itoh, K.: Command without a click: Dwell time typing by mouse and gaze selections. In: Proceedings of Human-Computer Interaction–INTERACT, pp. 121–128 (2003)
5. Kendon, A.: Gesture: Visible action as utterance. Cambridge University Press (2004)
6. Panger, G.: Kinect in the kitchen: testing depth camera interactions in practical home environments. In: Proceedings of the 2012 ACM Annual Conference Extended Abstracts on Human Factors in Computing Systems Extended Abstracts, pp. 1985–1990. ACM (2012)
7. Ruppert, G.C., Reis, L.O., Amorim, P.H., de Moraes, T.F., da Silva, J.V.: Touchless gesture user interface for interactive image visualization in urological surgery. World Journal of Urology 30(5), 687–691 (2012)
8. Salvador, R., Romao, T., Centieiro, P.: A gesture interface game for energy consumption awareness. In: 9th International Conference, ACE 2012, pp. 352–367 (2012)
9. Wilson, A., Pham, H.: Pointing in intelligent environments with the WorldCursor. In: INTERACT International Conference on Human-Computer Interaction (2003)

A Shadow Touching Technique for Interactive Projector Devices

Lan-Rong Dung and Ren-Yu Huang

National Chiao Tung University, Hsinchu 30010, Taiwan
lennon@faculty.nctu.edu.tw

Abstract. Touch devices have become one of the major elements in today's most electronic products. Touch technology can be divided into different types as resistive, capacitive, infrared, and so on. However, as the amount of detection sensors increases, most types of touch screen suffer from more cost and lower yield when the accuracy of touch location or larger size is required. Therefore, it is essential to design a different kind of touch technology with accurate detection and the cost is not proportional to its size. This paper proposed a kind of touch system using the distance between the object (eg. finger or stylus) and its shadow to determine whether the object touched the screen or not, and locate the touch point. It can be applied to any interactive projection system without using a lot of touch detecting sensor. Therefore, no additional costs are required for a large touch screen. The proposed touch system only requires one camera and one IR source, and cooperates with an interactive projector to detect the occurrence of touching and its location. The proposed system achieves an average detection rate of 97.53% if the tolerance of detected touch coordinates is in ± 10 pixels.

Keywords: Shadow touch, touch screen, interactive projector.

1 Introduction

Panels are quite popular due to its instinctive input method as a human-machine interface. There are three units in this kind of system. Most of them have sensors and coordinates calculation units, and some have the special signal transmission unit. The sensor unit is used to receive signal and generate information that can define the coordinates. The coordinates calculation unit transforms the information generated by sensor unit to coordinates or some other signals that can determine the location. There are some special touch system such as electromagnetic touch system must have additional transmission unit to generating specific signals for sensor unit.

The most common materials covered on the intermediate or small-sized touch panel are resistors and capacitors. However, as the panel size increases, the number of sensor units increases and leads to higher cost and lower yield rate. Therefore, these types of touch systems are not suitable for large-sized touch screen. On the contrary, ultrasonic, optical, electromagnetic, infrared, and vision-based

C. Stephanidis (Ed.): Posters, Part I, HCII 2013, CCIS 373, pp. 308–312, 2013.

touch system are more feasible to make a large or even extra large touch system since the sensor units will not increase with the panel size. However, these touch systems still have some drawbacks. For example, the cost of ultrasonic based touch system is relatively expensive. The electromagnetic based touch system requires an electromagnetic pen. The infrared and vision based system need more than one camera to locate the position.

This paper focused on developing a vision-based touch system with large-sized screen. The vision-based touch system is quite suitable for large touch screen. It has a camera that can catch images to calculate the location and decide the event of touching. There are many similar techniques of vision-based touch systems proposed by other researches [1]-[5]. The main issue of these touch systems is to determine whether the action of object really "touched" the screen or just a movement [2].

This paper proposed a vision-based touch technique that use the shadow information to detect the touch event and location. This system uses only one camera and does not use the gesture recognition to distinguish the touch event and movment. Hence it is more instinctive, user-friendly, and save more cost relative to two camera system.

2 Proposed System

The proposed touch system is shown in Fig. 1. The touch system includes an interactive projector with an infrared camera, an IR filter, a projection screen and an infrared light source. The interactive projector projects contents on projection screen, and the camera capture user's action in front of projection screen. The IR filter is installed in front of the camera lens to filter out interferences from the projection contents and other visible light. The infrared light source supply illumination to the system. The images captured by camera will be processed. Therefore, when the user touches projection screen, the system will detect the touches, and estimating the touching location.

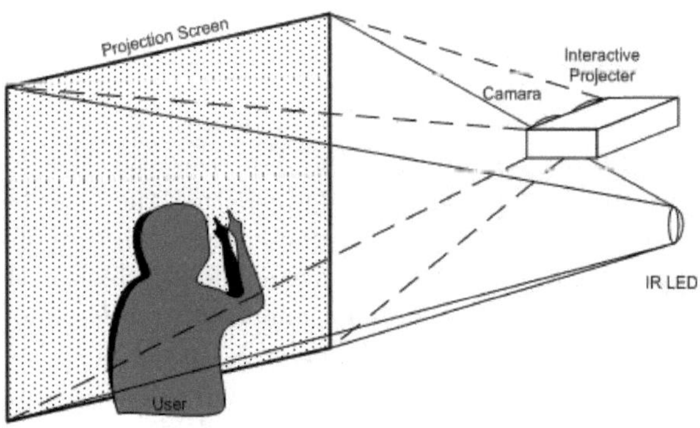

Fig. 1. Proposed System Framework

2.1 Shadow and Object Bi-level Images

After noise reduction and illumination correction, we can seperate the shadow pixels by using the threshold estimated in the initializaiton step. The preliminary bi-level image of shadow can be obtained by the following equation:

$$S(x, y) = \begin{cases} 1 \text{ ,if } f(x, y) < \theta_s(x, y). \\ 0 \text{ ,otherwise.} \end{cases} \tag{1}$$

Before segmenting the object from image, we first subtract current frame from the background image. Since the difference of two images in the same scene contains real object or noise. Hence we have to set a condition to reduce the noise effect. If the pixel absolute difference is greater than some pre-defined constant T_f, then set the pixel as the "foreground" pixel. This makes the system robust to segment the object from image. In our experiments, $T_f = 9$ is enough to distinguish the difference of object from difference of noise. The bi-level image of object can be obtained by:

$$O(x, y) = \begin{cases} 1 \text{ ,if } f(x, y) > \theta_o(x, y) \text{ and} \\ \quad |f(x, y) - bg(x, y)| > T_f \\ 0 \text{ ,otherwise.} \end{cases} \tag{2}$$

2.2 Tips Detection

After extracting the bi-level images of object and shadow, we have to find the possible locations of fingertip or stylus tip. We detect the tips of object and shadow by checking the four boundary of a 16x16 scanning mask, as shown in Fig. 2. If there is only one boundary contains the object or shadow pixels, then the tip is detected; otherwise, there is no tip in the mask. When the tip is detected, we calculate height and width of the tip. If the height is large enough and the width is small enough, then calculate and record the direction and coordinates of the tip.

2.3 Touch Judgement

After detecting the tips of object and shadow, we use the information of tips to determine touch-timing and touch-point. We trace the tips for more than one frame, and use four parameters to judge whether the object's tip touches the projection screen or not. The four parameters are *direction* of tips, the *distance* between object tip and shadow tip, *frame counts* which is the number of frames that include the same tip, and the *approaching velocity* of object's tip and shadow's tip. If the object's tip and shadow's tip are in the same direction and close enough, the the object's tip might be the peak of finger or stylus. If two successive frames have the same close object's tip and shadow's tip, the *frames counts* will increase by one. Then we calculate the *approaching velocity* of the object's tip and shadow's tip, if the object's tip and shadow's tip are getting closer in two successive frames, the approaching distance is added by the

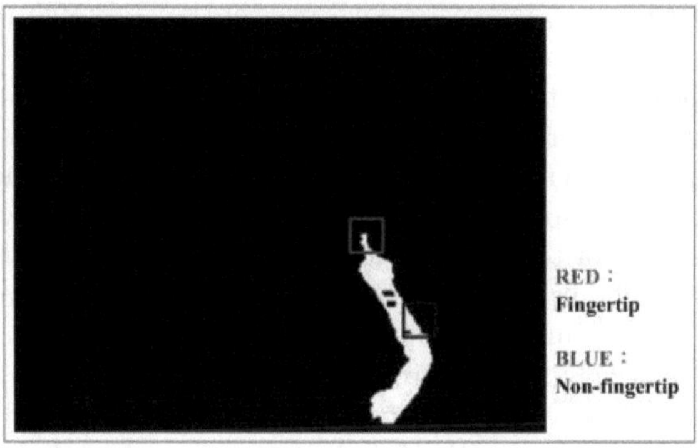

Fig. 2. Tip detection

Table 1. Detection rate and False Alarm Ratio

Test Pattern	Touch Number	Hits	Detection Rate (DR)	False Alarms	False Alarm Ratio (FAR)
1	81	81	100.00%	0	0%
2	122	119	95.90%	0	0%
3	51	49	96.08%	0	0%
4	72	72	100.00%	0	0%
5	104	101	97.16%	0	0%
6	83	79	95.18%	0	0%
7	87	84	96.55%	0	0%
8	58	58	100.00%	0	0%
9	59	59	100.00%	0	0%
10	61	58	95.08%	0	0%
11	73	70	95.89%	0	0%
Total	851	830	97.53%	0	0%

difference of the distance between object's tip and shadow's tip in two frames. *Approaching velocity* is approaching distance divided by *frames counts*, if the object's tip and the shadow's tip are getting closer in these successive frames, the *approaching velocity* will be positive. The formula for calculating *approaching velocity* is shown as Eq. (3).

$$V_{approach}(k) = \frac{D_{approach}(k)}{Frame\ Counts} \tag{3}$$

$$D_{approach}(k) = D_{approach}(k-1) + \Delta D$$

$$\Delta D = D(k) - D(k-1)$$

Where $D(k)$ is the Euclidean distance between object's tip and shadow's tip in the k-th frame, $D_{approach}(k)$ is the approaching distance, and $V_{approach}(k)$ is the *approaching velocity*.

3 Conclusion

This paper proposed an touch system which takes advantages of the relative relationship between finger or stylus and its shadow to determine whether a finger or stylus touches the screen. The touch system proposed in this paper needs only one camera and one IR source, and cooperate with an interactive projector to detect the occurrence of touches and locations. The proposed system does not using any touch detecting elements, hence no additional costs are needed for a greater touch screen. Comparing to other large-size touch panels, the proposed touch system is relatively low cost and portable.

We use 11 test sets to evaluate the performance of the proposed touch system. The test patterns are videos with 15 frames per second, and the frame size is 320x240 pixels. The performance of the proposed method is shown as Table 1. The proposed system achieves an average detection rate(DR) of 97.53% and false alarm ratio(FAR) of 0% if the tolerance of detected touch coordinate is in the range of ±10 pixels.

References

1. Mo, Z., Lewis, J.P., Neumann, U.: Smart Canvas: A Gesture- Driven Intelligent Drawing Desk System. In: 5th ACM symposium on Intelligent User Interfaces, pp. 239–243 (2005)
2. Bretzner, L., Laptev, I., Lindeberg, T.: Hand gesture recognition using multi-scale colour features, hierarchical models and particle filtering. In: Face and Gesture, pp. 423–428 (2002)
3. Chen, X., Koike, H., Nakanishi, Y., Oka, K., Sato, Y.: Two-handed drawing on augmented desk system. In: Working Conference on Advanced Visual Interfaces (May 2002)
4. Hall, D., Gal, C.L., Martin, J., Chomat, O., Crowley, J.L.: Magicboard: a contribution to an intelligent office environment. the International Symposium on Intelligent Robotic Systems 35(3), 215–223 (1999)
5. Wellner, P.: Interacting with paper on the digital desk. ACM Trans. on Communications 36(7), 86–97 (1993)
6. Hardenberg, C.: Fingertracking and Handposture Recognition for Real-Time Human-Computer Interaction, http://iihm.imag.fr/hardenbe
7. Tasdizen, T., Jurrus, E., Whitaker, R.T.: Non-uniform illumination correction in transmission electron microscopy. In: MICCAI Workshop on Microscopic Image Analysis with Applications in Biology (September 2008)
8. Otsu, N.: A Threshold Selection Method from Gray Level Histogram. IEEE Trans. on Systems, Man and Cybernetics 9, 62–66 (1979)
9. Wu, K., Otoo, E., Suzuki, K.: Optimizing two-pass connected-component labeling algorithms. Pattern Analysis & Applications 12(2), 117–135 (2009)
10. Barnes, L.R., Schultz, D.M., Gruntfest, E.C., Hayden, M.H., Benight, C.C.: Corrigendum: False alarm rate or false alarm ratio? Weather Forecasting (2009)
11. Gonzalez, R.C., Woods, R.E.: Digital Image Processing, 3rd edn. Prentice Hall (2008)

Modeling the Types of Interaction with Ambient Environment

DongJin Eun, Hark-Joon Kim, ChoonKyoung Moon, Pilseung Yang, Seonghoon Kang

Samsung Electronics Co.,Ltd, Suwon, Gyeonggi 443-742, Republic of Korea
{dj.eun,harkjoon.kim,ck11.moon,ps.yang,shoon.kang}@samsung.com

Abstract. This paper proposes a new modeling methodology about the interaction with the ambient environment such as tables, windows, physical objects and so on. We analyzed interaction factors in existing scenarios that involve the interaction, and then classified the result of analysis. We made modeling elements though the classification results and designed modeling method combining the elements. The modeling method can reduce the time to understand the existing interactions or the interactions that are designed by co-workers. Moreover, we believe that it can be useful when designers make a new scenario or modify the existing scenarios.

Keywords: Interaction Modeling, Pervasive Computing, Ambient Interaction, Interaction Categorization, Type of Interaction.

1 Introduction

Pervasive Computing opened the way that users get information or services from the ambient environment such as tables, windows, physical objects and so on. Therefore, many researchers have proposed a variety of scenarios based on Pervasive Computing and suggested scenarios that users interact with the ambient environment. [1-5]. Sixth Sense [1] is a typical study that makes user's ambient environment the interaction space using wearable system. Previous studies about modeling method of interaction have focused on expressing interaction flow [6-7]. The systematic approaches in modeling interaction type have been rarely studied. For the purpose of systemic ideation and analysis, we present a new modeling methodology about the interaction with the ambient environment by analyzing existing scenarios.

2 Interaction Analyze and Categorization

We analyzed the type of interfaces, the type of information, the presence of related digital devices and its relationship from the scenarios to figure out the category of the interaction with the ambient environment. As the result of the analysis, we classified the category as shown in the Fig.1. These categories are divided into two cases: the ambient environment used for 1) interfaces or 2) information. The former is categorized into two types. One is that the ambient environment always became an

C. Stephanidis (Ed.): Posters, Part I, HCII 2013, CCIS 373, pp. 313–316, 2013.

interface (we named this 'Static Ambient Interface'); another one is that the ambient environment temporarily became an interface depending on the related digital device (we named this 'Dynamic Ambient Interface'). The Dynamic Ambient Interface has five different types according to relationship between the device and the ambient environment. (1) Move: The interface of the device is moved to ambient environment. Therefore, the interface of the device becomes no longer available. (2) Expand: The interface of the device is expanded to ambient environment. (3) Divide: The interface of the device is functionally divided into ambient environment. (4) Duplicate: The interface of the device is duplicated in ambient environment. (5) Create: The interface on ambient environment is created by the digital device.

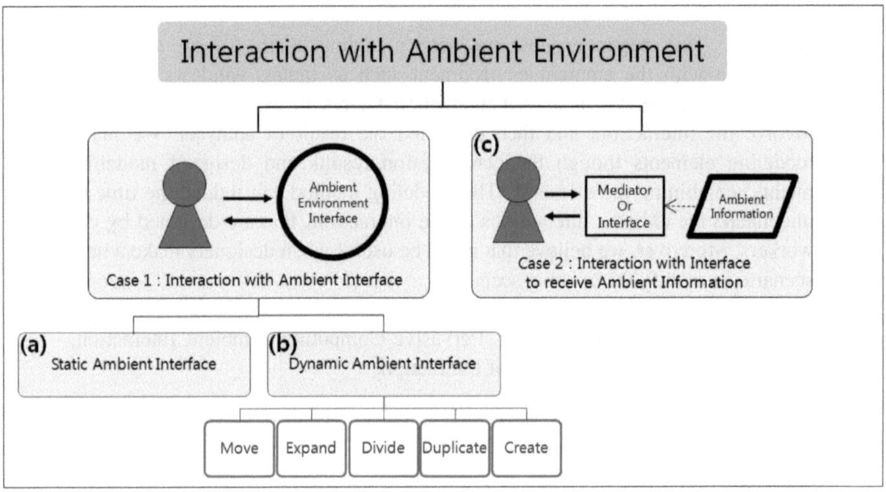

Fig. 1. Result of Classifications

(a) Environment/Real Objects always provide their own interfaces.

(b) Environment/Real Objects temporally provide their own interfaces depended on related digital devices.

(c) Information of Environment/Real Objects is inputted into interfaces.

3 Modeling Method Design

We made modeling elements (see Table.1) for designing interactions based on the result of the category in Fig.1. Then we designed a new method for modeling interactions by combining the modeling elements. The modeling elements categorized into four categories: 1) the interface/information factors, 2) the interface for user interaction, 3) the line that defines the relationship between factors, 4) the description about user actions in the relationship. 1) The *Factor* has three elements: Original Interface Device is the device that is made for the role of input/output interface (e.g., keyboard, mouse, display, and touch screen). Ambient Environment Interface is the original common thing, but become input/output interface by an embedded computer or a support device for ambient computing (e.g., projector, camera). Ambient Information is the information element of ambient environment received by input interface. 2) The *Interface* is divided between Input Interface and Output Interface, and each can contain elements of *Factor*. 3) The *Flow* defines the relationship in case of Dynamic Ambient Interface. The five elements of *Flow* (Move, Expand, Divide, Duplicate, Create) except for Input Information define the relationship between elements of *Factor*. And the Input Information of *Flow* defines the relationship between *Factor* and *Interface*.

Table 1. The modeling elements for designing interaction with ambient environments

1) Factor	Original Interface Device	Ambient Environment Interface	Ambient Information
2) Interface	*Elements* Input Interface	*Elements* Output Interface	
3) Flow	Move	Expand	Divide
	Duplicate	Create (Additional Option)	Input Information
4) User Activity	*Description* Description on User Action for Flow Process		

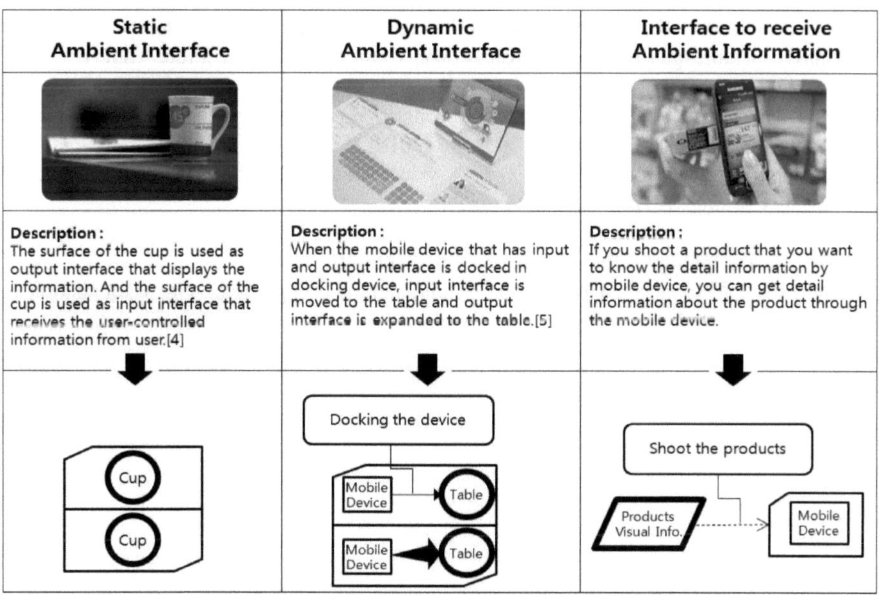

Fig. 2. Modeling examples

Elements in Table.1 can be expressed as one diagram in Fig.2 by combining elements. The *Interface* can have both input and output or have one of them. In case of having both, the Output Interface must be drawn under the Input Interface. Each of the *Interfaces* can contain elements of *Factor* except for the Ambient Information to indicate the interface composition. The contents of the *Factor* should be filled in the *Factor*. If the Interface has more than one *Factor*, *Factors* must be defined a relationship among elements of *Factor* by using elements of *Flow*. If Input Interface receives the Ambient Information, Input Interface must be linked to Ambient Information using Input Information of *Flow*. Therefore, Interaction designers can express only one diagram instead of a long and complicated description using the modeling method, as shown in Fig.2.

4 Conclusion and Future Work

The modeling method can reduce the time to understand the existing interactions or the interactions that are designed by co-workers. Moreover, we believe that it can be useful when novice designers make a new scenario or modify the existing scenarios.

Based on this study, we have a plan to apply the application of the method to other interaction theme, especially organic interaction.

References

1. Mistry, P., Maes, P.: SixthSense: a wearable gestural interface. In: Proc. ACM SIGGRAPH ASIA 2009 Sketches, Article No. 11 (2009)
2. Uriu, D., Namai, M., Tokuhisa, S., Kashiwagi, R., Inami, M., Okude, N.: Experience "panavi," Challenge to Master Professional Culinary Arts. In: Proc. CHI EA 2012, pp. 1445–1446 (2012)
3. Linder, N., Maes, P.: LuminAR: portable robotic augmented reality interface design and prototype. In: Proc. UIST 2010, pp. 395–396 (2010)
4. Microsoft's Future Concepts, http://www.youtube.com/watch?v=QL-zcUWwCZU
5. Samsung Corning "A Day Made of Glass2", http://www.youtube.com/watch?v=eOSJdQ3e6JE
6. Saffer, D.: Designing for Interaction, pp. 99–100 (2009)
7. Winograd, T., Flores, F.: Understanding computers and cognition: A new foundation for design, p. 65 (1986)

Interpret Human Gestures with a Time of Flight Camera Using Standard Image Processing Algorithms on a Distributed System

Bjoern Froemmer, Nils Roeder, and Elke Hergenroether

Hochschule Darmstadt, University of Applied Sciences,
Faculty of Computer Science
{bjoern.froemmer,nils.roeder,elke.hergenroether}@h-da.de

Abstract. The development of Human Computer Interfaces steadily moves away from peripheral devices like mouse and keyboard in certain areas, as is obvious when looking at the evolution of smart-phones, tablet-PCs and touch-enabled operating systems over the last few years. Nowadays we can even witness the transition from touch-based interfaces to touch-free interfaces. One common method to realize such interfaces is to incorporate new state-of-the art 3D cameras (often called "Time of Flight" cameras). The difficulty lies within the evaluation of the sensor-data, to achieve robust detection and tracking of people within the scene in real-time. We try to solve this task without using expensive knowledge-based approaches by employing standard image-processing algorithms because we wanted to keep the required manpower and development time, as well as costs, as low as possible.

Keywords: Natural User Interface, Human Computer Interface, Segmentation, 3D-Camera, Time-of-Flight, Region Growing, Edge Detection, Convexity Defects, Tracking, Gestural Interaction.

1 Introduction

The main research areas of this work have been as follows. What kind of image-processing methods can be used to segment and evaluate the sensor data of monocular 3D cameras in respect of tracking and evaluating human gestures? How fast (in terms of calculation time) can this be done? How reliable can we analyze and interpret human motions to achieve gestural interaction without using knowledge-based approaches?

To evaluate these questions we made use of a ToF[1] camera to record humans from the front (see figure 1). We then used the OpenCV Framework and some of it's standard image processing algorithms like edge detection, region growing and geometrical classification to segment and interpret the measured 3D data. We intentionally wanted to refrain from utilizing knowledge-based approaches like human-pose-databases in combination with classifiers that need to be trained (see [16] for example).

[1] ToF stands for Time-of-Flight and will be used as an abbreviation in this paper from here on.

C. Stephanidis (Ed.): Posters, Part I, HCII 2013, CCIS 373, pp. 317–321, 2013.

2 System and Algorithm

The implemented system consists of three main modules. These involve a camera-data server, a processing module and the client application. The camera server polls the data of the ToF camera and distributes it to the local network. The distributed data can then be accessed and processed by any number of so-called tracker-modules. This modular structure allows to disassemble complex tasks into partial solutions and distribute the computational load of the system onto multiple machines if needed. For example, it is conceivable that several trackers work cooperatively at the same or at completely different tasks within the same scene. The processing-module itself is divided into three distinct areas: segmentation, classification and tracking of objects.

Our goal is the segmentation of objects solely based on their depth information. The first step of the algorithm is to perform a pre-segmentation of the recorded depth-data to extract relevant areas for the subsequent main segmentation. This is achieved by the removal of static (unmoving) areas from the actual recorded depth-data. The next step is to remove depth-values with poor signal quality (values with low amplitudes). This ensures a solid basis for the subsequently described main-segmentation. After the aforementioned steps are done, only depth-values relevant to our goal remain and a region growing algorithm is utilized to clusterise spatially connected 3D points depending on their depth data. Based on the size of these clusters, areas of interest are identified which can then be processed further. Clusters that contain only few pixels, for example, will be eliminated using a threshold function. Depending on the application, it may be advantageous to select this threshold relative to the distance of an object. One of the possible reasons to do this is that the ratio of the areas between corresponding hands and torsos of people stays roughly the same, no matter how great the distance is between the user and the camera.

To realize hand-based interaction it is important to classify the identified objects, which remain after the segmentation, as certain body-parts. The goal here is to distinguish hands from other segmented body parts. For this task (the recognition of hands) we use geometrical classifiers based on convex hull polygons and so-called convexity defects as seen in figure 1 (image 9). The system later on basically tracks all segmented areas, but the intended human-computer-interaction should be made possible exclusively with the users hands. If a segmented area is identified as a hand, this classification will remain in the system as long as this body-part is visible to the camera, even though the hands pose might be changing. Following that preamble, a segmented area can either belong to the super-class *body-part* or to the derived class *hand*.

After this step is done, we can now track the classified body-parts (hands in this example) over time and send this data to multiple client applications, where the tracked data (movement paths of the detected hands, number of visible fingers on each hand and detected hand-pose) is processed.

3 Results and Discussion

The nature of monocular Time-of-Flight cameras allows the use of simple but efficient algorithms like region growing and edge detection to segment the measured data. Objects which are spatially connected in the 3D point-cloud will be clustered together and can then be classified as described in the foregone chapter. The Results of our implementations are visualized below:

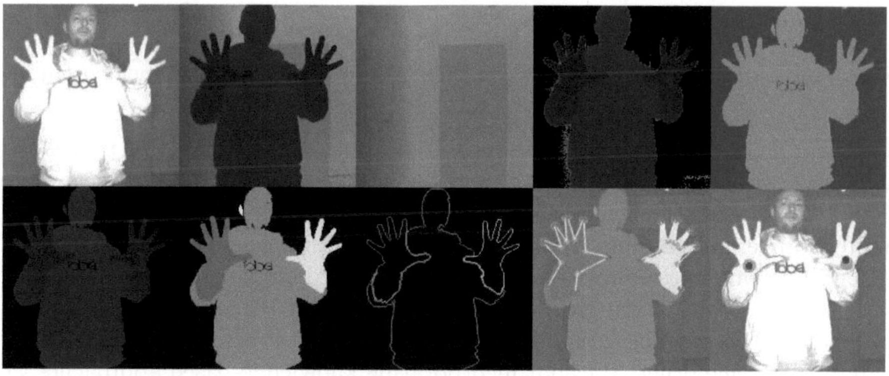

Fig. 1. Image processing chain of the segmentation algorithm

Images in Figure 1 (from left to right, top to bottom):

1. Intensity values (2D greyscale image)
2. Actual depth data (3D floating point image)
3. Initial depth data for background subtraction
4. Background subtraction result
5. Signal quality check
6. Remaining depth data after signal quality check
7. Region growing results
8. Edge detection results
9. Body-part classification through geometrical classifiers
10. Augmented intensity image with tracking results

The ToF camera we used[2] is capable of 3D-data-capturing with 25 frames per second. ToF cameras still have a relatively small resolution compared to state of the art 2D sensors (the camera we used has a sensor-resolution of 204 x 204 pixels) and limited operating range (the model we incorporated is capable of measuring 3D data in a range from 0.3 to 7 meters). As we can see in figure 2, the calculation-time progression of our algorithm directly depends on the number of segmented objects and its time-incrementation is nearly linear. With 9 segmented objects visible in the frame, a number common for our task as

[2] PMD CamCube 2.0, `http://www.pmdtec.com`

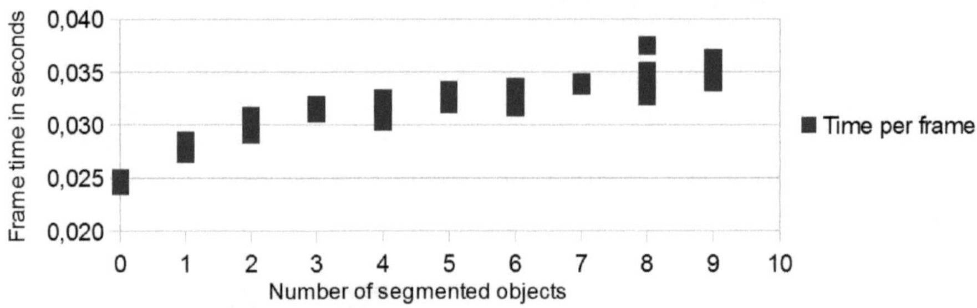

Fig. 2. Statistical analysis of calculation time in correspondence to segmented objects

empirical data shows, our yet un-optimized approach is capable of processing at least 28 frames per second. In a realistic situation we should not have more than 2 users inside the field of view of the camera because of it's aforementioned limited range and resolution. This shows that the implemented system is fast enough for real-time interaction under the described circumstances.

The main problem we encountered was based on the occlusion of objects within the 3D scene, for example when two persons visible in the scene stand or walk behind each other. Without incorporating knowledge-based approaches we were not able to eliminate these occlusion problems for now.

References

1. Parvizi, E., Wu, Q.M.J.: Real-Time 3D Head Tracking Based on Time-of-Flight Depth Sensor. In: 19th IEEE International Conference on Tools with Artificial Intelligence, pp. 517–521 (2007)
2. Parvizi, E., Wu, Q.M.J.: Multiple Object Tracking Based on Adaptive Depth Segmentation. In: Canadian Conference on Computer and Robot Vision, pp. 273–277 (2008)
3. Parvizi, E., Wu, Q.M.J.: Real-Time Approach for Adaptive Object Segmentation in Time-of-Flight Sensors. In: 20th IEEE International Conference on Tools with Artificial Intelligence, pp. 236–240 (2008)
4. Bing, L., Jesorsky, O., Kompe, R.: Robust Real-Time Multiple Object Tracking in Traffic Scenes using an Optical Matrix Range Sensor. In: Intelligent Transportation Systems Conference, pp. 742–747. IEEE (2007)
5. Fan, T.-J., Medioni, G., Nevatia, R.: Recognizing 3-D Objects using Surface Descriptions. IEEE Transactions on Pattern Analysis and Machine Intelligence, 1140–1157 (1989)
6. Bab-Hadiashar, A., Gheissari, N.: Range Image Segmentation using Surface Selection Criterion. IEEE Transactions on Image Processing, 2006–2018 (2006)
7. Powell, M.W., Bowyer, K.W., Xiaoyi, J., Bunke, H.: Comparing Curved-Surface Range Image Segmenters. Sixth International Conference on Computer Vision, 286–291 (1998)
8. Satoshi, S., Keiichi, A.: Topological Structural Analysis of Digitized Binary Images by Border Following. Computer Vision, Graphics, and Image Processing, 32–46 (1985)

9. Heckbert, P.: A Seed Fill Algorithm. Graphics Gems I, 275–277 (1990) ISBN-13: 978-0122861666
10. Shaw, J.R.: QuickFill: An efficient Flood Fill Algorithm, `http://www.codeproject.com/gdi/QuickFill.asp`
11. Wobbrock, J.O., Wilson, A.D., Li, Y.: Gestures without Libraries, Toolkits or Training: A 1-Dollar Recognizer for User Interface Prototypes. In: UIST 2007 Proceedings of the 20th Annual ACM Symposium on User Interface Software and Technology, pp. 159–168 (2007)
12. Kaltenbrunner, M., Bovermann, T., Bencina, R., Costanza, E.: TUIO: A Protocol for Table-Top Tangible User Interfaces. In: Proceedings of the 6th International Workshop on Gesture in Human-Computer Interaction and Simulation (GW 2005), Vannes, France (2005)
13. Welch, G., Bishop, G.: An Introduction to the Kalman Filter. University of North Carolina at Chapel Hill, NC (1995)
14. Ringbeck, T.: A 3D Time of Flight Camera for Object Detection. Optical 3-D Measurement Techniques, ETH Zürich (2007)
15. Sklansky, J.: Measuring Concavity on a Rectangular Mosaic. IEEE Trans. Comput., 1355–1364 (1972)
16. Shotton, J., Fitzgibbon, A., Cook, M., Sharp, T., Finocchio, M., Moore, R., Kipman, A., Blake, A.: Real-Time Human Pose Recognition in Parts from a Single Depth Image, Microsoft Research. In: IEEE Conference on Computer Vision and Pattern Recognition (CVPR), pp. 1297–1304 (2011)

Audio-Only Augmented Reality System for Social Interaction

Tom Gurion[1] and Nori Jacoby[1,2]

[1] Bar-Ilan University, Ramat Gan, Israel
{nagasaki45,nori.viola}@gmail.com
[2] Hebrew University, Jerusalem, Israel

Abstract. We explore new possibilities for interactive music consumption by proposing an audio-only augmented reality system for social interaction.

We designed and built an Android application that measures the relative position of the device from freely moveable Bluetooth beacons. Based on this information, an algorithm dynamically changes the music that the users hear in their earphones.

We assessed the interactive component of the system in the context of a silent rave party in a controlled experiment by comparing the system positioning readings in interactive and non-interactive control segments. We also directly assessed the user experience using self-report pre/post surveys. Our results suggest that the system facilitated higher levels of user movement in space and enhanced social interactions, thereby displaying the potential of using audio-only augmented reality in future mobile applications.

Keywords: Interactive Music System, Social Interaction, Augmented Reality, Indoor positioning system.

1 Introduction and Framework

In the past 60 years the development of new technology has fundamentally transformed music creation and consumption [1]. Today, interactive music systems are used in many different contexts ranging from instrument design [2] to socially interactive installations [3]. With the emergence of modern mobile devices, interactive music systems have become accessible to non-musicians (for example AutoRap by Smule [4], and RjDj [5]) as well as facilitating a shared process of music creation between different users in social context [6-7].

Meanwhile, the emergence of location-based services for mobile devices led to new demands for indoor positioning technologies [8]. Most indoor positioning systems for mobile devices today use Wi-Fi or Bluetooth communication and require external infrastructure [9]. In order to eliminate the need for external infrastructure, researchers have suggested relative indoor positioning systems using Bluetooth technology [10] or a device's built-in accelerometer and compass [11].

The main goal of our research is to propose an audio-only augmented reality system for social interaction based on relative indoor positioning Bluetooth technology. We implemented and evaluated the proposed system in the context of a

C. Stephanidis (Ed.): Posters, Part I, HCII 2013, CCIS 373, pp. 322–326, 2013.

silent rave party [12]. More generally, our work explores the potential for a new way of music consumption through mobile devices, considering their effect on social behavior, location-based services and augmented reality concepts.

2 System Description

Figure 1 shows a schematic diagram of our system, which consists of a mobile application developed for Android OS [13] and six specially designed Bluetooth beacons [14]. Participants can freely move the beacons that are installed on physical objects, thereby changing the structure of the music in the virtual space. The Android application repeatedly searches for nearby Bluetooth beacons (see figure 1, BB_1-BB_6). Received signal strength indication (RSSI) is used as an estimation of the distance between the user and the beacon. This is then sent to a Pure Data (Pd) patch [15] through the libpd API [16]. The Pd patch plays an audio loop corresponding to the nearby beacon. Every audio loop, played by the sound zone players SZP_1-SZP_6, is identified by a distinct musical style, and uses the RSSI value differently; for example by controlling volume, filter and granularity of the sound zone. In addition, the different sound zones are modules which can be rhythmically and harmonically synchronized with each other in almost endless combinations.[1]

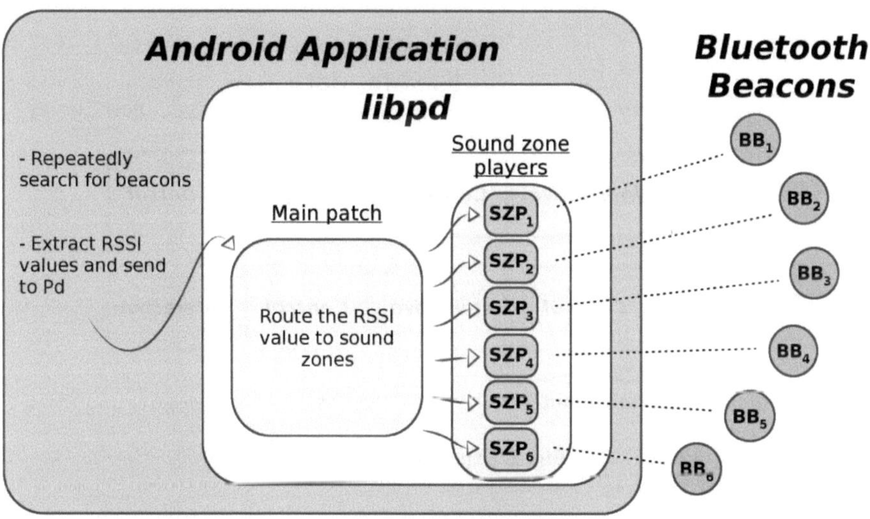

Fig. 1. System architecture

3 Experiment

According to Azuma, one of the main motivations for augmented reality (AR) systems is to enhance the user's interaction with the real world [17]. However, most of

[1] The interactive music composed for the system by the author T.G.

the research in AR nowadays does not describe a formal user evaluation of the interactive elements of the system [18].

In order to evaluate our system we invited eighteen volunteers to participate in an interactive silent rave party. Each participant installed the Android application on his or her phone and filled pre/post party surveys that included questions regarding their musical background and preferences as well as system evaluation feedback. The participants could freely move the six Bluetooth beacons which were installed on colored balloons. The party consisted of four alternating interactive/control blocks of duration 5:40 minutes each (see figure 2). The participants were randomly assigned to two groups: A and B, comprising the interactive and control blocks respectively.[2] They were generally informed that the experiment consists of interactive and control segments, however they were not informed about the exact schedule and timing of the blocks or the group assignments. Both groups started the experiment together. In the interactive blocks, the application generated music as described above, whereas in the control blocks the participants heard recorded non-interactive music created in advance using the musical material of the interactive system.[3]

Interaction with the system's components was assessed by counting the number of Bluetooth device discoveries made by each participant's phone during both the interactive and the control blocks. In order to eliminate edge effects, we analyzed only the two middle blocks of the experiment.

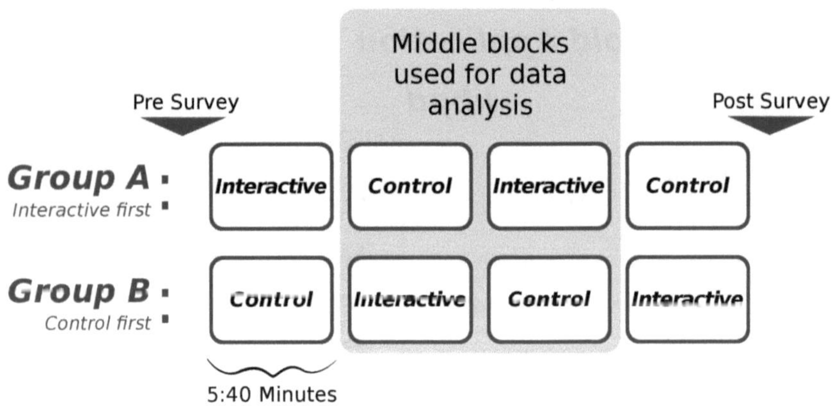

Fig. 2. Experiment design

4 Results and Conclusions

In the post-party survey, participants self-reported significantly higher levels of movement (paired t-test, $t(15)=3.9$, $p<0.01$) using the system, compared with their

---

[2] Group A (interactive first) consists of 8 participants (4 females and 4 males) with mean age of 36.7 (s.d=12.3); group B (control first) consists of 10 participants (3 females and 7 males) with mean age of 29.6 (s.d=10.2). Participants had a diverse musical background with 4.7 mean years of musical training (s.d=5.2).

[3] The control block music composed by Noam Elron (`http://www.noamelron.com`).

behavior on other parties as reported in the pre-party survey. Figure 3a shows that there was a significant difference (unpaired t-test, $t(33)=6.2$, $p<0.01$) in the mean response to these questions (at a scale of 1-3).

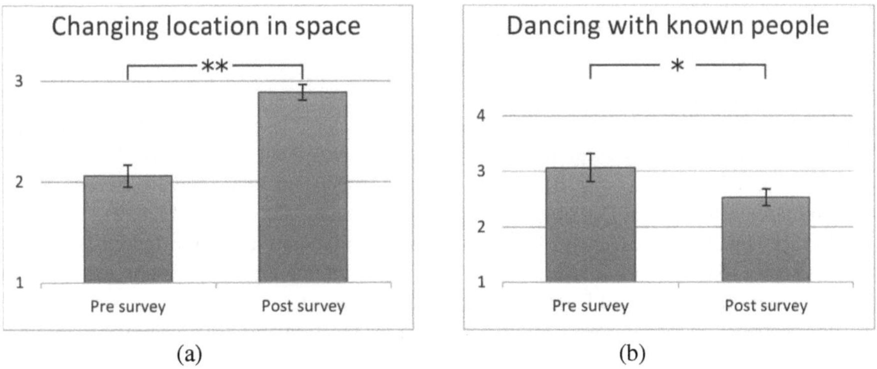

Fig. 3. Results from experiment surveys

In order to objectively assess if participants moved more in space, we measured the counting of Bluetooth discoveries made by the application's relative positioning system. Our results show slightly higher counts (paired t-test, $t(16)=1.7$, $p=0.06$, n.s) during the interactive blocks of the party compared with the control blocks. This suggests that the interactive components of the system facilitate greater participant movement in space, thereby offering more frequent opportunities for social interactions. Indeed, in the post-party survey participants reported that they danced significantly less with people that they knew in advance, compared with their usual behavior (paired t-test, $t(14)=-2.5$, $p=0.01$). Figure 3b shows that there was also a significant difference in the mean response to these questions in the pre/post surveys. Overall, participants showed a slightly stronger tendency (paired t-test, $t(16)=1.46$, $p=0.08$, n.s) to participate in an interactive party in the post-party survey, compared with their answer to identical questions in the pre survey.

Our preliminary results demonstrate the potential for audio-only augmented reality to significantly enrich the experience of music consumption and its attendant social interaction. We also show that this can be validated in a controlled experiment using both direct reports of subject and indirect objective measurements. In future research we plan to extend the evaluation of the system using live video tracking and accelerometer readings.

References

1. Winkler, T.: Composing Interactive Music: Techniques and Ideas Using Max. The MIT Press, Massachusetts (2001)
2. Jordà, S., Geiger, G., Alonso, M., Kaltenbrunner, M.: The reacTable: exploring the synergy between live music performance and tabletop tangible interfaces. In: Proceedings of the 1st International Conference on Tangible and Embedded Interaction, pp. 139–146. ACM, New York (2007)

3. Drummond, J.: Understanding Interactive Systems. Organised Sound 14(2), 124–133 (2009)
4. AutoRap by Smule, http://www.smule.com/autorap
5. Sonic Experiences – RjDj, http://rjdj.me/
6. DistributeDJ: Mobile Group Interaction Toolkit, http://crel.calit2.net/dj.html
7. DistributedDJ, http://ece842.com/S13/projects/S11/S11_ProjectReport_Team1.pdf
8. Zickuhr, K.: Three-Quarters of Smartphone Owners Use Location-Based Services. Technical report, Pew Research Center's Internet & American Life Project (2012)
9. Agrawal, R., Vasalya, A.: Bluetooth Navigation System using Wi-Fi Access Points. International Journal of Distributed and Parallel Systems 3(2), 185–192 (2012)
10. Rao, H., Fu, W.T.: A General Framework for a Collaborative Mobile Indoor Navigation Assistance System. In: Proceedings of the 3rd International Workshop on Location Awareness for Mixed and Dual Reality, pp. 21–24 (2013)
11. Pombinho, P., Afonso, A.P., Carmo, M.B.: Indoor Positioning Using a Mobile Phone with an Integrated Accelerometer and Digital Compass. In: Proceedings of the 2nd INForum Simposio de Informatica, pp. 443–446 (2010)
12. Silent Disco, http://en.wikipedia.org/wiki/Silent_disco
13. Android, http://www.android.com/
14. Bluetooth Technology Website, http://www.bluetooth.com/
15. Puckette, M.: Pure Data: another integrated computer music environment. In: Proceedings of the 2nd Intercollege Computer Music Concerts, pp. 37–41. Kunitachi College of Music, San Diego (1996)
16. Brinkmann, P.: Making Musical Apps. O'Reilly Media, Sebastopol (2012)
17. Azuma, R.T.: A Survey of Augmented Reality. Presence-Teleoperators and Virtual Environments 6(4), 355–385 (1997)
18. Swan, J.E., Gabbard, J.L.: Survey of user-based experimentation in augmented reality. In: Proceedings of the 1st International Conference on Virtual Reality, pp. 1–9. Lawrence Erlbaum Associates, Las Vegas (2005)

Calibrating Screen Coordinates of Tabletop Display Using Shadow-Cursor

Makio Ishihara[1] and Yukio Ishihara[2]

[1] Fukuoka Institute of Technology, 3-30-1 Wajiro-higashi, Higashi-ku, Fukuoka, 811-0295 Japan
m-ishihara@fit.ac.jp
http://www.fit.ac.jp/~m-ishihara/Lab/
[2] Kyushu University, 3-1-1, Maidashi, Higashi-ku, Fukuoka, 812-8582 Japan
iyukio@redoxnavi.med.kyushu-u.ac.jp
http://hyoka.ofc.kyushu-u.ac.jp/search/details/K004222/english.html

Abstract. This manuscript conducts an experiment in usability of shadow cursor for calibrating screen coordinates of tabletop displays. Shadow cursor is a mouse cursor without any visual feedback or an imaginary mouse cursor. To calibrate the screen coordinates properly, users have to move the shadow cursor in an indicated direction correctly. The experiment shows that its accuracy is about ± 5 degrees and the calibration is completed within about 700 milliseconds.

Keywords: shadow cursor, screen coordinates calibration, tabletop display, interaction design.

1 Introduction

A tabletop display is a horizontal display which multiple users sit down around and use together. The tabletop display is suitable well for collaborative work, so that it leads to a strong demand for a large screen space. One of key issues around large tabletop displays is how to make a pointing interface in the case that users cannot reach the contents by their own hands.

There have been three major ways of how a pointing interface is made for large tabletop displays. The first one uses sophisticated pointing sensors such as 6DOF magnetic ones, which may be used in CAVE systems. This often leads to expensive and cumbersome equipment. The second one uses a handheld camera to capture the quadrilateral of the entire screen so that the center of the camera performs a graphical cursor. Nintendo Wii remotes take this way. This way however works as far as the camera captures the quadrilateral of the entire screen. The third one uses invisible gray-code for the camera to capture not the entire screen but a position on the screen to locate it. Gray-code binary patterns appear on the screen in order then the temporal pattern at a position of the screen uniquely represents its own position. This way requires the screen to display invisible data to users like infrared one.

C. Stephanidis (Ed.): Posters, Part I, HCII 2013, CCIS 373, pp. 327–331, 2013.

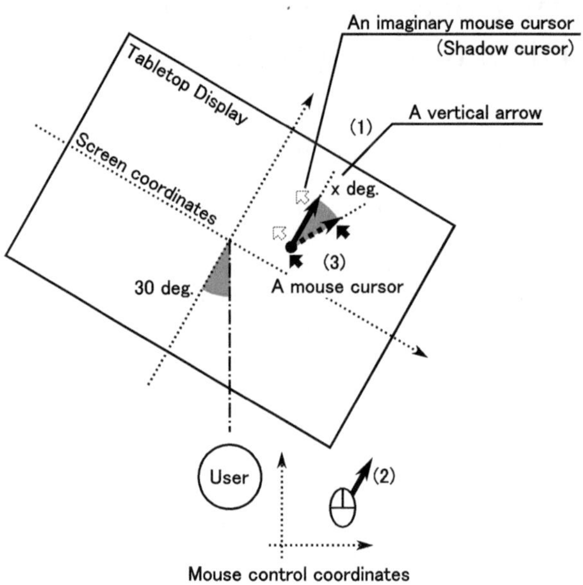

Fig. 1. Screen coordinates calibration with shadow cursor

Our pointing interface uses a common mouse. It is inexpensive and requires no infrared technique. One of major problems is that the coordinates of the screen (screen coordinates) are not always aligned with the coordinates of the mouse control space (mouse control coordinates). The first attempt to align the screen coordinates with the mouse control coordinates used a reflex in eye-hand coordination [1]. The experiments showed that the reflex would take about 4 seconds to align them and it was impractical. This manuscript reports on the second attempt which relies on the basic idea of shadow cursor. Shadow cursor allows users to perform a simple mouse-manipulation to align them, so that the calibration is expected to be completed in less than a second.

2 Shadow Cursor

A shadow cursor is an imaginary mouse cursor. Figure 1 shows how the shadow cursor works to align the screen coordinates with the mouse control coordinates. In the figure, there is the angular distance of 30 degrees between the screen coordinates and the mouse control coordinates. First, (1) a vertical arrow to the screen appears on it and (2) the user moves the mouse in the direction indicated by the vertical arrow and then (3) the mouse cursor will move at an angle of x degrees. In this case, x equals 30 degrees. At the step (3), the mouse cursor will move in the direction that the user does not expect, so that the mouse cursor is hopefully set invisible (invisible mouse cursor). The user needs to move the mouse without seeing the mouse cursor. In other words, the user needs to move

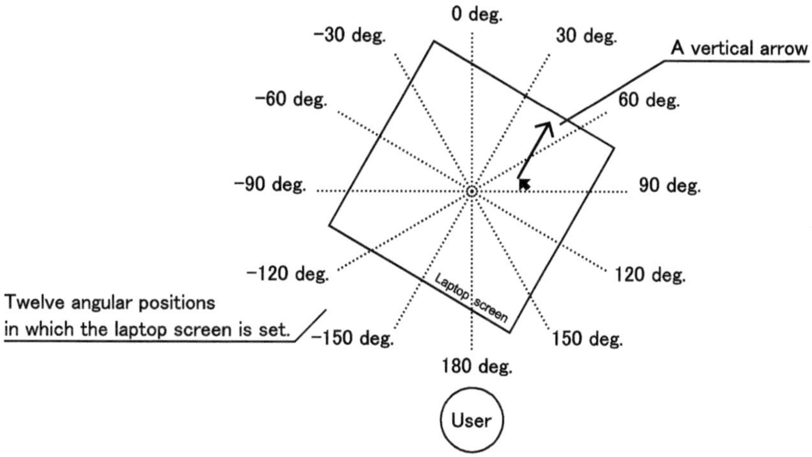

Fig. 2. Experiment settings

the mouse so that an imaginary mouse cursor (shadow cursor) moves in the direction indicated by the vertical arrow, where the user normally expects the invisible mouse cursor to move.

3 Experiment in Usability

We conducted an experiment in how accurately and fast the shadow cursor aligns the screen coordinates with the mouse control coordinates. Figure 2 shows the design of the experiment. The rectangle represents a laptop screen of Dell XPS L702X, which is 385mm wide and 215mm high (1600x900 pixels in resolution). The laptop has a quad-core processor of 2.40GHz. It is also equipped with a graphics card of nVidia GT 555M. The laptop screen is set in an angular position of -150 to 180 at 30 degree intervals and a vertical arrow appears where the subject right-clicks on the screen. Then the mouse cursor becomes invisible and the subject is asked to move the shadow cursor in the direction indicated by the vertical arrow. After that, the angular distance between the screen coordinates and the mouse control coordinates is calculated when the invisible mouse cursor goes out of the circle of 10 mm radius as shown in Figure 3. The screen coordinates are rotated by the observed angular distance.

There were 10 subjects between the ages of 22 and 36. All were right-handed and had an experience working with a mouse. Each subject had 10 trials for each angular position, resulting in 1200 trials. To avoid learning effects, the sequence of trials is in random order but it is the same between subjects.

$$10 \text{ subjects} \times 12 \text{ angular positions} \times 10 \text{ trials} \;=\; 1200 \text{ total trials} \qquad (1)$$

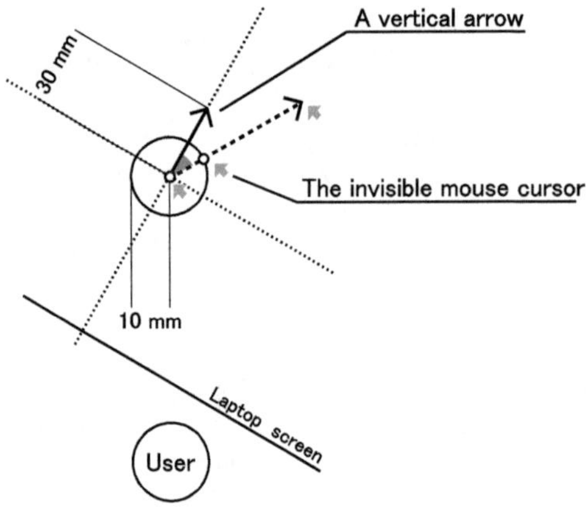

Fig. 3. Detecting the angular distance

4 Results

Figure 4 shows the result on calibration accuracy. The horizontal axis shows the initial angular position of screen and the vertical one shows accuracy of the observed angular position at each initial angular position across all the subjects. From the figure, there seems to be a certain positive correlation between the initial angular position and accuracy. This could be due to what the subjects' dominant hand is: They all are right-handed. There is also an increase in the center and two decreases around ± 30 to 60 degrees, two increases again at both sides. This could be due to directions where users think they move the

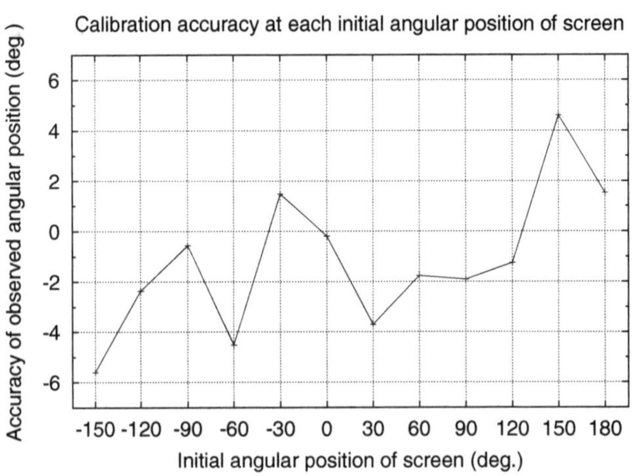

Fig. 4. Result of calibration accuracy

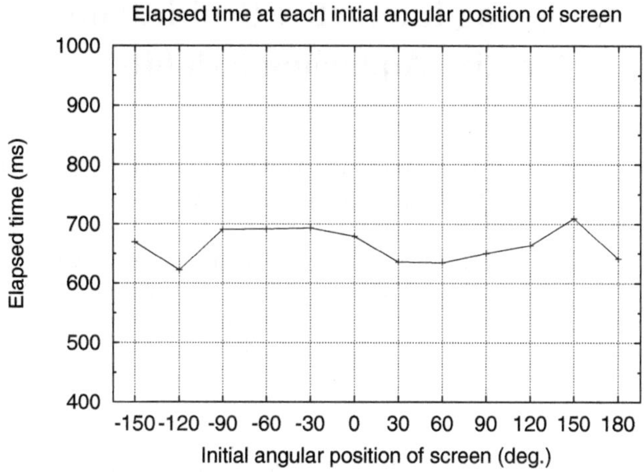

Fig. 5. Result of time efficiency

mouse comparatively easily: 0 and ±90 degrees. Analysis of variance shows that there is a significant impact of the initial angular position on calibration accuracy [F(11,1188)=4.91 at p=0.001]. The accuracy is however within about ± 5 degrees. Figure 5 shows the result on time efficiency. The vertical axis shows the elapsed time to complete the calibration across all the subjects. From the figure, all the calibration is completed within about 700 milliseconds. The time efficiency is improved by 17% as compared to the previous way [1].

5 Conclusions

This manuscript conducted an experiment in usability of shadow cursor for calibrating screen coordinates of tabletop displays. The results showed that the shadow cursor presents a good performance in accuracy and time efficiency.

Reference

1. Ishihara, M., Ishihara, Y.: Calibrating coordinates of a tabletop display with a reflex in eye-hand coordination. IEICE Trans. on Information and Systems e93-d(10), 2862–2865 (2010)

Designing Interactive Sonification for Live Aquarium Exhibits

Myounghoon Jeon[1], Riley J. Winton[2], Ashley G. Henry[2], Sanghun Oh[2], Carrie M. Bruce[2], and Bruce N. Walker[2]

[1] Mind, Music & Machine Lab, Michigan Technological University, Michigan, USA
[2] Sonification Lab, Georgia Institute of Technology, Georgia, USA
mjeon@mtu.edu, {rjwinton,ashleyghenry,soh72,carrie.bruce, bruce.walker}@gatech.edu

Abstract. In response to the need for more accessible and engaging informal learning environments (ILEs), researchers have studied sonification for use in interpretation of live aquarium exhibits. The present work attempts to introduce more interactivity to the project's existing sonification work, which is expected to lead to more accessible and interactive learning opportunities for visitors, including children and people with vision impairment. In this interactive sonification environment, visitors can actively experience an exhibit by using tangible objects to mimic the movement of animals. Sonifications corresponding to their movement can be paired with real-time animal-based sonifications produced by the existing system to generate a musical fugue. In the current paper, we describe the system configurations, experiment results for optimal sonification parameters and interaction levels, and implications in terms of embodied interaction and interactive learning.

Keywords: Embodied interaction, interactive learning, interactive sonification, interactivity, tangible objects.

1 Introduction

To improve the accessibility of exhibits and promote universal design in aquariums, researchers have studied real-time animal-based interpretive sonification as a strategy for translating visual aspects of live animal exhibits [1-2]. The Accessible Aquarium Project has focused on designing sonifications for individuals with vision impairment that convey the informational (e.g., animal type, location, movement, and facts) and aesthetic aspects (e.g., the "feeling" or mood perceived by visitors) of live exhibits. This enables visitors with vision impairment to experience an exhibit in both cognitive and affective aspects, and it also provides a shared experience so that all visitors could discuss their understanding and impressions of the exhibit. One way to accomplish this is through music that communicates both information and feeling. Previous studies [1-2] showed that we could match musical features such as pitch and tempo with animal information such as height in tank and swimming speed to facilitate understanding of exhibit dynamics. To fulfill and strengthen those aspects, a

C. Stephanidis (Ed.): Posters, Part I, HCII 2013, CCIS 373, pp. 332–336, 2013.

new, interactive sonification project attempts to enrich visitors' experiences in aquariums by combining and harmonizing animal-and audience-inspired sonifications. By increasing interactivity among animals and audience, it is expected that visitors will have richer experiences.

Interactivity. The Accessible Aquarium Project has contained coherent *reactivity* with a consistent feedback loop between animals and sounds, but it does not allow for *interactivity* [3] between the animals and audience. Rafaeli [3] has suggested a distinction between quasi interactivity (e.g., two way communication or reactive communication) and full interactivity depending on the nature of the communication responses. Both reactive and fully interactive communications require that communicants respond to each other. However, with quasi interactivity the content of response might have just a reaction to previous messages, whereas with full interactivity responses should incorporate references to the content already exchanged and conjure up memorable interactive exchanges. Based on Rafaeli's discussion, the initial sonification system can be categorized as quasi-interactive communication (Fig. 1. A (a)). Once the animal moves (M1), the sonification system creates music (M2) based on that movement. However, when the animal moves again, it is autonomous and not a response to the previous messages (M1 or M2). Thus, the previous system does not enable interactive communication between the animal and the visitor. In the latest interactive sonification configuration, communicants respond to each other in full interactivity (Fig. 1. A (b)). Once the animal-based sonification system generates melody 1 (M1), the audience (or audience-based sonification system) will generate counter-melody 1 (M2) based on the melody 1. Because melody 2 (M3) is not only based on the newer movement of animal, but also structurally based on M2, which is based on M1, the melody 2 incorporates references to all of the previous messages and responses. Thus, this new work adds full interactivity to the sonification of live exhibits by communication exchange between animal–and audience–based sonifications.

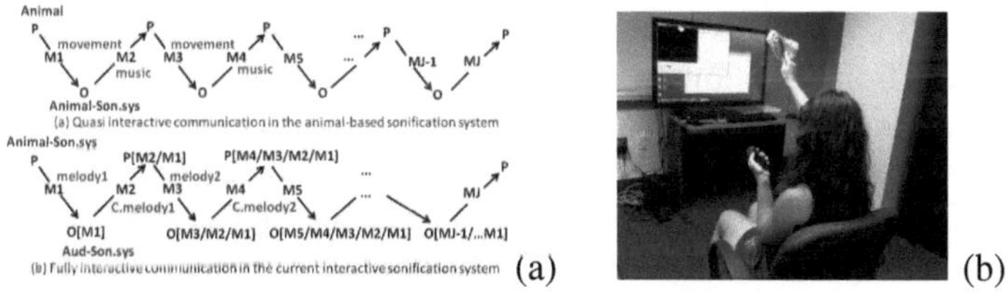

Fig. 1. A. Different communications in (a) the fish-based sonification system and (b) the interactive sonification system. B. View of the experiment

2 System Configuration and Experiment

System Configuration. Our first attempt at building an interactive system leveraged the existing real-time animal-based interpretive sonifications to enable a collaborative sonification. Consequently, visitors were able to contribute to a cooperative sonification of the live exhibit by generating a counter melody. For the rapid prototyping of the interactive sonification system, we took a simple movement-to-sound mapping approach to complement the real-time interpretive sonification of live animal movement. Based on the results of the preliminary pilot study [4], we enhanced the system configuration in several ways and conducted a lab experiment to identify optimal sonification parameters such as mapping, polarity, and interaction levels. First, we changed our tracking system from reacTIVision and TUIOs into Microsoft Kinect™ for better detection in terms of resolution and degree of freedom in users' movement. Second, we changed our graphical dataflow program from Max/MSP into Pure Data, which is an open source version of Max/MSP. Finally, instead of sequencing software, we employed a standalone virtual instrument to set up a lighter system platform. In this experimental system, the y-axis of space represented the pitch of the notes, and consisted of four different musical scales: major chord arpeggio (C3-E3-G3-C4), pentatonic scale (C3-D3-E3-G3-A3-C4), diatonic scale (C3-D3-E3-F3-G3-A3-B3-C4), and chromatic scale including all the semi tones in one octave (C3-C#3-D3-D#3-E3-F3-F#3-G3-G#3-A3-A#3-B3-C4). The x-axis represented panning of the sound, but was not used in the experimental task for control purposes. For the virtual instrument, LegacyCell patch 116: Poly Pad was used. A 40″ TV was used as a monitor and sounds were generated from the TV speakers with volume level 25.

Procedure. A total of 51 people participated in this study. 42 people were undergraduate students (27 male, 15 female; mean age = 20) and 9 were children (5 male, 4 female; mean age = 8). Of the 42 undergraduates, 36 had musical experience (23 male, 13 female; 21 mean age = 20; 2 with absolute pitch). Of the 9 children, 7 had musical experience (4 male, 3 female; mean age = 9). After the informed consent procedure, participants had a short practice session (1-2 minutes) to become familiar with how to control the toys and generate sounds. For this practice, the pentatonic scale was used, which was not included in the experimental session. Then, they were randomly presented with different polarity mapping (ascending and descending) between the movement of animal and sounds and asked to assess which they preferred. For example, in ascending mapping, if the toy animal moves up, the sound was generated from the lower note to the higher note and vice versa. Next, participants assessed an appropriate frequency range based on the size of the two fish toys of the same type (a small and large ray). They could select the frequency range among 36 (C1 range), 48 (C2 range), 60 (C3 range), 84 (C5 range), and 108 (C7 range). They were given the chance to hear each frequency range with a large animal and small animal. After completing polarity and size mapping tasks, participants were asked to perform a pitch-matching task. The overall goal of this task was for participants to generate the same sound as the target sound, which consisted of a successive three-note motif. The participant would move the toy until the target note was heard and then click the clicker to select the note. The experiment included three different scale conditions (major chord arpeggio, diatonic, and chromatic scales) and each condition had two blocks, which was composed of three different trials. Each condition was counterbalanced across participants and each trial was randomized in a block. With children participants, the conditions were not counterbalanced; thus, all children performed the major arpeggio, the diatonic, then the chromatic condition. This was done to help remove frustration when initiating the task. In the experiment, frequency range 60 (C3 range) was always used. After each condition, participants rated how 'difficult' and 'fun' the task was using seven-point Likert type scales.

Results. Overall, there was no difference based on musical experience or training. However, there were some interesting differences between adults and children participants. For the polarity of the sounds, the majority of the undergraduates (28/42) preferred the ascending direction. They wanted the sounds to go up in pitch when they moved the toy animal upwards, whereas most of the children (6/9) preferred the opposite ($p < .05$). For the size mapping, the undergraduates favored the large animal to be mapped onto lower frequency ranges ($M = 60$) and the small animal onto higher frequency ranges ($M = 63.7$) ($p < .05$), which confirms previous research [1-2]. Surprisingly, the children oppositely favored mapping the large animal onto higher frequency ranges ($M = 76$) and small animal onto lower frequency ranges ($M = 65.3$). In terms of pitch-matching task, both subjective and objective data revealed a challenging "cut-off" point in the interaction. As expected, as the scales increased in complexity, so did the reported difficulty. The major chord arpeggio scale ($M = 3.7$, $SD = 1.6$) was easier than the diatonic scale ($M = 4.7$, $SD = 1.4$), which was easier than the chromatic scale ($M = 4.9$, $SD = 1.3$). Somewhat similar results were shown in the fun rating with the least complex, major chord arpeggio scale ($M = 5.1$, $SD = 1.3$), being the most fun. However, there was no significant difference between the fun rating of the diatonic scale and chromatic scale (Both: Ms = 4.9). This tendency was similarly reflected in objective data. The more complicated scale yielded longer task completion time and lower accuracy (chromatic: 19.3s, 9.1%; diatonic: 17.9s, 18.7%; chord: 13.8s, 61.1%) (ps < .05). In short, the major chord arpeggio scale was the easiest and most fun. The diatonic scale was more difficult and less fun and although the chromatic scale was rated at the same level, it was too difficult to enjoy. Taken the results together, matching specific pitches might not be a desirable way of interaction. Therefore, a further analysis of "pattern matching" instead of exact pitch matching was performed. For example, if the given melody was note 1, 10, then 6 of a given scale, then the required pattern would have been "Up 9," (1 → 10) "Down 4" (10 → 6). Over all scale conditions, the undergraduates matched the exact pitch sequence 29.6% of the time. However, they matched the pattern direction of the sequence 87.7% of the time (chromatic: 86.1%, diatonic: 76.1%; chord: 79.4%). In cases where these users made errors in the magnitude of movement, they showed to differ by an average of only 1.9 notes (chromatic: 2.3 notes, diatonic: 1.6 notes, chord: 1.2 notes), which is promising for this type of approximate pattern matching interaction design. The pitch-matching task with children resulted in intriguing data. Both the difficulty and fun ratings did not follow the expected pattern. Interestingly, the difficulty rating of the major chord arpeggio scale ($M = 4.3$ $SD = 1.9$) was the highest compared to that of the diatonic scale ($M = 3.9$, $SD = 2.1$) and the chromatic scale ($M = 3.8$, $SD = 2.4$). The fun rating showed the opposite of what was expected with an increase in fun from the major chord arpeggio scale ($M = 5.7$, $SD = 1.6$) to the diatonic scale ($M = 5.9$, $SD = 1.3$). The fun rating then decreased for the chromatic scale ($M = 5.7$, $SD = 1.2$). However, these differences were not statistically different and might reflect innate order effects.

3 Discussion

The present work serves to approximate the ideal levels of interaction for various users. Parameter recommendations for polarity, pitch range, animal size, and note resolution have been derived from these experimental results. Given that most participants showed relatively low accuracy when matching specific pitch sequences, but a high ability to match the pattern of the movement, the next iteration of this system will allow visitors' approximate movement to automatically generate musically harmonized sounds with the animal-inspired sonification. The interaction between animals (or animal-based sonification system) and audience could further evolve into the interaction between audience and audience, which will lead to interactive learning [5]. Additional users could create 3rd or 4th counter-melodies by interacting with their fellow visitors. These multifaceted efforts could create innovative and engaging soundscapes in aquariums that attract diverse visitors, regardless of their age, visual, or musical abilities. It is clear that flexibility according to users' different preferences and abilities must always be considered. More specific recommendations and discoveries are likely to result from further research in this continuing project.

References

1. Walker, B.N., Godfrey, M.T., Orlosky, J.E., Bruce, C.M., Sanford, J.: Aquarium sonification: Soundscapes for accessible dynamic informal learning environments. In: 12th International Conference on Auditory Display, London (2006)
2. Walker, B.N., Kim, J., Pendse, A.: Musical soundscapes for an accessible aquarium: Bringing dynamic exhibits to the visually impaired. In: International Computer Music Conference, Copenhagen (2007)
3. Rafaeli, S.: Interactivity: From new media to communication Sage Annual Review of Communication Research: Advancing Communication Science, Sage, Beverly Hills, 16 pp. (1988)
4. Jeon, M., Winton, R.J., Yim, J.-B., Bruce, C.M., Walker, B.N.: AquariumFugue: Interactive sonification for children and visually impaired audience in informal learning environments. In: 18th International Conference on Auditory Display, Atlanta (2012)
5. Chi, M.T.H.: Active-constructive-interactive: A conceptual framework for differentiating learning activities. Topics in Cognitive Science 1, 73–105 (2009)

Emotional Speech Conversion Using Pitch-Synchronous Harmonic and Non-harmonic Modeling of Speech

Kwang Myung Jeon and Nam In Park

School of Information and Communications
Gwangju Institute of Science and Technology (GIST)
1 Oryong-dong, Buk-gu, Gwangju 500-712, Korea
{kmjeon,naminpark}@gist.ac.kr

Abstract. In this paper, an emotional speech conversion method using pitch-synchronous harmonic and non-harmonic (PS-HNH) modeling of speech is proposed. The proposed method converts neutral speeches into expressive ones by controlling emotional parameters for each syllable of the neutral speech. To this end, the proposed method first carries out syllable labeling by Viterbi decoding using acoustic hidden Markov models of the neutral corpus. Next, the PS-HNH analysis is performed on the neutral speech to modify the emotional parameters by the linear modification model of target emotion in a syllable-wise manner. Finally, the modified parameters are synthesized back into the emotional speech by the PS-HNH synthesis. The performance of the proposed method is evaluated by a subjective AB preference test for four types of target emotions (fear, sadness, anger, and happiness). It is shown from the preference test that the proposed method give better speech quality than the conventional method that is based on speech transformation and representation using adaptive interpolation of weighted spectrum (STRAIGHT).

Keywords: Emotional speech, speech conversion, pitch-synchronous, harmonic and non-harmonic modeling.

1 Introduction

Speech and audio processing are the major tasks to improve sound user interface (SUI)-based human computer interaction (HCI) applications [1]. Various studies have been performed to improve the SUI experience by expressing emotional speech [2][3], reducing unwanted signals [4][5], providing sound-based emotional interaction functionality [6][7], and improving the robustness of speech transmission [8][9]. Among these research fields, the expression of emotional speech by converting neutral speech into emotional speech is particularly important for the SUI to give emotional feedback to users [2][3].Recent studies related to emotional speech conversion techniques have commonly applied speech transformation and representation using adaptive interpolation of weighted spectrum (STRAIGHT) to control emotional parameters such as fundamental frequency (F0), duration, and intensity of neutral speech segments [2][3]. Due to its flexible speech modification

C. Stephanidis (Ed.): Posters, Part I, HCII 2013, CCIS 373, pp. 337–341, 2013.

property, STRAIGHT is suitable for the emotional speech conversion task [10]. However, it can cause the quality degradation of the modified speech due to the lack of phase information [11]. Thus, the quality of the emotional speech conversion can be further improved by applying a more sophisticated speech modification technique.In this paper, a novel emotional speech conversion method based on pitch-synchronous harmonic and non-harmonic (PS-HNH) modeling is proposed. The proposed method expresses various emotional speech signals by controlling four emotional parameters such as intensity, pitch, frequency, and duration of each syllable of the neutral speech. To this end, the proposed method first performs syllable labeling by Viterbi decoding using acoustic hidden Markov models (HMMs) that are trained by using the neutral corpus. The PS-HNH analysis is then performed to decompose the neutral speech of the syllable unit into the harmonic and non-harmonic components [11]. Further, the emotional parameters for both the harmonic and non-harmonic components are modified as specific factors by the linear modification model (LMM) of the target emotion, which is defined in [2]. Finally, the prosody-modified harmonic and non-harmonic components are synthesized back into the emotional speech by using pitch-synchronous overlap-and-add (PSOLA) and pseudo-random overlap-and-add (PROLA), respectively [11]. Following this introduction, Section 2 proposes an emotional speech conversion method based on PS-HNH modeling. Section 3 then evaluates the performance of the proposed method. Finally, Section 4 concludes this paper.

2 Proposed Emotional Speech Conversion Method Using PS-HNH Modeling of Speech

Fig. 1 shows the framework of the proposed emotional speech conversion method. As shown in the figure, syllable labeling is first performed by concatenating the phoneme sequence that is obtained from Viterbi decoding using the acoustic HMMs of the neutral corpus [12]. Specifically, for a given neutral speech, s, and its acoustic model, λ, the phoneme of s for the neutral speech, $\overline{w}$, is estimated by maximizing the likelihood as $\overline{w} = \arg\max\{p(w \mid s, \lambda)\}$. From $\overline{w}$, syllable labeling is conducted using the context-dependent label format that is used in statistical speech synthesis [12]. Second, the proposed method decomposes the syllable units of the neutral speech signal into harmonic and non-harmonic parts by PS-HNH analysis [11] for the syllable-wise prosodic modification. In other words, the syllable unit of the neutral speech, $s^j(n)$, is represented as $s^j(n) = s_h^j(n) + s_{nh}^j(n)$, where $s_h^j(n)$ and $s_{nh}^j(n)$ represent a harmonic signal generated by vibrating vocal folds and a non-periodic signal having noise-like characteristics, respectively. Note that j denotes the syllable unit index. In fact, $s_h^j(n)$ is modeled by the sum of harmonically related sinusoidal components within each analysis frame, which is written as

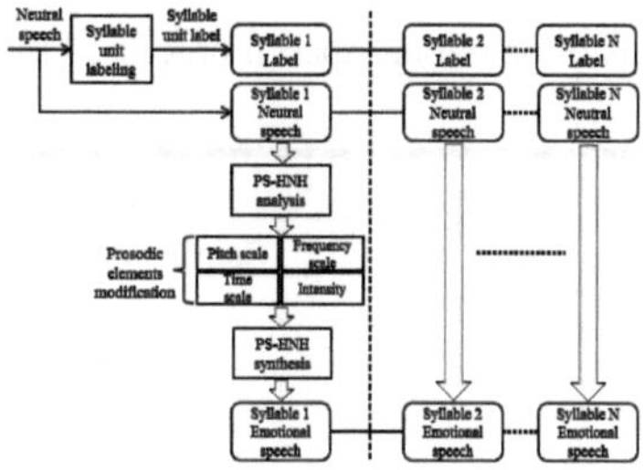

Fig. 1. Framework of the proposed emotional speech conversion method

$$s_h^j(n) = \begin{cases} \sum_k \sum_{l=1}^{L_k} a_k(l) \cos\left(2\pi l (n-m) f_{0k}\right), & if \ f_{0k} > 0 \\ 0, & otherwise \end{cases} \tag{1}$$

where $L_k = \lfloor f_s / f_{0k} \rfloor$ is the number of harmonic sinusoids at the k-th analysis frame and $a_k(l)$ is an amplitude of the l-th harmonic sinusoid at the k-th analysis frame. In addition, f_{0k} is the fundamental frequency of the k-th analysis frame, f_s is the sampling frequency, and, m indicates a frame shift that is defined as $m = L_k$. and In Eq. (1), f_{0k} is obtained by applying the F0 extraction technique in STRAIGHT [10], and $a_k(l)$ is estimated by using the least-square method introduced in the harmonic plus noise model [13].

Similarly to $s_h^j(n)$, $s_{nh}^j(n)$ is represented by the sum of sinusoids with pseudo-randomized frequencies, such as

$$s_{nh}^j(n) = \begin{cases} \sum_k \sum_{l=1}^{L} a_k(l) \cos\left(2\pi \ l (n-m)(1+r(k)) f_{nh}\right), & if \ f_{0k} > 0 \\ \sum_k \sum_{l=1}^{L} a_k(l) \cos\left(2\pi \ l (n-m')(1+r(k)) f_{nh}\right), & otherwise \end{cases} \tag{2}$$

where $L = \lfloor f_s / f_{nh} \rfloor$ is also the number of non-harmonic sinusoids and f_{nh} acts as a fundamental frequency for non-harmonic modeling but is set to a constant value. In this paper, f_{nh} is set to 50 Hz. Moreover, $r(k)$ in Eq. (2) is a pseudo-random number whose value ranges from -0.1 to 0.1. Note that $r(k)$ in the analysis step must be identical to that in the synthesis step. In addition, $m' = L$ is a frame shift for $s_{nh}^j(n)$. Finally, syllable-wise prosodic modification is conducted in PS-HNH synthesis [11]. Specifically, four emotional parameters such as intensity, pitch, frequency, and duration of $s_h^j(n)$ and $s_{nh}^j(n)$ are modified as

$$\hat{s}_h^j(n) = \begin{cases} \sum_{T(k)} M_i \sum_{l=1}^{L_k} a_k(l) \cos\left(2\pi l (n - m / M_p) f_{0k} M_f\right), & if \ f_{0k} > 0 \\ 0, & otherwise \end{cases} \tag{3}$$

Table 1. Preference test results of emotional speech processed by the conventional conversion method and the proposed one

Target Emotion	Preference Score (%)	
	Conventional	Proposed
Fear	18.18	81.82
Sadness	27.27	72.73
Anger	36.36	63.64
Happiness	9.09	90.91
Average	22.73	77.27

and

$$\hat{s}_{nh}^{j}(n) = \begin{cases} \sum_{T(k)} M_i \sum_{l=1}^{L} a_k(l)\cos\left(2\pi l(n - m/M_p)(1+r(k))f_{nh}M_f\right), & \text{if } f_{0k} > 0 \\ \sum_{T(k)} M_i \sum_{l=1}^{L} a_k(l)\cos\left(2\pi l(n - m'/M_p)(1+r(k))f_{nh}M_f\right), & \text{otherwise} \end{cases} \quad (4)$$

where $T(k) = \lfloor k(K-1)/(M_t M_p K - 1) + 0.5 \rfloor$ is a warping function with the total number of synthesized frames of K. In addition, M_i, M_t, M_f, and M_p are intensity, time, frequency, and pitch modification parameters, respectively. In this paper, all the modification parameters are differently selected for each syllable by the LMM of the target emotion to be converted [2].

3 Performance Evaluation

The performance of the proposed emotional speech conversion method was evaluated by carrying out an AB preference test, where the proposed method was compared with a conventional method based on STRAIGHT [10]. In the test, neutral speech clips of 10 males and 10 females were selected from the CMU US ARCTIC database [11]. Next, each neutral speech clip was converted into four different ones representing target emotions by the proposed method and the conventional one. Then, 11 listeners without any auditory disease, all between 20 and 30 years old, were asked to choose their preference between the emotional speech obtained by the proposed method and that obtained by the conventional one. Note that the participants were not informed of which method was used to obtain the emotional speech clips for the test. Table 1 compares relative preference of the proposed method to the conventional method for all target emotions. It was shown from the table that the proposed method gave better emotional speech quality than the conventional method.

4 Conclusion

In this paper, a PS-HNH-based emotional speech conversion method was proposed. The proposed method modified the prosodic parameters of the neutral speech signals to obtain emotional speech signals in a syllable-wise manner. In other words, the proposed method consisted of syllable labeling, PS-HNH analysis, prosodic parameter modification, and PS-HNH synthesis. The proposed method was evaluated by an AB preference test for the various target emotions, and the test demonstrated that the proposed method converted neutral speech into emotional speech with more favorable quality than the conventional method based on STRAIGHT.

Acknowledgments. This work was supported in part by the National Research Foundation of Korea (NRF) grant funded by the Korea government (MEST) (No. 2012-010636).

References

1. Jaimes, A., Sebe, N.: Multimodal human-computer interaction: a survey. Computer Vision and Image Understanding 108(1–2), 116–134 (2007)
2. Tao, J., Kang, Y., Li, A.: Prosody conversion from neutral speech to emotional speech. IEEE Transactions on Audio, Speech, and Language Processing 14(4), 1145–1154 (2006)
3. Aihara, R., Takashima, R., Takiguchi, T., Ariki, Y.: GMM-based emotional voice conversion using spectrum and prosody features. American Journal of Signal Processing 2(5), 134–138 (2012)
4. Kim, S.M., Kim, H.K., Kim, M.B., Kim, S.R.: Probabilistic spectral gain modification applied to beamformer-based noise reduction in a car environment. IEEE Transactions on Consumer Electronics 57(2), 866–872 (2011)
5. Park, J.H., Kim, H.K., Kim, M.B., Kim, S.R.: A user voice reduction algorithm based on binaural signal separation for portable digital imaging devices. IEEE Transactions on Consumer Electronics 58(2), 679–684 (2012)
6. Oh, Y.R., Yoon, J.S., Kim, H.K., Kim, M.B., Kim, S.R.: A voice-driven scene-mode recommendation service for portable digital imaging devices. IEEE Transactions on Consumer Electronics 55(4), 1739–1747 (2009)
7. Kang, J.A., Chun, C.J., Kim, H.K., Kim, M.B., Kim, S.R.: A smart background music mixing algorithm for portable digital imaging devices. IEEE Transactions on Consumer Electronics 57(3), 1258–1263 (2011)
8. Kang, J.A., Kim, H.K.: An adaptive packet loss recovery method based on real-time speech quality assessment and redundant speech transmission. International Journal of Innovative Computing, Information and Control 7(12), 6773–6783 (2011)
9. Kang, J.A., Kim, H.K.: Adaptive redundant speech transmission over wireless multimedia sensor networks based on estimation of perceived speech quality. Sensors 11(9), 8469–8484 (2011)
10. Kawahara, H.: Speech representation and transformation using adaptive interpolation of weighted spectrum: vocoder revisited. In: Proceedings of IEEE International Conference on Acoustic, Speech, and Signal Processing (ICASSP), Munich, Germany, pp. 1303–1306 (1997)
11. Jeon, K.M., Kim, H.K.: High-quality speech modification based on pitch-synchronous harmonic and non-harmonic modeling of speech. Advanced Science and Technology Letters 14, 176–179 (2012)
12. Zen, H., Tokuda, K., Black, A.W.: Statistical parametric speech synthesis. Speech Communication 51(11), 1039–1064 (2009)
13. Stylianou, Y.: Applying the harmonic plus noise model in concatenative speech synthesis. IEEE Transactions on Speech and Audio Processing 9(1), 21–29 (2001)
14. Kominek, J., Black, A.W.: The CMU ARCTIC speech databases. In: Proceedings of the 5th ISCA Tutorial and Research Workshop on Speech Synthesis (SSW-5), Pittsburgh, PA, pp. 223–224 (2004)

Lyricons (Lyrics + Earcons): Designing a New Auditory Cue Combining Speech and Sounds

Myounghoon Jeon

Mind, Music & Machine Lab, Michigan Technological University, Houghton, Michigan, USA
mjeon@mtu.edu

Abstract. To complement visual displays, auditory researchers have developed various auditory cues such as auditory icons, earcons, spearcons, and spindex cues. Even though those auditory cues were successfully applied to a number of electronic devices, they still require some improvements. From this background, the present work introduces more intuitive and fun auditory cues, "Lyricons (Lyrics + Earcons), which integrate the benefits of speech (i.e., accuracy) and earcons (i.e., aesthetics). We categorized functions of electronic products into meta-functional groups and devised a plausible earcon set for each functional group. Nine students conducted the sound card sorting task to match earcons with functional groups and brainstormed to generate lyrics for each functional group. Based on the results, several lyricon sets were created and improvements and application directions were discussed in focus group sessions. The use of lyricons is expected to increase accessibility to electronic devices for multiple users, including novices, older adults, children, and people with vision impairment.

Keywords: Auditory displays, lyricons, speech sounds, non-speech sounds.

1 Introduction

For two decades, auditory displays have been actively studied to complement or even replace visual displays for both visually impaired and sighted users. The most obvious means of using auditory representation is speech. However, speech is not the entirety of auditory displays. Just as visual icons allow users for quick scan, auditory icons [1] (representative part of sounds of objects) have been introduced and followed by earcons [2] (ear + icons, short musical motives as symbolic representations of objects). As compensating for their innate issues (e.g., practicality of auditory icons and arbitrariness of earcons), researchers have returned to speech and tweaked it for glance purpose, which led to creation of spearcons [3] (compressed speech) and spindex [4] (speech + index). Both auditory cues were successfully applied to various mobile and vehicle contexts. Yet spearcons require minimum learning and spindex cues can be applied to only the menu with an alphabetical order. Based on these backgrounds, the current paper introduces new auditory cues, "Lyricons", which combine the benefits of speech (i.e., accuracy) and earcons (i.e., aesthetics). Lyricons are composed of two parallel layers including earcons (e.g., "Do-Re-Mi") and corresponding lyrics of the designated function (e.g., "Func-Tion-On").

C. Stephanidis (Ed.): Posters, Part I, HCII 2013, CCIS 373, pp. 342–346, 2013.

2 Function Analysis and Earcon Design

Because using auditory cues for every function of electronic products might result in auditory pollution, we categorized functions of electronic products (appliances, mobile devices, and in-vehicle devices) into meta-functional groups [5-6] using preliminary function analysis. Then, a professional sound designer created a plausible earcon set for each functional group (see Table 1). For the experimental purpose, all sounds were uniformly played as the same timbre, piano sound.

Each meta-functional group represents several functions of electronic products. For example, the "Cancel" group includes 'cancel', 'back', and 'magnitude change limit'. The "Function off" group includes 'pause/stop', or 'end function'. The "Function on" group includes 'play' or 'start cycle'. Likewise, the "Power off" group includes 'terminate products', 'turn off', or 'power off'. The "Power on" group includes 'initiate products', 'turn on', 'power on', or 'boot up'. The "OK" group includes 'accept', 'select', or 'check'. The "Touch" group includes 'basic control', 'press', 'enter', or 'touch on screen'. The "Unavailable" group includes 'unavailable button', 'unavailable touch area', etc. In addition to short auditory feedback, there is relatively longer auditory feedback: "reminder" for prospective memory (e.g., mom's birthday or meeting time) and "informing" (e.g., cycle completed" in washing machine) as neutral information, and "alarm", which means danger happens now, (e.g., fire alarm) and "warning", which means danger will happen if user action is not taken (e.g., door open in oven while cooking) as negative information.

Table 1. Meta-functional group and corresponding earcon designs

No.	Meta-Functional Group (Musical Notes of Earcons)
1	Cancel/ Back/ Magnitude Change Limit (G5G5).wav
2	Function Off (E4D4C4).wav
5	Function On (C4D4E4).wav
8	Informing or reminder ("Over the rainbow").wav
9	Informing or reminder ("Unfamiliar Melody").wav
10	Magnitude Change Down (A4G4).wav
11	Magnitude Change Up (G4A4).wav
12	OK (G5E5).wav
16	Power Off (C5G4E4G4C4).wav
17	Power On (C4G4E4G4C5).wav
21	Touch (G5).wav
22	Unavailable (G1).wav
23	Warning or alarm (C5D5C5D5C5D5).wav
24	Warning or alarm (C5D5C5E5F5E5).wav

3 Sound Card Sorting Task and Lyricon Design

To identify how intuitively users can match earcons with intended functions, the sound card sorting task [7] was used. In total, nine graduate students (male 5; female 4) participated in the subsequent sessions. Each participant was given four sound cards, each containing a recording of one experimental sound stimulus and four index cards, each containing a functional description. First, an experimenter explained the meaning of each function to participants. Before they start a sorting task, participants were told to listen to all of the sound recordings. Then, participants paired each sound stimulus with the function that best relates. Participants were allowed to have as much time as they wanted to complete the sorting task. Upon completion, responses were recorded by the experimenter. The session consisted of two blocks (i.e., sets 1 and 2, 1 and 3, or 2 and 3 for each participant), and thus all participants paired eight sound cards with the eight functions in total. At the end of the session, they were urged to label (i.e., making lyrics of) each sound.

Table 2 shows the sound card sorting task results. Even though all of the sounds were created by a sound designer, based on the guidelines which have been used in industry (e.g., Samsung Electronics, LG Electronics, and General Electric), the average of the matching accuracy was less than 60%. Only "unavailable" and "power-on" sound attained 100% accuracy as a designer's intention. Even neutral auditory signals such as reminder and informing and negative signals such as alarm and warning were confusing with each other, which implies that although non-speech sounds are carefully designed, it is still hard for users to intuitively match those sounds with the intended functions, which led to the design of lyricons.

Table 2. Participants' responses from the Sound Card Sorting Task. The intended response is bold.

	Participant1	Participant2	Participant3	Participant4	Participant5	Participant6	Total (%)
Function On	16	**5**	**5**	16	16	12	33%
Power Off	5	**16**	**16**	12	12	16	60%
OK	**12**	**12**	**12**	5	5	5	50%
Unavailable	**22**	**22**	**22**	**22**	**22**	**22**	100%

(a) Set 1

	Participant1	Participant2	Participant3	Participant7	Participant8	Participant9	Total (%)
Function On	21	**2**	**2**	**2**	**2**	**2**	83%
Power Off	**17**	**17**	**17**	**17**	**17**	**17**	100%
OK	2	1	**21**	**21**	1	1	33%
Unavailable	**1**	21	**1**	**1**	21	21	50%

(b) Set 2

	Participant4	Participant5	Participant6	Participant7	Participant8	Participant9	Total (%)
Reminder	**9**	**9**	**8**	23	24	24	50%
Informing	24	24	24	**8**	**9**	**9**	50%
Alarm	**23**	**23**	**23**	9	8	8	50%
Warning	8	8	9	**24**	**23**	**23**	50%

(c) Set 3

Based on participants' naming, the following sets of lyricons were designed. Lyricons for the reminder, informing, alarm, and warning functions were not created in this study. Lyrics can be classified largely into two categories: words imitating sounds (e.g., TaDaDong) and functional names (e.g., FuncTionOff).

Table 3. Functional groups and Lyrics for each group

No.	Functional Groups (Musical Notes)	"Lyrics"
1	Cancel/ Back/ Magnitude Change Limit (G5G5).wav	PiDing/ Back/ Ceiling
2	Function Off (E4D4C4).wav	FuncTionOff/ SleePing Mode/ TaDaDong
5	Function On (C4D4E4).wav	FuncTionOn/ WaKingUp/ TaDaDing
10	Magnitude Change Down (A4G4).wav	DaDong/ DeScend/ Down/ GoDown
11	Magnitude Change Up (G4A4).wav	DaDing/ Ascend/ Up/ GoUp
12	OK (G5E5).wav	OKay/SuCess
16	Power Off (C5G4E4G4C4).wav	DaRaDaRaDong/ TurnItOff
17	Power On (C4G4E4G4C5).wav	DaRaDaRaDing/ TurnItOn
21	Touch (G5).wav	Ping/ Tink
22	Unavailable (G1).wav	Bumb/ Dumb/ Nope

4 Focus Group

Using the lyricon sets, successive focus group sessions were conducted with a total of 6 participants (male 2; female 4). They discussed plausible usage, advantages, and improvements of several designs of Lyricons. Out of the two types of lyricons, they encouraged researchers to apply functional names over words imitating sounds to train users to be familiar with sound patterns and their meanings. One commented, "It would be helpful for my grandma." The other said, "It seems to give the machine identity and users would not throw away their *'speaking'* or *'singing'* mobile phone." Participants agreed that this auditory user interfaces could be more appropriate to mobile phones and in-vehicle technologies because those systems are more privately attached to users and this humanization (adding human voice) would facilitate such relationship. Moreover, participants reported that they are already familiar with human voices from the navigation devices in their car. One participant pointed out that the lyric part is sometimes hard to understand due to the earcon part. This balance issue should be addressed in the next design iteration.

5 Discussion

The present work provides a novel approach to devising auditory cues, lyricons, in electronic products by combining the two layers of earcons and speech. This new approach is expected to enhance accessibility of auditory user interface for children, visually impaired users, older adults and even sighted users. Moreover, this idea can contribute to auditory user interfaces in terms of the implementation of *funnology* (fun

+ technology) and the improvement of interface aesthetics. More practically, once users get familiar with this type of auditory user interface and automatized in using it, then they may use only "earcons" part without the "lyrics" part just as in the spearcons case – once users are familiar with "spearcons + text-to-speech", they can use "spearcons-only" mode without text-to-speech part [8]. We plan to conduct experiments using lyricons in various mobile contexts including in-vehicle infotainment.

References

1. Gaver, W.W.: Auditory icons: Using sound in computer interfaces. Human-Computer Interaction 2, 167–177 (1986)
2. Blattner, M.M., Sumikawa, D.A., Greenberg, R.M.: Earcons and icons: Their structure and common design principles. Human-Computer Interaction 4, 11–44 (1989)
3. Walker, B.N., Lindsay, J., Nance, A., Nakano, Y., Palladino, D.K., Dingler, T., Jeon, M.: Spearcons (speech-based earcons) improve navigation performance in advanced auditory menus. Human Factors 55(1), 157–182 (2013)
4. Jeon, M., Walker, N.B.: "Spindex" (Speech Index) improves acceptance and performance in auditory menu navigation for visually impaired and sighted users. ACM Transactions on Accessible Computing 3(3), 10:1–10:26 (2011)
5. Lee, J.H., Jeon, M., Ahn, J.H., Han, K.H.: Developing the design guideline of auditory user interface for domestic appliances. In: Korean Conference on Human Computer Interaction, Kangwon (2006)
6. Jeon, M.: Tow or three things you need to know about AUI design or designers. In: International Conference on Auditory Display, Washington, D.C (2010)
7. Bonebright, T., Jeon, M.: Information research methods for evaluating auditory displays. In: International Conference on Auditory Display, Atlanta (2012)
8. Suh, H., Jeon, M., Walker, B.N.: Spearcons improve navigation performance and perceived speediness in Korean auditory menus. In: 56th Annual Meeting of the Human Factors and Ergonomics Society, Boston (2012)

The Difference of the Emotional Communication by Movement on the Digital Contents

Jieun Lee and Hayashi Mitsuko

Hokkaido University of Education, Humanities and Regional Science, hachimancho 1-2, hakodate-shi, Hokkaido, Japan
jeentwo@gmail.com, hayashi.mitsuko@h.hokkyodai.ac.jp

Abstract. In this paper, a sensitivity evaluation of digital contents with dynamic motion, including linguistic and visual functions, and musical and visual rhythms was performed. In order to improve student's expressive and utilizing skills by using digital contents with dynamic representations and to support of the design education in the new environment of media, it is necessary to understand sensitivity evaluation of digital contents with motion as the most new form of communications. As a result, it was confirmed that static content with music and content displayed a similar change in sensitivity than music's in the static digital content with music.

Keywords: Digital contents, Music, Contents, Movement, Emotion.

1 Introduction

Through the preliminary study and this paper, investigations aimed at understanding the sensitivity of digital contents which include linguistic and visual functions, and musical and visual rhythms in the new environment of media. To understand the influence which music and content bring to digital content, the difference in sensitivity towards a) music as the focus on emotional communication, b) static digital content (poem) with music and c) content (using b) were compared in the preliminary study. It was confirmed that static digital content with music and content displayed a similar change in sensitivity than music. However in another preliminary study using the digital contents with dynamic motion (kinetic typography) and music, some inquiries have revealed that kinetic typography with music and music which was produced by are considerably influenced by sensitivity evaluation of music then the content which was used. Therefore, this research was conducted in order to understand the influence of the motion in kinetic typography carefully for the next step.

2 Purpose and Method of Study

In the preliminary studies, stimulus material of static digital contents with music and kinetic typography with music were used to the identity contents and music. Therefore, to make it easy to understand and to carry out the emotion measurement, positive music, positive contents, negative music, and negative contents were used.

C. Stephanidis (Ed.): Posters, Part I, HCII 2013, CCIS 373, pp. 347–351, 2013.

For this study, based on the result of the preliminary study, the AVSM (affective value scale of music: It was introduced by Taniguchi in 1995), was used to understand the emotion of kinetic typography. The emotion measurement was conducted with adjectives of 24 items after watching stimulus materials. Then the positive emotion was determined by the average measure score of the 'Uplift' factor. It gained 16 or more and 'Depression' factor gained 6 or less, also negative emotion was determined the average measure score of the 'Depression' factor gained 16 or more and 'Uplift' factor gained 6 or less using AVSM.

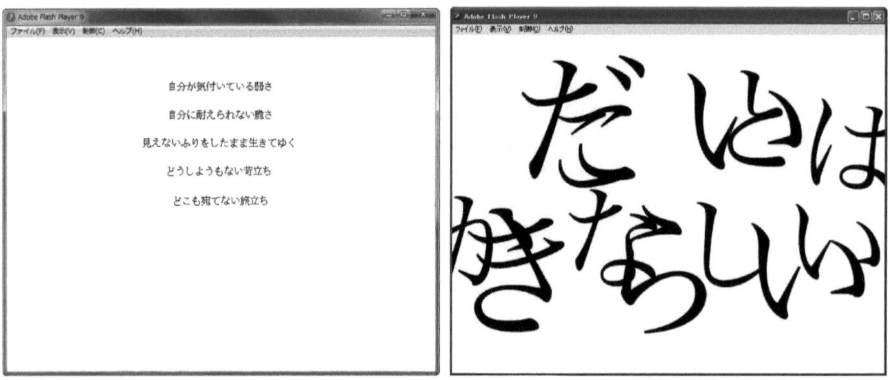

Fig. 1. Left Stimulus material (Survey 1): "music" which is auditory information and "contents" with a semantic action overlap except for a "motion" with positive emotions or negative emotions, Right Stimulus material (Survey 2): dynamic typography as a preceding paragraph story for inquiring about a musical and visual rhythm with a semantic action.

3 Survey Participant

The participants were 102 students for the Survey 1(static digital contents with music), emotion values were measured in 53 male and 51 female student volunteers (the average age: 20.39). Then, the participants were 91 students for the Survey 2(kinetic typographies with music), emotion values were measured in 44 male and 47 female student volunteers (the average age: 20.16).

4 Result of Research

It was investigated whether three groups (music, digital content with music, and content) would have a statistical significant difference for each factor. The results were shown in Table 1.

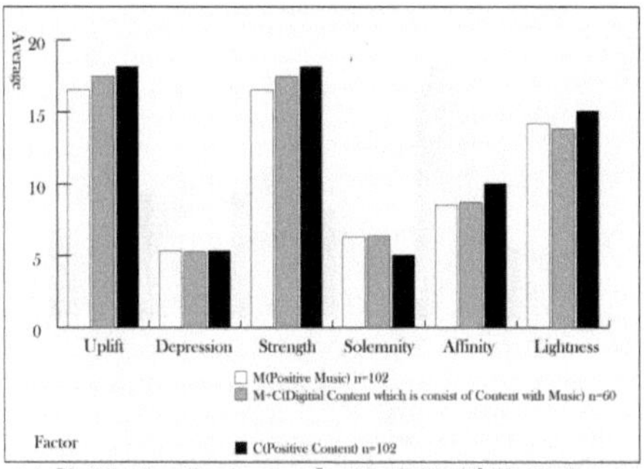

Music: 『The Kicker』 (Horace Silver), Content:part of 『mainichi happi! rakkimaido!』 (Takeshi Suzuki)

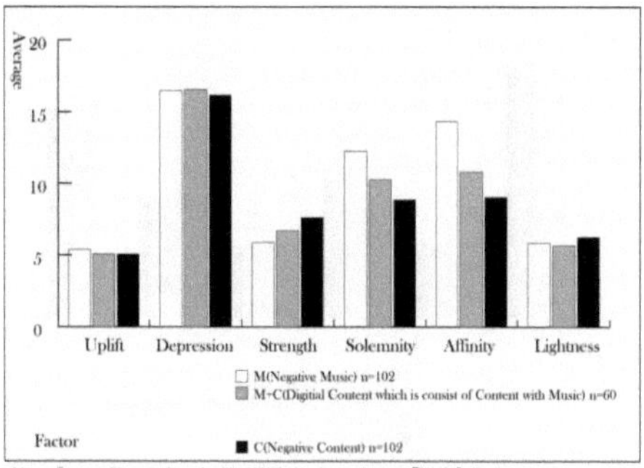

Music: 『Ame no Merry-Go-Round』 (Taro HAKASE), Content: part of 『Hiroki』 (Do As Infinity)

Fig. 2. This figures shows the result of the investigation 1. The left figure is the results of positive emotion values and the right figure is the results of negative emotion values. Both figures were similarly compared in the order of music, digital content with music, and content.

Table 1. Statistical significant difference of each factor among music, digital content with music, and content

Positive	PM_PMPC_PC	Negative	NM_NMNC_NC
Uplift	$F_{(2,261)}$=12.07, *p<.01*	Uplift	$F_{(2, 261)}$=0.65, *ns*
Depression	$F_{(2, 261)}$=1.16, *ns*	Depression	$F_{(2, 261)}$=0.40, *ns*
Strength	$F_{(2, 261)}$=20.65, *p<.01*	Strength	$F_{(2, 261)}$=10.15, *p<.01*
Solemnity	$F_{(2, 261)}$= 8.08, *p<.01*	Solemnity	$F_{(2, 261)}$= 19.87, *p<.01*
Affinity	$F_{(2, 261)}$= 5.72, *p<.01*	Affinity	$F_{(2, 261)}$= 63.68, *p<.01*
Lightness	$F_{(2, 261)}$=1.81, *ns*	Lightness	$F_{(2, 261)}$=1.59,*ns*

As Table 1 shows, some factors in positive or negative emotion had a significant difference among 3 groups. Then, to understand the significant difference between two means (static digital contents with music and content) and another two means (static digital contents with music and music)were calculated by LSD test.

In case of positive emotion, it was confirmed that there were no significant difference in Uplift(MSe=5.77, p<.05), Strength(MSe=14.52, p<.05), Solemnity(MSe=5.20, p<.05) between static digital contents with music means and content means. On the contrary, there were no significant difference in Affinity(MSe=11.95, p<.05) between static digital contents with music and music. Also, in case of negative emotion, there were no significant difference in Solemnity(MSe=15.14, p<.05) between static digital contents with music and content, in Strength(MSe=7.66, p<.05) between static digital contents with music and music.

As a result, it was confirmed that static content with music and content displayed a similar emotion than music.

It was investigated whether a significant difference would be in three groups (music, kinetic typography with music, and content) in Survey 2 like the Survey 1. The result is summarized in Table 2.

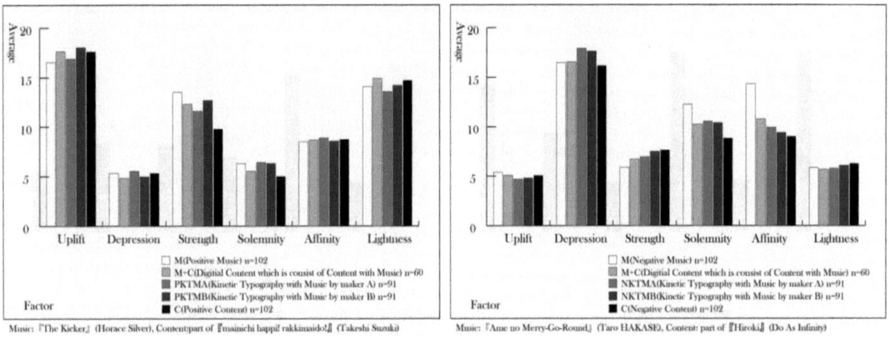

Fig. 3. This figures shows the result of the investigation 2. The left figure is the results of positive emotion values and the right figure is the results of negative emotion values. Both figures were similarly compared in order of music, kinetic typographies with music by maker A, kinetic typographies with music by maker B, and content.

Table 2. Statistical significant difference of each factor among music, kinetic typographies with music and content

Positive	PM_PKTM_PC	Negative	NM_N KTM_NC
Uplift	$F_{(2,\,383)}$=6.27 *p<.01*	Uplift	$F_{(2,\,383)}$=3.17 *p<.05*
Depression	$F_{(2,\,383)}$=0.05,*ns*	Depression	$F_{(2,\,383)}$=12.30, *p<.01*
Strength	$F_{(2,\,383)}$=18.25, *p<.01*	Strength	$F_{(2,\,383)}$=9.06, *p<.01*
Solemnity	$F_{(2,\,383)}$= 8.92, *p<.01*	Solemnity	$F_{(2,\,383)}$= 15.86, *p<.01*
Affinity	$F_{(2,\,383)}$= 6.41 *p<.01*	Affinity	$F_{(2,\,383)}$= 68.12 *p<.01*
Lightness	$F_{(2,\,383)}$=3.44, *p<.05*	Lightness	$F_{(2,\,383)}$=0.97, *ns*

As Table 2 shows, some factors in positive or negative emotion had a significant difference among 3 groups. Then, to understand the significant difference between two means (kinetic typography with music and content) and another two means (kinetic typography with music and music) were calculated by LSD test.

In case of positive emotion, there were no significant difference in Uplift (MSe=10.87, p<.05) between kinetic typography and content. On the contrary between kinetic typography and music, there were no significant differences in Solemnity (MSe=7.07, p<.05) and Affinity (MSe=11.66, p<.05). Even Lightness(MSe=15.01, p<.05) had a statistical significant, however in post-hoc analysis, there were no significant difference between kinetic typography and content, and kinetic typography and music. In case of negative emotion, there was no significant difference in Uplift (MSe=4.14, p<.05), Affinity (MSe=13.41, p<.05) and Strength (MSe=9.66, p<.05) between kinetic typography and content.

5 Conclusion

In order to understand how music and content influence in kinetic typography, the authors investigated whether a significant difference would be in three groups (music, kinetic typography with music, and content) in this paper. As a result, it was

both physical and cognitive actions. Our body responds biologically to external stimulus and we somehow interpret that into a particular emotion. That biological response changes the way we deal with different situations and this has an impact on the way we interact with computer systems. [1] In this paper, we tested the Smart TV usability in four different interfaces; emotion based facial expression recognition interface, the TV remote control unit (RCU) based interface, the voice recognition interface, gesture recognition interface. We found several research papers on our study and extracted important theoretical background from those papers.

2 Theoretical Backgrounds – Motivation

Most of the people watching TV consume contents according to their emotions and characters. Thus, the more complex the user centered interface, the higher the demand for user centered smart devices in HCI.[4] People should not change radically to "fit in with the system", rather the system should be designed to match their requirements (Brooke et al, 1990).[5] The purpose of watching TV is to get information or get entertained [3], and the latter is especially important in watching TV. Thus, in order to attain the representativeness and universality of contents of different genre, pilot TESTs were taken and programs and genres were set based on the results. We can clearly see that emotion plays a significant role in selecting contents.

Different Methods of User Interface. 1) Remote controller 2) voice recognition 3) Emotional recognition 4) Gesture recognition systems

3 Emotion Based Facial Expression Recognition Interface

People usually use their facial expressions, gestures, verbal pitches, and postures to express their emotional state.[7] Emotions can be divided into two layers: momentary emotion and mood. Momentary emotions are the behaviors that we display briefly when interacting to events (e.g., angry, happy, or sad). Ekman's six emotional expressions [8] show happiness, sadness, anger, surprise, fear, and disgust/ contempt. Emotions and moods are displayed in our bodily movement more apparently than in personality. The attitude toward other people displays the interpersonal relationship.

Different Emotion of Sadness contents in Gender. Males and females understand, interpret, and regulate the emotion of sadness differently in accordance with gender-specific social norms. Sadness is stereotypically perceived as a Feminine emotion associated with weakness and lack of control (Brody, 1985).

4 Structure of Emotion Recognition Detection

The research focused on improving the accuracy of emotion recognition for accurate measure of tendency of personality. The camera receives a fixed image of a participant's face which is automatically sent to the software. Then, the software detects the facial expression of the participant. The image is then used to recognize emotion expression. According to the categorization of data, four emotions are displayed.

5 Research Question

Emotion recognition through individualized facial expression on Smart TV

RQ1) Which user interface was more effective to males and females, and in terms of emotion recognition user interface, which gender responded more effectively?
RQ2) What is the most satisfactory user interfaces among emotion recognition interface, remote control, voice recognition interface and gesture recognition interface on Smart TV?
RQ3) Is the user satisfied with the customized contents based on the recognition of the happy & sadness of emotion through individualized facial expression?

6 Method of Experiment

Experiment #1. Emotion recognition from facial expression on Smart TV

Participant. Sample size: 40 people (20 males and 20 females) Age: Between 20 and 30

Procedure. 40 people will randomly experience 4 types of user interfaces, which are emotion recognition interface, remote control, voice recognition interface and gesture recognition interface on Smart TV. With each interface, participants will use Smart TV for 20 seconds. They have to choose and watch the contents they want with remote control, voice recognition and gesture recognition interface. However, with emotion recognition interface, their emotion will be detected automatically by their facial expression, and they will be shown specific contents according to the detected emotion. If the emotion is detected as happy or surprising, the programs of TV will shift to funny or interesting shows (Gangnam style) whereas if sad or angry mode is detected it will change to moving or touching shows(Titanic).[6] After 10minutes, the feeling of response from the user is defined. (The idea is already protected by the patent law at home, and the patent is in process overseas.)

Measure. A questionnaire with a scale of 1-7 was used to measure the level of satisfaction of Smart TV in each user interface.
Statistical Analysis / T-TEST & Correlations Test
DV: UI type 1) remote controller 2) voice recognition 3) emotion recognition 4) gesture recognition systems CV: Contents (Sad Dramas Comedies Game Shows)
IV: Sex (male, Female)

Analyses within Design. Emotion Recognition Interface. Fraunhofer IIS SHORE™ [9] Emotion recognition software base on the tested for cognitive TV models as below.

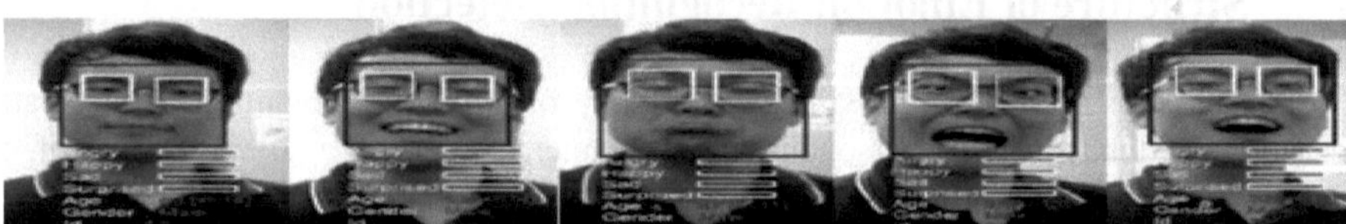

Fig. 1. Recognition of participants' emotion through the Software

From Ekman's six basic categories of emotion (i.e. happy, sad, angry, fearful, disgusted, and surprised) [8].

7 Results

Remote Controller Unit (RCU) Based Interface. All of the result is not significant.

Voice Recognition Based Interface. All of the result is not significant.

Gesture Recognition Based Interface. Most of the results may not be significant, but the results for expectation is significant (T(38)= -3.78,P <0.05). In addition, the level of perceived (Mmale = 5.45, SE = .35) was the highest for men when experiment with gesture recognition was con-ducted, and women had the highest expectation (Mfemale = 5.95, SE = .26). Men had the lowest satisfaction level (Mmale = 4.27, SE = .41) using the remote control and usefulness (Mfemale = 4.37, SE = .35) was at the lowest for women.

Emotional Recognition Based Interface. Most of results may not be significant, But evaluation is significant (T(38)= -2.134,P <0.05) and satisfaction is significant (T(38)= -3.388,P <0.05) In addition, perceived level (Mmale = 5.25, SE = .29) was the highest for men when experiment with gesture recognition was conducted, and women had the highest satisfaction (Mfemale = 5.85, SE = .28). Men had the lowest usefulness (Mmale = 3.88, SE = .32) using the remote control and usefulness (Mfemale = 4.53, SE = .26) was also at the lowest for women.

8 Conclusions

In this study, in order to find out the most satisfactory user interface, we experimented with 20 men and 20 women of ages between 19 and 31, average age of 25 and they spend one hour in average, on watching smart TV.

Among the four user interfaces, Gesture recognition interface had the highest level of expectation (T(38)= -3.78,P <0.05). However, the overall satisfactory level of gesture recognition was at the lowest. Especially, the emotion recognition interface had the highest evaluation and satisfaction level (Mean= 4.96) (T(38)= -3.38,P <0.05) when compared to other user interfaces. Overall, the satisfaction level was the highest on emotion based recognition interface and next came voice recognition (Mean = 4.85). The next was the remote control (Mean= 4.82) and the next was gesture recognition (Mean=4.08). Especially, women were very satisfied with emotion recognition interface (Mean=5.85). Men's satisfactory level on emotion recognition interface was (Mean=4.08). In terms of QUIS (Questionnaire for User Interaction Satisfaction) satisfaction, those who were highly satisfied with remote control also had high level of satisfaction of voice recognition, and those who were highly satisfied with voice recognition also had high levels of remote control and gesture recognition. Those who were satisfied with gesture recognition were also satisfied with voice recognition and those who were highly satisfied with emotion recognition interface were also highly satisfied with gesture recognition.

With the experiment on emotion recognition user interface, we also found out that in terms of preferences of contents, those who had negative feelings preferred watching sad dramas. (Mean=5.25). Those who had positive feelings preferred entertaining contents. (Mean=4.28). Since women tend to be more sensitive to emotion when watching the contents, ways to approach women in a different way is needed.

Thus, this paper proposes the most appropriate user centered interface since the way to approach and use contents on Smart TV is very complicated. In terms of approaching media contents, we cannot ignore the mood of the viewers. Thus, it is important to provide the right content according to different moods and it holds significant influence on the satisfactory level of the user. Although emotion recognition may not be applied universally, it may be very effective when applied at the right spot. Thus, recommendation of the user centered interface and appropriate contents will present the future direction of an innovative user interface.

References

1. Dix, A., Finlay, J., Abowd, G.D., Beale, R., et al.: Human-Computer Interaction (2005)
2. Asimakopoulos, S.: New Human Computer Interaction Trends Focus on User Experience, pp. 6–3 (2012)
3. Haridakis, P.M., Rubin, A.M.: Motivation for Watching Television Violence and Viewer Aggression. Mass Communication & Society 6(1), 29–56 (2003)
4. Stephanidis, C.: User Interfaces for All: New perspectives into Human-Computer Interaction. In: Stephanidis, C. (ed.) User Interfaces for All - Concepts, Methods, and Tools, pp. 3–17. Lawrence Erlbaum, Mahwah (2001) (ISBN 0-8058-2967-9, 760 pages)
5. Lekakos, G., Chorianopoulos, K., Spinelis, D.: Information Systems in the living room: A case study of personalized interactive TV design. In: Global Co-Operation in the New Millennium The 9th European Conference on Information Systems Bled, Slovenia, June 27-29 (2001)
6. Kim, J.: Do we improve, disrupt, or embrace sadness? Exploring sadness-based media choice and its anticipated effects on coping. Submitted in Partial Fulfillment of the Requirements for the Degree of Doctor of Philosophy, Pennsylvania State University (August 2007)
7. Sharon OviattIncaa Designs, Human-Centered Design Meets Cognitive Load Theory: Designing Interfaces that Help People Think (2006)
8. Ekman, P.: An Argument for Basic Emotions. In: Stein, N., Oatley, K. (eds.), pp. 169–200. Lawrence Erlbaum (1992)
9. Fraunhofer IIS SHORE^{TM}, `http://www.iis.fraunhofer.de/bf/bsy/produkte/shore/`

Effects of Plane Mapping on Sound Localization in a Virtual Auditory Environment

Kyla A. McMullen[1,2] and Gregory H. Wakefield[1]

[1] The University of Michigan, Ann Arbor, MI 48109-2121
[2] Clemson University, Clemson, SC 29634
kyla@clemson.edu, ghw@umich.edu

Abstract. Virtual auditory environments (VAEs) can be used to communicate spatial information, with sound sources representing the location of objects. A critical factor in this type of immersive system is the degree to which the participant can interact with the virtual environment. Our prior work has demonstrated that listeners can successfully locate virtual spatialized sounds, delivered over headphones, in a VAE using a mouse and screen to navigate the virtual world. The screen indicates the avatars position on the vertical plane. The present study seeks to determine the effects of plane mapping on listener performance. In the horizontal-plane interface, the listener used a WACOM tablet and pen to navigate the VAE on the horizontal plane. Results suggest that there is no significant performance difference when locating a single sound source. In the multi-source context, it was observed that the time taken to locate the first sound was significantly larger than the time taken to locate the remaining sounds.

1 Introduction

Digital sounds can be processed, creating auditory cues that convey spatial information within a virtual auditory environment (VAE). In this type of environment, locations are indicated by sound sources. To increase immersion, a user needs to explore this VAE as naturally as possible. A challenge in developing VAEs is choosing the proper mediation through which the user will interact with the environment. An interface that allows the listener to easily explore the world, while minimizing potential perceptual overhead is desirable.

Generally speaking, most people are familiar with using a mouse interface and receiving locational feedback through a standard computer monitor. On the surface, one might assume that using a mouse driven interface to navigate a VAE is ideal since it is inexpensive, does not present calibration issues, can be used by virtually any computer application, and requires little training to be used by most people. On the other hand, the use of a mouse and screen also requires the perceptual overhead of mapping horizontal mouse movements to vertical locations on the screen.

The present experiment assessed the effects of horizontal to vertical plane mapping on the listener's ability to find a virtual sound source. Listener performance was assessed as they searched for sounds in an interface that required

C. Stephanidis (Ed.): Posters, Part I, HCII 2013, CCIS 373, pp. 357–361, 2013.

plane mapping and compared to an interface that did not require such mapping. In the non-mapping interface, the listener navigated the environment by moving a pen on a WACOM tablet (on the horizontal plane) while absolute position was indicated by the pen's location on the tablet.

2 Methods

An experiment was designed to determine the performance effects of using a mapping vs. a non-mapping interface during a search task in a VAE. The VAE was comprised of acoustic sources arranged along a circle in an otherwise anechoic environment. In the search task, listeners were asked to find a sound source by moving to the location of that source. Participants moved through the VAE by physically moving the pen on the WACOM tablet or by using the mouse to change position, presented on a vertical display. Henceforth, the mouse and vertical screen display will be referred to as the mouse mediation and the WACOM tablet and pen will be referred to as the tablet mediation. A training task was used to acclimate participants to each mediation. During training, each user practiced locating a single sound source as quickly as possible. Next, in the test phase, listeners were presented with four sound sources and asked to locate each in a prescribed sequence.

2.1 Procedure

In the training and test phases, each trial began with a source (or sources) positioned randomly along a fixed circle placed horizontally on the ear-level plane and the participant positioned in the center of that circle. Participants moved to the sound source and were notified with a diotic auditory cue when they arrived within a fixed radius of the source. Training continued until a participants current and past four search times had a standard deviation of 2.5 seconds or less.

Four sound sources were used in the test phase of the four-source environment. At the beginning of a trial, participants were cued with the source they should search for. Then, all four sources were presented and the participant began their search. Upon successfully locating the first source, the sources were turned off, the second cue was presented, and all sources were turned back on. This sequence continued until all four sources were cued and located. Once a participant finished the test and training phases for one modality, they repeated for the alternate modality.

The four sources were selected from a publicly available database of audio recordings [1]. Recordings of a typewriter, street crowd, brook, and electronic sounds, as might be heard in a piece of computer music were selected.

Eight paid volunteers participated in the experiment. These students were chosen from the undergraduate Performing Arts Technology Program at the University of Michigan. Half began using the mouse mediation while the other half began using the tablet mediation.

3 Results

3.1 Training

The scatter plot in Figure 1 displays the mean search times, once optimality was reached, for each subject. The mouse-first subjects are labeled "M-subject Number" and tablet-first subjects are labeled "T-subject Number". The mouse interface search time is on the x-axis and the tablet mediation search time is on the y-axis. The 45 ° diagonal line indicates where each subject's time would be plotted if there were no difference between either mediation. During optimal performance, listeners took significantly more time to search in the mouse mediation than the tablet mediation [$F_{1,78}$=4.14, p<0.05].

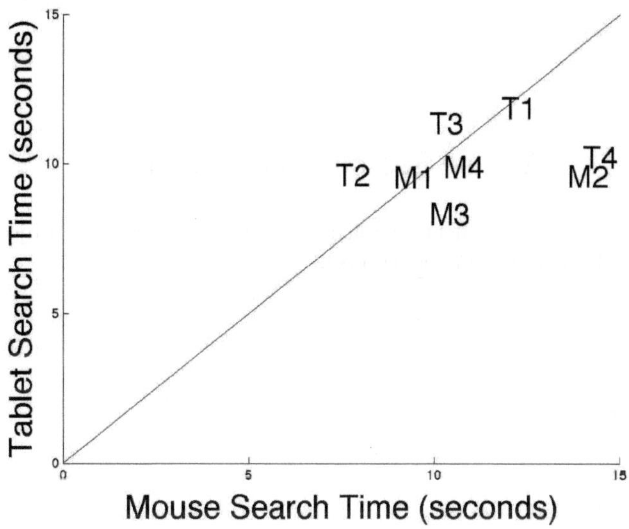

Fig. 1. Mean search times are shown for mouse-first (M-subject number) and tablet-first (T-subject Number) subjects during the training phase

3.2 One Source Context

Figure 2 shows the mean search times for each subject while searching for one source in the single-source environment. There was no significant difference observed as an effect of mediation type [$F_{1,318}$=0.84, p=0.33].

3.3 Four Source Context

Figure 3 shows the mean search times for each subject while searching for the first source in the four-source environment. Search time for one source in the four-source environment was significantly higher than the single-source condition

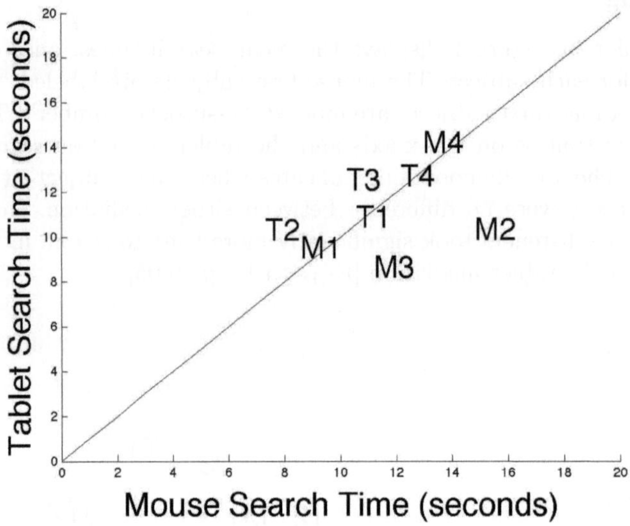

Fig. 2. Single-source environment search times for mouse-first (M-subject Number) and tablet-first (T-subject Number) subjects

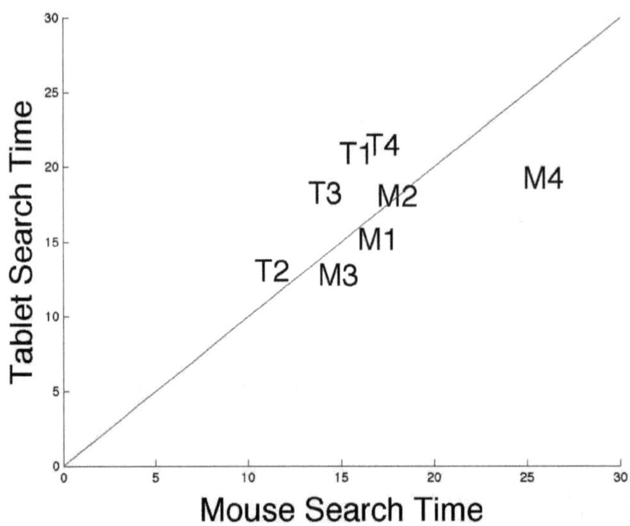

Fig. 3. Search times for the first source within the 4-source context for mouse-first (M-subject Number) and tablet-first (T-subject Number) subjects.

[$F_{1,638}$=70.58, $p<0.01$]. Collapsed across subjects, no significant difference was observed as an effect of interface type [$F_{1,318}$=0.21, $p=0.65$]. It should also be noted that tablet-first subjects had a significantly lower search time with the mouse mediation than the tablet mediation [$F_{1,158}$=4.92, $p<0.05$].

4 Discussion

The present work examined the effect of plane mapping on a listener's search time while looking for a sound in a VAE, with and without competing sources. Overall, training and testing results suggest that search performance is not affected by mediation type.

During training, it was observed that listeners needed significantly more time when using the mouse mediation, however, once the listener performed more trials in the one-source and four-source context, the increase in time for mouse mediation was not observed.

It was also observed that listeners needed significantly more time to search for one source in the four-source context than in the one-source context. This finding suggests that competing sources in the background may create a distraction for the listener, perhaps making the task a bit more challenging. This observation could also be attributed to the subjects' need to spend additional time orienting to the environment.

Tablet-first listeners performed significantly better using the mouse interface than with the tablet interface, in the four-source context. This could possibly be due to the four-source task presenting more of a challenge, which resulted in better performance with the more familiar interface.

The key finding of our experiment is that overall, there is no significant difference in search time for listeners interacting with a VAE using mouse mediation or tablet mediation. Once the participants are adequately trained, they appear to use both interfaces equally as effectively.

Reference

1. Begault, D.: 3-D sound for Virtual Reality and Multimedia (2000)

Automatic Facial Expression Recognition Using Modified Wavelet-Based Salient Points and Gabor-Wavelet Filters

Nooshin Nabizadeh and Nigel John

Department of Electrical and Computer Engineering, University of Miami, Miami, FL
{n.zadeh,nigel.john}@miami.edu

Abstract. In this paper, we present an automated approach for recognizing seven facial expressions including the neutral expression. The approach is based upon efficient feature extraction, feature compression, and an artificial neural network (ANN) classification. In the proposed method, the basic components of face, eyes, eyebrow, and mouth, are first segmented from the whole face using modified Wavelet based salient points. Then, the features of the eye and the mouth are extracted using Gabor-wavelet filters. Afterwards, the dimension of the features is reduced using principal component analysis (PCA). Finally a multi layer perceptron neural network is used to classify the facial expressions. The simulated results show high recognition rate as well as the low computational complexity that makes the proposed algorithm remarkable for accurate and fast facial expression recognition.

Keywords: Facial expression recognition (FER), Wavelet-based salient point, Gabor-wavelet filters, Multi layer perceptron neural network.

1 Introduction

Psychological and social research indicates that facial expression provides as much as 55 percent of the context of a spoken message [1]. Research has also shown that from a behavioral cognition point of view, intrinsic emotions and facial expression have a strong relationship [2]. Hence, facial expression recognition has become an important part of many scientific fields such as behavioral science, psychological studies, robotics, security and anti-terrorism systems, and human-computer interaction. Ekman et al. categorized facial expressions into six basic expressions namely sadness, happiness, fear, anger, disgust, and surprise. These are called universal expressions [3]. All the methods that have been used for facial expression recognition have similar steps. After face detection and segmentation, the next step is feature extraction and feature selection. The final step is feature classification. The differences between methods are based on the variety of features selected, the feature extraction method and the feature classification method.

Feature extraction methods are categorized as either analytic or holistic techniques. Holistic methods include model-based techniques that analyze the entire face, making one pattern without decomposing the face to sub components [4, 5]. Analytic methods

C. Stephanidis (Ed.): Posters, Part I, HCII 2013, CCIS 373, pp. 362–366, 2013.

or geometric feature-based methods divide the face into smaller components or sub sections from which the expression can be identified. The number of sub-sections and the extraction method used has a direct effect on the speed and accuracy of the system. Therefore a simple, fast, and accurate method that is invariant to noise, illumination, brightness and individual change is needed. Though much progress has been made, recognizing facial expression with a high accuracy remains a difficult problem due to the complexity and variety of facial expressions. In this work, after brief preprocessing, the eyes and the mount area are segmented by a modified wavelet based salient point method, because extraction of proper face component strongly affects recognition rate and decreases the computational volume. After that, Gabor filters are employed to extract discriminative feature vectors from the segmented areas. In order to reduce the dimensions of the feature vectors, PCA is then used. The preferred classifier is neural network, which results in significant computational efficiency without decreasing of the recognition rate. So, the reduced dimension feature vectors are classified utilizing a multi-layer perceptron neural network.

2 Modified Wavelet-Based Salient Points

Salient points are conceptually the components of an image, which a person would remember when looking at an image for a brief moment [2]. For saliency point detection, the multi-resolution wavelet decomposition is implemented for several levels to decompose the original image into several levels. The subset of points at level j is called the children of C_{j+1} where the child with great gradient value has the most critical role in the saliency measure of an image. These subsets at C_j are known as the salient points of the C_{j+1}. The saliency point selection is started from last level. At this level the entire coefficient values higher/lower than the two predefined thresholds are selected from the coefficient set, equation (1).

$$Saliency(k) = \langle\, |C_k| > T_{1(k)} \,|\, |C_k| < T_{2(k+1)} \;\&\; \textstyle\sum_j^k N_k < N_m \rangle + |\nabla C_0| \tag{1}$$

Where ∇ denotes the gradient operator, N_m is the total number of preselected saliencies, $\sum_j^k N_k$ is the cumulative number of saliencies. k denotes the index of the level. j is the index of last level. Attention is given the proper selection of T_{1j} and to prevent the $\sum_j N_k > N_m$at the last level. The values outer this boundary is set to zero. The selected coefficients are then reconstructed up to the level zero. The same selection and reconstruction mechanism is used for the coefficient at lower levels to extract other saliency points at level zero. The total saliency is the sum of all saliencies obtained from all levels. The total number of saliencies should not exceed a specified value. In order to accelerate finding the coarsest level, an entropy criterion is used. The determination of the proper number of levels by entropy criterion depends on the shape of mother wavelet and the original image as well. A correlation coefficient for finding a particular relationship between the image and the mother wavelet function is used. It is noted that the density of salient points in eyes and mouth area is greater than for other parts of the face. Based on this, eye and lip areas are segmented using a window, which sweeps the image. The location of the sweeping window with most concentration of salient points indicates right and left eyes and the mouth areas.

3 Feature Extraction on Facial Components Using Gabor Filter

Gabor features analysis is one of most effective and successful techniques in the facial recognition fields, facial features extraction, and facial expression analysis [6]. Various resolution information, very critical in face and facial expression recognition, is provided by Gabor features. Frequency locality, spatial locality, and orientation selectivity for a given facial images can be represented by set of multi-frequency, different orientation Gabor features [7]. Here, Gabor filter kernels in six orientations and two stages are applied to the segmented main face components to extract expression discriminative features. Experiments show that the features extracted by just two first frequency channel decompositions can reach discriminatively good performance and require much less computations.

4 Experimental Results

The JAFFE data set including 213 images of Japanese female facial expressions is used [8]. Initially, salient points of an image are extracted using modified wavelet based salient points. In the next step, Gabor filter kernels are applied to the segmented eye and lip segmented areas. Experiments show that the features extracted by just two first frequency channel decompositions and six orientations in 0, 60, 120, 180, 240, 300 degrees can reach discriminatively good performance and require much less computations. The output of Gabor filter kernels for happy and sad lip, and also surprised left eye and feared left eye, are shown in the figures (1) and (2). Afterward, applying PCA, feature vector length is reduced to 40. The result of PCA convergence is shown in figure (3). In figures (4), a specific representation of mapping of happy lip feature vector and disgusted lip feature vector on lip subspace are shown. With side-by-side comparison of the result of mapping feature vector on forty PCA Eigen vectors, it is recognizable that our goal to acquire obviously different and discriminative features is elevated.

Finally, extracted feature vectors are classified using a neural network classifier, which is a back propagation feed forward multi-layer perceptron with 40 input nodes, 3 hidden layer nodes and 1 output node. The advantage of multilayer perceptron is that it makes no prior assumptions regarding the data distribution. Moreover, it can model highly non-linear functions and can be trained to accurately generalize when presented with new, unobserved data [9]. In this work, using 10 fold cross validation, 80% of data are chosen to train the ANN and the remaining unseen subjects are used to test it. The classification accuracy is 93.2±2.1% and 90.4±2.3% when just lip feature vectors and just eye feature vectors are applied, respectively. The classification accuracy increases up to 95.8±2% when the combination of the lip and eye feature vectors is applied. Comparison of recognition rate of our study and some other studies is presented in Table 2 [10-15]. The confusion matrix of seven-class FER results is shown in Table 1. Two expressions joy and anger have the highest classification accuracy, and fear and sadness have the lowest one. Fear is highly confused to neutral and disgust and sadness is highly confused to neutral and fear.

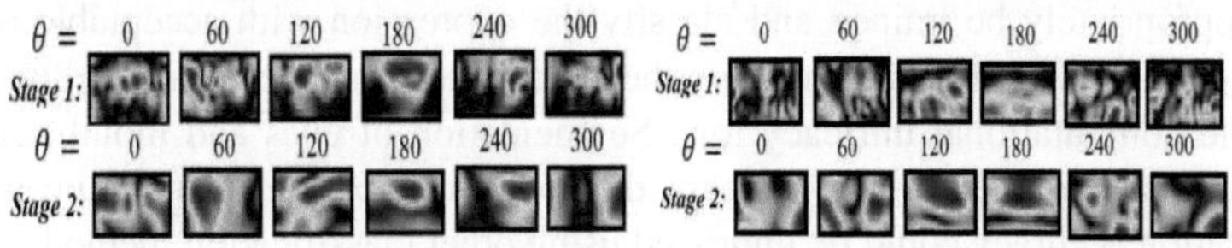

Fig. 1. Twelve Gabor filter kernels applied on a happy lip (left), and a sad lip (right)

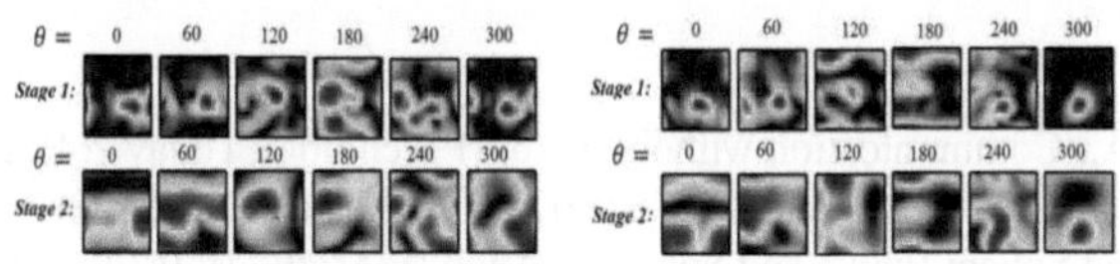

Fig. 2. Twelve Gabor filter kernels applied on a surprised left eye (left), and a feared left eye (right)

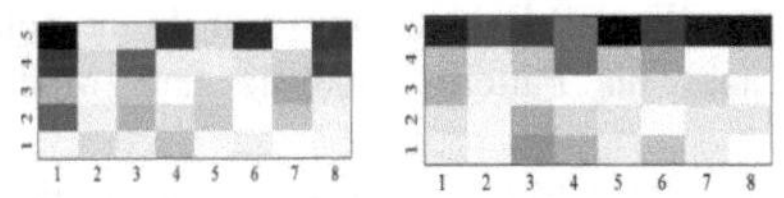

Fig. 3. Result of mapping of feature vector of a happy lip (left) and a disgusted lip (right) on forty PCA vectors

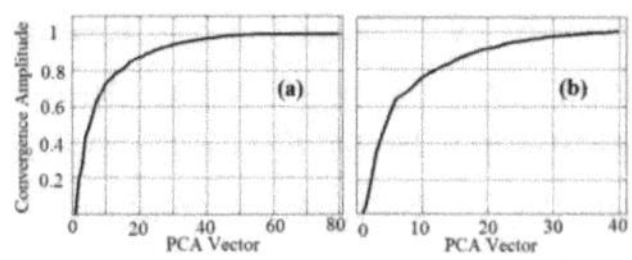

Fig. 4. Convergence of PCA Eigen-vector on 40th vector, lip (a), eye (b)

Table 1. Confusion matrix of seven class facial expressions recognition using lip & eye

	Anger (%)	Disgust (%)	Fear (%)	Joy (%)	Sadness (%)	Surprise (%)	Neutral (%)
Anger	**97.4**	1.0	0	0	1.4	0	0.2
Disgust	0.6	**96.3**	1.1	0.4	1.6	0	0
Fear	0	1.9	**93.4**	0.2	0.9	0.5	3.1
Joy	0	1.0	0.5	**97.6**	0	0.3	0.6
Sadness	1.2	0	1.8	0	**93.8**	0.6	2.6
Surprise	0.3	0.4	1.5	0	0	**96.9**	0.9
Neutral	0.9	0.4	1.2	0.4	1.8	0	**95.3**

Table 2. Comparison of recognition rate of different studies for the JAFFE database

Study	Z. Zhang et al_1998	X. Feng et al_2005	M.J. Lyons et al_1999	I. Buciu at al_2004	S. Liao et al_2006	Y. Shinohara et al_2004	Our Study
Accuracy	92.3%	93.8%	92%	91%	90.54%	69.4%	**95.8%**

5 Conclusion

The facial expression recognition based on modified wavelet-based salient points, Gabor filters, principle component analysis, and neural network was proposed. It can be seen that the combination of modified wavelet-based salient point method and Gabor transform help to acquire effective feature vector for a successful classification. The multi-layer perceptron neural network with three hidden layer could appropriately be trained and classify the expression with acceptable accuracy. The proposed method could increase the recognition rate up to 95.8±2% while it keeps the computational intricacy low. Segmentation of eyes and mouth reduce the computational complexity and increase the speed in next steps. In future work, the classification accuracy could be improved using other classification methods.

References

1. Mehrabian, A.: Communication without words. Psychology Today 2(4), 53–56 (1968)
2. Hosseini, I., Shams, N., Amini, P., Sadri, M.S.: Facial Expression Recognition Using Wavelet-based Salient Points and Subspace Analysis Methods. IEEE (2006)
3. Ekman, P., Friesen, W.V.: Unmasking the Face. Prentice Hall, New Jersey (1975)
4. Huang, C.L., Huang, Y.M.: Facial Expression Recognition using Model-Based Feature Extraction and Action Parameters Classification. Journal of Visual Communication (1997)
5. Yacoob, Y., Davis, I.S.: Recognition Human Facial Expression from Long Image Sequences using Optical Flow. IEEE Trans. on Pattern Analysis and Machine Intelligence 18(6), 636–642 (1996)
6. Trujillo, L., Olague, G., Hammoud, R., Harnandez, B.: Automatic feature Localization in Thermal Images for Facial Expression recognition. In: IEEE Computer Society Conference on Computer Vision (2005)
7. Yang, D., Jin, L., Yin, J., Zhen, L., Huang, J.: Facial Expression Recognition with Pyramid Gabor Features and Complete Kernel Fisher Linear Discriminate Analysis (2005)
8. Lyons, M., Akamatsu, S., Kaamachi, M., Gyoba, J.: Coding Facial Expression with Gabor Wavelets. In: Proc. 3rd IEEE Int. Conf. Automatic face & Gesture Recognition, Japan (1998)
9. Gardner And, M.W., Dorling, S.R.: Artificial Neural Network-A Review, p. 1352. Elsevier Science Ltd. (1998)
10. Zhang, Z., Lyons, M., Schuster, M.: Comparison Between Geometry-Based And Gabor-Wavelets-Based Facial Expression Recognition Using Multi-Layer Perceptron (1998)
11. Buciu, I., Pitas, I.: Application Of Non-Negative And Local Non Negative Matrix Factorization To Facial Expression Recognition. In: ICPR 2004. IEEE (2004)
12. Shinohara, Y., Otsu, N.: Facial Expression Recognition Using Fisher Weight Maps. IEEE (2004)
13. Liao, S., Fan, W., Chung, A.C.S., Yeung, D.-Y.: Facial Expression Recognition Using Advanced Local Binary Patterns, Tsallis Entropies and Global Appearance Features. IEEE (2006)
14. Feng, X., Pietikäinen, M., Hadid, A.: Facial Expression Recognition with Local Binary Patterns and Linear Programming. Pattern Recognition and Image Analysis 15(2) (2005)
15. Lyons, M.J., Budynek, J., Akamatsu, S.: Automatic Classification of Single Facial Images. IEEE Trans. on PAMI 21 (1999)

Virtual Flying Experience Contents Using Upper-Body Gesture Recognition

Jae-wan Park, Chi-min Oh, and Chil-woo Lee

Dept. of Electronics and Computer Engineering,
Chonnam National University, Gwang-ju, Korea
cyanlip@naver.com, sapeyes@gmail.com, leecw@jnu.ac.kr

Abstract. In this paper, we describe an algorithm and an interactive content using the idea to experience feeling of bird's flying by using gesture recognition of a user's upper body. In the algorithm we assume that gesture is composed of several key poses. So, in order to recognize the user's gesture, we firstly classify the user pose into the several predefined key poses and then analyze the sequence of the poses. In the key pose recognition procedure, the information of upper-body configuration is estimated by using joint locations of depth image from a Kinect camera. If the user performs a consecutive motion, the content recognizes the key poses and then synthesizes a gesture according to the order of the key poses. The stage of the content is consisted with three parts in order to enjoy the various flight experiences.

Keywords: Virtual Flight Experience, Gesture Interface, pose recognition.

1 Introduction

Body Gesture is one of the most important non-verbal communication methods for human being. Since it does not need direct contact and any physical channel, it has been used as a key technology for constructing multi-modal information system. However, it is very difficult to use gesture for real-time interaction system because human body is a very complicated object with many limbs and the gesture is composed of articulated motion with very high degree of freedom. In this paper, we present an algorithm and interactive content using that idea for animating bird's flying motion synchronized by user's gesture. Using the predefined gestures on our system, the users can vividly enjoy various feeling of bird's flying in real time.

Recently, KINECT camera is very popular in constructing interactive system such as game. It can easily segment moving region of human body by using depth information and produce sequential information of the joint locations of the user. However, even though the camera gives good information about a motion or human pose, it is another thing to recognize sequential static poses as a gesture. That means that gesture recognition needs some specific knowledge and procedures.

C. Stephanidis (Ed.): Posters, Part I, HCII 2013, CCIS 373, pp. 367–371, 2013.

In this research we assume that a gesture is composed of sequential specific poses, and we call it key poses. Therefore if we sequentially classify the poses captured with camera in correct order, we can recognize the meaning of the motion as the gesture. That implies if we are able to set a certain scenario which ruling the user's pose as we can meet in simple situation of interactive game, and then gesture recognition becomes more convenient and effective one to be used in various applications. In this paper, we suppose such simple situation of animating flying motion and gesture of upper-body would be applied to make a dynamic motion of a flying object.

2 The Plot of the Flying Animation

In the beginning of the animation, a user can see an avatar having a shape of human bird in virtual world, and the avatar waits for admission from the user. As the user comes on the playing stage, it gets a signal to start and animation is executed according to user's gesture. While the user is watching the scene of the virtual world with two bare eyes makes specific gestures to control the speed, direction, and height of avatar. Flapping of the both arms of the user can produce beat of flying motion; speed of the flight, and the height difference of the arms decides the direction of the flight. All the behavior of the both arm and upper-body is mapped onto the motion of the avatar.

When user makes slow swing in steady speed, the avatar flies upward from standing position and it continues the flying animation according to user's gesture. The flapping speed of user's arm determines the acceleration or deceleration condition. Namely that speed is calculated from the number of the flapping arms per a second. During the simple flying animation, we cannot have immersive feeling of real flight, so we insert some missions of avoiding obstacles and taking coins. When the avatar arrives the fixed landing position, a specific routine for landing motion is executed. Otherwise, the animation ended with failure.

Avatar used in the contents utilizes only predefined particular gestures and as the player's response is requested, it imitates the motion of the player in the virtual world. Using this animation repeating the player's motion, we can have the feeling of free flight with the virtual object which can overcome the space limitation.

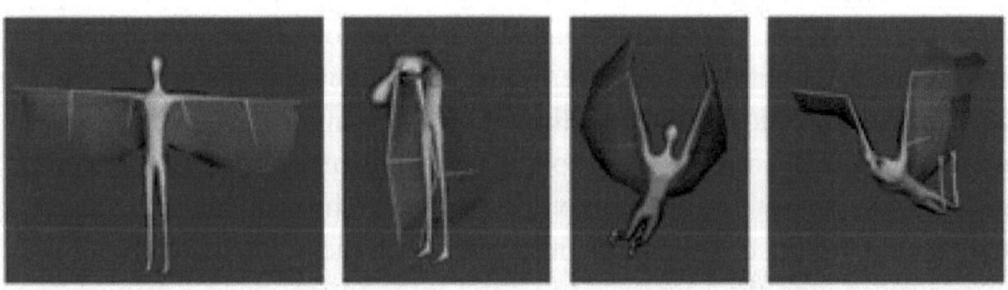

Fig. 1. The 3D Avatar used in the content and some examples of specific pose

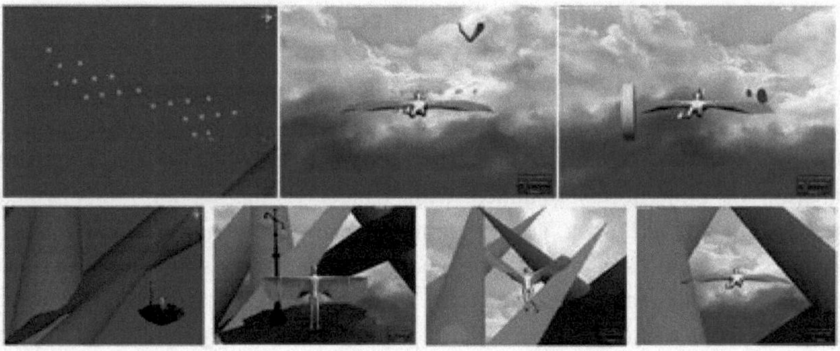

Fig. 2. The objects which are used for special missions: obstacle avoidance, coin collection, and etc

The animation routines which are used in the content are shown in figure 3. It is a sequential motion of taking-off, steady flying(flying without flapping), flying, turning, and landing motion as we can suppose. These animation routines are invoked by particular gestures which are defined as key poses, and consequently user can execute animations of flight by using only simple upper-body motion.

The whole experience of the content is divided into three stages. In the first stage, it makes the user to learn flapping motion which is needed for the continuous flight by acting the taking-off gesture. In the second stage, user can enjoy the experience of specific mission; avoiding obstacles by using the "steady flying" and "turning" gesture as already mentioned.

In the third stage, we can collect coins scattered in the virtual space to experience feeling of immersive interaction. When the user arrives the finish point, user should stop flapping to make landing at the finishing point.

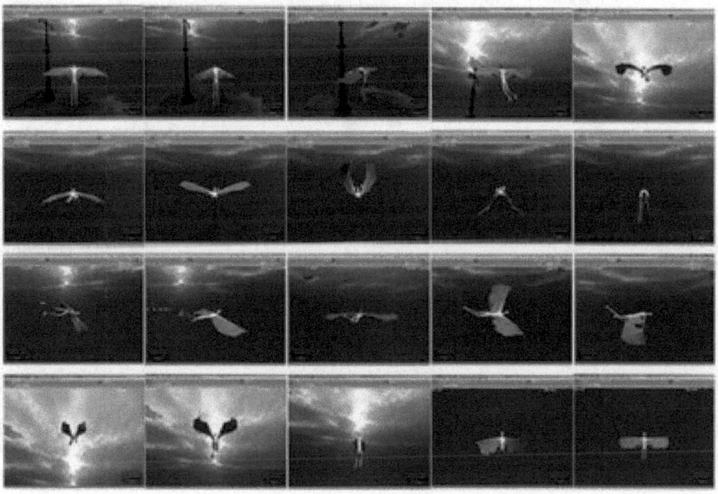

Fig. 3. Some examples of animated scene using gesture recognition

3 Key-Pose Definition and Gesture Recognition

In figure 4, we show the key-poses which are used for the "taking-off" gesture, "right or left movement", and "flight maintaining" gestures. All gesture of upper-body is judged by these key-poses. In order to recognize the gestures we compare the information of body joints obtained with Kinect to the model joints which are previously constructed as a gesture template for the individual key-poses. The advantage of our approach is that joints configuration is very simple, and so that pose estimation is very fast because joint locations are estimated by sequential transformation for a base joint. In order to compare the configuration of the joints, it is needed to estimate the angle between the joints. In this step, we use only major joints; red joints in figure 5, which determine important appearance of the body. In the right image of figure 5, it shows one example of the angle estimation of the left elbow joint.

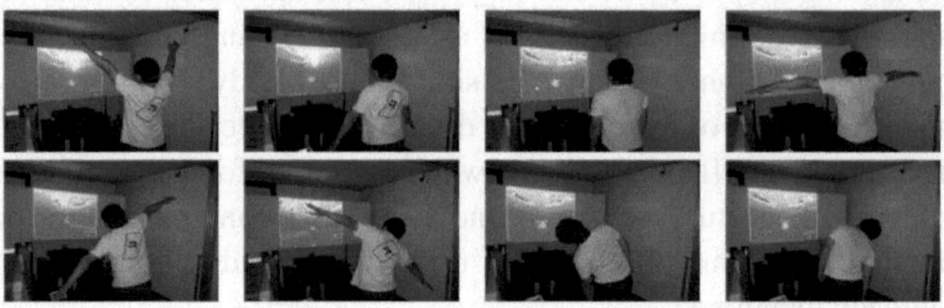

Fig. 4. Key-Poses used in Contents

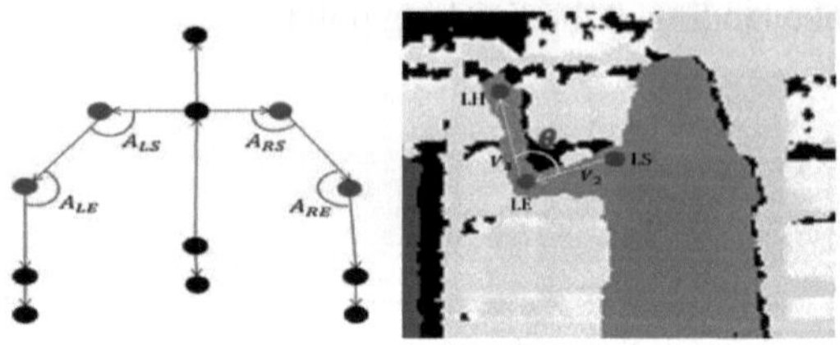

Fig. 5. Some examples of animated scene using gesture recognition

In Equation (1), V1 is the left shoulder joint vector and V2 is the left elbow joint vector. The angle of the left elbow joint can be extracted by using these two vectors. The angle of the two vectors can be extracted by projecting the two vectors onto the x-y, y-z, and z-x plane respectively.

$$|V'_1| = \sqrt{(x'_1 - x'_2)^2 + (z'_1 - z'_2)^2} \quad (1)$$

$$|V'_2| = \sqrt{(x'_3 - x'_2)^2 + (z'_3 - z'_2)^2} \quad (2)$$

$$V'_1 \cdot V'_2 = (x'_{v1} \times x'_{v2}) + (z'_{v1} \times z'_{v2}) \quad (3)$$

$$\theta_{zx} = \cos^{-1}(V'_1 \cdot V'_2) \quad (4)$$

In above equations, x, y, and z are used for expressing 3D location of joints in camera space. After obtaining the inner product of two vectors with equation (3), we determine the angle between two vectors by using the equation (4). We can obtain three angles per one joint if we repeat these processes to each projection plane. These angle values are used for evaluating matched level of the joints. Each pose template is composed of the joint vectors of 11 joints. It means one pose template has 10 vectors as feature information. When user makes some pose, it recognizes gesture to compare to closest pose template.

4 Conclusion

In this paper, we describe an algorithm and an interactive content using the idea to experience feeling of bird's flying by using gesture recognition of a user's upper body. In the algorithm, a gesture is previously defined as a set of some sequential poses. And a pose is estimated with difference of joint angles between models and input joints coming from Kinect camera. Combining the consequential pose estimation, we can recognize the meaning of user's motion as a gesture. Using this result we can animate the player's motion with the avatar, and then we can experience the feeling of free flight of virtual object.

Acknowledgment. "This research was supported by the MKE(The Ministry of Knowledge Economy), Korea, under the ITRC(Information Technology Research Center) support program (NIPA-2013-H0301-13-3005) supervised by the NIPA(National IT Industry Promotion Agency)".

References

1. Haritaoglu, I., Harwood, D., Davis, L.S.: Ghost: A human body part labeling system using silhouettes. In: Proc. of the 14th International Conference on Pattern Recognition, pp. 77–82 (1998)
2. Iwasawa, S., Ebihara, K., Ohya, J., Morichima, S.: Real-Time Estimation of Human Body Posture from Monocular Thermal Images. In: Proc. of 1997 IEEE Computer Society Conference on computer Vision and Pattern Recognition, pp. 15–20 (1997)
3. Goldberg, D.E.: Genetic Algorithm in search, optimization, and machine learning. Addison-Wesley (1989)
4. Micilotta, A.S., Ong, E.-J., Bowden, R.: Real-Time Upper Body Detection and 3D Pose Estimation in Monoscopic Images. In: Leonardis, A., Bischof, H., Pinz, A. (eds.) ECCV 2006. LNCS, vol. 3953, pp. 139–150. Springer, Heidelberg (2006)
5. Gavrila, D., Davis, L.: 3-D model-based tracking of humans in action: a multi-view approach. In: Proc. of IEEE Conference on Computer Vision and Pattern Recognition, san Francisco, pp. 73–80 (1996)

Adaptive Multimodal HCI with Uncertain Data by Collaborative Fission and Fusion

Felix Schüssel, Frank Honold, and Michael Weber

Institute of Media Informatics, Ulm University, Ulm, Germany
{felix.schuessel,frank.honold,michael.weber}@uni-ulm.de

Abstract. Multimodal systems that adapt their interface to the surroundings and the user shall be able to handle uncertain data provided by ubiquitous sensors. This has to be realized for the complete communication cycle and therefore demands collaboration between the system's output and input processes. In this article we demonstrate how dedicated fission and fusion components that handle uncertainty can be connected via an additional interaction content management component. We present the overall architecture of the resulting adaptive system and discuss the status quo of our implementation.

Keywords: Adaptive HCI, Multimodal Interaction, Fission, Fusion, Collaboration of Output and Input Processing.

1 Introduction

While interacting, human beings continuously adapt their way of communication to their surroundings and their communication partner. Although present context-aware ubiquitous systems gather a lot of information to maximize their functionality, they predominantly use rather static ways to communicate. In order to fulfill the user's communication needs and demands, ubiquitous sensors' diverse information can be used to dynamically adapt the user interface. Until now, reasoning algorithms used for that purpose are bound to clearly defined information, often ignoring the uncertain and sometimes ambiguous nature of information provided by diverse sensors. This means that the way of how different user input information fragments are fused should consider this uncertainty. In the same way the method of how a system represents its communicable information has to respect the same contextual real-world decision knowledge that is fraught with uncertainty.

In this paper we demonstrate, how multimodal fusion based on evidential reasoning and probabilistic fission with adaptive reasoning can act together to form a highly adaptive and model driven interactive system. A special component, called interaction content management facilitates this. The resulting system can handle uncertain or ambiguous data throughout the complete interaction cycle with a user.

2 Importance of Uncertainty in HCI

In order to realize flexible, adaptive interactive systems, a model-based procedure can be seen as the de facto standard approach in HCI. Starting from abstract models of tasks,

C. Stephanidis (Ed.): Posters, Part I, HCII 2013, CCIS 373, pp. 372–375, 2013.

users, dialog, information, and context knowledge, refinement steps automatically lead to a final user interface that is realized on the end use devices. The incorporation of uncertainty in this process is important, because only this allows for informed decisions in any situation, where non-perfect sensors gather user and context data. This not only holds true for the observed user actions containing possible inputs, but also for the information output, that shall be adapted to uncertain contextual knowledge. Although many approaches for each direction of communication exist, integrated systems, which offer the best of both worlds, are virtually non-existent. To fill this gap, and to form a highly dynamic and adaptive user interface, we introduce a so-called interaction content management, as explained in the next section.

3 Own Approach

The simplified overall architecture of our adaptive multimodal system is depicted in Figure 1. In order to realize a complete interaction loop, an abstract description of a dialog output is handed over from the application/dialog management to the multimodal fission component. Using an extensible set of decision functions, the best way to output the given information in the current situation and the currently available devices is computed and realized [5]. Our model-based implementation extends the often theoretical approaches of the state of the art [1-4] and introduces probabilistic reasoning to integrate uncertain and ambiguous knowledge [5]. It is designed to easily integrate new reasoning knowledge at runtime. With respect to the reasoning time, the approach is qualified to be used without any noticeable time lag while interacting.

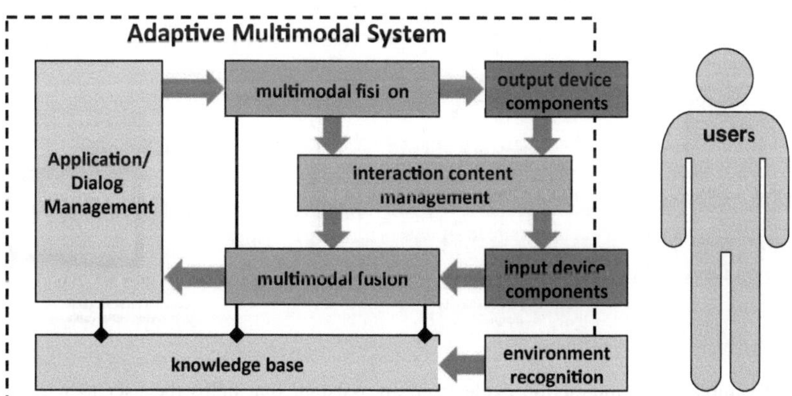

Fig. 1. Architectural overview of our adaptive multimodal system where the interaction content management mediates between the fission and fusion components

Once the concrete final user interface is realized on the assigned device components, the interaction content management (ICM) provides an interaction description of the realized output to the multimodal fusion component. This description is generated automatically from the fission's interaction output and the linked output device components' models. It contains information about all possible multimodal inputs the system may encounter. In addition, the ICM's information can be used as configuration data for the input device components. The fusion component then uses the approach described in [6] to receive uncertain observations from the available input device components, fuses them and decides on the most likely input. At the same time the robustness of input recognition is increased by the combination, disambiguation, reinforcement, and conflict detection capabilities of the adapted Transferable Belief Model (TBM) when compared to existing approaches [7-9]. This input is then handed back to the application/dialog management to finally proceed in the application logic. The aforementioned approaches, which only focus on one direction of interaction (input or output), are extended by the ICM, facilitating the full collaboration of both directions. Figure 2 shows an example for one complete interaction cycle of an assistant that helps users wiring up a home cinema system.

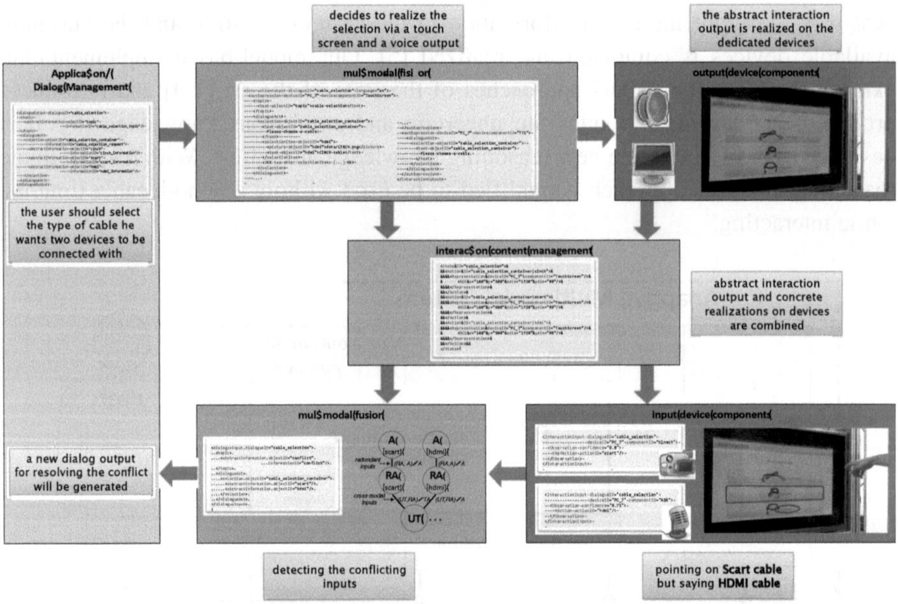

Fig. 2. Example of an interaction cycle from an assistant that helps the user to wire a home cinema system. The content management provides the necessary information, so that the multimodal fusion component can correctly detect a conflicting user input. As the graph shows, the action for scart "A [scart]" and the reference to hdmi "RA [hdmi]" are not directly connected via an edge and therefore yield a conflict if observed at the same time. All components communicate via XML messages, from which the most relevant are shown.

4 Discussion

The presented architecture and the embedded components represent a complete implementation of Norman's action cycle [10] on the side of the multimodal system. Both directions of interaction (fission and fusion) are realized via new methods yielding unprecedented capabilities compared to other approaches [5, 6] and are connected via the addition of the dedicated ICM component. Besides, our system is fully functional as presented in [11]. At this stage, the implementation allows for a user and context adaptive system of dialog navigation and selection tasks. Currently we are working on the full utilization of the fission and fusion capabilities in collaboration to allow a broader range of application domains. For the future, we plan to conduct a case study emphasizing the architecture's functionality and the ICM's benefit.

References

1. Costa, D., Duarte, C.: Adapting multimodal fission to user's abilities. In: Stephanidis, C. (ed.) Universal Access in HCI, Part I, HCII 2011. LNCS, vol. 6765, pp. 347–356. Springer, Heidelberg (2011)
2. Foster, M.E.: State of the art review: Multimodal fission. University of Edinburgh, Edinburgh (2002)
3. Rousseau, C., Bellik, Y., Vernier, F., Bazalgette, D.: A framework for the intelligent multimodal presentation of information. Signal Processing 86(12), 3696–3713 (2006)
4. Hina, M.D., Tadj, C., Ramdane-Cherif, A., Levy, N.: A Multi-Agent based Multimodal System Adaptive to the User's Interaction Context. In: Alkhateeb, F. (ed.) Multi-Agent Systems – Modeling, Interactions, Simulations and Case Studies, pp. 29–56. InTech (2011)
5. Honold, F., Schüssel, F., Weber, M.: Adaptive Probabilistic Fission for Multimodal Systems. In: Proceedings of the OzCHI 2012, pp. 222–231. ACM, New York (2012)
6. Schüssel, F., Honold, F., Weber, M.: Using the Transferable Belief Model for Multimodal Input Fusion in Companion Systems. In: Schwenker, F., Scherer, S., Morency, L.-P. (eds.) MPRSS 2012. LNCS, vol. 7742, pp. 100–115. Springer, Heidelberg (2013)
7. Holzapfel, H., Nickel, K., Stiefelhagen, R.: Implementation and evaluation of a constraint-based multimodal fusion system for speech and 3d pointing gestures. In: Proceedings of the 6th International Conference on Multimodal Interfaces, ICMI 2004, pp. 175–182. ACM, New York (2004)
8. Pfleger, N.: Context based multimodal fusion. In: Proceedings of the 6th International Conference on Multimodal Interfaces, ICMI 2004, pp. 265–272. ACM, New York (2004)
9. Dumas, B., Ingold, R., Lalanne, D.: Benchmarking fusion engines of multimodal interactive systems. In: Proceedings of the 2009 International Conference on Multimodal Interfaces, ICMI-MLMI 2009, pp. 169–176. ACM, New York (2009)
10. Norman, D.A.: Psychology of Everyday Things. Basic Books, New York (1988)
11. Honold, F., Schüssel, F., Nothdurft, F., Kurzok, P.: Companion Technology for Multimodal Interaction. In: Proceedings of the 14th ACM International Conference on Multimodal Interaction, ICMI 2012, pp. 67–68. ACM, New York (2012)

A Design on Gestural User Interaction Techniques for Tiled Displays Using Kinects

Ki-Young Seo[1], Seokhwan Kim[2], Yongjoo Cho[3], Soyon Park[4], and Kyoung Shin Park[5]

[1] Department of Computer Science, Dankook University
[2] Department of Computer Science, University of Tsukuba
[3] Division of Digital Media, Sangmyung University
[4] Department of Media Art, Jeonju University
[5] Department of Multimedia Engineering, Dankook University
windzard@empas.com

Abstract. With increased popularity of large tiled displays, a range of user interaction techniques have been explored in HCI, but gesture-based interaction mechanisms for tiled displays are still under investigation. This paper presents the design and implementation of gestural interaction techniques using Kinect sensors, designed for supporting natural user interaction for tiled display system. In particular, the Kinect interaction manager aggregates user skeleton data from the sensors, analyzes positions and changing user postures to recognize user gestures and triggers the Kinect handler to generate gestural interaction events that can be used for tiled display applications. We have built two tiled display applications with this interaction mechanism and it shows promising results in terms of user experience and performance.

Keywords: Tiled Display, Natural User Interaction, Gestural Interface, Kinect sensors.

1 Introduction

Nowadays public display devices tend to become increasingly large and high-resolution as the cost of display hardware has fallen and consumers prefer high-quality images. However, current public displays (composed of a single large display or tiled displays) are primarily used for information delivery. With the fast growth of emerging technology, multiple user interaction with contents on large public displays has received more growing attention. Large and scalable high-resolution tiled displays have been used in scientific visualization and analysis of multidimensional complex data sets allowing visual detection of patterns that increases user performance. Now they are used in many other application domains such as virtual reality, game and digital signage. However human-computer interaction on tiled displays is challenging as it leads to more physical user movements.

Clearly, tiled display user interaction is not well supported by traditional desktop computer interfaces such as mouse and keyboard due to the screen size and resolution. Typically the tiled display is too wide so that users cannot perceive all

C. Stephanidis (Ed.): Posters, Part I, HCII 2013, CCIS 373, pp. 376–379, 2013.

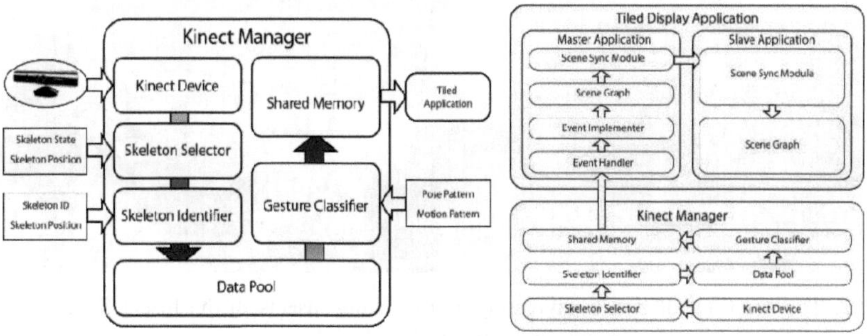

Fig. 1. The overall system architecture design

contents at a glance. It is also inconvenient to keep track of a mouse cursor and to move the cursor across the large screen [1]. Hence it is necessary to develop new input mechanisms for more natural user interaction from any point and distance on the tiled display. While a variety of interaction techniques for tiled display have been investigated in HCI [2, 3, 4], gestural user interaction mechanisms have not yet been thoroughly explored. In this research, we therefore exploit gestural user interaction techniques using Kinect sensors which address the mobility requirement but also provide natural user interaction with the tiled display system.

The current research and development of tiled display interfaces is widely ranged including physical movement, laser-pointer, multi-touch, mobile device, 3D gyro mouse, motion sensor based interface like Nintendo Wii remote controller and vision-based gesture interface like Microsoft Kinect [2,3,4]. However, there is no single user interface standard for the tiled display existed yet and there are several systematic challenges needed to be addressed. One challenge is how to help users interact with the contents (such as navigating the virtual world or selecting, moving, scaling, and rotating objects) on the large tiled display viewing from a distance.

In this paper, we present the design and implementation of the Kinect gestural user interaction system using Kinect sensors on the tiled display. This system is designed to support natural user interaction for a high-resolution and scalable tiled display by the Kinect Manager and the Event Implementer for the tiled display application module.

2 Design and Implementation

Fig. 1 shows the overall architectural design of the Kinect gesture-based user interaction system for the tiled display. This system design is divided into two components: the Kinect Manager and the tiled display application module consisting of the Event Implementer. The Kinect Manager processes user skeleton data aggregating from Kinect sensors to recognize meaningful user gesture data (such as swipe, wave, walk, etc) and to generate gesture types and event messages for the tiled display applications. This mechanism enables sharing user gestural controls to interact with any tiled display applications.

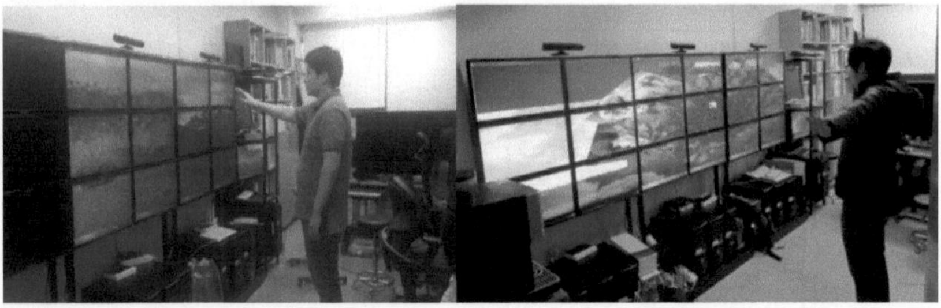

Fig. 2. The snapshot of user's navigating and catching insects in the Insect Safari (left) and selecting and manipulating images in the ImageWorld (right)

Microsoft's Kinect sensor consists of RGB camera, depth sensor (IR projector and camera) and multi-array microphone configuration. Kinect SDK library provides the color image, grayscale depth image, and the users' skeleton information (twenty-one points in 3D coordinates) using RGB camera and depth sensor through two-dimensional face recognition and three-dimensional depth value.

In the Kinect manager, each Kinect adapter collects raw user skeleton data obtained from the Kinect device. The Skeleton Selector analyzes raw data received from the Kinect adapter to classify the valid data and the Skeleton Identifier assigns the identification number for the valid skeleton data. Then, these data are accumulated in the Data Pool. The Gesture Classifier recognizes the position of user skeletons and the pattern of changing user posture. For example, when a user moves knees high above the ground, "walk-in-place" gesture is recognized. Finally, such recognized gestures are stored in the shared memory to be used as inputs to the tiled display application.

The gesture types and events are then used by the Event Handler to generate events in the master's tiled display application. Only the necessary gesture information is processed and sent to the Event Implementer of the tiled display application. The event implementer is defined to suit the characteristics of each tiled display application to handle the event of the user's gesture. A separate event implementer is used for each tiled display application depending on the user's gesture interaction design. For example, "Swing-Right-Hand" gesture recognized by the Kinect Manager can be processed to throwing a ball in the baseball game or wielding a fist in the fighting game.

Fig. 2 shows the photograph of user's standing in front of the tiled display and interacting with the application using hand and body gestures without the need for any interface devices. This tiled display system has a high quality resolution of 2456x12288 pixels (42.5 M pixels). In the Insect Safari (on the left image of Fig. 1), the player's "walking-in-place" and "twisting shoulder" gestures are used for 3D navigation in the virtual world and "swiping-hand" or "shaking-hand" gestures for catching flying or ground insects. In the ImageWorld (on the right image of Fig. 1), the users can freely move their hands in mid-air to select images directly by "pushing" gesture and then translate, rotate and scale the images by two-hands "sliding", "turning", "pinch-and-stretch" gestures.

3 Conclusions

In this paper, we presented the design and implementation of gesture-based user interaction techniques using Kinect sensors designed for supporting natural user interaction on a scalable high-resolution tiled display. Unlike other user interaction technologies, this gesture-based user interaction mechanism allows users to freely interact with the tiled display applications without having to use separate input devices. We developed two applications built using this interaction method, demonstrating the possibility of using various kinds of gestural user interactions for the tiled display. The proposed method meets the scalability of tiled display system while allowing multiple users to interact with tiled display applications in a certain distance from the screen. Thus, we expect that it will contribute to increase the utilization of tiled display system.

Acknowledgments. This work was supported by the National Research Foundation of Korea (NRF) grant funded by the Korean Ministry of Education, Science and Technology (MEST) (No. 2012-003462).

References

1. Robertson, G., Czerwinski, M., Baudisch, P., Meyers, B., Robbins, D., Smith, G., Tan, D.: The Large-Display User Experience, pp. 2–9. IEEE CG&A (2005)
2. Badillo, B., Bowman, D.A., McConnel, W., Ni, T., Silva, M.: Literature Survey on Interaction Techniques for Large Displays. Technical Report TR-06-21, Computer Science, Virginia Tech. (2006)
3. Daniel, D., Hagen, T.-M.S., Bjorndalen, J.M., Anshus, O.J.: Gesture-Based, Touch-Free Multi-User Gaming on Wall-Sized, High-Resolution Tiled Displays. Journal of Virtual Reality and Broadcasting 5(10) (2008)
4. Davis, J., Chen, X.: Lumipoint: Multi-user laser-based interaction on large tiled displays, Displays 2002, vol. 23, pp. 205–211. Elsevier (2002)

The Shaking Screening Desktop Interaction Types Based on Tablet Computer

Shasha Wang and Dong Han

School of Computer Software, Tianjin University, P.R. China
ytsasatj@163.com, winter1976@hotmail.com

Abstract. Though the human-computer interaction (HCI) design of mobile devices and various applications become diversified, the HCI design of the tablet computer desktop no longer satisfies the needs of users. This paper describes a new Shake-Screening Human-Computer Interaction Type (SSHIT) for solving these problems. The aims of SSHIT are to optimize the management and selection mode of applications on the tablet computer desktop and propose a 3D virtual environment facilitates user interaction in ambient intelligence environments. Meanwhile, SSHIT can be also adapted for screening function for various mobile devices and applications.

Keywords: Shaking screening, Human-computer interaction (HCI), Natural, 3D desktop environment.

1 Introduction

The improving mobile communication capability and faster processing speed allow people to access a large amount of information on mobile devices. What's more, varieties of input and output technology of the software and hardware provide abundant expressions for the interaction design of tablet computers, but effective supports for interaction design on tablet computer desktop are not so advanced.

At present, the management and selection mode of applications on the desktop is usually inefficient or not intuitive. In this condition, interaction design limitations, especially in tablet computers desktop, could be the potential detriments for the expressiveness, effectiveness and appropriateness of the interaction design methods of tablet computers desktop. Therefore, an innovative method is required to optimize the interaction design of the management and selection mode of tablet computer desktop.

2 Related Work - Current Interaction Design on Tablet Computer Desktop VS. SSHIT

Take iPad as an example. According to the latest user surveys, many users would like to arrange the application icons reach 5 to 9 pages, indeed, lots of users make it more than 10 pages through external software. Currently, the management mode uses page

C. Stephanidis (Ed.): Posters, Part I, HCII 2013, CCIS 373, pp. 380–384, 2013.

show and folder classification. Users feel that it is usually not intuitive or not easy to operate. But SSHIT can maximize the screen usage, and more icons can be arranged in table space.

The current selection mode of applications uses paging navigation and the searching tool, it is monotonous and significantly decreasing the efficiency of selection operations. Therefore, we provide SSHIT to decrease the number of interactions when a user finding an application. The target application can be easily located.

Table 1. Current Status‘ Interaction times and SSHIT’s Interaction times

The page number of the target icon	3	5	9
Current Status‘ Interaction times	> 3	> 5	> 9
SSHIT’s Interaction times	>2/4		

3 Results - Characteristics and Operation Steps

3.1 The Management of Applications

SSHIT creates a real hierarchy by piling up all the application icons in the desktop naturally. (Figure 1)

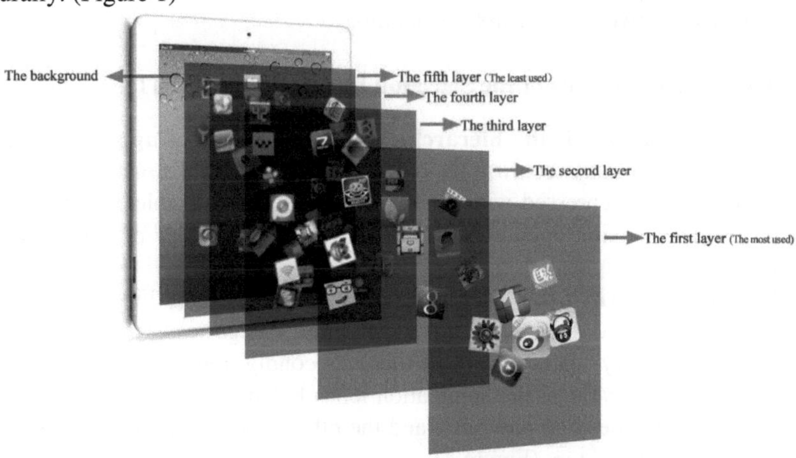

Fig. 1. Hierarchical structure

Hierarchical Structure. According to “recently used”, “used frequency”, “applications category” or “download time”, all the application icons are arranged hierarchically. The default status is “recently used”, and users can set or switch any category of hierarchical structure based on their needs or using habits.

The icons in the hierarchy simulate the objects’ form in real space. The size of the icons on the first layer is the largest, with clearest and closest shadows. The size of the icons on the least layer is the least, and the shadows are the blurriest and the furthest. (Figure 2)

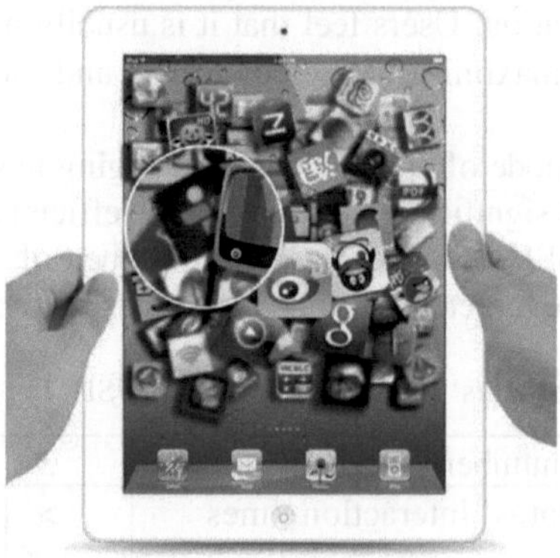

Fig. 2. The 3D virtual environment

3.2 The Selection Mode of Target Applications

3.2.1 Convert the Application Icons as the Navigation Elements

SSHIT allows the users to easily find a target application by sliding the repositioning icons on the desktop. When users shaking the tablet computer for screening the target application icons, the icons simulate how objects move in the real space. In other words, the icons are given inertia and acceleration.

3.2.2 The Operation Steps of the Selection Interaction of SSHIT

- **Step1: Choose or switch the hierarchical structure type of application icons through shaking.** Firstly, confirm the category of hierarchical structure, then keep the category button depressed with the thumb, and shake the tablet computer with both hands. The shaking operations as the way of simulate how people screening objects in real life. (Figure 3)
- **Step2: Choose or switch the filter category through shaking.** Firstly, choose the filter category. There are three types of filter categories: "use frequency", "applications category" and "download time". Secondly, repeat the above shaking action. After the operations, the application icons belonging to the target category are arranged on the desktop naturally, and the other types of application icons are screened out of the desktop. (Figure 4)
- **Step3 (optional step): Further options.** Due to the natural characteristic of the hierarchical structure, some of the icons may be arranged in large angle or overlap each other. These cases may be in low recognition for users to select and identify the target icons. Therefore, SSHIT provides the following process:
  - **Step1**, circle the target area with a finger on the desktop.
  - **Step2**, slide other icons out of the desktop by fingers.
  - **Step3**, shake the tablet computer with both hands, then icons which are in the target area are arranged on the desktop naturally. (Figure 5)

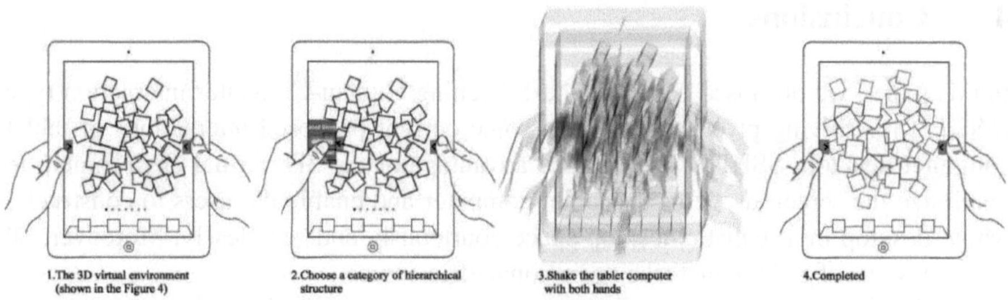

Fig. 3. Choose the hierarchical structure category of application icons

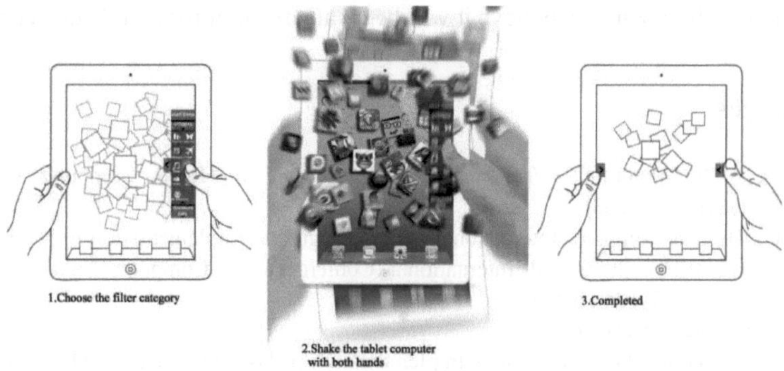

Fig. 4. Choose the filter type through shaking

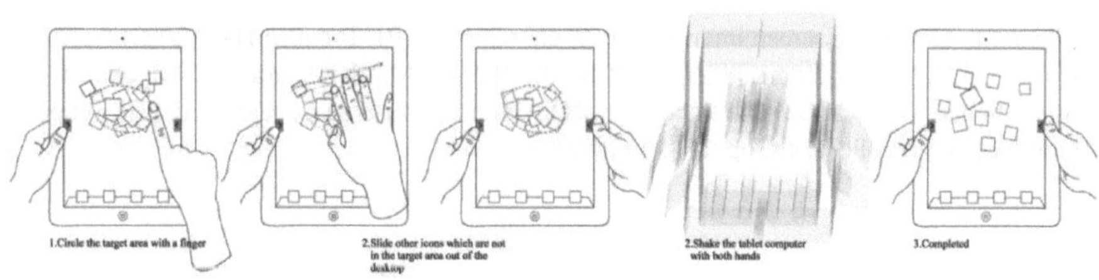

Fig. 5. Further options

3.2.3 Technical Support

SSHIT takes advantage of the accelerometer or/and three-axis gyroscope to analysis the motion of tablet computer in X axis, Y axis, and Z axis, and measure the direction of motion and the dynamic acceleration t in detail to get the needed data. The running Platform uses IOS, development language uses Objective-C, development tool is iOS SDK, development environment is the VMWare virtual machine in Windows System, Install Mac OS X System. We use an engine called Ogre enabling 3D graphics applications.

4 Conclusions

In this paper, we proposed a new Shake-Screening Human-Computer interaction type (SSHIT) for solving problems found in some current proposed interactions of tablet computer desktop. SSHIT can also take advantage of the 3D Virtual environment to maximize the screen usage of the tablet computer and enable the users to construct a whole desktop in a realistic desktop space courteously and seamlessly. Moreover, all of the designs of SSHIT increase operational efficiencies.

SSHIT can be used in academic research as well as a direct human-computer interaction testing method of tablet computers. SSHIT also can be used in smart phone, MP4, and information selection type of applications. Although this technique is still under refinement, we believe it will be a valuable tool for mobile devices.

References

1. Pan, Y.: The Naturalness Tendency in the Design of Human-Computer Interface. ZHUANGSHI (6) (2008)
2. Pan, C.: Human-Computer Interaction System Design and Implementation in Network. In: Proc. 2012 IEEE, 2010 2nd International Conference on Computer Engineering and Technology, p. V7-105 (2012)
3. http://www.apple.com/
4. Goyal, D., Chong, P.H.J.: Design & Implementation of User Interface for Mobile Devices. In: ICICS-F'CM 2003, pp. 155–156 (2003)
5. Ouchi, Y., Nishino, H.: A Tangible 3D Desktop Environment with Force Feedback. In: 2011 International Conference on Network-Based Information Systems, pp. 349–350. IEEE (2011)
6. Pinson, J.: Designing screen interfaces in C, ch. 6, pp. 64–91. Prentice Hall (2000)
7. Bowman, D.A., Coquillart, S., Froehlich, B., Hirose, M., Kitamura, Y., Kiyokawa, K., Stuerzlinger, W.: 3D User Interfaces: New Directions and Perspectives. In: IEEE Computer Graphics and Applications, pp. 20–36 (2008)

Arm Gesture Recognition Using Continuous DP for User-Defined Gestures

Kohei Yamazaki, Hidetoshi Miyao, and Minoru Maruyama

Computer Science and Engineering, Shinshu University, Nagano, Japan
{miyao,maruyama}@cs.shinshu-u.ac.jp

Abstract. The purpose of our study is to construct a system where a user can register his/her own arm gestures as templates and entered gestures are recognized precisely on a real-time basis. In order to realize them, we propose the following method: (1) 3D positions of both user's wrists are captured by using a Kinect sensor. (2) Sequences of motion vectors of both wrists are detected from the time series 3D position data. (3) The entered gesture is recognized based on the similarity between the entered gesture and each template. The similarity can be calculated by applying continuous DP matching to the sequences of motion vectors of them. The templates are gestures which are recorded by the user before the recognition process. In our experiments, good results were obtained.

Keywords: gesture recognition, continuous DP matching, Kinect.

1 Introduction

In most of gesture recognition systems, users have to enter gestures in accordance with pre-defined system constraints which are rules for how to move their hands. In other words, the users can not register their own gestures and the systems can cope with only gestures which are pre-defined for the systems [1],[2]. In these systems, there are the following disadvantages:

- Users have to learn how to enter the system-defined gestures.
- The system-defined gestures would be suitable for most of users, but they would not be for some of users.

As a result, they would lack of both usability and intuitive operation. Therefore, in order to improve the operability, we propose a system where a user can register his/her own gestures and entered gestures are recognized precisely on a real-time basis.

To realize gesture recognition, an arm tracking system is required. In some of the existing systems, a Wiimote equipped with an acceleration sensor, is used to get positions of a hand [3],[4]. However, it would be a burden on users since they have to handle it or wear it. To reduce user's burden, we use a sensor camera 'Kinect for Windows' [5] produced by Microsoft. By using the camera, we can acquire the 3D positions of a human skeleton without users wearing any devices.

C. Stephanidis (Ed.): Posters, Part I, HCII 2013, CCIS 373, pp. 385–389, 2013.

Many gesture recognition methods have been proposed. Murakami et al. proposed a method by using recurrent neural networks [6] and Chen et al. proposed a method using hidden Markov models (HMM) [7]. In these approaches, it is necessary to prepare a large number of gesture samples to train the identifiers. In other words, users have to enter a large number of gestures before use. To reduce the tedious user inputs, we use continuous DP matching method [8], [9] which can recognize gestures by using only a small number of template gestures.

2 Arm Gesture Recognition

In our system, a user has to register his/her arm movements as user-defined gestures (template patterns) before use. After the registration process, when the user inputs an arm gesture, the system compares the gesture with each of the template patterns successively, if a similar pattern is found, the system outputs a recognition result corresponding to the pattern. In this section, we will describe the representation of gestures and the gesture recognition method by using the continuous dynamic programming matching (continuous DP matching).

An arm movement can be represented by sequences of motion vectors of user's wrist. The sequences for both arms are obtained as follows:

- 3D positions of both user's wrists are captured every 200ms by using a Microsoft Kinect sensor. In this process, the positions of both wrists are captured synchronously.
- A motion vector is calculated for 2 adjacent data in the captured time-series data. As a result, time-series motion vectors can be obtained for each arm movement.

Next, we describe a matching method between one of the template patterns and an input pattern. For template pattern c, time-series motion vectors of a user's right arm and ones of a left arm are represented by $J_{R1}^c, \cdots, J_{Rt}^c, \cdots, J_{RT}^c$ and $J_{L1}^c, \cdots, J_{Lt}^c, \cdots, J_{LT}^c$, respectively, where J_{Rt}^c and J_{Lt}^c are captured data at same time t. On the other hand, for the input pattern, time-series motion vectors of a right arm and ones of a left arm are represented by $I_{R1}, \cdots, I_{R\tau}$ and $I_{L1}, \cdots, I_{L\tau}$, respectively. For the input pattern, the time index '1' denotes the starting point of the input and 'τ' denotes the newest captured point. The comparison between the template pattern c and the input one is done by continuous DP matching [8]. If the τth motion vector of the input pattern coincides with the tth motion vector of the template pattern c, the local cost is calculated by the following equation:

$$d_c(t, \tau) = \|J_{Rt}^c - I_{R\tau}\|^2 + \|J_{Lt}^c - I_{L\tau}\|^2. \tag{1}$$

The accumulated distance $g_c(t, \tau)$ is calculated as follows:
Initial value:

$$g_c(t, -2) = g_c(t, -1) = \infty, (0 \leq t \leq T - 1) \tag{2}$$

Recurrence formula ($\tau \geq 0$):

$$g_c(1,\tau) = 3d_c(1,\tau) \quad (3)$$

$$g_c(2,\tau) = min\begin{cases} g_c(1,\tau-1) + 3d_c(2,\tau) \\ g_c(1,\tau) + 3d_c(2,\tau) \\ g_c(1,\tau-2) + 2d_c(2,\tau-1) + d_c(2,\tau) \end{cases} \quad (4)$$

$$g_c(t,\tau) = min\begin{cases} g_c(t-1,\tau-1) + 3d_c(t,\tau) \\ g_c(t-1,\tau-2) + 2d_c(t,\tau-1) + d_c(t,\tau) \\ g_c(t-2,\tau-1) + 3d_c(t-1,\tau) + 3d_c(t,\tau) \end{cases}, (2 < t \le T-1) \quad (5)$$

Using the above formulas, the minimum accumulated distance $g_c(T,\tau)$ is calculated. To reduce the effect of difference number of motion vectors, this value is normalized as follows:

$$G_c(T,\tau) = \frac{g_c(T,\tau)}{3T} \quad (6)$$

If the value is less than a certain threshold value, the system outputs a result corresponding to the template pattern c. However, if there are two or more template patterns which satisfy the above condition, the pattern which produce the minimum value, is adopted as the most similar pattern. After the output of the result, the starting point of the input pattern is reset for the following gesture recognition process.

3 Registration of Gestures

In order to accept the slight difference of wrist's positions in arm movements for same gestures, 3 template patterns are prepared for one gesture (recognition class). In this system, we call the first entered template 'basc template', and call the second and third entered templates 'auxiliary templates'. Each of the template patterns is registered by the following procedure:

1. A user holds his/her hands for a while at the starting point of the registration.
2. Motion vectors are calculated and registered while the one or two hands are moving.
3. The user also holds his/her hands for a while at the ending point.

To improve the recognition performance, the system does not allow a user the registration of the following patterns:

1. A pattern which is similar to one of already registered templates belonging to another recognition class
2. An auxiliary template pattern which is not similar to its base template.
3. A pattern which consists of low number of motion vectors.

In the constraints 1 and 2, a similarity measure among the patterns is calculated by the normalized accumulated distance $G_c(T,\tau)$ described in section 2.

4 Experimental Results

First, a test user registered the 8 gestures as shown in Table 1 following the procedure described in section 3. In this table, 'Right arm gesture' means that the user holds his/her left arm and move only his/her right one. The arrows represent the starting points of each right arm gesture. For the both arm gestures, the starting points are the same as those of the right arm gesture. 'Back and forth' gesture means that the user moves his/her right arm or both back and forth 3 times in parallel with a floor.

Next, to evaluate the recognition performance of the system, 20 patterns were entered in succession for each of 8 registered gestures by the user who entered the templates. Table 2 shows the recognition results. For total patterns, high recognition rate of 88.1 % was obtained. However, the recognition rate for both arm gestures (81.3%) is lower than that for right arm ones (95%). The reason is that the accumulated distance $G_c(T, \tau)$ for several both arm gestures were not less than the specified threshold value since the distance tends to be larger than that for one-handed gestures. Therefore, it is necessary to modify the calculation of the local cost for movements of both arms.

Finally, we will discuss about the processing time. The processing time from the user enters a gesture till the recognition result is obtained, was less than 1 second for all of the gestures by using a PC (CPU: Intel Core i7-740QM 1.73GHz). Therefore, the system can operate in real time. However, if there are a large number of target gestures, the processing time would be longer and we have to improve the processes.

Table 1. Target 8 gestures

	2	4	6	Back and forth
Right arm gesture	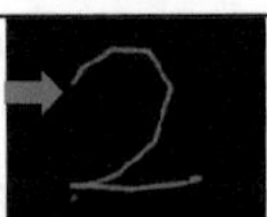	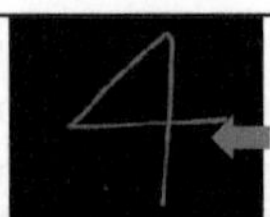	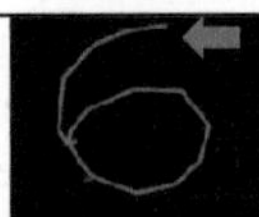	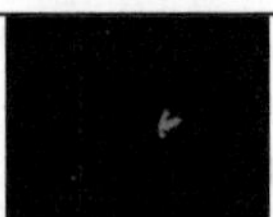
Both arm gesture	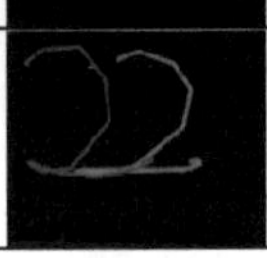	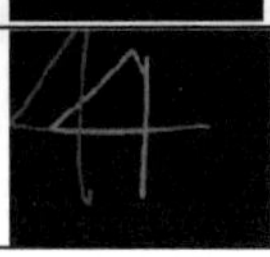	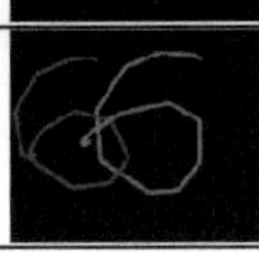	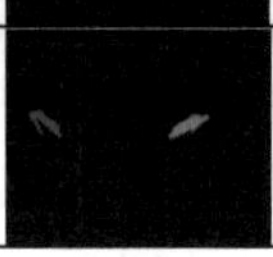

Table 2. Recognition results for 8 gestures [%]

	2	4	6	Back & forth	Total
Right arm	100	100	80	100	95.0
Both arms	95	85	85	60	81.3
				Total	88.1

5 Conclusion

To construct a system where a user can register his/her own gestures and entered gestures are recognized precisely on a real-time basis, we determined the rules for the registration process and have proposed the recognition methods based on continuous

DP matching. In the experiments, a test user registered 4 gestures with one arm and 4 ones with both arms, where 3 templates were prepared for each gesture (recognition class). In the recognition process, the same user entered 20 gestures continuously for each class. As a result, high recognition rate of 88.1% was obtained. The processing time from the user enters a gesture till the recognition result is obtained, was less than 1 second for all of the gestures. Therefore, the system can cope with the registration of new gestures and can recognize the user-entered gestures precisely and quickly.

The future works are as follows:

- The recognition rate for both arm gestures tends to be low. Therefore, we have to improve the calculation method of the local cost in DP matching for them.
- In our system, it cannot cope with registration of a pair of patterns which are similar to each other in the course of arm movements. For example, if a user wants to register Arabic numbers '2' and '3', they were not allowed to be registered since part of the arm movement for '3' is similar to that for '2' and the system cannot distinguish between them. It would cause to reduce a degree of freedom of the system. We are planning to remove the restriction.

References

1. Wu, J., Pan, G., Zhang, D., Qi, G., Li, S.: Gesture Recognition with a 3-D Accelerometer. In: Zhang, D., Portmann, M., Tan, A.-H., Indulska, J. (eds.) UIC 2009. LNCS, vol. 5585, pp. 25–38. Springer, Heidelberg (2009)
2. Kohn, B., Belbachir, A.N., Hahn, T., Kaufmann, H.: Event-driven body motion analysis for real-time gesture recognition. In: IEEE International Symposium on Circuits and Systems (ISCAS) 2012, pp. 703–706 (2012)
3. Schlomer, T., Poppinga, B., Henze, N., Boll, S.: Gesture Recognition with a Wii Controller. In: Proceedings of the 2nd International Conference on Tangible and Embedded Interaction, TEI 2008, pp. 11–14 (2008)
4. Kwon, D.Y., Gross, M.: A Framework for 3D Spatial Gesture Design and Modeling Using a Wearable Input Device. In: Proceedings of the 11th IEEE International Symposium on Wearable Computers, pp. 23–26 (2007)
5. Develop for Kinect | Microsoft Kinect for Windows, http://www.microsoft.com/en-us/kinectforwindows/
6. Murakami, K., Taguchi, H.: Gesture recognition using recurrent neural networks. In: Proceedings of the SIGCHI Conference on Human Factors in Computing Systems, CHI 1991, pp. 237–242 (1991)
7. Chen, F.S., Fu, C.M., Huang, C.L.: Hand gesture recognition using a real-time tracking method and hidden Markov models. Image and Vision Computing 21(8-1), 745–758 (2003)
8. Oka, R.: Spotting Method for Classification of Real World Data. The Computer Journal 41(8), 559–565 (1998)
9. Serra, B., Berthod, M.: Subpixel Contour Matching Using Continuous Dynamic Programming. In: Proceedings of CVPR 1994 IEEE Computer Society Conference on Computer Vision and Pattern Recognition, pp. 202–207 (1994)

Part V
Cognitive and Psychological Aspects of Interaction

Using EEG Biometric Feedback Devices to Investigate Interruption Impact on Multi-tasking Task Completion

Robert Beaton , D. Scott McCrickard, and Manuel Pérez-Quiñones

Virginia Tech, Department of Computer Science, Blacksburg, VA 24060 USA
{rbeaton,mccricks,perez}@cs.vt.edu

Abstract. This work explores ways to unobtrusively capture biometric data, calculate metrics important to the user, and deliver the metrics in ways that empower people to lead more mentally balanced lives. An initial experiment explored how one type of biometric data (EEG) could be unobtrusively collected and analyzed in real time to differentiate user task engagement for single and dual tasks. We found statistically significant differences in mean engagement values across tasks, with a higher engagement mean when participants were asked to monitor a constantly updating news-feed than when they were asked to complete a math test, or the two simultaneously. Similar biometric inputs could be used to explore mental state from cognitive variables like interruption. Future work focuses on how devices worn or carried by the user can provide on-demand information about daily mental activity, balanced by web dashboards that can provide a rich contextual viewport.

Keywords: Interruption, Engagement, Attention, Biometric Feedback, Encephalography (EEG), affective computing.

1 Introduction

Research in the last 10 years has shown how frequently knowledge workers are interrupted in their work day[5, 6, 8]. It is evident that increasingly more knowledge workers manage multiple digital projects in our regular work environment. This means that interruptions often cause not just a disruption of work but also constant change of context for work. This research explores the impact on "mental fitness" of interruptions and context switches. These types of activities used to be typical only on managerial level of workers, but today, with information technology facilitating the distribution of digital information, most knowledge workers face similar situations.

Today's mentally stimulating world presents a need for mental balance, which we describe as a cognitively-centered set of measures that can help guide a person's choices of activities. This work leverages the informed-user perspective seen in both industry and academia (e.g., [2-4]), with a focus on providing both short-term and long-term fitness information to users--empowering them to make decisions that best fit their goals and lifestyles. This approach is in contrast to affective computing and other AI-based approaches, in which decisions are made on behalf of the user based

C. Stephanidis (Ed.): Posters, Part I, HCII 2013, CCIS 373, pp. 393–397, 2013.

on measured data [2-4]. Affective computing is commonly known as computing that influences or influenced by emotion or other affective phenomena. The goal of this work is philosophically contrasting to that definition. This work is focused on providing data/information about a person's state in the moment, and displaying that information through physical/portable artifacts with the purpose of empowering the user to influence making decisions towards a positive state of wellness. In this case, wellness refers to cognitive activity. Affective computing relies on some core level of automation that detects and interprets emotion/stress before making recommendations or context sensitive switches. The difference here is a focus on providing information to the user to make a change to their current action, versus offloading such decision making to an outside source and having actions take place automatically.

Our approach enables the users to make informed decisions about their choices for tasks moving forward by creating models of the users' cognitive experiences through biometric monitoring, and by aggregating the data in a way that is meaningful to the end user. Much of the recent work in this area has proposed to automatically adjust aspects of an interface based on possible or perceived interruptors [5, 6]. This approach ignores the explicit desires of the user: perhaps the user is focused on a single critical task, or the user is working on several critical tasks that all require taxing cognitive attention. Often interfaces seek to do things for the user, e.g., to control when interruptions take place by limiting access to information when they could play a more supplemental role. This work seeks to make information available to users that can help them assess their current and temporal mental state--toward empowering the decision about whether to take a walk, turn off their email and messaging services, make a self-promise of an evening out, or carry on with their activities. Specifically, this project explores ways to unobtrusively capture biometric data, derive what information is important to the user to create a truly empowering interaction, and ways to appropriately share it with people that empower them to lead more mentally balanced lives.

2 Engagement and Affective Computing

Technology connects to humans through emotional inputs and outputs, seeking to understand the emotions of users in order to adapt behavior based on this understanding. There have been many researchers, practitioners, and philosophers that have worked on this topic [1, 7]. Perhaps the most concrete realization of the work is seen in the area of affective computing, as pioneered by Rosalind Picard and her colleagues at MIT. For example, in [8] Rosalind Picard says a mentor might detect frustration level as an indicator of when to intervene with a student. The frustration in that example is prompted by the problem that the student is solving unsuccessfully. It is not clear at which point student's stress (as indicated by EEG measures or other autonomic metrics) has reached a point that prompts an intervention by a tutor. But more importantly, and in particularly in situations outside of education, a user might decide to take a break on the problem if the stress produced by a problem reaches a point where productivity will decrease.

Also important in examining this prior work is considering how the information is communicated. Affective systems have used a wide range of techniques, including avatars, desktop notifications, cumulative dashboards, and email summaries. In addition, there's also a lot of "pop psychology" solutions that purport to be in the area of affective computing-things like mood rings, mood shirts, or emotive buttons-that lack scientific credibility but do reflect the types of "displays" that the people wearing them wish that they had. These approaches often seek to match emotion, show sympathy, and thus connect more deeply-even at the risk of disempowering the user. Our work certainly draws from one side of affective computing: the probing of emotive cues from people. But we seek a different goal in this work, choosing instead to focus on the cognitive cues that are best suited to help humans guide their own decision-making-cues that are often considered to guide or influence our emotions. We are considering the myriad ways that affective data is presented, but are doing so through the lens of providing data that empowers the user to emote rather than seeking to elicit any particular emotion. As EEG devices become more ubiquitous, they become viable tools for long period of non-intrusive cognitive data collection. In particular, this work uses a Bluetooth enables NeuroSky Mindset EEG device. The Mindset gathers EEG measurements from the FP1 region of the cortex. This cortex is commonly associated with visual working memory, mental states, learning, concentration, and problem solving. Grounding is achieved by connecting three nodes to the A1-T3 region. The device samples at a rate of 512Hz and is sensitive to frequencies in the range of 3-100Hz. It communicates wirelessly via Bluetooth and is capable of tracking alpha (high and low), beta (high and low), theta, gamma (high and low), delta, as well as two proprietary metrics: attention and meditation. Diagnostic data such as error rate, battery life, and raw signal can also be read in real time. Filtering is accomplished by passing the raw data through high- and low-pass filters to remove any EMG anomalies that were captured. The raw signal is converted into individual wave readings using Fast Fourier Transforms.

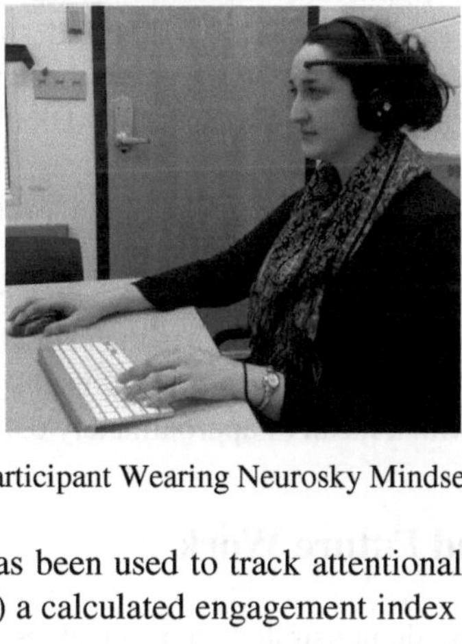

Fig. 1. Participant Wearing Neurosky Mindset EEG

The Mindset EEG device has been used to track attentional performance (referred to in this paper as engagement) a calculated engagement index ratio based on α, β, and θ waves [9, 10]:

$$E = \beta / (\alpha + \theta) \quad (1)$$

To investigate the impact of multi-tasking on multiple devices, we designed and conducted a laboratory experiment in which participants completed a set of multi-tasking and single tasks in succession. EEG data was used to calculate changes in activity engagement in real time, and questionnaires were used to collect subjective evaluations of the participant experience. Performance data was collected through numerical scoring and action rates.

3 Engagement Differences When Multi-tasking

We conducted a 3x1 within-participants study in which the activity that the participant completed was manipulated. The independent variable was the task type for each condition: conditions 1 and 2 were single mode tasks, condition 3 was a dual mode task. In condition 1, participants were asked to complete a 5-question math test consisting of questions taken from the 8th grade level Virginia Standards of Learning. In condition 2, participants were asked to actively monitor a top-to-bottom scrolling twitter-style ticker for approximately 6.5 minutes. They were asked to identify any headlines that related to "Virginia Tech Dining Services, specifically Turner Place" by clicking a "READ LATER" link directly under the headline. In condition 3, participants were asked to multi-task by completing a similar 6 question math test with questions from the 8th grade Virginia SOL while monitoring a scrolling headline twitter-style ticker for stories also related to Virginia Tech Dining Services. Each task was displayed on an individual 21.5" Apple iMac computer located directly next to each other. To help mitigate distraction, inactive computer monitors were turned off during single-mode tasks.

As expected, the EEG measurements of engagement showed that seemingly more engaging tasks (in this instance the continually updating ticker) evoke a higher level of engagement. There was a significant difference in the mean engagement scores of participants for dual-task (m=0.350, SD=0.0417) and single-task twitter-style ticker (m=0.407, SD=0.088) conditions, as well as in the mean engagement scores of participants for single-task math quiz (m=0.352, SD=0.060) and single-task twitter-style ticker (m=0.407, SD=0.088) conditions. A one-way analysis of variance found $F(2,34)=11.33$, $p=0.00017$. To determine which of the levels of Condition differed from one another, a pair-wise T-test with the Bonferroni correction for alpha inflation was computed. The pairwise t-test findings indicated that engagement scores for the twitter-style ticker condition were significantly higher than for the Math (p=0032) and dual-task (p=0.0098) conditions. The engagement mean results were in line with Szafir and Mutlu's recent work[17], with a mean of approximately 0.4 engagement units.

4 Conclusions and Future Work

The reported experiment demonstrated that changes in engagement could be successfully monitored with portable EEG devices, were complementary to traditional tools, and the context of the activity influenced the change. This was just one of several possible metrics that could be tracked in real time and displayed to the user. The next step is determining what users associate with the metric, and how they respond to it at a behavioral level.

Wearable devices could provide constant feedback about biometric measures to users during their daily lives, either implicitly or explicitly suggesting activities that will positively affect their mental well-being. Information dashboards could support the user's ability to delve into biometric measures, toward identifying healthier behavioral patterns that support a goal of better mental balance. An important design goal is to have the information consistently available, through smartphone apps and web dashboards. Additional metrics besides engagement need to be evaluated, with the possibility of increased modality by combining biometric device information.

The core work of novel information metric design needs to be completed. To date this work has focused on the collection of biometric data and analysis of its meaning. That information presentation must be meaningful and easily interpretable to truly impact users. This work has the potential to impact the way people view mental balance and the impact cognitive action has on their everyday lives.

References

1. Baddeley, A.D., Hitch, G.J.: Working Memory. In: Bower, G.H. (ed.) The Psychology of Learning & Motivation: Advances in Research & Theory, pp. 47–89. Academic Press, New York (1974)
2. Clark, D., Edmonds, C., Moore, A., Harlow, J., Allen, K., Winchester III, W., McCrickard, D.W., Estabrooks, P.: Android Application Development to Promote Physical Activity in Adolescents. In: Proceedings of the 2012 International Conference on Collaborative Technologies and Systems (CTS 2012), Denver, CO (2012)
3. Consolvo, S., Landay, J., McDonald, D.W.: Designing for Behavior Change in Everyday Life. IEEE Computer 42(6), 86–89 (2009)
4. Fitbit, `http://www.fitbit.com`
5. Fogarty, J., Hudson, S., Atkeson, C., Avrahami, D., Forlizzi, J., Kiesler, S., Lee, J., Yang, J.: Predicting human interruptibility with sensors. ACM Trans. Comput.-Hum. Interact. 12(1), 119–146 (2005)
6. Mark, G., Gudith, D., Klocke, U.: The Cost of Interrupted Work: More Speed and Stress. In: Proceedings of CHI 2008 (2008)
7. Norman, D.A.: Emotional Design: Why We Love (or Hate) Everyday Things. Basic Books (2004)
8. Picard, R.: Affective Perception. Communications of the ACM 43(3), 50–51 (2000)
9. Pope, A.T., Bogart, E.H., Bartolome, D.S.: Biocybernetic system evaluates indices of operator engagement in automated task. Biological Psychology 40, 187–195 (1995)
10. Szafir, D., Mutlu, B.: Pay Attention! Designing Adaptive Agents that Monitor and Improve User Engagement. In: Proceedings of CHI 2012 (2012)

Empirical Review of Challenge Design in Video Game Design

Michael Brandse[1] and Kiyoshi Tomimatsu[2]

[1] Graduate School of Design, Kyushu University
[2] Faculty of Design, Kyushu University
4-9-1 Shiobaru Minami-ku Fukuoka 815-0032, Japan
michaelbrandse@kyudai.jp, tomimatu@design.kyushu-u.ac.jp

Abstract. In this paper, we examine the concept of challenge in video games and argue that the current way of defining challenge is faulty in nature. Since challenge should be considered a core component to any digital video game, it is of importance that we understand the concept of challenge in-depth while designing games. With challenge being generally defined by its level of difficulty, we propose to define challenge by how challenge should be designed instead and have defined six characters by which a proper challenge should adhere. The goal of this paper is to clarify the concept of challenge and to redefine it according to the way challenge is created, not through the height of its difficulty.

Keywords: Mental model design, Patterns of DUXU solutions, Usability methods and tools, Challenge design, Video game design.

1 Introduction

Even within the design field, challenge is in many ways a unique concept. For design, the goal is generally to make experiences more accessible for users whereas challenge aims to achieve the opposite by making obstacles much more difficult to overcome. In the field of game design, challenge takes a very important role as most of a game revolves around overcoming challenges of various kinds. To games, challenge is a very important element to create a good user experience [1]. This is further confirmed by Johannes Huizinga, who stated that games are largely about overcoming something [2], giving further weight to the notion that challenge is integral to games. Juul, J., also heavily hints at this in his definition of what is a game, as games need to be "challenging" [3].

Since the earliest games like the famous Pong from the 1970's, games have developed into a huge industry that is now catering to millions of people. Within this timeframe, the industry has gone through many transformations and innovations. Not just in the sense of scope, but also in how games are being designed. One element that has not changed is how challenge remains a core component to the majority of games. However, while the need for challenge has not diminished, the ways challenges are designed has. Back in the earliest renditions of games, designers simply didn't know what made a good challenge. The result was a large variety of games that were too

C. Stephanidis (Ed.): Posters, Part I, HCII 2013, CCIS 373, pp. 398–406, 2013.

difficult, impossible even, an issue that remedied itself as designers gained more experience. Along with the experience gained, designers have found a large variety of ways to incorporate challenge into their games.

However, along with this experience, the definition of what is challenge in games has become vague, with a tendency of defining challenge through its difficulty. This is a particular trend for instance among game developers and players of games, as they often refer to challenge in games in how difficult they are [4][5][6][7]. The goal of this paper is to redefine challenge, in such a way that it can be properly designed and used for further research.

2 The Challenge Dilemma

Even though the challenge has become something of interest, the field remains largely unexplored and has led to an erroneous interpretation of what challenge entails. Game designers and Academics alike seem to agree that a good challenge is one that is not too difficult nor to easy. Game designers often use the term "easy to learn, hard to master", as an ideal to strive for [8][9]. This gives the impression a player should be eased into the game, giving the player enough instructions and practice for the player to master the basics. Through this definition, game challenge can be likened to the zone of proximal development.

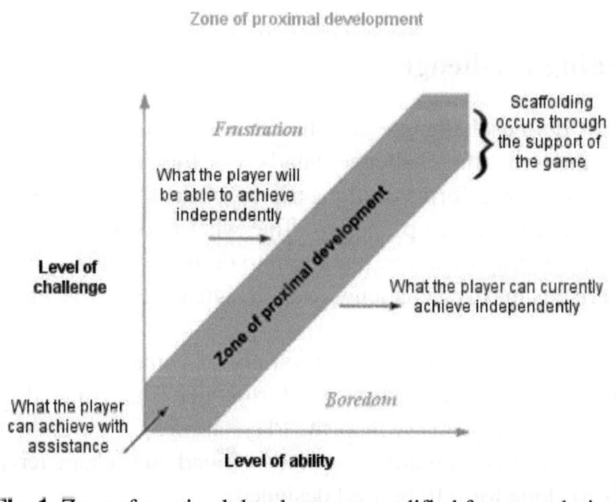

Fig. 1. Zone of proximal development, modified for game design

However, when looking at challenge, this is actually of little consequence. This is because no matter the difficulty level, there will always be players for whom the challenge is either well or ill-suited. Making a game too difficult will alienate new players of games, but making a game too easy will turn off experienced players as well. When defining challenge through the means of difficulty, we are not defining the nature of the challenge, but we are defining the user group for whom the challenge is intended. In other words, if one talks about challenge in the context of difficulty, challenge becomes very subjective.

Furthermore, when defining challenge through its difficulty, we are actively ignoring the existence of various forms of challenge. If we look at this in reverse that also means that we are not able to effectively determine the difficulty of a challenge if we are not able to distinguish between what form of challenge we are looking at. A player of a role playing game, where most often a core component is to strengthen the player's avatar through patient grinding[1], is experiencing a different form of challenge than someone who is playing a first person shooter, where the player needs to gain mastery of weapons in order to be competitive in the game.

Taking all of this into account, it makes a definition based on the difficulty of the challenge problematic. But why is defining challenge of such importance? In related research so far, it is hard to find a proper definition of what challenge truly is [10][11][12]. Crawford, C. has tried to define challenge, but defined it through its difficulty and concluded there is no objective answer to what challenge is [13]. However, by defining challenge, we will be able to better design one of the core components to a game. Furthermore, if we are to create a standard for genres within games, knowing what challenges there are within games becomes important, as a game cannot only be classified by its theme and setting, much like you would with a book or a movie. It is also a necessity for other challenge studies to have a base set of definitions in regards to challenge. For instance, in studies such as those for dynamic difficulty [14], to know what forms of challenge exist in order to create dynamic renditions from those.

3 Redefining Challenge

When looking to define challenge, we should not be looking at the height of the challenge, but rather what the challenge entails. For this paper, we will be looking at challenge in its most basic form; challenge is an obstacle in the game world for the player to overcome. In order to properly define what makes a good challenge rather than a bad design, we propose a new paradigm to define it; we are going to be looking at what characteristics makes a challenge well designed and define challenge based on those characteristics.

For this paper, we have played a large variety of games across a large variety of platforms, spanning from the earliest platforms like the Nintendo Entertainment System, to current day platforms such as the Playstation 3.

Through our empirical research, we have found six characteristics to which challenge needs to abide for it to be well designed.

3.1 Core Game-Play

A Challenge Should be Solvable through the Core Game-Play as Established by the Game. A game should clearly establish what core game-play the game offers and should not deviate from that established core. All challenges the player must solve

[1] Grinding is an activity where the player collects experience points through defeating enemies within the game world, in order to make the player's avatar grow stronger and become more competitive.

need to be solved through this core game-play. It should be noted that this does not refer to additions which complement the core game-play, but rather elements that completely differ from the core game-play.

An often recurring problem in Japanese Role Playing Games is that the game requires the player to complete a mini-game[2]. This becomes an issue when successfully completing that mini-game is a necessity in order to complete the game or gain important resources for progression that cannot be gained otherwise.

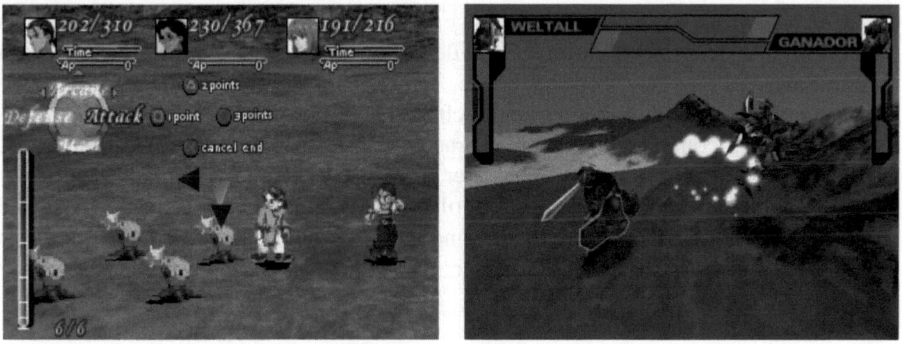

Fig. 2. Xenogears. The left part of the image shows the core game-play, where the right part shows a mini-game that needs to be completed to advance the game.

The core game-play of the game Xenogears[3] involves the player and enemies taking turns. When the turn arrives, the player can choose what actions the player's avatar has to take. However, during the game the player will have to play a mini-game called "battling," which is essential in advancing the game. This mini-game is the opposite of what is established during the core game-play, in that it does not have the turn mechanic and is thus much more action oriented.

3.2 Technical Implementation

Challenge Should Not Be Marred through Bad Technical Implementation. A challenge should not be dependent on a faulty control scheme or otherwise faulty elements that prevent the player from overcoming challenge encounters within a game, such as (game breaking) bugs. Overcoming challenges should only be made more difficult through the encountered challenge itself, e.g. by introducing additional obstacles to a challenge that was previously overcome by a player. We should note that these concern flaws that affect the actions the player can undertake.

A common example of this flaw is the player camera. Since a player camera influences how much the player can see at any given time, the role of a player camera is of utmost importance in a game. Especially in games where the game-play requires the player to make skillful maneuvers, it is important that the player has a good understanding of the area in which the player current resides in. However, what often

[2] A mini-game is a small game within the main game itself, with rules that often differ from those established by the core game-play of the game.

[3] Xenogears, 1998, Square Co., ltd.

happens in games is that the player camera cannot be controlled or the camera working against the player, thus making maneuvers needlessly complex and often even frustrating.

3.3 Player Actions

The Outcome of a Challenge Should Largely Be Determined through the Actions of the Player. A player should have the ability to contribute a reasonable amount of input in order to overcome a challenge. When the outcome of a challenge is predominantly determined through outside influences, such as luck, it becomes a design flaw.

A common example of this particular challenge design flaw is in games where co-operation with a computer controlled character is necessary in order to beat the game, especially when the loss of said character results in a game over for the player. In these events, the AI of the character is of utmost importance in order to make the game playable. In the event that it is not and the computer controlled character causes more work and frustration for the player, it becomes an example of this particular design flaw.

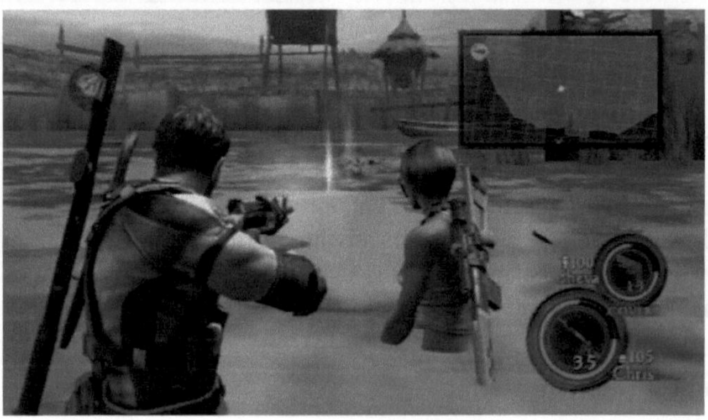

Fig. 3. Resident Evil 5

In Resident Evil 5[4], the player controls one character, whereas the other character is either controlled by a friend or by the computer. To finish the game, the player cannot lose this partner. However, if the partner is controlled by the computer, it will rush into enemies, fail to help the player or spend necessary items without any foresight thus creating a challenge where the player has little to no influence on the outcome.

3.4 Information

The Player Should Have at all Times all the Necessary Information in Order to Complete a Challenge. A game should provide all the necessary information required

4 Resident Evil 5, 2009, Capcom Co., Ltd.

to overcome the challenges in the game and should not require additional knowledge from outside of the game in order to complete it. This also refers to obscured content within the game that is essential for the player to see in order to effectively overcome it (such as an enemy sniper that can shoot the player from outside of the player camera's field of view).

An example of this design flaw regards platforming games[5], games where the player needs to control an avatar and make his way through an obstacle course to reach the end of the level. Often, in these games, there are so called endless pits, holes that mean instant death if you fall into them. Because of this, these holes are associated with certain death and give the impression that they should be avoided at all times. Certain games however, require you to dive into one of those holes in order to find exits or secrets. Since this goes contrary to the player expectations and the game never gives the information that these endless pits could contain secrets, it should be considered a design flaw.

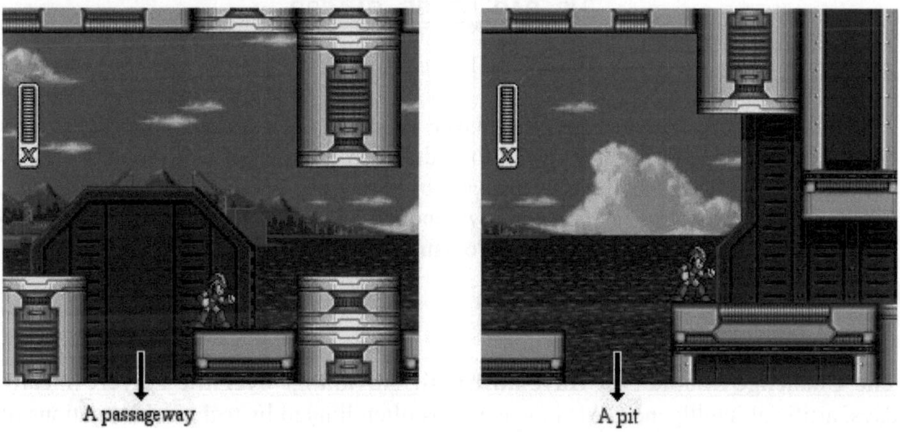

Fig. 4. Mega Man X 3

In Mega Man X3[6], the player needs to avoid pits, as falling in a pit means the player has to start over. However, oftentimes there are passageways that look identical to pits, thus requiring the player to make a leap of faith.

3.5 Effects on Future Challenges

The Player Should be Aware of the Ramifications Player's Actions can have on Future Challenges. A player should always be aware what he can expect to happen in the future course of the game, when it regards elements that can impede the player's progress.

A very common example consists out of so called "missables", which are items in a game that are only available for a limited amount of time. Oftentimes, the player is

[5] A platforming game is a particular type of game where a large part of the challenge comes from running and jumping over obstacles.

[6] Mega Man X 3, 1995, Capcom Co., ltd.

not informed about the limited available of the item, or even of the item itself. The player can often only find out by chance the player is missing an item, or needs to look up guides for help in order to find them. This is especially frustrating when the item needed for completion of the game was a miss-able item and the player becomes unable to complete the game.

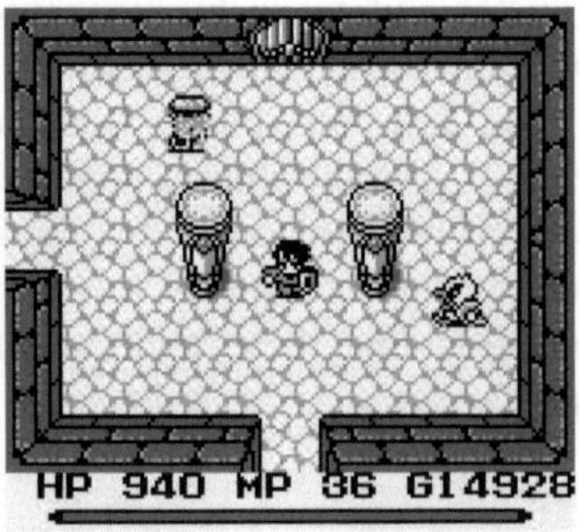

Fig. 5. Final Fantasy Adventure

In Final Fantasy Adventure[7], the player needs to open locked doors with keys bought in villages. After entering the final dungeon, the player will be unable to go back again. However, the player is unaware of how many keys the player will need in this dungeon. If the player does not have enough keys, the player will be unable to advance and will need to restart the entire game.

3.6 Challenge's Advantage

The Challenge Should Not Have an Unfair Advantage over the Player. In early days, artificial intelligence (AI) in games was often limited by technical limitations of the hardware. For that reason, designers would give the AI advantages over the player

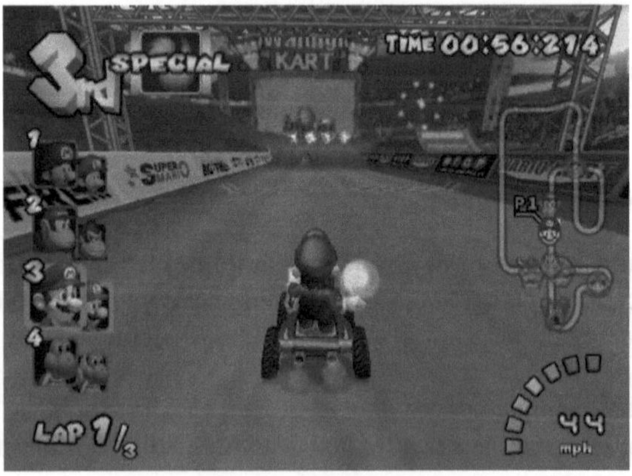

Fig. 6. Mario Kart: Double Dash!!

[7] Final Fantasy Adventure, 1991, Square Co., ltd.

in order to make the game more competitive to the player and to compensate for lacking processing power. This gave rise to a myriad of ways in which the AI could be "cheating" the player.

An example of this challenge design flaw is "rubber band AI," which is an AI often used in the Mario Kart series of racing games[8]. What this particular kind of AI does is that when computer controlled opponents are lagging behind the player, they are given advantages in order to remain competitive and thus keep the challenge interesting. However, in various games this causes the AI to gain abilities that were otherwise impossible to have (e.g. having cars that become faster than their supposed maximum speed in racing games). This in turn causes frustration for the player as the player is unable to overcome the odds even though technically, the player should be able to do so.

4 Conclusion

This paper has proposed a new paradigm of defining challenge for video game design. Instead of looking at challenge through its difficulty, we proposed to look at challenge through how it is designed, as difficulty is too subjective to be an effective definition. For this reason, we state the most basic of a challenge as an obstacle the player has to overcome, which has to abide to six characteristics by which a proper challenge should be designed.

Using this new way of defining challenge, we believe that this will open up new research possibilities not just when it comes to challenge in games, but also in other fields that have been hard to define before due to lack of any standards. For instance, genre study for game design is notorious for being difficult to research as everyone has their own genre definitions.

5 Future Works

Using the way of describing challenge as defined in this paper, we wish to distill forms of challenge from them that can be applied to design. The goal is to gain definitions of forms of challenge that are not dependent on the definition of difficulty. We are going to do research this through the same means we have come to the results of this paper, namely through empirical reviews of games.

References

1. Cox, A.L., Cairns, P., Shah, P., Carrol, M.: Not Doing but Thinking: The Role of Challenge in the Gaming Experience. In: CHI 2012 (2012)
2. Huizinga, J.: Homo Ludens: a Study of the Play Element in Culture. Beacon Press (1968)
3. Juul, J.: The Game, The Player, The World: Looking for a Heart of Gameness. In: Copier, M., Raessens, J. (eds.) Level Up: Digital Games Research Conference Proceedings, pp. 30–45. Utrecht University, Utrecht (2003)

[8] Mario Kart: Double Dash!!, 2003, Nintendo Co., ltd.

4. Kain, E.: Games are getting easier, 5 reasons why that's a bad thing, http://www.forbes.com/sites/erikkain/2012/06/28/games-are-getting-easier-5-reasons-thats-a-bad-thing/ (retrieved November 30, 2012)
5. Abbot, M.: Video Games Are Easier Than Ever, Yet Harder To Manage, http://kotaku.com/5887020/video-games-are-easier-than-ever-yet-harder-to-manage (retrieved November 30, 2012)
6. Etherington-Smith, J.: Are games getting easier?, http://mygaming.co.za/news/columns/9207-are-games-getting-easier.html (retrieved November 30, 2012)
7. Geoffrey, T.: FFD: are games getting too easy?, http://www.lazygamer.net/general-news/ffd-are-games-getting-too-easy/ (retrieved November 30, 2012)
8. Malone, T.W.: Heuristics for designing enjoyable user interfaces: Lessons from computer games. In: Thomas, J.C., Schneider, M.L. (eds.) Human Factorsin Computing Systems, Ablex Publishing Corporation, Norwood (1982)
9. Desurvire, H., Caplan, M., Toth, A.J.: Using Heuristics to Evaluate the Playability of Games. In: CHI 2004 (2004)
10. Salen, K., Zimmerman, E.: Rules of Play. MIT Press (2004)
11. Rabin, S.: Introduction to Game Development. Charles River Media, Inc. (2005)
12. Church, D.: Formal Abstract Design Tools. In: Salen, K., Zimmerman, E. (eds.) The Game Design Reader: A Rules of Play Anthology, pp. 366–380. The MIT Press, Cambridge (2006)
13. Crawford, C.: Chris Crawford on Game Design. New Riders (2003)
14. Hunicke, R.: The Case for Dynamic Difficulty Adjustment in Games. In: Proceedings of the 2005 ACM SIGCHI International Conference on Advances in Computer Entertainment Technology, Valencia, Spain, June 15-17, pp. 429–433 (2005)

Emotion-Cognition Interaction of Decision Making in the Social Context

Chongwook Chung, Jeounghoon Kim, and Chung-kon Shi*

Graduate School of Culture Technology
Korea Advanced Institute of Science and Technology (KAIST)
Daejeon 305-701, South Korea
{rachung,miru,chungkon}@kaist.ac.kr

Abstract. The goal of this study is to investigate how decision making takes place in social contexts by emotion and cognition. This study had two kinds of tasks; Need for Cognition (NFC) and Iowa Gamble Tasks (IGT/ modified IGT). The results show a significant main effect in the NFC conditions as well as interaction between types of NFC and types of IGT in significant ways. In other words, in the IGT, differences between types of NFC did not appear, whereas they did appear significantly in the mIGT, which was manipulated to include social contexts. These results can be used to estimate that when two types of NFCs make a decision, social contexts can work as a social facilitator (to the NFC-high) or as a social inhibitor (to the NFC-low) respectively.

Keywords: Decision making, Emotion, Cognition, Social context, Need for Cognition, Iowa Gamble Task.

1 Introduction

Decision making is a cognitive process through which choices are made from among several alternatives; this process occurs at every moment of daily life. In addition, all decision making leads to a resulting final selection [1] and this can affect life in large or small ways. From the perspective of cognitive psychology, decision making is a successive process that occurs while humans are continuously interacting with factors such as the environment and the context; therefore, it takes place through the interaction between individuals' characteristics and diverse contextual characteristics.

As mentioned above, decision making is context-dependent [2]. In particular, decision making in social contexts, which contexts are generated by the existence of others, inevitably involves interactions between emotion and cognition [3]. This is because the element of emotion, which is inherent in social relationships, coexists with cognitive elements, which seek to hold a more varied and prudent position. In other words, when one makes decisions in consideration of others rather than alone, one is bound to be more affected by emotional factors rather than by cognitive factors. According to previous research [4], emotional factors play important roles in individuals' decision making; therefore, it is natural that there is a strong impact of

C. Stephanidis (Ed.): Posters, Part I, HCII 2013, CCIS 373, pp. 407–411, 2013.

emotion, which affects decision making in social contexts that are generated by the presence of others or of social relationships. However, there has been not any research that has considered the impact of two factors on decision making at once. Thus, we conducted a study in order to verify the effect of cognition and emotion on decision making, particularly in social contexts.

Consequently, we used the Need for Cognition (NFC) scale and two types of Iowa Gamble Task (IGT) to achieve the aim of this study. First, the NFC is a concept that can explain individual differences in the degree to which circumstances requiring cognitive efforts are accepted and enjoyed, NFC has been used in numerous psychological studies [5] [6]. In addition, the IGT was developed to experimentally simulate real-life decision making [7]. Because emotions can be seen as important factors in decision making, and because IGT is frequently used in research into cognition and emotion [8], we used this as the tool of the decision making task; we also modified IGT to include social contexts.

2 Materials and Method

2.1 Participants

The present study was conducted on a total of thirty undergraduate and graduate students. The participants volunteered for the experiments through a website; 15 males and 15 females, aged 25.4 on average, received $5 for participation.

2.2 Need for Cognition (NFC)

In the present study, the NFC was used as a tool for measuring individuals' cognitive efforts, and it was expected that those with a high NFC would put more effort into cognitive processes such as decision making than would those with a low NFC and that those with a low NFC would make decisions based on more emotional elements.We used an eighteen-questioned version of the NFC scale [9].

2.3 Iowa Gamble Tasks (IGT)

Participants performed IGT as well as the modified IGT (mIGT), this second of which was modified to suit the purposes of the present study. The number of times a participant selected a card in each task amounted to 100; the rules followed those of the conventional IGT. In the case of the mIGT, however, a gray colored border as a guide was presented to create a circumstance involving social contexts. Through the explanation that this guide constituted opinion from others who had performed the same task earlier, the presentation of the guide served as a condition for the participants' decision making in the social context (examples of task are shown in Fig. 1).

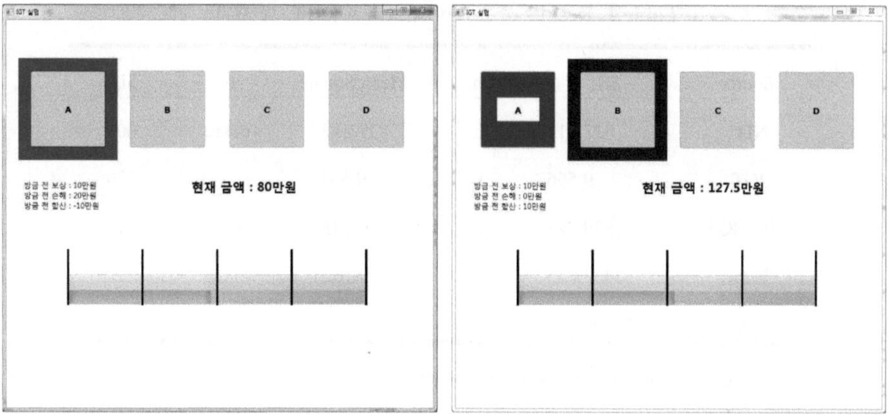

Fig. 1. IGT and mIGT

3 Results

3.1 NFC

For the thirty respondents who participated in the surveys, the male-female ratio was adjusted, and, by grading the responses to the questions, those with high scores and low scores were classified into NFC-high (17) and NFC-low (13) groups, respectively (seventeen NFC-high).

3.2 IGT and mIGT

The IGT consisted of two types: the original task and the modified task. The participants had to perform each of the tasks, which were presented randomly. In the IGT, with the difference between the number of times that the advantageous card decks were selected and the number of times that the disadvantageous card decks were selected making up the rationality score, differences between the NFC-high and NFC-low groups were verified. The converted scores, which had been turned into standard scores with an average of 50 and a standard deviation of 10, were used in this study.

The converted scores in the IGT were analyzed using a two-way analysis of variance (ANOVA) with two factors: NFC type (high or low within subject) and task type (IGT or mIGT between subjects). The main effect of the type of NFC was significant[$F(1,56)=10.450$, $p<.01$], and there was a significant NFC × task interaction[$F(1,56)=6.818$, $p<.05$], whereas no significant main effect in the type of task condition was found. The results are shown in Table 2, Fig 2.

Table 1. Results of 2-way ANOVA (NFC × IGT)

Source	SS	df	Mean Square	*F*	Sig.
NFC	827.212	1	827.212	10.450	.002
IGT	9.596	1	9.596	.121	.729
NFC×IGT	539.743	1	539.743	6.818	.012
Error	4433.045	56	79.162		
Total	155799.962	60			

a R Squared = .236 (Adjusted R Squared =.195)

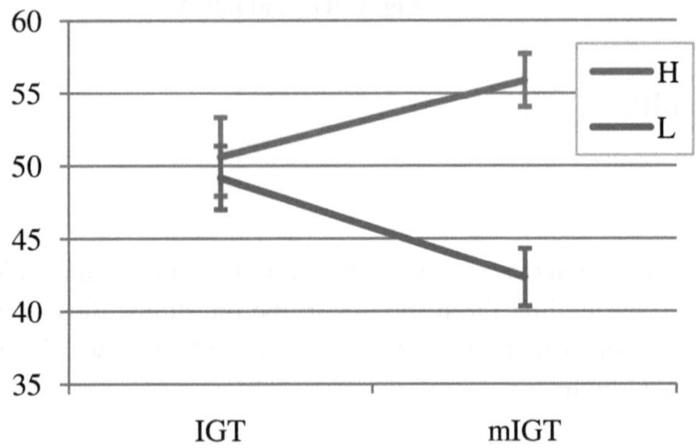

Fig. 2. NFC (high/ low) × task (IGT/ mIGT) interaction

4 Discussion

The present study was conducted to verify the effect of emotion and cognition on decision making in social contexts. As the scale for measuring individuals' cognitive efforts, the NFC was used. High NFC scores were assumed to be linked to the ability to make more rational decisions; low NFC scores were assumed to be linked to a tendency to make decisions based more on emotional factors. As for the decision making task, the IGT, which is known to reflect emotional decision making, was used, as was the mIGT, to which a social context condition was added. The results showed that, while differences between types of NFC did not appear in the original IGT, they did appear significantly in the mIGT which had been manipulated to involve social contexts. Such results indicate that when cues for making decisions increased, choices could change, in the present study, according to the social context and the NFC. In addition, it was possible to estimate that when people with the characteristic of NFC-high makes a decision in social contexts, some factor of social contexts works as a social facilitator, on the other hand, it worked as a social inhibitor for the NFC-low. These two mechanisms could possibly be used in future work, therefore, to consider new factors that have effect on decision making.

The present study has some limitations. First, in the statistical results of the present study, the standard deviation within groups was considerable. It is necessary to conduct controlled follow-up experiments to determine whether the characteristics of the groups classified through the NFC are clear. Second, because the experimental design was made without emotional manipulation, there were no results for emotional effect or for effect of interaction between emotion and cognition on decision making in social contexts. Thus, it is necessary to develop a way to measure how emotional factor affects decision making and to redesign the experiment to consider the effect of interaction between emotion and cognitive factors on decision making. In conclusion, in terms of conducting a follow-up study, this study was conducted as a pilot test with missing factors and imperfect experimental design, as mentioned above. Thus, future work should focus on the effect of interaction between emotion and cognition on decision making in social contexts in order to for the future experiment to be more elaborate.

Acknowledgements. This research was supported by the Converging Research Center Program funded by the Ministry of Education, Science and Technology (2012K001342).

References

1. Reason, J.: Human error: models and management. BMJ: British Medical Journal 320(7237), 768 (2000)
2. Kahneman, D., Thaler, R.H.: Anomalies: Utility maximization and experienced utility. The Journal of Economic Perspectives 20(1), 221–234 (2006)
3. Niedenthal, P.M., Winkielman, P., Mondillon, L., Vermeulen, N.: Embodiment of emotion concepts. J. Pers. Soc. Psychol. 96, 1120–1136 (2009)
4. Funke, J.: Solving complex problems: Exploration and control of complex systems (1991)
5. Cacioppo, J.T., Petty, R.E.: The need for cognition. Journal of Personality and Social Psychology 42, 116–131 (1982)
6. Cacioppo, J.T., Petty, R.E., Kao, C.F.: The efficient assessment of need for cognition. Journal of Personality Assessment 48, 306–307 (1984)
7. Bechara, A., Damasio, A.R., Damasio, H., Anderson, S.W.: Insensitivity to future consequences following damage to human prefrontal cortex. Cognition 50(1), 7–15 (1994)
8. Dunn, B.D., Dalgleish, T., Lawrence, A.D.: The somatic marker hypothesis: A critical evaluation. Neuroscience and biobehavioral reviews 30(2), 239 (2006)
9. Cacioppo, J.T., Petty, R.E., Feng Kao, C.: The efficient assessment of need for cognition. Journal of personality assessment 48(3), 306–307 (1984)

Evaluation of Subjective and EEG-Based Measures of Mental Workload

Gregory Funke, Benjamin Knott, Vincent F. Mancuso, Adam Strang, Justin Estepp, Lauren Menke, Rebecca Brown, Allen Dukes, and Brent Miller

Air Force Research Laboratory, Wright-Patterson AFB OH, USA
{Gregory.Funke,Benjamin.Knott,justin.estepp,becky.brown, lauren.menke.ctr,brent.miller,allen.dukes}@wpafb.af.mil, vincemancuso@gmail.com, adam.strang.ctr@us.af.mil

Abstract. Assessment of mental workload is an important aspect of many human factors and HCI applications. Not surprisingly, a number of workload measures have been proposed. This study examined the sensitivity, convergent and concurrent validity of several subjective self-report and EEG workload measures. Most measures displayed adequate sensitivity to task difficulty manipulations, but relatively modest convergent and concurrent validity. Overall, we believe these result serve to aid human factors practitioners in selecting measures of workload for varied applications.

Keywords: Mental, Workload, EEG.

1 Introduction

Most methodologies for assessing workload fall into three categories, performance-based, subjective, and physiological measures - with subjective and physiological measures receiving the most attention [2]. While several studies have compared the individual suitability of various subjective and physiological metrics [1, 3-10], to our knowledge no research has employed and examined them all in the same experiment. Without such an inquiry, it is difficult to know the capabilities of each measure, and the possible relations between them. Therefore, the purpose of the current study was to examine several subjective and EEG-based measures of workload for their intercorrelations and relationships with task performance. To this end, three psychometric properties will be specifically examined across measures: sensitivity (i.e., measurement response to changes in task difficulty), convergent validity (correlation of measures with each other), and concurrent validity (correlation of measures with performance).

2 Methods and Materials

2.1 Participants

Twenty-five participants (20 men and 5 women; $M_{Age} = 26.52$, $SD_{Age} = 5.36$) were recruited, all of who had normal (or corrected to normal) vision/hearing and were free of neurological disorders.

C. Stephanidis (Ed.): Posters, Part I, HCII 2013, CCIS 373, pp. 412–416, 2013.

2.2 Subjective Workload Measures

Four subjective workload measures were employed: NASA Task Load Index (TLX), Multiple Resource Questionnaire (MRQ), Workload Profile (WP), and Subjective Workload Dominance Technique (SWORD) [6-9]. For all multidimensional subjective measures, a global score was computed for each.

2.3 EEG-Based Workload Measures

EEG measures were collected using an Advanced Brain Monitoring (ABM) X-10 wireless headset. Signals were sampled at 256 Hz, band-pass filtered at 0.01 to 100 Hz, and decontaminated using ABM's proprietary software. Log power spectra were calculated from 1-second windows (for Fz, POz and P3, respectively) and averaged across each trial. Measurements of average band power were computed for each participant of the theta (4-7 Hz), alpha (8-12 Hz), and gamma (30-40 Hz) bands. In addition, a measure of EEG-based task engagement employed by Prinzel et al. [11] was included for evaluation.

2.4 Experimental Task

The Air Force Space Shooter (AFSS) simulation, a variant of videogame Atari Asteroids, was employed. In AFSS, participants control a spaceship (using a hand-held gamepad) in a simulated "asteroid field." The goal was to destroy as many asteroids as possible without colliding with them. Task difficulty was manipulated by changing the number of asteroids on the screen. The easy, medium, and hard conditions featured 10, 15, and 20 asteroids, respectively. A performance score was calculated as the number of asteroid destroyed (per trial) divided by the total number of asteroids featured in that trial (i.e., 10, 15, or 20).

2.5 Procedures

Upon arrival, participants were given written and verbal instructions concerning the study and how to play AFSS. Next, the X-10 headset was applied and calibrated. Participants were then given two practice trials, each lasting 10 minutes and featuring a reduced number of asteroids (2 and 5, respectively). During the second practice trial, participants were required to demonstrate sufficient proficiency with the task in order to proceed to experimental trials. Next, participants were assigned to an order of difficulty conditions and completed the three experimental trials. Each experimental trial lasted 15 minutes. Post-trial, participants completed the TLX and the MRQ; after concluding all trials, participants completed the WP and SWORD. EEG measures were recorded continuously during each trial.

3 Results

Performance scores were examined for sensitivity to task difficulty using a single factor (trial difficulty) repeated measures ANOVA. In this analysis an omnibus effect was detected, F (2, 48) = 45.56, $p < .05$. Post-hoc analyses indicated that performance scores decreased linearly from the easy (M = 60, SD = 18) to the medium (M = 49, SD = 14) and hard (M = 40, SD = 12) conditions. This confirmed that the task difficulty manipulation was effective in reducing task performance.

Analysis of the sensitivity of workload measures to task difficulty indicated that with the exceptions of average Fz theta and POz alpha power, each measure demonstrated a degree of sensitivity to the manipulation (Table 1). Notably, it appeared that the subjective measures were generally more sensitive to this effect compared to the EEG measures.

Table 1. Summary results of repeated measures ANOVAs and paired sample t-tests for each workload measure

		Paired sample *t*-tests		
Measure	Omnibus F	Easy vs. Med.	Easy vs. Hard	Med. vs. Hard
Subjective				
TLX	13.87*	-2.37*	-5.08*	-3.17*
MRQ	4.46*	-1.35	-2.65*	-2.20*
WP	28.34*	-5.78*	-6.49*	-2.32*
SWORD	29.94*	-5.60*	-6.93*	-3.63*
EEG				
Fz Theta	.96	- - -	- - -	- - -
POz Alpha	.17	- - -	- - -	- - -
P3 Gamma	3.39*	-.17	-2.31*	-2.26*
Engagement	5.79*	-2.03*	-3.03*	-1.56

* $p < .05$

Pearson correlations were calculated between the task performance score and each measure in each task difficulty condition. From these values mean correlations across conditions were computed (Table 2). With regard to correlations between each measure and the performance score (concurrent validity), values were generally low. Of the measures examined the MRQ, WP, and POz average alpha band power appear to demonstrate the greatest (though very modest) correlations with performance.

Regarding the correlation of measures with each other (convergent validity), correlations between TLX, MRQ, and WP were moderate and positive, suggesting modest convergence between those instruments. In addition, the WP was moderately correlated with POz alpha and P3 gamma, also indicating some degree of convergence between those measures. Several of the EEG measures displayed reasonable convergence including POz alpha and Fz theta and P3 gamma, and EEG task engagement and Fz theta and P3 gamma.

Table 2. Mean Peason correlations between the performance score and each workload measure

		Subjective				EEG			
Measure	1	2	3	4	5	6	7	8	9
1. Score	- - -								
Subjective									
2. TLX	-.019	- - -							
3. MRQ	-.001	.251	- - -						
4. WP	-.195	.437*	.332	- - -					
5. SWORD	.240	.078	-.111	-.016	- - -				
EEG									
6. Fz Theta	-.076	.078	.029	.102	-.147	- - -			
7. POz Alpha	-.172	.148	.229	.193	-.178	.594**	- - -		
8. P3 Gamma	.140	.009	-.061	-.338†	.016	.056	.314	- - -	
9. Engagement	.037	.227	-.038	-.098	.058	-.290	.072	.634**	- - -

†$p < .10$. *$p < .05$. **$p < .01$.

4 Discussion

The purpose of the study was to examine the sensitivity, convergent validity, and concurrent validity of several subjective and EEG-based metrics of mental workload.

Regarding sensitivity, most of the metrics displayed some degree of responsiveness to the task difficulty manipulation. Overall, subjective measures performed more consistently, with most exhibiting significant differences in perceived workload across task difficulty conditions. In addition, P3 average gamma band power and EEG task engagement demonstrated sensitivity comparable to the subjective metrics. With reference to convergent validity, most workload measures exhibited only modest correlations with each other. Broadly, subjective multidimensional measures (i.e., TLX, WP and MRQ) exhibited stronger correlations with each other as compared to their respective individual correlations with EEG measures. Likewise, the EEG measures demonstrated some convergence with each other. Of the metrics examined, the WP exhibited the highest convergent validity, though the strengths of those correlations were moderate. The poor convergence observed between the subjective and EEG-based measures is not necessarily an unexpected outcome. For example, others [12, 13] have found little correlation between subjective and physiological workload measures. This may support the suggestion that physiological workload measures are more responsive to moment-to-moment changes in workload, and post-trial/post-experiment subjective measures index aggregate or trial-average workload levels [13].

Finally, analysis of concurrent validity suggested some dissociation between the included workload measures and performance. However, the observed correlations are within the range those reported in other experiments examining workload and performance in complex tasks [1, 14]. SWORD displayed the highest correlation with performance, followed by the WP and POz average alpha band power, respectively. The results of the current study tend to support the utility of the WP, and to a lesser extent, the SWORD, over the other examined subjective measures. Additionally, P3 average gamma band power and EEG task engagement both exhibited favorable qualities. Overall, we believe the results of this study will help human factors and HCI practitioners make informed decisions when selecting measures of workload.

References

1. Rubio, S., Diaz, E., Martin, J., Puente, J.M.: Evaluation of Subjective Mental Workload: A Comparison of SWAT, NASA-TLX, and Workload Profile Methods. Applied Psychology: An International Review 53, 61–86 (2004)
2. Tsang, P.S., Vidulich, M.: Mental Workload and Situation Awareness. In: Salvendy, G. (ed.) Handbook of Human Factors and Ergonomics, 3rd edn., pp. 243–268. Wiley, New York (2006)
3. Hill, S.G., Iavecchia, H.P., Byers, J.C., Bittner, A.C., Zaklade, A.L., Christ, A.E.: Comparison of Four Subjective Workload Rating Scales. Human Factors 34, 429–439 (1992)
4. Finomore, V.S., Warm, J.S., Matthews, G., Riley, M.A., Dember, W.N., Shaw, T.H., Ungar, N.R., Scerbo, M.W.: Measuring the Workload of Sustained Attention. Proceedings of the Human Factors and Ergonomics Society Annual Meeting 50, 1614–1618 (2006)
5. Vidulich, M.A., Tsang, P.S.: Absolute Magnitude Estimation and Relative Judgment Approaches to Subjective Workload Assessment. Proceedings of the Human Factors and Ergonomics Society Annual Meeting 31, 1057–1061 (1987)
6. Hart, S.G., Staveland, L.E.: Development of NASA-TLX (Task Load Index): Results of Empirical and Theoretical Research. In: Hancock, P.A., Meshkati, N. (eds.) Human Mental Workload, pp. 239–250. North Holland Press, Amsterdam (1988)
7. Tsang, P.S., Velazquez, V.L.: Diagnosticity and Multidimensional Subjective Workload Ratings. Ergonomics 39, 358–381 (1996)
8. Vidulich, M.A.: The Use of Judgment Matrices in Subjective Workload Assessment: The Subjective Workload Dominance (SWORD) Technique. Proceedings of the Human Factors and Ergonomics Society Annual Meeting 33, 1406–1410 (1989)
9. Boles, D.B., Adair, L.P.: The Multiple Resources Questionnaire (MRQ). Proceedings of the Human Factors and Ergonomics Society Annual Meeting 45, 1790–1794 (2001)
10. Gevins, A., Smith, M.E.: Neurophysiological Measures of Cognitive Workload During Human-Computer Interaction. Theoretical Issues in Ergonomics Science 4, 113–131 (2003)
11. Prinzel, L.J., Freeman, F.G., Scerbo, M.W., Mikulka, P.J., Pope, A.T.: A Closed-Loop System for Examining Psychophysiological Measures for Adaptive Task Allocation. The International Journal of Aviation Psychology 10, 393–410 (2000)
12. Myrtek, M., Deutschmann-Janicke, E., Strohmaier, H., Zimmermann, W., Lawerenz, S., Brügner, G., Müller, W.: Physical, Mental, Emotional, and Subjective Workload Components in Train Drivers. Ergonomics 37, 1195–1203 (1994)
13. Wilson, G.F., Hankins, T.: EEG and Subjective Measures of Private Pilot Workload. Proceedings of the Human Factors and Ergonomics Society Annual Meeting 38, 1322–1325 (1994)
14. Braarud, P.O.: Subjective Task Complexity and Subjective Workload: Criterion Validity for Complex Team Tasks. International Journal of Cognitive Ergonomics 5, 261–273 (2001)

Self Soothing by Reviewing Favorite Memories: An Exploration of Mobile Application Prototypes, Which Facilitate Positive Wellbeing via Reminiscing

Alice Good, Claire Ancient, Georgiana Postolache, Alexandru Socianu, and Adam Afghan

University of Portsmouth, PO1 3AE UK
{alice.good,claire.ancient}@port.ac.uk

Abstract. The premise of this paper is to promote the results from a small study which sought to evaluate the effectiveness of three different prototype mobile applications, in promoting well being by the reminiscing of positive memories. Interviews were carried out with mental health professionals, including psychotherapists and psychiatric nurses, who were questioned on their opinions as to the effectiveness of the proposed app after using the prototype. The results indicate a significant interest in the proposed tool, with all professionals recognizing the effectiveness of positive reminiscing and indicating a willingness to take part in subsequent prototype evaluation developments.

Keywords: Wellbeing, Mobile Applications, Reminiscing.

1 Introduction

There is potential for using mobile applications as a means to facilitate the process of reminiscing, and this is the focus of the presented research. Whilst there are now a vast range of apps to support physical health, supporting mental health is still a new area, particularly in the area of behavioral therapy.

Mobile applications could be used to facilitate positive reminiscing, and as such, be utilized as a self soothing or distraction tool, for people experiencing low moods or anxiety (Good et al, 2012). The theory is based upon Reminiscent Therapy (RT), designed for people with dementia and involves using meaningful prompts, including photos, music and recordings as an aid to remembering life events (Norris, 1986). Some research states that it has been useful in reducing depression (Scogin F & McElreath, 1994) as well as being an important tool to facilitate socialization. Positive reminiscing can also promote a sense of wellbeing.

The process of reminiscing as a self soothing tool is relatively under explored area. Whilst it has been predominantly utilized in people with dementia, there could be scope for applying the theory of RT in other mental health conditions, particularly where depression and general low mood are common Good et al, 2013). This could potentially induce a 'self soothing' process which could lend itself well to people who struggle with day to day living as a result of low mood, or indeed who experience the

C. Stephanidis (Ed.): Posters, Part I, HCII 2013, CCIS 373, pp. 417–421, 2013.

occasional 'off-day'. The act of 'self soothing', that is calming us down, is in fact one of the most difficult things to achieve when you have mental health problems. Yet the capability to be able to calm oneself down, to essentially self soothe, would be hugely advantageous to people with mental health problems, and could potentially prevent problems from escalating further, if only by means of a distraction. It is the premise of this research to develop apps that can help facilitate positive reminiscing.

2 Mobile App Prototypes for Reminiscing

This research presents examples of reminiscent applications. Three alternative prototype mobile applications were designed on IOS and Android platforms, to display meaningful memorabilia which could be used to promote positive wellbeing.

2.1 I Remember When

'*I Remember When*' (Ancient et al, 2013) is designed as a tablet application, originally intended for people with dementia, but with potential to be utilised by wider user groups (See Figure 1). Users have the option of reminiscing with personal memories or memories through different eras. The latter option would be particularly suitable for people with dementia, for promoting discussion (Norris, 1984).

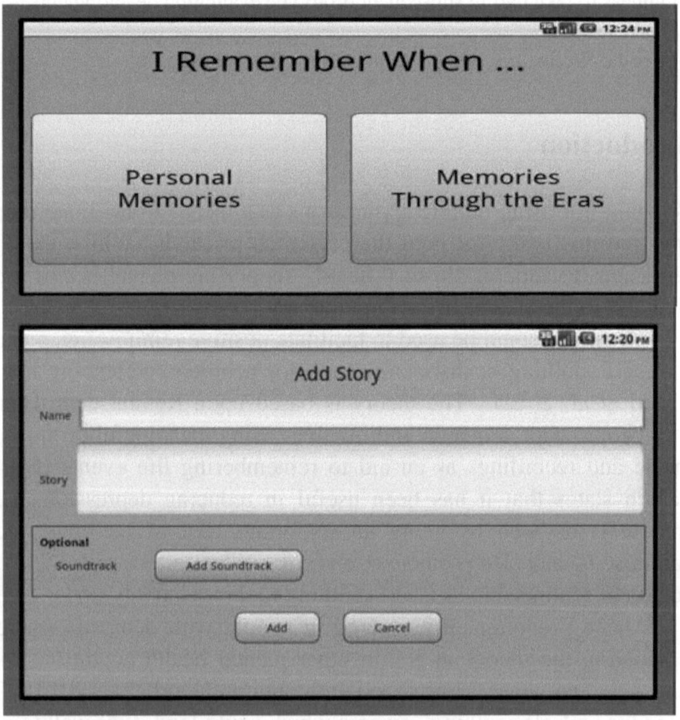

Fig. 1. Mobile App: *I remember when*

The app also provides the facility for users to add personal stories about their lives, which could be related to certain events that triggered positive memories. There is also the facility to assign a relevant sound track to this story, which could enhance the reminiscence process.

2.2 Remember Me

The second prototype – '*Remember Me*' was designed for IOS phones. Users can upload their favourite pictures, videos, audio and notes into the app. There is the facility to assign meaningful comments/notes to the memorabilia. In addition, users could copy and paste content from texts, emails and other files into the 'notes' section, for example poems or special messages (see figure 2).

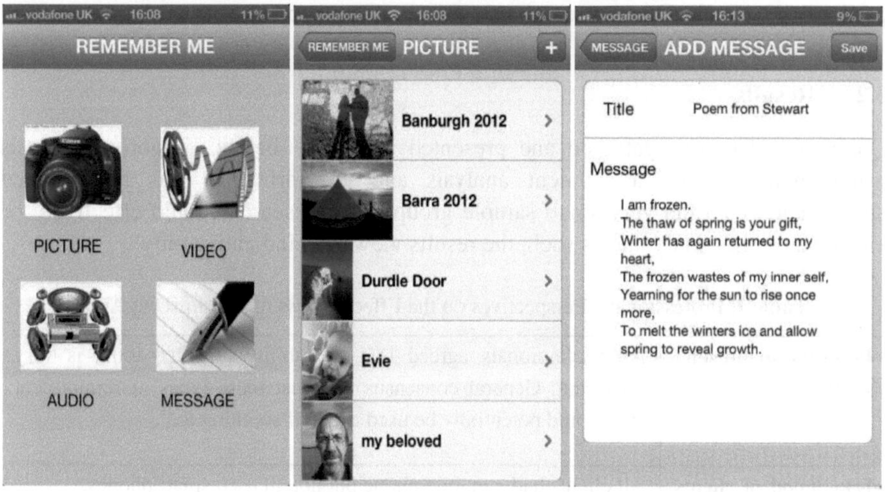

Fig. 2. Mobile App: *Remember Me*

2.3 My Favourite Memories

The final prototype, entitled '*My Favourite Memories*' (see figure 3), was also designed as a tablet application but can also be used on Android phones. With this app, users can store favorite photos and music as well as meaningful notes. As with the previous apps, users can add descriptions or positive notes in the form of prompts to the uploaded media.

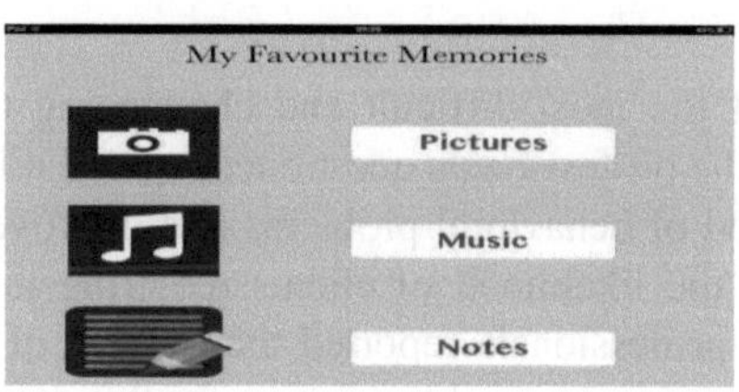

Fig. 3. Mobile App: My Favourite Memories

3 Evaluation Study

3.1 Method

In adopting a user-centered approach to design, the researchers carried out an evaluation of the prototype applications with six experienced professionals who support people with a range of psychiatric disorders, including anxiety, depression and personality disorder. These professionals, who were interviewed separately, were presented with prototypes of the three apps. They were then questioned on the following criteria: whether they thought the app would be suitable in promoting self soothing; likelihood of their clients using these types of apps; likelihood of clients becoming stressed using the app and lastly, whether they would be interested in participating in subsequent research using the proposed apps.

3.2 Results

Qualitative data was gathered and presented in table 1 below. Rigorous analysis using methods such as content analysis and categorization was not deemed appropriate given the very small sample group. This research should effectively be viewed as a pilot study and as such, the results viewed as indicative only.

Table 1. Professionals' Perspectives on the Effectiveness of Reminiscent Apps

Potential to aid self soothing	All professionals agreed that the ability to self soothe is very important. General consensus was that these types of reminiscent apps could potentially be used as a self soothing tool.
Likelihood of clients using app	All clients had a mobile phone but not all used smart phones.
Likelihood of clients becoming stressed whilst using app	Some issues with regards to getting started and maintaining the usage of the app.
Interest in involvement in subsequent research	Five out of six indicated an interest in becoming involved in any subsequent research and trials using the app.

4 Discussion

Self soothing is one of the most difficult and challenging things to achieve when feeling stressed. All of the professionals questioned, agreed it is an important skill and can reduce the likelihood of behavioral problems and improve mental health, as well as potentially reducing the likelihood of clients requiring intervention from mental health services. Some professionals reported that not all of their clients had smart phones, others were not sure. A possible solution for this could be to ensure the apps could be used via laptops or desktop computers. Two professionals voiced concern in relation to clients becoming stressed using the app, but this was more in relation to the likelihood of clients requiring encouragement to get started and to maintain usage. Whilst the application can be set up by individuals, it could also be set up with the support of service providers, for example community nurses/support workers. Five out of the six professionals indicated an interest in becoming involved in related research which involved user testing for effectiveness and usability.

The results of the study suggest that mobile applications could be an effective, as well as accessible method to facilitate positive emotional wellbeing, when used as a self soothing tool. Further research is required to address design issues, particularly in relation to usability and user experience. The apps will need to be designed in such a way that they not only promote self soothing, but also a positive user experience, as clients could potentially be stressed prior to usage and will require an intuitive, easy to use app. Furthermore, studies will be required with end users to evaluate effectiveness. This study is part of a larger research project which focuses on the development of mobile applications for promoting self soothing and wellbeing.

References

1. Ancient, C., Good, A.: Can Ubiquitous Devices Utilising Reminiscence Therapy be Used to Promote Well-being in Dementia Patients? An Exploratory Study. In: Universal Access in Human-Computer Interaction, part of HCI International 2013, Las Vegas, July 21-25 (2013) (in press)
2. Good, A., Sambhantham, A., Panjganj, V.: Looking back at Facebook content and the positive impact upon wellbeing: Exploring reminiscing as a tool for self soothing. In: Online Communities and Social Computing, part of HCI International 2013, Las Vegas, July 21-25 (2013) (in press)
3. Good, A., Wilson, C., Ancient, C., Sambhanthan, A.: A Proposal to Support Wellbeing in People with Borderline Personality Disorder: Applying Reminiscent Theory in a Mobile App. In: The ACM Conference on Designing Interactive Systems (2012)
4. Norris, A.D.: Reminiscence with Elderly People. Winslow, London (1986)
5. Scogin, F., McElreath, L.: Efficacy of psychosocial treatments for geriatric depression: a quantitative review. Journal of Consulting & Clinical Psychology 62, 69–74 (1994)

The Effects of Information Format and Reading Task on Mobile User's Reading Behavior: A Cognitive Fit Perspective

Tse-Ming Tsai, Shih-Chun Chou, Bo-Fu Liu, and Yuting Lin

Institute for Information Industry, Taipei, Taiwan
{eric,benchou,bofuliu,ytlin}@iii.org.tw

Abstract. The ownership of mobile devices rapidly expand which results to the behavior of reading is transformed. A central feature to the success of mobile publications is the design of an effective interface to link text to image information. However, the suitability of the prevalent information formats in supporting various mobile reading tasks is not known. Using the cognitive fit theory as the theoretical framework, we developed a research model to investigate the fit between information format and reading task, and examined its influence on mobile user's reading performance and perceptions of reading experience. As the information format has been shown to affect readers' mobile reading behavior, even when the information content is held constant, the practical implications for mobile publication designers include providing both types of information format on their mobile publications and matching the appropriate information format to the individual reader's task.

Keywords: cognitive fit theory, interface design, mobile publication, multi-touch gesture, reading experience.

1 Introduction

Ownership of mobile devices (also known as pad, tablet and smart phone) are growing. In order to seize widespread business opportunities, individuals such as designers, traditional media publishers, ad agencies, and companies of all sizes want to create, distribute, monetize, and optimize engaging content and publications for mobile devices [1]. A central feature to the success of mobile publications is the design of an effective interface to link text to image information. However, the specification of mobile publication is totally different from web or even paper. Moreover, the suitability of the prevalent information formats in supporting various mobile reading tasks is not known. Therefore, in this research, our objective is to present a research model to investigate the fit between information format and reading task, and examine its influence on mobile user's reading performance and perceptions of reading experience. Grounded on our research, mobile publication designers could match the appropriate information format to the different purpose of the publications based on reader's tasks in order to provide complete reading experience.

C. Stephanidis (Ed.): Posters, Part I, HCII 2013, CCIS 373, pp. 422–426, 2013.

2 Theoretical Background

2.1 Cognitive Fit Theory

The cognitive fit theory was developed to help understand how the fit between the presentation format and the decision-making task can influence individuals' problem solving performance [2]. It basically argues that the performance of problem solving depends on both the problem representation (hereinafter referred to as "information format") and the nature of the task. Different information formats, such as tables and graphics, emphasize different types of information and problem-solving processes. Similarly, different problem-solving tasks, such as trend detection and data value retrieval, also emphasize different types of information and problem-solving processes [3]. The cognitive fit theory suggests that when both the information format and the task emphasize the same types of information and processes, a cognitive fit will occur, which produces a consistent mental representation for problem solving. However, when there is a mismatch between the information format and the task, cognitive fit will not take place. Problem solvers will then need to transform some of the mental representation, inducing additional effort and resulting in relatively lower performance than when there is a cognitive fit.

2.2 Reading Tasks: Searching versus Browsing

The most important feature of content is segmentation due to the different preferences fulfilling various tasks. Take a female teenager as an example, she prefers scanning a gossip magazine to take some rest rather than skimming businesses journal because distinct readership has own interest on the specific type of publications. While searching and browsing are deemed to be distinct activities on the e-publications, researchers also recognized that they represent two ends of a continuum rather than a strict dichotomy [4]. Prior research mainly focus on e-commerce domain which means readers will act differently when they have different reading tasks in mind. [3] However, e-publications on mobile devices should renew an outstanding perspective. We differentiate between searching tasks and browsing tasks by the degree to which readers are specific about their studying objectives.

2.3 Information Format: Tap versus Swipe

Information format is defined as the presentation and organization of information about the available alternatives and their attributes [5]. Not mention to the mobile devices has already revolutionized the way that how people perceive the content presentation. The existence of multi-touch gesture or device sensors such as tap, swipe, gyroscope, and accelerator brings more playfulness for readers to have immersive reading experience. Take automobile chassis for an example, as Figure 1, readers can understand more detail about the structure of the car. These two presentations are used extensively in the present mobile publication applications including catalogs and magazines (which we will refer to as App in this paper).

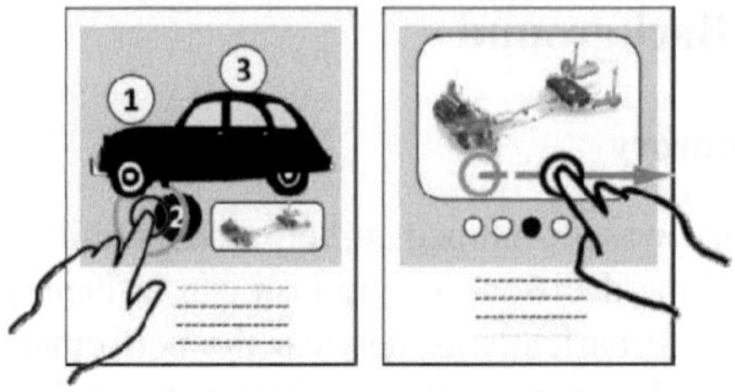

Fig. 1. Screen demonstrations of tap and swipe format

3 Research Model and Hypotheses

The research model is presented in Figure 2. According to prior research in reading behavior and human-computer interaction, users read books online for both goal-oriented and experiential reasons [6]. Therefore, two types of measures can be included when studying users' reading behavior. The first type is performance measures, including reading efficiency (as reflected by the time used) and communicative effectiveness (as reflected by the text/image information that readers can recall from the App). The second type is related to reading experience, such as readers' perceptions of cognitive effort in completing the reading tasks and their attitude toward using the App. Based on the prior theoretical background, we propose that when there is a match between the information formats (tap versus swipe) and the reading tasks (searching versus browsing), more positive outcomes in terms of the two types of measures will result. We firstly conducted a convenience subject in order to sketch the whole picture of the mobile reading experience, then in the next phase of our study we will collect more samples to evaluate the model.

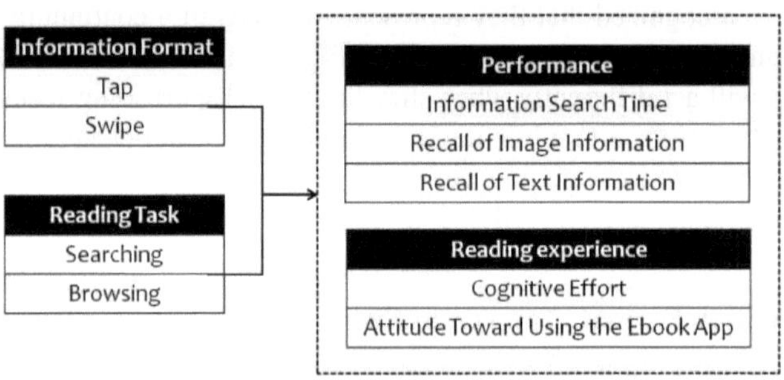

Fig. 2. Research model

3.1 Performance

Time is often used as an indicator of performance in certain tasks involving different information formats. [7] Less time indicates more efficient operation and better interface design, which are desirable to both system designers and system users. Recall is another dependent variable that is frequently adopted in IS research to indicate the effectiveness of communication by different information formats [8]. Readers' recall of text/image information on the publication App can be used as an indication of the degree to which the publication App is successful in conveying ideas to the readers.

According to the earlier analysis, we propose an interaction effect between the information format and the reading task on performance measures. When there is a match between the two, readers will perform better in their reading processes, because effort expended on adjusting any mismatched mental representation can be minimized. Specifically, we expect that the swipe format, which supports local scanpaths, matches the browsing task, and the tap format, which supports global scanpaths, matches the searching task. As a result, not only will the readers' information search time be shorter (H1), but their recall of text/image information will be higher(H2).

- H1: Information search time will be shorter when the information format matches the reading task (i.e., the swipe information format matches the browsing task, and the tap information format matches the searching task).
- H2: Recall of text/image information will be higher when the information format matches the reading task (i.e., the swipe information format matches the browsing task, and the tap information format matches the searching task).

3.2 Reading Experience

The cognitive fit theory suggests that when there is a mismatch between the information format and the reading task, the readers will invest more effort in reading processes. Hence, we propose that cognitive effort will be lower when the information format matches the reading task (H3). Similarly, a more positive attitude from the reading experience will be formed if the readers' reading tasks are well supported by the information formats. Due to the matches between the swipe format and the browsing task and between the tap format and the searching task, we expect that attitude toward using the publication Apps will be more positive when the swipe format is provided for the browsing task and the tap format is provided for the searching task (H4).

- H3: Cognitive effort will be lower when the information format matches the reading task (i.e., the swipe information format matches the browsing task, and the tap information format matches the searching task).
- H4: Attitude towards using the publication Apps will be more positive when the information format matches the reading task (i.e., the swipe information format matches the browsing task, and the tap information format matches the searching task).

4 Discussions and Conclusions

Current study has proposed the role of information format in influencing readers' reading behavior. Utilizing the cognitive fit theory as the theoretical framework, our analysis suggests that mobile users' reading performance is influenced by both the presentation and tasks. By matching the information formats of an App page interface with mobile users' reading tasks, the time that readers spend searching for desired information can be shortened while their recall of text/image information on the App page site can be improved. Furthermore, readers may not consciously be aware of these effects, suggesting that editors or publishers can influence readers in a desired way by manipulating the information format to suit readers' reading tasks.

Future research can build on the findings of this study in other settings using different intervening variables. For example, they can examine whether the findings still hold when the content is in varied domains such as education, retail, travel, health or fashion. Moreover, the effects of other interface characteristics, such as animation of images or text and use of device sensor, can be examined. The predictive power of the cognitive fit theory and vision research in investigating the effects of the App page interface on readers' reading behavior can also be further explored. Continuing research will contribute to a better understanding of the role of the information format in improving reading performance in mobile cyberspace.

Acknowledgement. This study is conducted under the "III Innovative and Prospective Technologies Project" of the Institute for Information Industry which is subsidized by the Ministry of Economy Affairs of the Republic of China.

References

1. Bringhurst, B.: Design Decisions for Digital Publishing Apps. In: InDesign Docs, `http://blogs.adobe.com/indesigndocs/` (retrieved March 13, 2013)
2. Vessey, I.: Cognitive fit: A Theory-based Analysis of the Graphs versus Tables Literature. Decision Sciences 22, 219–240 (1991)
3. Hong, W., Thong, J.Y.L., Tam, K.Y.: The Effects of Information Format and Reading Task on Readers' Reading Behavior: A Cognitive Fit Perspective. Journal of Management Information Systems archive 21, 149–184 (2004)
4. Murphy, J.: Surfers and Searchers. Cornell Hotel and Restaurant Administration Quarterly 40, 84–95 (1999)
5. Cooper-Martin, E.: Effects of Information Format and Similarity among Alternatives on Consumer Choice Processes. Journal of the Academy of Marketing Science 21, 239–2463 (1993)
6. Chen, R., Rose, A., Bederson, B.B.: How People Read Books Online: Mining and Visualizing Web Logs for Use Information. In: European Conference on Research and Advanced Technology for Digital Libraries, pp. 364–369 (2009)
7. Benbasat, I., Dexter, A.S.: An Experimental Evaluation of Graphical and Color-Enhanced Information Presentation. Management Science 31, 1348–1364 (1985)
8. Umanath, N.S., Scamell, R.W., Das, S.R.: An Examination of Two Screen/Report Design Variables in An Information Recall Context. Decision Sciences 21, 216–240 (1990)

Experiment on How Type A and Type B Behavior Pattern Affect Decision-Making

Yichun Luan, Hongjun Xue, and Liwei Ding

School of Aeronautics, Northwestern Polytechnical University, Xi'an 710072, China
{zylyc,Xuehj}@nwpu.edu.cn, 362061894@qq.com

Abstract. Individual decision-making behaviors are affected by context probability, success experiences and individual difference. Experiment on difference of individual decision-making behaviors is designed to explore the rules. Subjects are tested as type A or B behavior pattern before participated in experiment. Decision-making tendency is main analyzed option. The conclusions show that given probability leads subjects' decision-making behaviors in extreme probability states, last outcome and individual differences also impact subjects in average probability states. The causations about subjects' decision-making behaviors match choice's probability, correct-unchanged tendency was more than other tendencies, and difference with type A or B behavior pattern are discussed.

Keywords: decision-making behaviors, probability matching, decision-making tendency, type A and B behavior pattern, last outcome.

1 Introduction

Kahneman found choices of individual decision-making matching with given probability but deviated from the rational choice, pointed those unrational deviation from typical model was followed some rules and could be predicted [1]. Anderson pointed given probability, successful experience and individual difference was main affection factors and simulated individual decision-making by ACT-R model in 1998[2].

Personality will affect decision-making and Phineas Gage was the first sample due to brain injures inducing decision-making [3, 4]. We would explore whether type A and B behavior pattern will affect individual decision-making, whether individuals with different type pattern will make different choice in different probability, and how given probability and successful experience affect decision-making. Type A Behavior Pattern (TABP) was defined by Rosenman and Friedman, which included two type pattern: A and B [5]. Individuals with type A behavior pattern were impetuous, unsteadily emotion, emulative, high efficiency, impatience and high time pressure etc, on the contrary, individuals with type B were peace and quiet, relaxed, comfortable, less ambition, obedient, reticent, cogitative, deep-voiced, costive etc.

Subjects with type A or B behavior pattern are invited to test difference of decision-making behavior to prove those hypotheses:

C. Stephanidis (Ed.): Posters, Part I, HCII 2013, CCIS 373, pp. 427–431, 2013.

1. In extreme probability states given probability would be dominant subjects decision-making behaviors, in average probability states last outcome and individual differences would all impact subjects.
2. In average probability difference of subjects with type A or B behaviors pattern would be remarkable.

Decision-making tendency is main analyzed option. Decision-making tendencies are choices after the last outcome. Last outcomes include correct and error and choices includes changed and unchanged, so there are four tendencies: correct-unchanged, correct-changed, error-unchanged, and error-changed.

2 Difference of Individual Decision-Making Behaviors Experiment

2.1 Testing of Type A or B Behavior Pattern

Testing of type A or B behavior pattern mostly uses questionnaires, those questionnaires include Structure interview (SI), Jenkins activity survey (JAS), Common life scale (CLS) and Type A behavior pattern questionnaire (TABPQ). We use DXC psychometrical instrument, which was developed by the Fourth Military Medical University, and embodied a type A behavior pattern questionnaire which was self-presentation and edited by Zhang Boyuan in 1984.There are 23 students as subjects to be invited to identify type behavior pattern. Table 1 is the outcome. One subject' lie detector exceeded seven, and then his questionnaire was eliminated.

Table 1. The outcome of type A and B behavior pattern identification

type behavior pattern	A（36~50）	A-（28~35）	M（27）	B-（19~26）	B（1~18）
amount	3	10	0	5	4

2.2 Methods

The test process is developed by E-Prime software.

Subjects: 22 students of College of Aeronautics.

Material: There are two alarm lamps, master caution lamp and master warning lamp in the experimental interface. One lamp will light in each test, and the probability is 10%, 20%, 30%, 40%, 50%, 60%, 70%, 80%, 90%, then another will reverse. There are nine groups, and each group has fifty tests. Experimenters forecast and choose which one lamp will light between two alarm lamps. Software will give probability clue of one lamp will light for subjects before starting and correct or error clues after they each choose. The probability of lamp lighting is random and no name. Correct or error clue will show on the interface. Subjects will modify their choices according to clues and probability of lamp light.

3 Results and Discussions

3.1 Affection of Given Probability

Individual chooses according with option' right proportion is defined as Probability Matching. The probability of subjects' choices is gradually close to the given probability, as Fig.1 presents. This result consists with former' experiments.

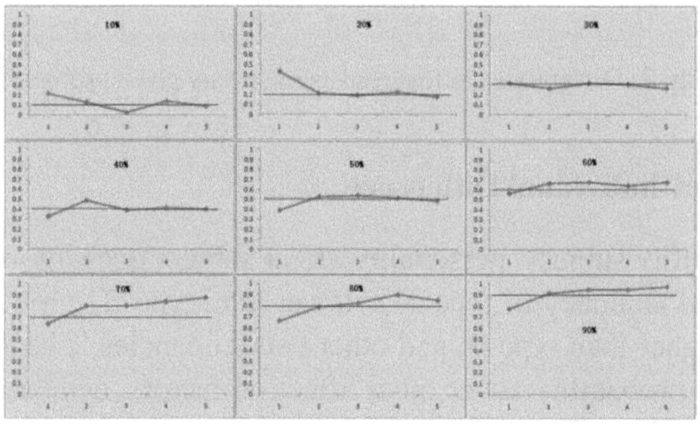

Fig. 1. Subjects' choices matching given probability

Given probability is dominant subject decision-making in extreme probability such as 10%, 20%, 80%, 90% and subject prefers former option and ignores last outcome; in average probability such as 40%, 50%, 60% each choice option has near probability and subject adjusts choice according of last outcome, finally probability of subjects' choices is also close to given probability, from another point of view, it affects subject. In significant level $\alpha = 0.05$, difference of unchanged tendency and changed tendency is significant in all extreme probability state, and insignificant in all average probability state.

3.2 Affection of Last Outcome

Subject' decision-making tendencies are mainly affected by last outcome in average probability, as Fig.2 shows. In extreme probability last outcome is ignored by subjects. In average probability if last outcome is correct, subject will prefer correct option and correct-unchanged tendency is higher than correct-changed; if last outcome is error, subject will change their choice, then error-changed tendency is higher than error-unchanged.

Correct-unchanged tendency is higher than other tendencies and correct-changed is lower than other tendencies in all probability. That is subject will prefer former option if last outcome is correct and weaken affection of given probability. For example, four tendencies would be same in 50% probability, but correct-unchanged tendency is highest, and correct-changed is lowest. Then last outcome is another main factor to affect subject decision-making. Literature 2 described subject choice was affected by last outcome and last last outcome, for example, the probability of A option was chosen lower in turn from AA, BA, AB, BB.

In significant level $\alpha = 0.05$, difference of correct-unchanged tendency and other three tendencies is significant in all given probability.

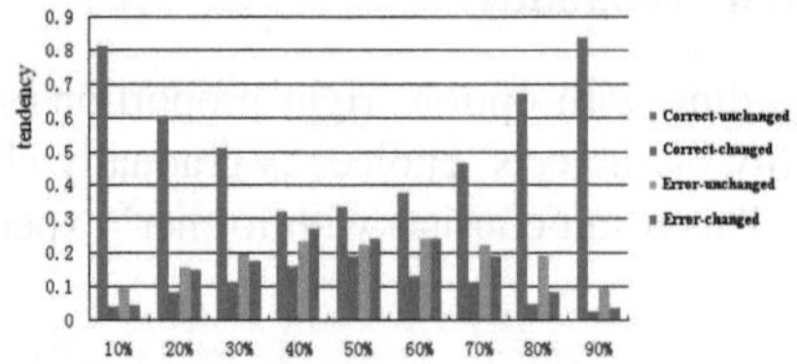

Fig. 2. Differences of four tendencies in vary given probability

3.3 Affection of Individual Difference

In average probability subject' personality affect subject decision-making liked Fig.3. Correct-unchanged tendency of type A is lower than type B, correct-changed tendency of type A is higher than type B, and other two tendencies is nearly. But in extreme probability, given probability cover other affection factors, and subject' tendencies of type A and B is nearly, as Fig.4 showed.

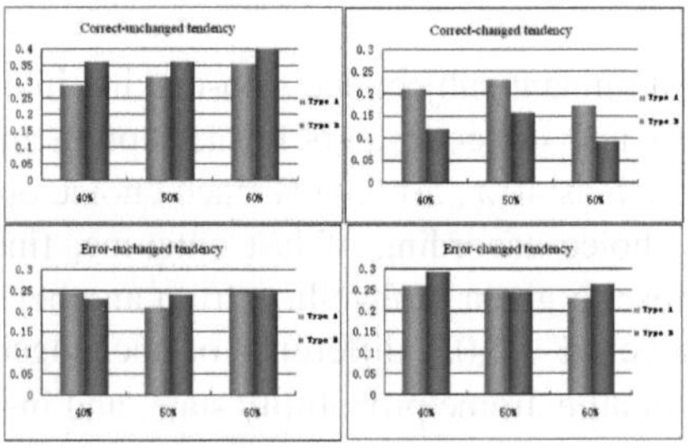

Fig. 3. Differences of subjects with type A or B behavior pattern in average probability

In significance level $\alpha = 0.05$, correct-unchanged tendency of subjects with type A is significantly lower than subjects with type B in average probability; correct-changed tendency with type A is significantly higher than type B; two error tendencies aren't significant in average probability and differences of four tendencies of two types aren't significant in extreme probability.

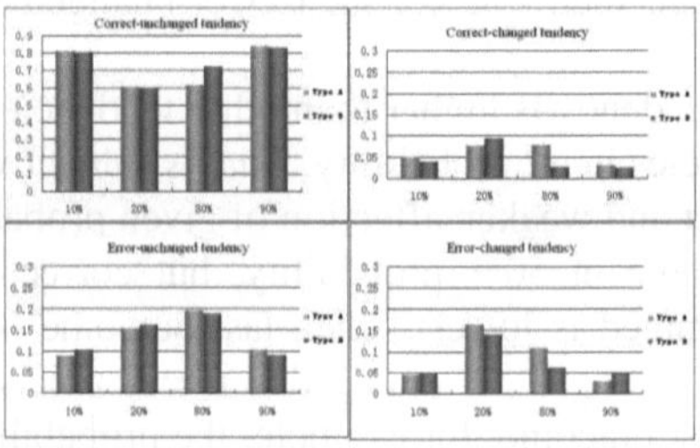

Fig. 4. Differences of subjects with type A or B behavior pattern in extreme probability

3.4 Discussions

1. Explaining probability matching in psychology could be considered that individual adjusts choices according to given probability for most incomes. Affections of last outcome and individual difference for subjects are unnoticed in extreme probability and very clearly in average probability. Explaining correct-unchanged tendency is more than other tendencies could be consider that there is subconscious inertia affecting subject's choices. This inertia is contrary with rational decision-making. When the last outcome is correct, subject prefers the former option, even though accurate rate of that option isn't higher than other options. Hypothesis one is tenable.
2. In average probability difference of subjects with type A or B behaviors pattern are remarkable: Correct-unchanged tendency of subjects with type A is significantly lower than subjects with type B; correct-changed tendency with type A is significantly higher than with type B. Hypothesis two is tenable. That could be considered subjects with type B are more affected by subconscious inertia, and more obedient than type A.

4 Conclusions

Individual decision-making behaviors adjust mainly according to options' given probability and also are affected by last outcome and individual difference. Affection of given probability results in probability matching, affection of last outcome results in correct-unchanged tendency is more than other tendencies, and affection of individual difference results in significant difference of subjects with type A or type B in average probability. But whether correct-unchanged tendency is more than other tendencies, whether difference type pattern behavior results in different decision-making behaviors, those would be proved by more experiments.

Acknowledgments. This research was supported by National Basic Research Program of China (973 Program) (Number: 2010 CB734101).

References

1. Kahneman, D., Tversky, A.: Choice, Values, and Frames. American Psychologist 39(4), 341–350 (1984)
2. Anderson, J.R.: Atomic Components of Thought. Erlbaum, Mahwah (1998)
3. Sanfey, A.G., Hastie, R., Colvin, M.K., Grafman, J.: Phineas gauged: Decision-making and the Human Prefrontal Cortex. Neuropsychologia 41(9), 1218–1229 (2003)
4. Anderson, J.R.: Cognitive Psychology and Its Implication, 7th edn. Worth Publishing, New York (2010)
5. Sanfey, A.G., Hastie, R., Colvin, M.K., Grafman, J.: Phineas gauged: Decision-making and the Human Prefrontal Cortex. Neuropsychologia 41(9), 1218–1229 (2003)

The Error Prevention Mechanisms of Pointing: Eye Focusing and/or Memory Enhancing?

Takayuki Masuda[1], Masayoshi Shigemori[2], Yasuhiro Kitamura[1], and Naohiro Akiu[1]

[1] Human Science Division, Railway Technical Research Institute, 2-8-38 Hikari-cho, Kokubunji-shi Tokyo, 185-8540, Japan
[2] Department of Contemporary Communication, Shizuoka Eiwa Gakuin University Junior College, 1769 Ikeda, Suruga-ku, Shizuoka-shi, Shizuoka-ken, 422-8545, Japan
{Masuda,kitamura,akiu}@rtri.or.jp, gemo@h9.dion.ne.jp

Abstract. The error prevention effects of "point and call checks (P&C Checks)" are known and used in several industries in Japan. We investigated whether or not "pointing" had an error prevention effect and if the effect is due to eye focusing. Participants performed tasks under different experimental conditions: (1) with pointing, (2) without pointing. The density of the dots were controlled (high or low). This task had two subtasks. One, focusing on the only target dots and two, remembering the dots which have been counted. The result indicated that only in low density condition the number of counting error in "with pointing" conditions was significantly fewer than that in "without pointing" condition. The result supported the memory enhancing effect of pointing.

Keywords: "point and call checks", human error, error prevention.

1 Introduction

In various industries, human error is indicated as the main cause of accident. For the purpose of preventing human error, several tangible and intangible countermeasures have been developed. Although both countermeasures are important for enhanced safety, tangible countermeasures usually get most attention. Intangible measures are also important for safety. "Point and call checks (P&C Checks)" is one form of intangible countermeasure broadly used in various industrial fields in Japan. Various workers, for example train drivers, factory workers, plant workers and nurses use P&C Checks in complicated perceptual situations or when operating complicated systems in order to prevent errors. In the railway field, various workers, not to mention train drivers and conductors, use P&C Checks in Japan. For example, train operators check a railway signal while pointing at it with their finger and calling out its state. Maintenance workers check project status with P&C Checks, too. P&C Checks is a method for confirming an action or status by pointing at the object or task with index finger and calling out its state or status [1]. Several studies have demonstrated that the P&C Checks have error prevention effects, but the error prevention mechanisms of P&C Checks have not been verified sufficiently. Therefore we need to confirm each mechanism in detail.

C. Stephanidis (Ed.): Posters, Part I, HCII 2013, CCIS 373, pp. 432–436, 2013.

In this paper we focus on the mechanism of eye fixation with pointing. We experimentally investigated whether or not "pointing" had an error prevention effect and if the effect is due to eye focusing. We compare the error rate in the task of counting dots on the PC display in high and low density conditions. This task had two subtasks. One, focusing on only target dots and two, remembering the dots which have been counted. For the purpose of confirming the eye focusing effect of pointing, eye movements were recorded. Because of the deterioration of the data due to the head movement of the participants, the data was not analyzed. Details of the results of the eye tracker data will therefore not be fully described.

2 Procedure

2.1 Participants

Forty people (nineteen male, twenty one female) participated in the study; they had the mean age of 21.35 years. All participants were aware of their right to withdraw from the study at any time and had a full debriefing about the aims of the study.

2.2 Equipment

We collected data using the experiment software (developed with Microsoft Visual Basic 2010). Experiment software was installed to the PC (FUJITSU FMVDE2A0L1). Output was shown on the 17in. display (Mitsubishi RDT1713LM) at 1024 × 768 pix. The responses of participants were recorded with a keyboard connected to the PC. The display was positioned 60 cm from the participants.

2.3 Task

The task was to count the dots on the display. This experiment consisted of two sessions. The first session was a trial session. Participants performed the task under different experimental conditions: (1) with pointing, (2) without pointing. The density of the dots was controlled (high or low: Figure 1). In the trial session, participants experienced one high density trial and one low density trial without pointing, and the order was randomly selected. One session consisted of twelve trials: six high density trials and six low density trials in each experimental condition. Each trial was selected randomly. With or without tests alternated. The dot density was controlled not to be the same in the six consecutive trials. In the trial session, forty dots on the screen in one trial. In one session, the number of the dots on the screen was selected from 37, 38, 39, 41, 42, 43 (average 40).

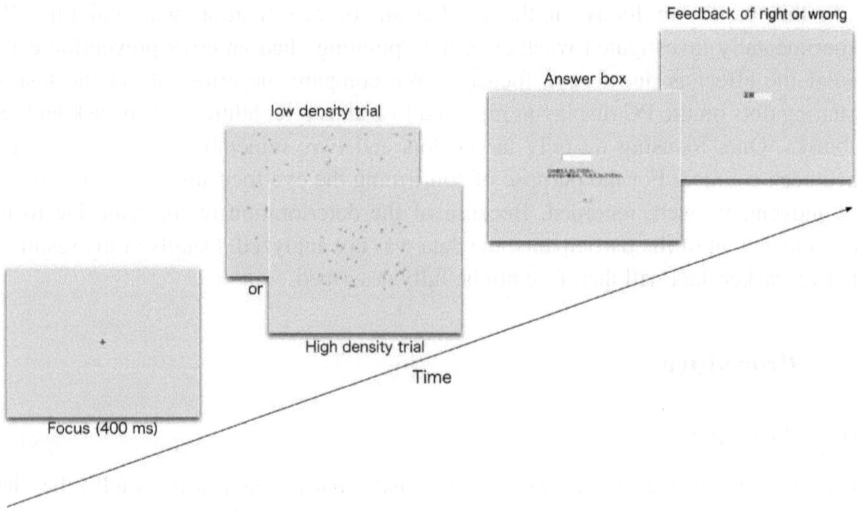

Fig. 1. Flow of experiment

The screen was divided into the 70 x 50 arrays of cells. In high density trials, the locations of the dots presented on the screen were selected from all cells. On the other hand, in low density trials, the locations of the dots presented on the screen were selected from limited cells (from rows eighteen to fifty three and from columns thirteen to thirty eight).

The dots were presented for 400ms per each dot. When forty dots were presented, dots were presented for 16000ms.

3 Hypothesis

If the error prevention effect of pointing is due to the effect of eye focusing, the error prevention effect should be revealed more clearly in high density condition than in low density condition, because focusing on only target dots is more difficult. On the contrary, if the error prevention effect was revealed more clearly in low density conditions than in high density conditions, then pointing may have memory enhancing effect. The result indicated that only in low density condition the number of counting error in "with pointing" conditions was significantly fewer than that in "without pointing" condition. The result supported the memory enhancing effect of pointing.

4 Results

4.1 Control of the Density of Dots

In order to confirm the control of the density of dots, analysis of variance was conducted. The results indicated that the main effect of the density and the average distance between dots in high density condition was fewer than that in low density condition (F (1, 39) = 23358.28, p < .01). There was no main effect of with/without pointing and interaction between with/without pointing and density of dots. These result validated the control of the density of dots.

4.2 Error Rate

Analysis of variance (ANOVA) was conducted to examine the effects of with/without pointing and density of dots. The results indicated that the main effect of with/without pointing and the number of wrong count in with pointing condition was significantly fewer than that in without pointing condition (F (1, 39) = 4.20, p < .05). There was no significant interaction between with/without pointing and density of dots (F (1, 39) = 1.20, n.s.).

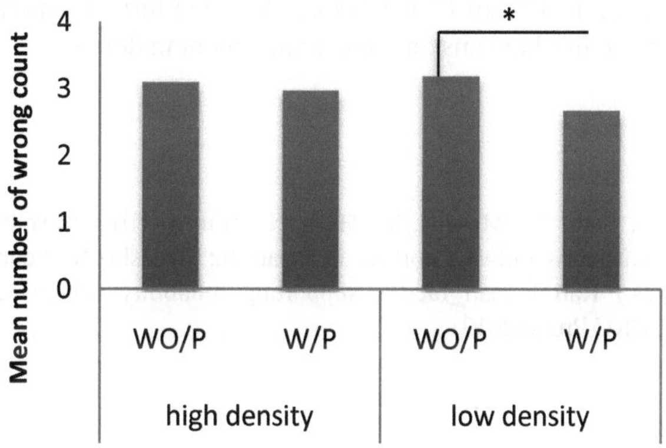

Fig. 2. Error rate in each experimental condition (*: *p*<.05)

Although, significant interaction between with/without pointing and density of dots was not seen, a t-test was conducted to examine the effects of with/without pointing in each density conditions. The result indicated that the number of wrong count with pointing condition was significantly fewer than that without pointing condition in low density condition (t = 2.07, df = 39, p<.05). There was no difference between with pointing condition and without pointing condition in high density condition (t = 0.54, df = 39, n.s.).

5 Discussion

Although, significant interaction between with/without pointing and density of dots was not seen, the result of t-test indicated that error prevention effect of pointing was seen only in low density condition.

One interpretation of this result is that error prevention effect of pointing is not only due to the effect of eye focusing, but may be due to other error prevention mechanism. One possibility is that pointing has the memory promoting effect. Pointing accompanying physical movement may prompt spatial memory. Consequently, error prevention effect of pointing was seen only in low density condition. In order to count the dots accurately, remembering what dots have already been counted is important. Therefore, it can hardly be assumed that eye fixation have no relation with error prevention effect. Because of the deterioration in the accuracy of the eye tracker calibration, we couldn't test the difference in eye fixation between each experimental condition. As a result, we can't test to what extent eye fixation has relation with prompting memory and error prevention. We need to perform further experiments under various density conditions and to research using eye camera.

Identifying the error prevention mechanisms is important not only in terms of academic progress, but also in terms of application to the field. One application is to education. Intangible counter-measures such as P&C Checks are easy to lose popularity. Learning the mechanisms of P&C Checks may contribute to enhanced understanding and retention of P&C Checks. We need further experiments to identify the error prevention mechanisms and to examine them in detail.

Reference

1. Shigemori, M., Sato, A., Masuda, T., Haga, S.: Human error prevention effect of point and call check used by railway workers in Japan. In: Dadashi, N., Scott, A., Wilson, J.R., Mills, A. (eds.) Rail human factors supporting reliability, safety and cost reduction, pp. 599–608. CRC Press (2013)

A Novel Approach to Cognitive Engineering: Manipulating Access Cost

Phillip L. Morgan[1,*], Victoria Smy[2], Helen Seeby[2], and John Patrick[2]

[1] School of Psychology, Counselling, and Early Years, University of South Wales, Caerleon Campus, Newport, NP18 3QT, UK
[2] School of Psychology, Cardiff University, Tower Building, Park Place, Cardiff, CF10 3AT, UK
phillip.morgan2@newport.ac.uk,
{smyva,seebyh,patrickj}@cardiff.ac.uk

Abstract. The traditional approach to cognitive engineering involves reducing workload by providing operators with immediately accessible relevant information. We suggest that such immediate access may not always improve human performance. Somewhat counter-intuitively, making some information harder to access by slightly increasing the time, physical and mental effort to view it can induce a more memory-based planning strategy that can improve performance. Studies are described that find increasing access cost leads to improved recall, more efficient problem solving, and resilience to interruption. Implications for cognitive engineering are discussed.

Keywords: Information access cost, cognitive engineering, display design, soft constraints, memory, planning, problem solving, task interruption.

1 Introduction

Rapid developments in information technology have far outstripped our ability to develop corresponding intellectual technology concerning its optimal use. Advances in computer processing speed, computer memory capacity, and networking capabilities, have afforded software engineers the scope to design interfaces that allow operators unprecedented access to large volumes of information. Operators of complex safety-critical systems such as aircraft, process control plants, and command centers, are increasingly flooded with immediately available information from multiple sources. The question is how should these technological developments be harnessed to design interfaces that optimize human performance?

1.1 Traditional Approach to Cognitive Engineering

The traditional assumption is that fast access to relevant information will reduce workload and improve performance [1, 2, 3]. Interface design has been driven by human processing capabilities and limitations when humans interact with systems [4].

* Corresponding author.

C. Stephanidis (Ed.): Posters, Part I, HCII 2013, CCIS 373, pp. 437–441, 2013.

Its main goals are to develop systems that: are easy to learn and use [5]; support effective cognitive functioning (e.g., attention, memory); improve performance, and reduce errors and accidents [6]. Consequently the traditional approach to cognitive engineering provides operators of complex systems with immediately available relevant information by taking advantage of human perception, attention, and psychomotor abilities. For example, Ecological Interface Design proposes that complex relationships between data should be made directly accessible to operators in a manner that allows effortless extraction of information from an interface [7]. Similarly, information fusion attempts to present operators with a more coherent 'situational' picture [2]. Essentially, both methodologies assume that reducing cognitive workload when operators access and extract information from complex displays will always benefit performance. The present paper challenges this assumption by demonstrating how a brief delay in accessing important information can induce a more cognitively-oriented processing strategy that can improve performance in some specific situations.

1.2 The Theory of Soft Constraints and Information Access Cost

The theoretical underpinning for the effect of manipulating access cost comes from Anderson's seminal work on adaptive cognition [8], and the theory of 'soft constraints' [9]. These approaches emphasize that any cognitive strategy is developed on the basis of its perceived benefits and costs. Increasing the millisecond cost of accessing information from an interface can affect the selection between a display-based and more memory-intensive strategy [9]. The idea is that operators attempt to avoid small time delays in accessing information by adopting a more memory-based strategy. In display-based interaction, the interface is used as an external memory resource, thus minimizing the need for internal memory. Consequently information may not be deeply processed as it is easily available at the interface. However, increasing the cost of accessing information results in the operator trying to avoid this cost, with a powerful shift to a more memory-based strategy [9]. Thus, somewhat counter-intuitively, small delays in information accessibility can encourage deployment of a more cognitively intensive strategy that may subsequently improve task performance.

Information access cost is defined as the time, physical and mental effort involved in accessing task critical information (e.g., the goal-state in a problem solving task). In the following studies, access costs were varied among three levels. With a Low access cost, the goal-state was permanently visible. With a Medium cost, the goal-state was covered with a mask that disappeared immediately when a mouse cursor was moved into the goal area and reappeared when the cursor was moved out of that area. A High cost had an extra second or two lockout time for the mask to disappear.

2 The Effect of Increasing Information Access Cost

First, increasing access cost can improve recall. The Blocks World Task (BWT, Figure 1) involves copying a target pattern of colored blocks in a target window to a workspace window by dragging and dropping colored blocks from a resource palette.

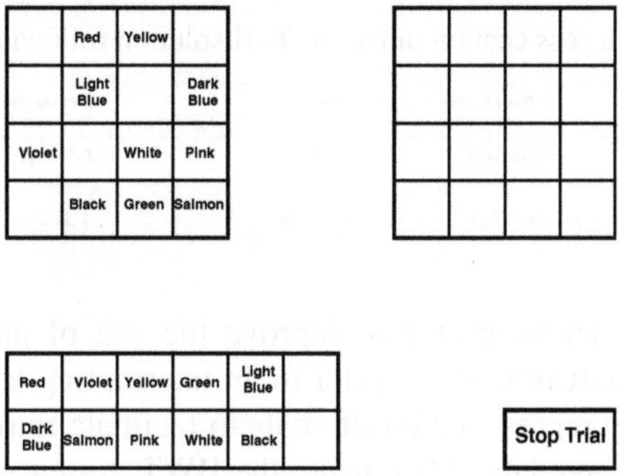

Fig. 1. Example of a Low Goal Access Cost Start-state (BWT). Squares were presented as actual colors with no overlaying text as in Figure 1, and all blank squares were grey.

Access costs for viewing the target pattern (Low, Medium, & High) were manipulated by Waldron, Patrick, Morgan and King [10] and participants had to recall the target pattern in a surprise recall test. A display-based strategy was adopted in the Low access condition and a more memory-based strategy in higher cost conditions, with more blocks correctly recalled in the Medium and High cost conditions (Table 1).

Second, increasing access cost can improve planning, which is notoriously difficult to encourage. Better recall and better planning go hand-in-hand. A study by Waldron, Patrick & Duggan [11], using a problem solving variant of the BWT, investigated the effect of varying access cost on the nature of planning (memory- or display- based) and when planning occurred (before or during action). In a High access cost condition (i.e., 2.5 second cost to access the goal-state), more planning before action was observed and less during action. This was evidenced by longer first-move latencies and more moves per goal-state visit. A further study by Morgan & Patrick [12] investigated whether increasing access cost improved planning in the Tower of Hanoi problem solving task. Performing the task under a High access cost resulted in fewer moves to solution and more perfect solutions, as a consequence of better planning.

Table 1. Effect of goal-state access cost on recall in the BWT [10]

High access cost		Med access cost		Low access cost	
Mean	SD	Mean	SD	Mean	SD
9.00	1.78	9.00	4.37	4.70	1.95

Third, increasing access cost can also improve memory-based planning that helps recovery from interruption. Interruptions have many detrimental effects on performance including delays in resuming a primary task and forgetting goals [13]. Inducing a more memory-based planning strategy by manipulating access cost can mitigate the effect of forgetting goals after different types of interrupting task [13]. In problem solving studies by Morgan & Patrick [12, 14] High access cost conditions not only promoted more efficient problem solving, in terms of the number of moves to solution, but participants also maintained this efficiency following interruption (Table 2).

Table 2. Effect of access cost on moves to ToH solution following interruption [14]

High access cost		Med access cost		Low access cost	
Mean	SD	Mean	SD	Mean	SD
9.87	.39	10.20	.35	11.27	.44

Finally, increasing access cost can improve the use of an interruption lag. An interruption lag is a short time delay prior to an interrupting task that can be used to strengthen the memory representation of goals to facilitate retrieval after interruption [15]. Morgan, Patrick and Tiley [16], using the BWT, tested whether a 5-second lag was sufficient to recall planned moves and whether any beneficial effect was dependent upon the strength of the memory-based strategy used to perform the task. Prospective memory was very poor with and without an interruption lag when the task was performed under Low and Medium access costs (Figure 2). However, prospective memory was not only improved under High access cost without an interruption lag, but this improvement was substantial with an interruption lag (Figure 2).

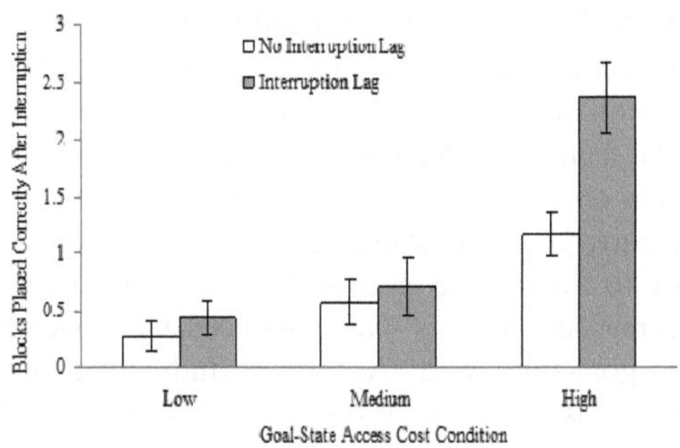

Fig. 2. Effect of access cost and an interruption lag on recall following interruption [16]

3 Conclusions and Implications

The findings demonstrate that delaying access to information within a display, albeit only over a second or two, can induce a more memory-based planning strategy that can improve performance in terms of memory recall, problem solving, and recovering from interruption. We do not advocate that information access is always delayed but we do suggest that the traditional assumption of immediate access to information may not be the optimal solution in some situations where recall and planning are important aspects of performance. Thus, manipulating access cost could be used to complement the traditional cognitive engineering approach when more intensive cognitive processing of information is crucial to improve performance, such as when recall is required or when tasks are prone to being interrupted. Furthermore, access costs are intrinsic to everyday computer interactions, e.g., when opening applications, emails, or documents and when navigating menus. It is possible that these intrinsic costs could be exploited to obtain powerful changes in task strategy and subsequent improvements in performance akin to those discussed within the current paper.

References

1. Rasmussen, J., Pejtersen, A., Goodstein, L.: Cognitive Systems Engineering. John Wiley & Sons, New York (1994)
2. Vicente, K.J.: Ecological Interface Design: Progress and Challenges. Human Factors 44, 62–78 (2002)
3. Woods, D.D., Roth, E.M.: Cognitive Systems Engineering. In: Helander, M. (ed.) Handbook of Human-Computer Interaction, 1st edn. North-Holland, New York (1988)
4. Wickens, C.D., Hollands, J.G., Banbury, S., Parasuraman, R.: Engineering Psychology and Human Performance, 2nd edn. Pearson Education, New Jersey (2012)
5. Roth, E.M., Patterson, E.S., Mumaw, R.J.: Cognitive Engineering: Issues in User-Centered System Design. In: Marciniak, J.J. (ed.) Encyclopedia of Software Engineering, 2nd edn. John Wiley & Sons, New York (2002)
6. Gersh, J.R., McNeely, J.A., Remington, R.W.: Cognitive Engineering: Understanding Human Interaction with Complex Systems. Johns Hopkins APL Tech Digest 26(4), 377–382 (2005)
7. Dasarathy, B.V.: Information Fusion – What, Where, Why, When, and How? Information Fusion 2, 75–76 (2001)
8. Anderson, J.R.: The Adaptive Character of Thought. Erlbaum, Hillsdale (1990)
9. Gray, W.D., Sims, C.R., Fu, W.-T., Schoelles, M.J.: The Soft Constraints Hypothesis. A Rational Analysis Approach to Resource Allocation for Interactive Behaviour. Psychological Review 113, 461–482 (2006)
10. Waldron, S.M., Patrick, J., Morgan, P.L., King, S.: Influencing Cognitive Strategy by Manipulating Information Access. The Computer Journal 50, 694–702 (2007)
11. Waldron, S.M., Patrick, J., Duggan, G.B.: The Influence of Information Access Cost on Planning during Problem Solving. Quarterly Journal of Experimental Psychology 64(3), 485–503 (2011)
12. Morgan, P.L., Patrick, J.: Paying the Price Works: Increasing Goal Access Cost Improves Problem Solving and Mitigates the Effect of Interruption. Quarterly Journal of Experimental Psychology 66(1), 160–178 (2012)
13. Morgan, P.L., Patrick, J., Waldron, S.M., King, S.L., Patrick, T.: Improving Memory after Interruption: Exploiting Soft constraints and Manipulating Information Access Cost. Journal of Experimental Psychology: Applied 15(4), 291–306 (2009)
14. Morgan, P.L., Patrick, J., Patrick, T.: Increasing Information Access Costs to Protect against Interruption Effects during Problem Solving. In: Proceedings of the 32nd Annual Conference of the Cognitive Science Society, pp. 949–955. Erlbaum, Hillsdale (2010)
15. Altmann, E.M., Trafton, G.J.: Memory for Goals: An Activation-Based Model. Cognitive Science 26, 39–83 (2002)
16. Morgan, P.L., Patrick, J., Tiley, L.: Improving the Effectiveness of an Interruption Lag by Inducing a Memory-Based Strategy. Acta Psychologica 142(1), 87–95 (2013)

Role of Metacognition in Basic Electric Circuit Problem Solving Process

Atsuo Murata, Yukio Ohta, and Takehito Hayami

Graduate School of Natural Science and Technology, Okayama University, Okayama, Japan
murata@iims.sys.okayama-u.ac.jp, ohtayuki@wine.plara.or.jp

Abstract. Metacognitive ability demonstrated in algebra word problem solving for primary school pupil is directly not applicable to more complicated and advanced problem solving such as electronic circuit. The aim of this study was to analyze the metacognitive process when solving basic problems concerning electronic circuit. In spite of mastering scientific knowledge and formula necessary for the solution, the lower performance group could not reach a higher score like higher performance group. We judged that this difference of performance must be due to the lack in metacognitive ability, especially the plan and the control and execution abilities. Thus, the importance of metacognitive ability, especially the plan ability was identified in the problem solving of basic electric circuit.

Keywords: metacognition, problem solving, plan, monitior, basic electric circuit.

1 Introduction

When solving a science problem such as a mathematical or a basic electric circuit problem, in spite of mastering knowledge and formula necessary for the solution, we sometimes encounter a situation where we cannot reach the correct answer. The reason can be contributed to the lack in metacognitive abilities. "Metacognition" refers to one's knowledge on one's own cognitive processes and products and products related to them. The role metacognition plays in mathematical performance is explored [1-4]. It has been conceptually shown that successful problem solving depends on not only adequate knowledge related to the problem but also sufficient awareness and control of the cognitive process during problem solving, that is, metacognition.

Lawanto [5] developed a lecture system using enhanced guided notes (EGN) in an electric circuit course for beginners. The difference between the traditional lecture system and the proposed one was that the proposed one made an attempt to prompt students to evaluate their metacognitive knowledge. Although he showed that the proposed lecture system led to higher performance of students, the problem solving process was not analyzed at all.

C. Stephanidis (Ed.): Posters, Part I, HCII 2013, CCIS 373, pp. 442–446, 2013.

In general, metacognitive abilities consist of (1) comparing the difficulty of problem with own ability, (2) proper plan of solution process, (3) conscious monitoring of solution process, and (4) control of solution process. Although Lawanto [5] suggested the importance of metacognitive knowledge in the problem solving process, he did not explore how the metacognitive knowledge contributed to the enhanced performance in each of the processes (1)-(4) above. In this study, we judged that this difference of performance must be due to the lack in metacognitive ability.

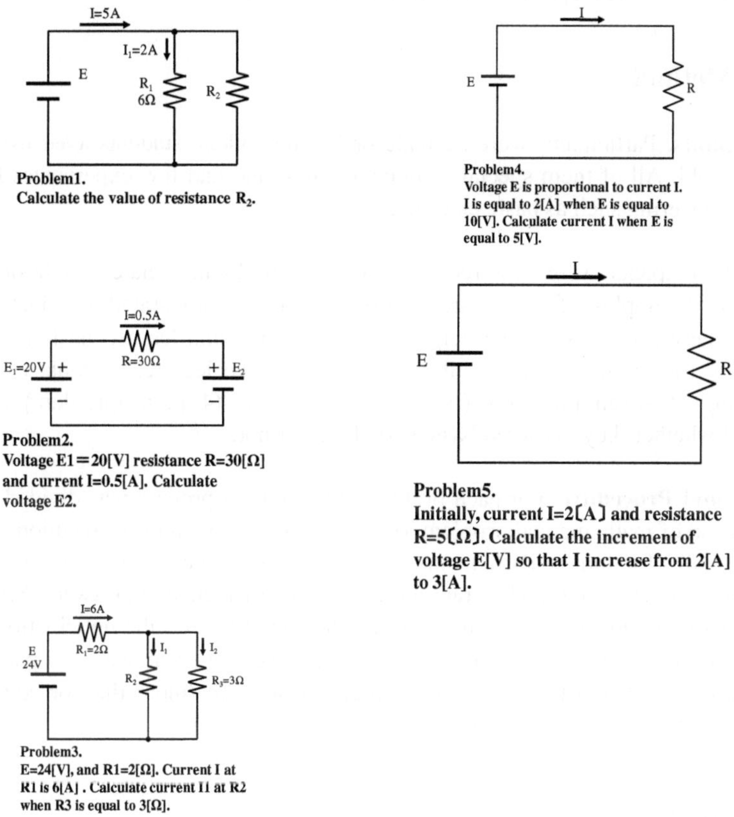

Fig. 1. Problems1-5 used in this study

The role and importance of metacognitive ability mainly in algebra word problem solving for primary school pupil was explored [2-4]. These results are directly not applicable to more complicated and advanced problem solving such as linear algebra, differential calculus, integral calculus, or electronic circuit. The aim of this study was to analyze the metacognitive process when solving basic problems concerning electronic circuit.

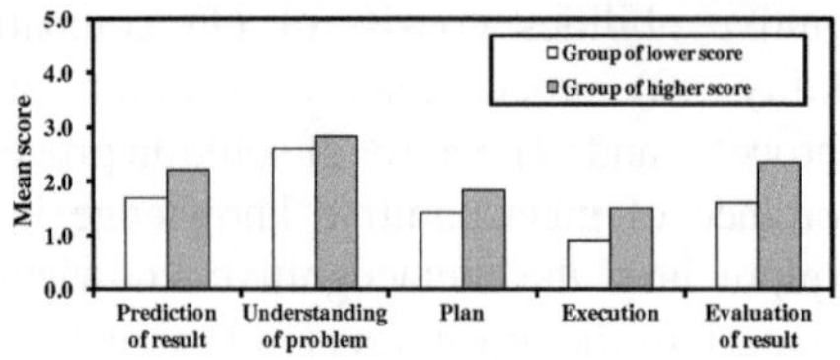

Fig. 2. Mean score of five basic electric circuit problems as a function of cognitive process and classification of score (upper and lower score groups)

2 Method

Participants. Participants were 22 male or female college students aged from 19 to 20 years old. All of them specialize in economics, and had few experiences learning basic engineering such as basic electric circuit.

Task. Participants were required to solve five problems related to basic circuit problem. Examples of basic circuit problems are demonstrated in Fig.1. Before solving these problems, the participants took a lecture and learned basic knowledge necessary for solving basic circuit problems. After the lecture, all took a brief test consisting of seven problems (full mark: 28 points (4 points/problem) and was checked whether they mastered basic knowledge or not.

Design and Procedure. For each problem, the solution process was divided into (a) recognition of mathematical problem, (b) plan of solution, and (c) execution (monitor and control) of solution. Participants were required to rate the anticipation whether they can solve it or not, and to rate the confidence of their own answer. Participants were also required to describe the reason why they selected the anticipation rating. According to the total score of preliminary test mentioned above, the participants were categorized into the group of the higher test score (more than or equal to 14 points) and the group of the lower test score (below 16 points).

3 Results

In Fig.2, the mean score of five basic electric circuit problems is compared among cognitive process and between high and low score groups. In Fig.3, the mean score of problems 1 and 5 during the prediction process of result is compared between higher and lower performance groups. Similar results for the understanding of problem, the plan of solution, the execution of solution, and the evaluation of result of problem solving are depicted in Figs. 4-7. Figs.8, 9, and 10 plot the mean score as a function of cognitive process and classification of score (upper and lower score groups) for problems 2, 3, and 4, respectively.

4 Discussion

As shown in Fig.2, as a whole, statistically significant differences were detected between the high and low score groups, especially at the plan and the execution processes. As for the rating on the anticipation of result and the confidence of own answer, significant differences were found between both groups. Moreover, the relationship between the score of plan process and the score of execution process was

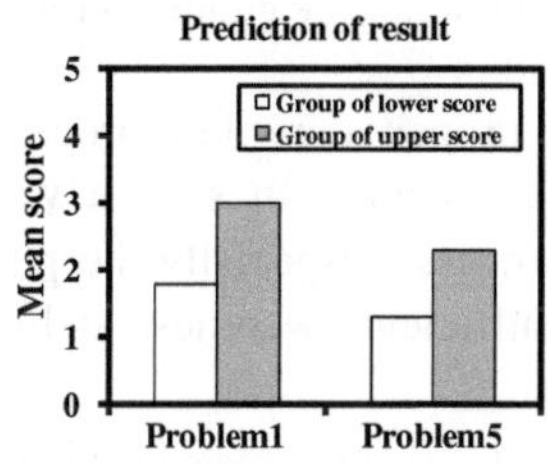

Fig. 3. Mean score of problems 1 and 5 during the prediction processes whether he or she can correctly solve the problem compared between classification of score (upper and lower score groups)

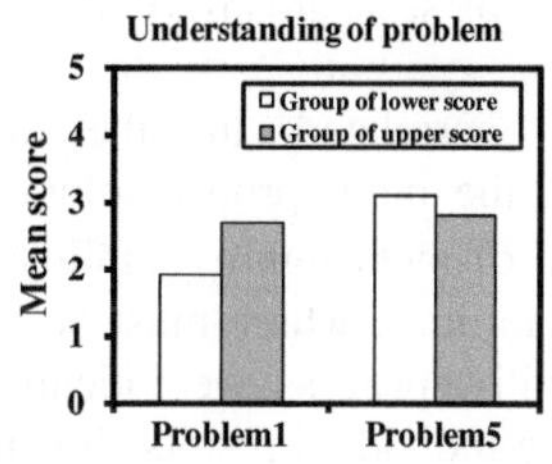

Fig. 4. Mean score of problems 1 and 5 during the understanding processes of the problem compared between classification of score (upper and lower score groups)

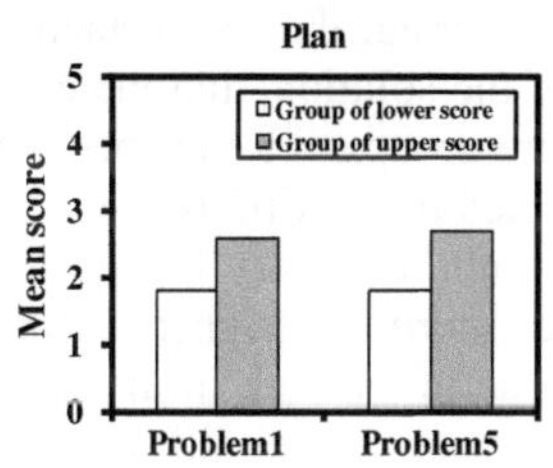

Fig. 5. Mean score of problems 1 and 5 during the plan processes of the solution between classification of score (upper and lower score groups)

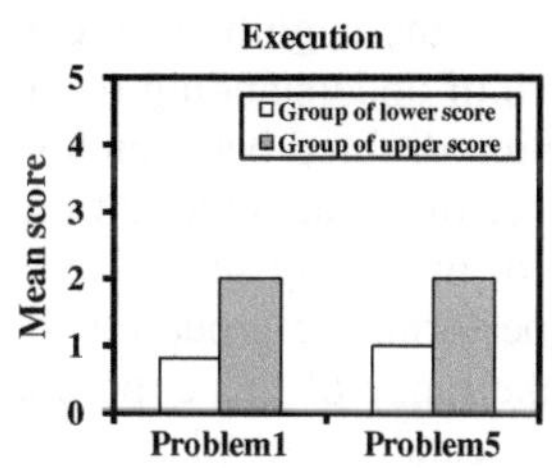

Fig. 6. Mean score of problems 1 and 5 during the execution processes of the solution between classification of score (upper and lower score groups)

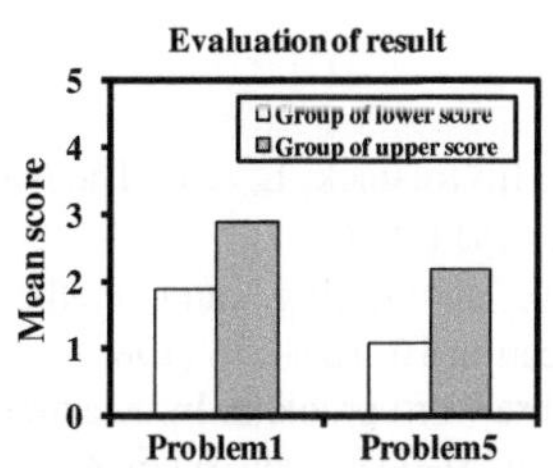

Fig. 7. Mean score of problems 1 and 5 during the evaluation of result between classification of score (upper and lower score groups)

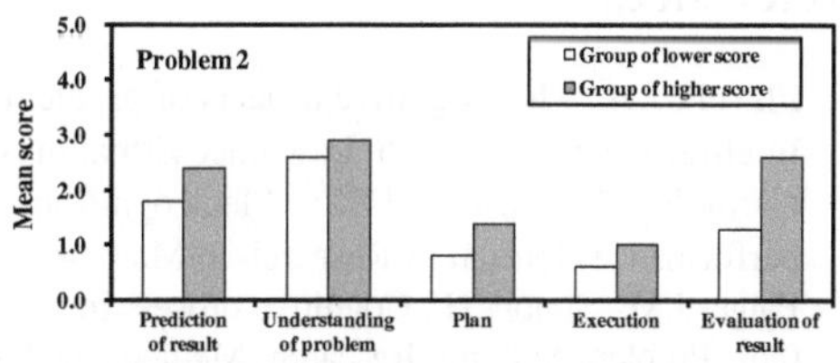

Fig. 8. Mean score as a function of cognitive process and classification of score (upper and lower score groups) (Problem2)

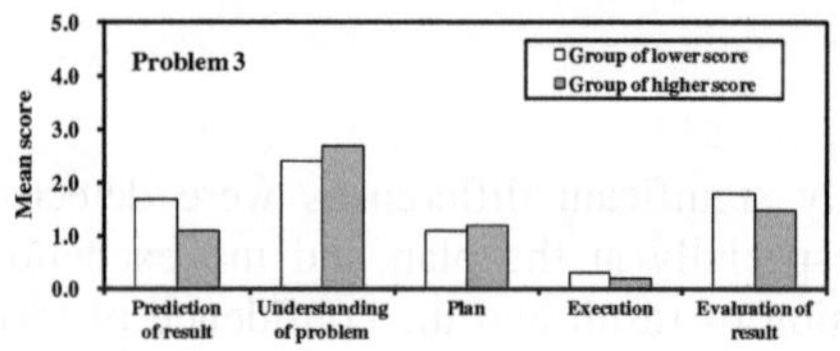

Fig. 9. Mean score of as a function of cognitive process and classification of score (upper and lower score groups) (Problem3)

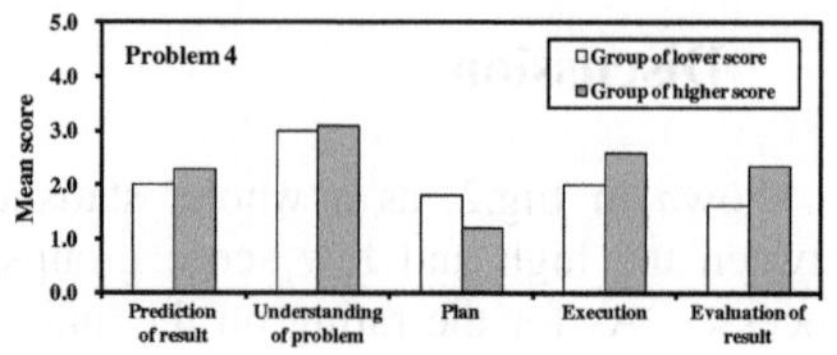

Fig. 10. Mean score as a function of cognitive process and classification of score (upper and lower score groups) (Problem4)

statistically correlated. In other words, the more proper the plan process was conducted, the more proper solution the participants reached. In such a way, the importance of metacognitive ability in the solving process, especially the plan and execution abilities, which must be accompanied by sufficient awareness and control of the cognitive process, were identified.

From the individual results shown in Figs. 3-7, similar results were observed. The higher performance group tended to be superior to the lower score group in the plan and the execution abilities.

Metacognition is one of mind works related to knowledge, monitoring, and control of own cognitive processes. It is believed that metacognition plays an important role in a variety of problem solving. In other words, successful problem solving depends on not only adequate knowledge related to the problem but also sufficient awareness and control of the cognitive process during problem solving, that is, metacognition. As the score of understanding of the problem, plan of the solution, and the execution of the solution differed between high and low test score groups, we can speculate that the difference of metacognitive function must be reflected in this difference.

In spite of mastering scientific knowledge and formula necessary for the solution, the lower performance group could not reach a higher score like higher performance group. In the range of this experiment, this must be due to the lack in metacognitive abilities, especially the plan and the control and execution abilities. Thus, the importance of meta-cognitive ability, especially the plan ability was identified in the problem solving of basic electric circuit. Future research should propose a lecturing method that enhance the metacognitive ability of students and lead to higher test performances (scores).

References

1. Flavell, J.H.: Metacognitive aspects of problem solving. In: Resnick, L. (ed.) The Nature of Intelligence, pp. 231–235. Lawrence Erlbaum Associates, NJ (1976)
2. Garofalo, J., Lester, F.K.: Metacognition, cognitive monitoring, and mathematical performance. Journal of Research in Mathematical Education 16, 163–176 (1985)
3. Paige, J.M., Simon, H.: Cognitive process in solving algebra word problem. In: Kleinmunts, B. (ed.) Problem Solving: Research, Methods, and Theory, pp. 51–119. John Wiley & Sons, NY (1966)
4. Rosenthal, D.J.A., Resnick, L.B.: Children's solution processes in arithmetic word problems. Journal of Educational Psychology 66, 817–825 (1974)
5. Lawanto, O.: The use of enhanced guided notes in an electronic circuit class: An exploratrory study. IEEE Trans. on Education 55(1), 16–21 (2012)

Evaluating the Attention Devoted to Memory Storage Using Simultaneous Measurement of the Brain Activity and Eye Movements

Akiko N. Obata , Takusige Katura, Hirokazu Atsumori, and Masashi Kiguchi

Central Research Laboratory, Hitachi, Ltd., Saitama, Japan
{akiko.obata.rg,takusige.katura.ny,hirokazu.atsumori.et, masashi.kiguchi.py}@hitachi.com

Abstract. Our study indicates that combined measures of brain activity and eye movement are useful parameters for quantifying the attention devoted to memory storage. We measured eye movements with an Eye Tracker and prefrontal cortex activity using a wearable Optical Topography in 18 participants performing a visual working memory task. We used these measures to calculate a combined index of brain activity and eye movement, which revealed that increased brain activity and higher fixation counts were related to improved task performance.

Keywords: memory, attention, eye movement, brain activity.

1 Introduction

Eye movements can indicate where others direct their gaze and focus their atten-tion, but they cannot indicate whether an item is stored into memory. Therefore, we used simultaneous measurements of brain activity and eye movement to develop an index that quantifies the attention devoted to memory storage. Our index is a useful parameter for optimizing memory-learning systems and for designing advertisements.

2 Methods

Participants. Eighteen subjects (twelve male and six female: mean age 37.2 years) participated in this study. All subjects provided informed consent after they received an explanation of the experiments.

Measurement Settings. The WOT-220 system (Hitachi) measured changes in cerebral blood volume at 22 positions (channels) in the prefrontal cortex [1]. Eye movements were measured with the TX300 eye tracker system (Tobii). WOT system had a black rubber sheet that shaded light from the eye tracker system.

Task Paradiam. Participants performed a working memory task that was similar to those used in previous studies [2]. A single task trial was performed in three periods:

C. Stephanidis (Ed.): Posters, Part I, HCII 2013, CCIS 373, pp. 447–449, 2013.

memorization, maintenance, and retrieval (Fig. 1). In the memorization period, the participants memorized four pictures that were presented simultaneously on a display for 8 s. In the maintenance period, the participants had to maintain in memory the contents and positions of the four pictures for 4 s. In the retrieval period, a colored target appeared at one of the four previous picture positions (target picture), and the participants were allowed 5 s to correctly select the corresponding picture from four pictures presented at the bottom of display. Each participant performed 20 task trials, with a 20-s rest period between each trial. During the rest period, the participants were instructed to push a keyboard button according to a left or right arrow presented on the monitor. The arrows appeared every 0.5 s with a 1-s duration. Eye movements, brain activity, reaction time, and task response were recorded for each participant. The pictures presented in the task were randomly selected from 32 pictures for each subject. The eye tracker system was calibrated for each subject prior to beginning the task.

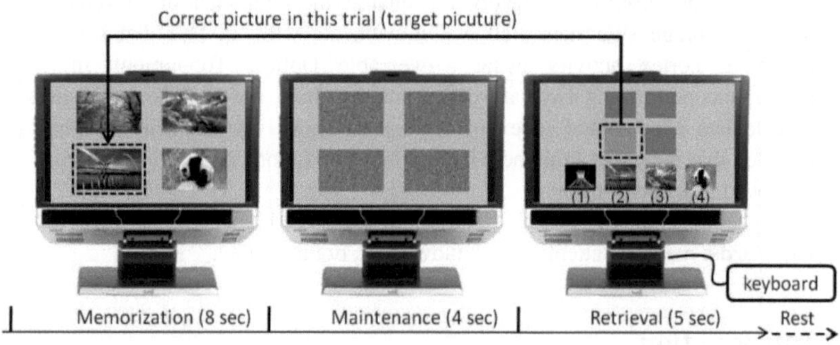

Fig. 1. Task paradigm

3 Results and Discussion

The time, duration, and locations of gaze fixations, as well as the number of fixa-tions counted (fixation count), were calculated for the target picture in the memoriza-tion period by using Tobii Studio. The fixation count was used as an index for eye movements. The WOT signals were translated into oxy- and deoxy-hemoglobin (Hb) signals by Platform for Optical Topography Analysis Tools [3]. Six channels (3 on each side) were excluded because of the noise from the analysis. We corrected the Oxy-Hb signal with a three-degree fitting, channel exception (over 0.3 mM*mm in one sampling or over 0.8 mM*mm in maximum amplitude), band pass filtering (high pass: 0.02 Hz, low pass: 0.80 Hz), and by averaging over an 18-s period that began 5 s before each task trial. We confirmed significant changes in brain activity in each participant by comparing the rest and task periods with t-tests (Fig. 2-1). The index of brain activity was determined by the average activity across the channel that showed the most significant change from the rest period.

The correct task rate was determined for each participant from the answers they provided during the task. All trials were divided into four groups on the basis of the fixation count and Hb averages. The four groups were as follows: high brain activity, high fixation number (H:brain-H:eye); high brain activity, small fixation number (H:brain-S:eye); low brain activity, large fixation number (L:brain-H:eye); and low brain activity, small number of fixation (L:brain-S:eye). Criteria for determining high or low activity or high or small numbers were based on the percentile among all trials: the upper 25% were considered high and the lower 25% were considered low or small. After the trials were categorized, we compared the correct rate among the four groups. We found that the high brain activity and the high fixation number group (H:brain-H:eye) demonstrated the highest correct rate (Fig. 2-2). This suggests that the combination of brain activity and eye movement is useful in quantifying the amount of attention devoted to memory storage, more so than eye movement or brain activity alone. Our future studies will aim to validate this combination index.

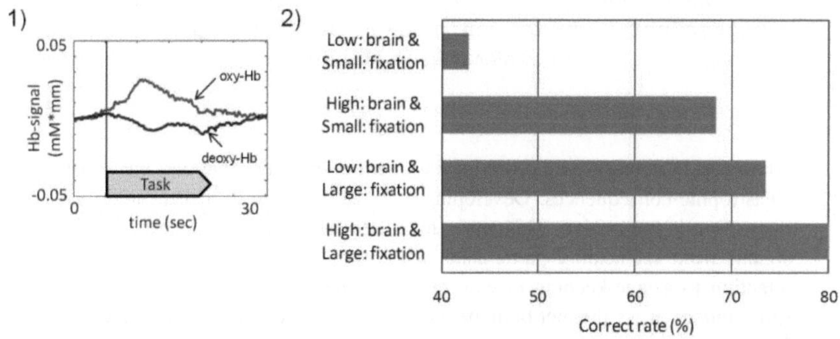

Fig. 2. Data analysis and correct rate for the four trial groups

1) Time course of Hb-signals (red:oxy-Hb, blue: deoxy-Hb).
2) Correct rate for each trial group.

4 Conclusion

We examined the relationship between brain activity and eye movements in sub-jects performing a working memory task. A high correct rate in the task was related to a combined index that revealed high brain activity and a high fixation number.

Acknowledgments. This study received generous support from Social Innovation Business Project Division, Hitachi, Ltd. and Tobii technology.

References

1. Atsumori, H., Kiguchi, M., Obata, A., Sato, H., Katura, T., Funane, T., Maki, A.: Development of wearable optical topography system for mapping the prefrontal cortex activation. Rev. Sci. Instrum. 80(4), 43704 (2009)
2. D'Esposito, M., Detre, J.A., Alsop, D.C., Shin, R.K., Atlas, S., Grossman, M.: The neural basis of the central executive system of working memory. Nature 378(6554), 279–281 (1995)
3. Platform for Optical Topography Analysis Tools (POTATOs), `http://www.hitachi.co.jp/products/ot/study/kaiseki.html`

Tracking Attention Based on EEG Spectrum

Yu-Kai Wang[1,2], Tzyy-Ping Jung[1,4], Shi-An Chen[1,3],
Chin-Sheng Huang[1,3], and Chin-Teng Lin[1,2,3]

[1] Brain Research Center, National Chioa Tung University, Hsinchu, Taiwan
[2] Department of Computer Science, National Chiao Tung University, Hsinchu, Taiwan
[3] Department of Electrical Engineering, National Chiao Tung University, Hsinchu, Taiwan
[4] Swartz Center for Computational Neruoscience, Institute for Neural Computation, University of Callifornia San Diego, San Diego, CA, USA

yukaiwang@cs.nctu.edu.tw, jung@sccn.ucsd.edu, sachen@nctu.edu.tw, chih.sheng.huang821@gmail.com, ctlin@mail.nctu.edu.tw

Abstract. Distraction while driving is a serious problem that can have many catastrophic consequences. Developing a countermeasure to detect the drivers' distraction is imperative. This study measured Electroencephalography (EEG) signals from six healthy participants while they were asked to pay their full attention to a lane-keeping driving task or a math problem-solving task. The time courses of six distinct brain networks (Frontal, Central, Parietal, Occipital, Left Motor, and Right Motor) separated by Independent Component Analysis were used to build the distraction-detection model. EEG data were segmented into 400-ms epochs. Across subjects, 80% of the EEG epochs were used to train various classifiers that were tested against the remaining 20% of the data. The classification performance based on support vector machines (SVM) with a radial basis function (RBF) kernel achieved accuracy of 84.7±2.7% or 85.8±1.3% for detecting subjects' focuses of attention to the math-solving or lane-deviation task, respectively. The high attention-detection accuracy demonstrated the feasibility of accurately detecting drivers' attention based on the brain activities. This demonstration may lead to a practical real-time distraction-detection system for improving road safety.

Keywords: Distracted Driving, Attention, Safety.

1 Introduction

Driving is a skill that requires drivers pay full attention to control cars and respond to the events on the road [1]. Distraction while driving has become a leading cause to many catastrophic motor vehicle crashes [2]. As mobile devices and automotive electronic devices such as dashboard Internet become increasingly commonplace and accessible while driving, the drivers' attention is easily shifted away from the primary driving task to others [3], causing a serious and growing threat in the daily life. Developing a countermeasure to detect the drivers' attention is imperative. This study explores the feasibility of detecting the focus of attention of a driver based on brain

C. Stephanidis (Ed.): Posters, Part I, HCII 2013, CCIS 373, pp. 450–454, 2013.

activities collected noninvasively from the scalp. The goal of this study is to develop a closed-loop system that can accurately detect driver distraction continuously and deliver warning signals to alert the driver.

2 Methods

2.1 Experiment and Subjects

Ethical concerns would prohibit exposing subjects to physical danger of distraction while driving an automobile on the road. This study thus developed a virtual-reality (VR) dynamic motion simulator as a test bed for studying the EEG dynamics associated with distraction during driving. The driving simulator includes 3D surround scenes, consisting of seven projectors projecting highway and driving scenes in 360° (see Fig. 1). Two tasks were randomly displayed on the screen in this experiment. These two tasks included a lane-keeping driving task [4] and a math problem-solving task. During the lane-keeping driving task, the car cruised with a fixed velocity of 100 km/hr on the VR-based highway scene and randomly drifted either to the left or to the right away from the cruising position with a constant velocity. Participants needed to steer the vehicle back to the center of the cruising lane as quickly as possible when they detected a drifting event. During the math problem-solving task, mathematic equations were haphazardly displayed one at a time on the screen (Fig. 2a). The participants had to validate the mathematic equations by pressing a 'right' or a 'wrong' buttons on the wheel (Fig. 2b). The allotment ratio of correct-incorrect equations was 50-50.

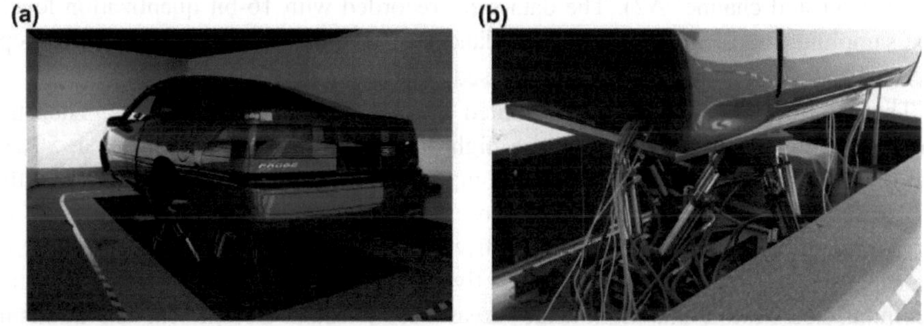

Fig. 1. A virtual-reality driving simulator consists of (a) Am immersive 360° VR-based highway and driving scenes projected from 7 LCD projectors. (b) A real car mounted on a 6-DOF dynamic Stewart motion platform, which provides the kinesthetic stimulus to the participants.

Six healthy young (20-28 years of ages; mean, 24.3) participants were recruited from National Chiao Tung University in this study, and all of them owned valid driver's licenses. Before the experiments, they were asked not to drink coffee, smoke, drink wine, or take medicine, because all of which might influence the central and

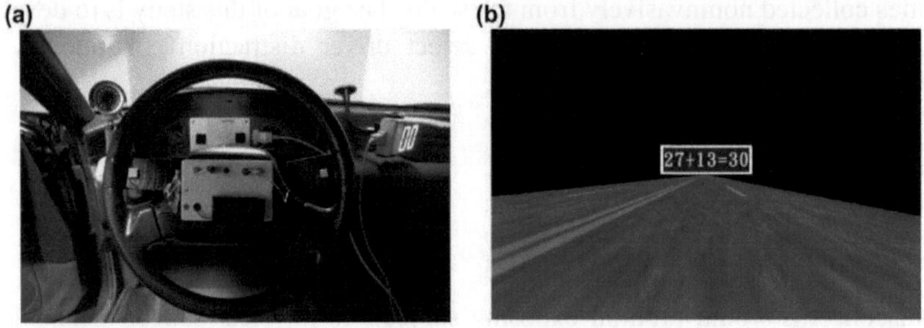

Fig. 2. The steering wheel and the tasks (a) The participants can interact with virtual driving by the steering wheel in the car. Two buttons are assembled on the both sides of the steering wheel. (b) The mathematic equation is displayed randomly at the center of the screen. The participants need to calculate it and response through the buttons on the steering wheel.

autonomic nervous system. The participants had to pay their full attention to the assigned tasks and respond as quickly as possible during the experiment. Every participant needed to finish four runs, separated by 10min rest, to complete an experiment, and each run lasted 15 minutes.

2.2 Data Processing and Feature Extraction

Continuous EEG signals were acquired by a 32-channel EEG system ((Neuroscan, Compumedics Ltd., Australia). Scalp electrodes were placed according to the modified International 10-20 system and referred to the linked mastoids (average of channel A1 and channel A2). The data were recorded with 16-bit quantization levels at a sampling rate of 500 Hz. The impedances of skin-electrode interfaces were kept below 5 kΩ through injecting a NaCl-based conductive gel.

The recording data were down-sampled into the 250 Hz sampling rate. Then the data were filtered by a low pass and a high pass filtering with frequencies at 50 Hz and 0.5 Hz, respectively. Independent Component Analysis (ICA) was applied to the pre-processed EEG data to separate source activities arising from different brain or extra-brain areas. The separated sources from each subject were selected according to the scalp maps. Six brain components activated in or near Frontal, Central, Parietal, Occipital, Left Motor, and Right Motor areas were selected. Component activations in each trial were segmented by 400 ms overlapping window, and the time latency between two segments was 50 ms, resulting in a total of 17 epochs from each 1.2-sec trial. Fast Fourier Transform (FFT) was then applied to each epoch to obtain estimated power spectra at 20 frequency bins between 1 to 20 Hz. The Wilcoxon signed-rank test (signrank, Matlab statistical toolbox, Mathworks) was used to test if the spectral difference between driving and math tasks was significant.

This study then focuses on investigating the feasibility of using EEG spectra from the driving and math tasks and machine-learning methods to detect the attention of the subjects (to the driving or problem solving). The EEG spectra of the six selected independent components were used to build the distraction-detection model. Across subjects, 80% of EEG data and their labels (driving vs math) were used to train the various classifiers which were then used to test the remaining 20 % of EEG data. It is worth noting that the training or testing data were selected on the trial basis. If one trial was the training data, all 400ms segments extracted from the trial were grouped as the training data.

3 Results

Fig. 3 shows the averaged spectra time series of six components. The spectra were calculated from the EEG data 1.2 sec after the onsets of math equation or lane deviation. The spectra were significantly different between the two tasks in all six component clusters. These results suggested the possibility of using EEG spectra to detect the focus of attention of the participants.

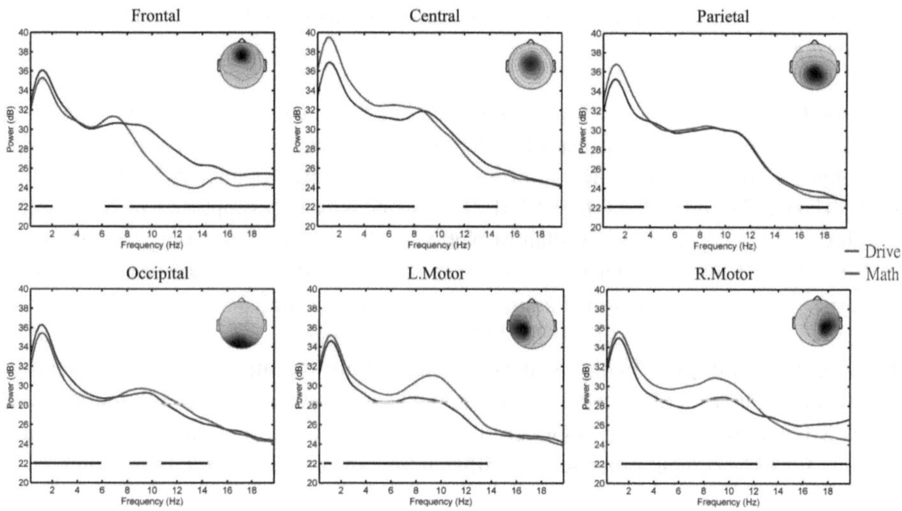

Fig. 3. The power spectra of distinct brain areas in two task conditions. The red and blue curves are the averaged spectrum related to driving and math, respectively. The black horizontal lines mark the frequency bins where spectral differences between driving and problem solving were statistically significant.

Table 1 lists the classification performance of different machine-learning classifiers across all the subjects. All results were repeated 100 times for reliability and stability. Most classifiers reached the accuracy of 80%. Particularly, support vector machines (SVM) with the radial basis function (RBF) kernel achieved accuracy of 84.7±2.7% and 85.8±1.3% for detecting subjects' focuses of attention to the problem-solving (math) or lane-deviation (driving) task, respectively.

Table 1. The accuracy of various classifiers

	LDA	NMSC	13NN	PARZEN	PERLC	DRBMC	SVM
Math	80.9±3.5	81.3±5.0	77.2±3.1	73.6±2.9	81.0±2.8	83.0±1.9	84.7±2.7
Drive	81.8±2.2	79.2±5.1	71.7±5.5	69.0±5.2	82.6±2.7	82.8±1.7	85.8±1.3

4 Conclusions and Future Work

This study demonstrated the feasibility of accurately tracking subject's attention through the noninvasively recorded brain activities. The best performance of the distraction-detection model is based on the SVM with the RBF kernel. Our future work includes testing the distraction-detection system on EEG data in a dual task, which involves shifts of attention between two different tasks, to correlate the predicted attention and task performance. Presumably, if participants were distracted from the math (or driving) task, their task performance would impair. This demonstration may lead to a practical real-time distraction-detection system for improving road safety.

Acknowledgement. This work was supported in part by the UST-UCSD International Center of Excellence in Advanced Bioengineering, which is sponsored by the Taiwan National Science Council I-RiCE Program under Grants Number NSC-101-2911-I-009-101 and NSC-101-2911-I-010-101. This work was also supported in part by the Aiming for the Top University Plan of National Chiao Tung University, the Ministry of Education, Taiwan, under Grant Number 102W963. Research was also sponsored in part by the Army Research Laboratory and was accomplished under Cooperative Agreement Number W911NF-10-2-0022. The views and the conclusions contained in this document are those of the authors and should not be interpreted as representing the official policies, either expressed or implied, of the Army Research Laboratory or the U.S Government. The U.S Government is authorized to reproduce and distribute reprints for Government purposes notwithstanding any copyright notation herein.

References

1. Carr, D.B., Ott, B.R.: The older adult driver with cognitive impair-ment. The Journal of the American Medical Association 303(16), 1632–1641 (2010)
2. Wilson, F.A., Stimpson, J.P.: Trends in fatalities from distracted driving in the United States 1999 to 2008. American Journal of Public Health 100(11), 2213–2219 (2010)
3. Jacobson, P.D., Gostin, L.O.: Reducing Distracted Driving Regulation and Education to Avert Traffic Injuries and Fatalities. The Journal of the American Medical Association 303(14), 2213–2219 (2010)
4. Huang, R.-S., Jung, T.-P., Makeig, S.: Tonic changes in EEG power spectra during simulated driving. In: Schmorrow, D.D., Estabrooke, I.V., Grootjen, M. (eds.) FAC 2009. LNCS, vol. 5638, pp. 394–403. Springer, Heidelberg (2009)

Measurement of Useful Field of View during Ocular Following Response

Kimihiro Yamanaka and Atsushi Minochi

Tokyo Metropolitan University, Tokyo, Japan
{kiyamana,minochi-atsushi}@sd.tmu.ac.jp

Abstract. There have been numerous studies related to useful field of view with regard to ensuring safety during activities and preventing recognition failures that can result in human error. As a result, the form of the useful field of view has been determined and methods for its measurement have been proposed. Most studies have assumed a fixed gaze, however, thus failing to consider the useful field of view during eye movement. The present research takes an experimental approach toward discovering the effects of eye movement speed and direction on useful field of view, limiting eye movement speed to 30°/s. As a result, the direction of gaze movement, increases in speed, and the direction of the recognized object with respect to the focal point cause variation in the narrowing of the useful field of view.

Keywords: useful field of view, eye movement, effects of binocular summation.

1 Introduction

Visual information processing is performed on information obtained from not only the center of the field of view, but also along its periphery. The range of visual information collection that can be effectively used during visual cognitive tasks is called the useful field of view (UFOV), and is an important visual characteristic for recognition of, for example, obstacles and markers [1,2]. There have been numerous studies related to UFOV with regard to ensuring safety during activities and preventing recognition failures that can result in human error. As a result, the form of UFOV has been determined and methods for its measurement have been proposed. Most studies have assumed a fixed gaze, however, thus failing to consider UFOV during eye movement [3-5]. Yet in actual working environments there are few tasks that workers perform with a fixed gaze; in most cases, necessary visual information will be collected during eye movement. It is therefore important to better understand the features of UFOV in unrestrained situations.

The present research takes an experimental approach toward discovering the effects of eye movement speed and direction on UFOV, limiting eye movement speed to 30°/s (the accepted maximal speed at which perception can occur).

C. Stephanidis (Ed.): Posters, Part I, HCII 2013, CCIS 373, pp. 455–459, 2013.

2 Experimental Outline

Fig.1 shows a diagram of the experiment and the path of the tracking markers. A participant was seated with the head secured by a chin rest (HE285, Handaya Co., Ltd.), and visual stimuli were presented via a rear projector (HD70MH700, Victor) at a point located 225 cm in front of the eyes. A program developed by us in Microsoft Visual Basic 2008 generated the visual stimuli. In the presentation, a white, circular marker with 1.25° diameter moves randomly in horizontal, vertical, and diagonal directions, and upon reaching the center of the screen a Landolt ring is randomly shown in the screen center and at the screen edge in one of three directions (horizontal, diagonal, vertical) at one of five distances (between 1.25° and 3.25°) from the center. The participant then presses arrow keys on a keyboard to indicate the direction of the center and edge Landolt rings. The tracking marker moved at one of three speeds (10, 15, or 20°/s) in one of three directions (horizontal, diagonal, or vertical). Lighting in the participant's visual area was 122.2 lx, verified according to the 5-point method in JIS C7612 (Methods for Measuring Illumination).

Ten university students aged 23.7 ± 1.1 with corrected or uncorrected vision of 0.8 or better participated in the experiment. An eye tracker (EMR-8, NAC Image Technology) monitored whether participants continued visual tracking during the experiment, and those who did not were excluded from analysis. We also simultaneously performed experiments with an unmoving focus point as a measure of UFOV with a fixed gaze.

3 Measurements of Useful Field of View

The purpose of this experiment is to measure the threshold of recognition when the response category changes from "possible to detect" to "impossible to detect" or vice versa. It is well known that the function linking the possibility of detection and the strength of the stimulus can be obtained as a psychometric curve [6]. Since the

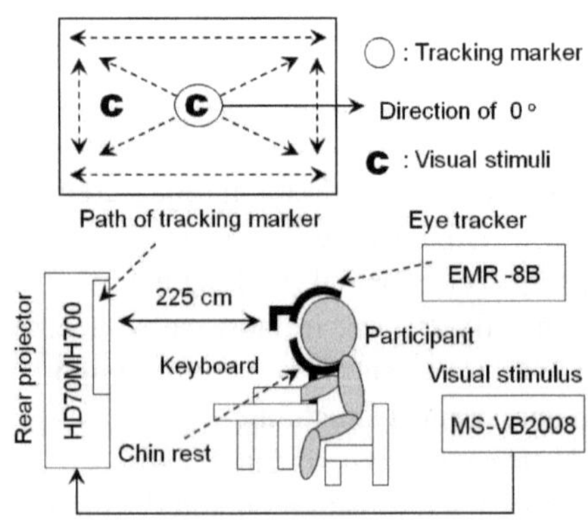

Fig. 1. Experimental setup

distance of the boundary between the "possible to detect" and "impossible to detect" categories indicates the threshold of recognition, the latter can be estimated by using a psychometric curve. Therefore, it may be possible to obtain the psychometric curves in any direction from the fixation point, and it is also known that the stimulus threshold can be obtained as a probabilistic percentile of this psychometric curve. One of the examples of this threshold with a 50% probability is the point of subjective equality (PSE), which is equivalent to the threshold of recognition. As shown in Fig.2, if we can assume that the region plotted within these stimulus thresholds is defined as UFOV, then the outer limit of the region connected with PSE for each angle is also defined as UFOV [7].

4 Experimental Results and Discussion

Table 1 shows average values for the edge of UFOV for all participants during eye movement in each direction. The results in that table show that for all directions, the range of UFOV decreases as tracking speed (eye movement speed) increases. Two-way analysis of variance with eye movement speed and direction with respect to focus point as factors reveals that as focal point movement speed increases, the visual field narrows in all directions.

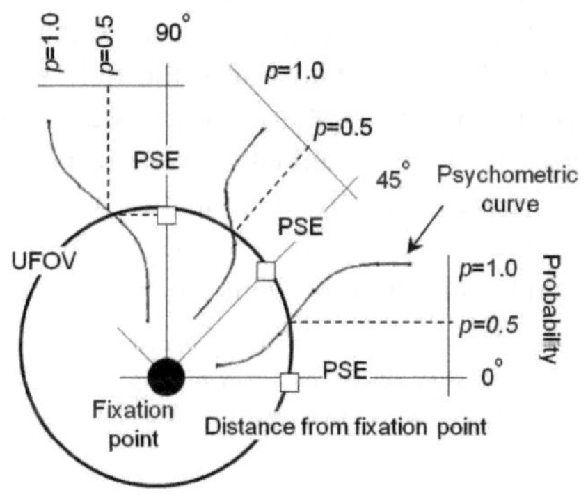

Fig. 2. Definition of UFOV

Table 1. Average values of UFOV (°)

		Horizontal eye movements			Diagonal eye movements			Vertical eye movements		
Eye movement speed (°/s)		10	15	20	10	15	20	10	15	20
Directions from fixation	Horizontal	7.74	6.23	5.44	6.77	5.94	4.43	6.46	4.75	3.75
	Diagonal	5.37	4.64	4.85	5.22	4.59	3.89	5.03	4.01	2.21
	Vertical	6.07	5.15	5.13	5.30	4.40	3.50	4.90	3.67	3.09

We next focused on the amount of narrowing of the effective visual field for each eye movement direction. Fig.3 shows eye movement speed and area of UFOV as estimated according to direction of the focus point. Fig.3(a)–(c) respectively show values during horizontal eye movement, diagonal eye movement, and vertical eye movement. The figures indicate that UFOV is reduced most during vertical eye movement, and least during horizontal eye movement, suggesting that the reduction of field of view varies with the direction of eye movement.

We next consider reasons for this remarkable narrowing during vertical eye movement. Numerous previous studies have reported that the forward field of view in humans has a greater horizontal range than vertical range. The reason for this remains unclear, but one possible explanation is the horizontal positioning of the eyes, which may broaden the range in which objects can be detected. While only one of the left or right eye detects objects near the horizontal periphery of the field of view, both eyes are involved in detection of objects near the vertical periphery. This means that detection thresholds are lower due to the effects of binocular summation. In other words, at the edge of the field of view for a single eye one can expect a higher sensitivity for object detection by both eyes in the vertical direction than in the horizontal direction. The effects of binocular summation means that functionality is increased for a pair of eyes rather than one alone, and there have been reports that when corresponding points in the retinas of both eyes are given equal stimuli the functioning of both is high, and that the functioning of both eyes decreases with increased imbalance in sensitivity between the nasal retina and the temporal retina [8,9]. This supports the idea that the expansion of the field of view may be greater in the vertical direction than in the horizontal direction due to the effects of binocular summation. In other words, for a given reduction with respect to the field of view for a single eye regardless of direction, vertical reduction of the field of view for both eyes may be more significant, because there was a larger increase in that direction due to The effect of binocular summation. This may also explain the remarkable narrowing of the field of view when the view is shifted vertically: the vertical rotational speed of the eye would increase, imparting a greater control load for eye movement than if the movement were horizontal. Verification of this hypothesis is a topic for future research.

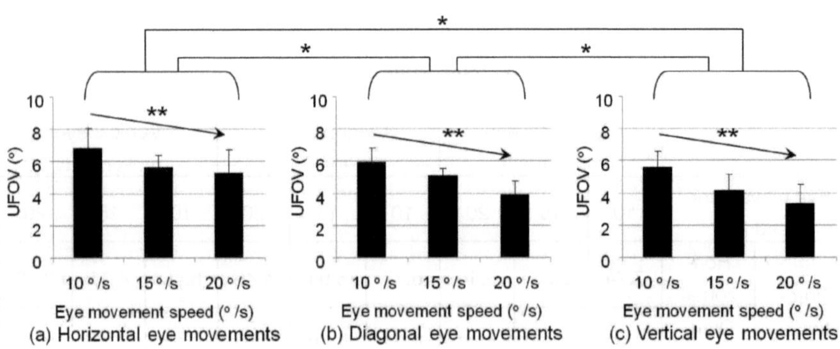

Fig. 3. Eye movement speed and area of UFOV (*:p<0.05, **:p<0.01)

5 Conclusions

In this research, experiments were conducted to investigate the effects of the speed and direction of eye movement on the effective field of view during ocular following response. Our investigation resulted in the following conclusions:

1. The direction of gaze movement, increases in speed, and the direction of the recognized object with respect to the focal point cause variation in the narrowing of the effective field of view.
2. The effect of binocular summation likely explain the phenomenon of remarkable narrowing of the field of view in the vertical direction.

References

1. Hill, F.S., Walker, S., Gao, F.: Interactive image query system using progressive transmission. Computer Graphics 17(3), 323–330 (1983)
2. Vivek, D.B.: Ergonomics in the automotive design process, pp. 105–126. Taylor & Francis Group, LLC (2012)
3. Ball, K., Owsley, C.: The useful field of view test: a new technique for evaluating are-related declines in visual function. Journal of the Optical Society of America 64(1), 71–79 (1993)
4. Owsley, C., Ball, K., Keeton, D.M.: Relationship between visual sensitivity and target localization in older adults. Vision Res. 35(4), 579–587 (1995)
5. Alan, H.S., Chan, D.K.T.: Measurement and quantification of visual lobe shape characteristics. International Journal of Industrial Ergonomics 36, 541–552 (2006)
6. Dixon, W.J., Mood, A.M., Ameri, J.: A method for obtaining and analyzing sensitivity data. Journal of American Statistical Association 43, 109–126 (1948)
7. Kimihiro, Y.: A model of human behavior based on visual information processing mechanism for reliability-based system design. Psychology and Behavioral Sciences 2(2), 20–27 (2013)
8. Pirenne, M.H.: Binocular and Uniocular Threshold of Vision. Nature 152, 698–699 (1943)
9. Wood, J.M., Collins, M.J., Carkeet, A.: Regional variation in binocular summation across the visual field. Ophthalmic & Physiological Optics 12(1), 46–51 (1992)

Part VI
Perception and Interaction

Visual Perception Modeling on Sense of Material of Object Surface

Yoshiki Aoyama[1] and Toshikazu Kato[2]

[1] Industrial and System Engineering, Graduate School of Science and Enginnering, Chuo University
cat.aoyama@gmail.com, n72001@educ.kc.chuo-u.ac.jp
[2] Industrial and System Engineering, Chuo University
kato@indsys.chuo-u.ac.jp

Abstract. Human can quickly recognize the state of object surface. This sensation is called "Sense of Material". When simulating materials with CG, the method of complex physical model is mainstream. However, this method causes large production time and cost so we propose simple material models based on human visual characteristics called "Tri-Contrast Perception Model" and "Binocular Parallax Model". The results of discriminant analysis to some material samples, we found that binocular parallax is important affect for sense of material.

Keywords: CG, Texture, Visual Characteristic.

1 Introduction

Human can quickly recognize the state of object surface such as smooth or rough. This sensation is called "Sense of Material" and it is said significant sensation to recognize outside world. When simulating materials with CG, the method of complex physical models is mainstream. However, this method is effective for only skilled person of CG drawing and causes production time and cost. We supposed human could finally perceive sense of material processing in the brain. However, the perception process of sense of material is still unknown. By simulating the process of this perception, we thought it be possible to express the state more effectively and simply. In this paper, we propose a visual model based on our hypothesis that describes sense of materials.

2 Previous Works of Sense of Materials

Human can perceive light reflection characteristics as simple information of brightness in the brain. Motoyoshi, et al said brightness is an important reason of sense of material. [1] They revealed that global feature using brightness parameter could explain glossiness and semi-transparency of object. Humans have photoreceptor

C. Stephanidis (Ed.): Posters, Part I, HCII 2013, CCIS 373, pp. 463–467, 2013.

cells that reacts prominently not only global brightness but also changes in local brightness contrast. Retinal ganglion cells (RGC) have a mechanism to properly recognize human brightness and color contrast. [2][3] When we see something, it is naturally happen. Therefore, we have developed a visual characteristic model based on local contrast perception stimulation.

3 Methods

3.1 Tri-Contrast Perception Model

As one of the models to quantify the human visual stimuli, Michelson Contrast is known. [4] This is a model that represents the amount of human stimulus received from the local brightness contrast in the image. Based on this visual stimulation model, we have developed a perceptual model of the material texture. [5]

3.2 Binocular Parallax Model

Human eyes are set part from one another; also visual images reflected several retinas are different. Human eyes have mechanism that can determine the distance to the target by adjusting the angle of convergence. [Fig.1]; therefore our brain can perceive distance and depth. [6] Human can determine whether the target is three-dimensional or not by binocular parallax. Also human can perceive state of surface, such as ruggedness, roughness and so on. Therefore, We have defined as Binocular Parallax Model to add feature vector left image to right image. (1)

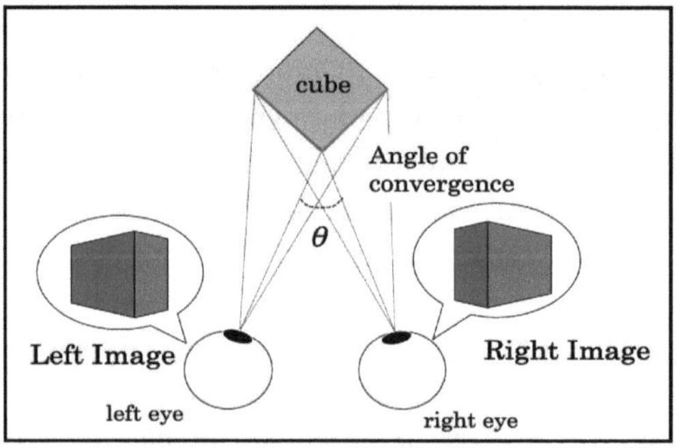

Fig. 1. Binocular Parallax

$$B.P^{(i)} = \left| f_{left}^{(i)} + f_{right}^{(i)} \right| \quad (i = 1, \ldots, n) \tag{1}$$

4 Experiment

In order to evaluate our methods, we extracted feature of texture images from eight different samples (Table 1), and verified the classification accuracy by using a liner discriminant analysis. In chapter 4.1, we explain how to convert "real" texture samples into image "data" to extract features from samples. In chapter 4.2, we show the results of the classification accuracy.

Table 1. Texture Samples

Texture Sample	Counts
Carpet	4
Felt	4
Paper File	4
Leather	4
Stone – Rugged	5
Stone – Smooth	5
Wood	5
Wool	4

4.1 Photographing Samples

To prevent avoid noises and to suppress decreasing amount of real data, we used High-Resolution Cooled CCD Camera [Fig. 2]. We put the camera away from the sample 300mm and then rotate the sample 8 degrees to left and right. Also we took three image data per 1 sample.

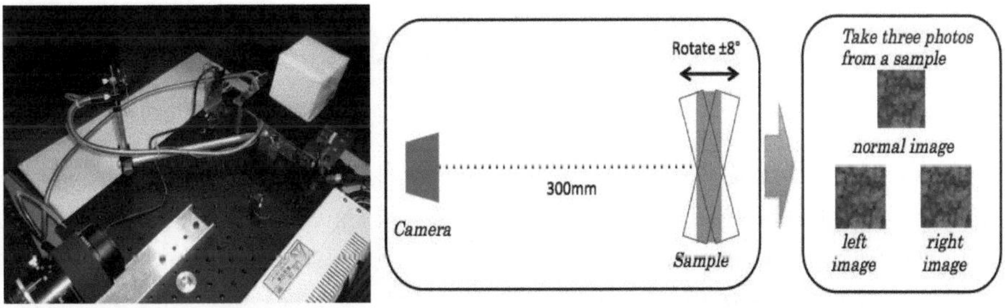

Fig. 2. High-Resolution Cooled CCD Camera & The Way of Photographing Samples

4.2 Result

The results are shown below (Fig. 3).

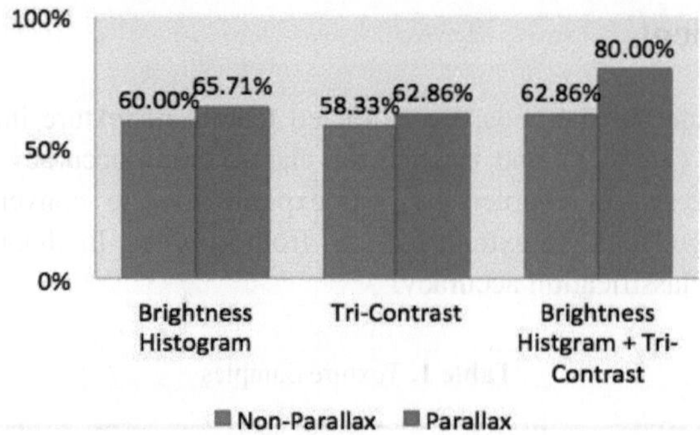

Fig. 3. Comparison of Average of Discrimination Accuracy

We found that when considering parallax, discrimination accuracy increased in all models. Among them, "Brightness Histogram and Tri-Contrast" model is the highest accuracy. As a result, binocular parallax is important affect for sense of material.

4.3 Consideration

We examined factors of discrimination to "Brightness and Tri-Contrast" model by using the random forest [7] for. We converted feature vector to five scalar values (median, mean, variance, skewness, kurtosis). As a result, we found that mean of Tri-Contrast, median of Tri-Contrast and variance of Brightness Histogram are affecting the discrimination of sense of material. (Fig.4). In other words, sense of material can be classified by intensity of the brightness contrast in the image.

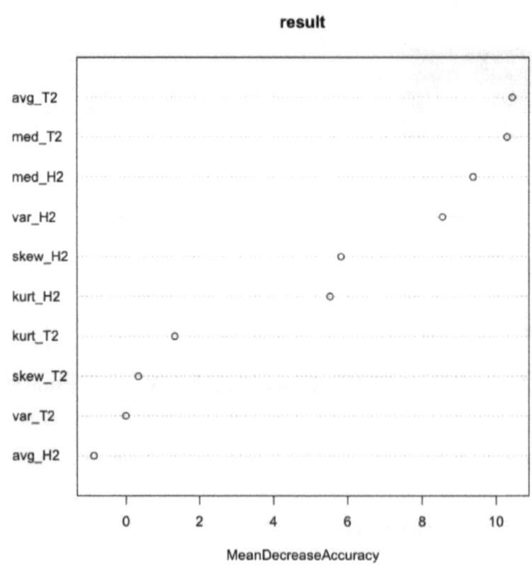

Fig. 4. Mean Decrease Accuracy

5 Prospects

In this paper, we proposed "Binocular Parallax Model" to modeling sense of material. We found binocular parallax is important for classification of sense of material. As a result of examining influence of the feature, sense of material can be classified by intensity of the brightness contrast in the image. In the other hand, we assume there are two residual problems. First, we must develop rigorous models on binocular parallax and second, we should develop a new perceptual model of intensity of the contrast.

Acknowledgements. This work was partially supported by JSPS KAKENHI grants, "Effective Modeling of Multimodal KANSEI Perception Processes and its Application to Environment Management" (No. 24650110), "Robotics modeling of diversity of multiple KANSEI and situation understanding in real space" (No. 19100004) and TISE Research Grant of Chuo University, "KANSEI Robotics Environment".

References

1. Motoyoshi, I., Nishida, S., Sharan, L., Aselson, E.H.: Image statistics and the perception of surface qualities. Nature 447 (2007)
2. Spillmann, L., Werner, L.S.: Visual Perception. Academic Press (1990)
3. Schwartz, S.H.: Visual Perception: A Clinical Orientation, 4th edn., ch. 12, pp. 271–276. McGraw-Hill (2009)
4. Ibid, ch. 7, pp. 169-173
5. Tada, M., Kato, T.: Visual Impression Modeling Using SVM for Automatic Image Classification. Knowledge Sci. Lab. 1, 872–877 (2006)
6. Schwartz, S.H.: Visual Perception: A Clinical Orientation, 4th edn., ch. 10, pp. 236–237
7. Svetnik, V., Liaw, A., Tong, C., Culberson, J.C., Sheridan, R.P., Feuston, B.P.: Random Forest: A Classification and Regression Tool for Compound Classification and QSAR Modeling. Chem. Inf. Comput. Sci., Vol 43, 1947–1958 (2003)

Eye Gaze and Mouse Cursor Relationship in a Debugging Task

Monchu Chen[1] and Veraneka Lim[1,2]

[1] Madeira Interactive Technologies Institute, Funchal, Portugal
[2] Eindhoven University of Technology, Eindhoven, The Netherlands
monchu@m-iti.org, v.lim@tue.nl

Abstract. This study evaluates the relationship between eye gaze and mouse cursor movements in a debugging task. 9 students with relevant programming experience participated in this study. Debugging difficulty was manipulated (error types; lexical, logical and syntactic) in order to measure the effects on debugging performance (accuracy and reaction time), eye gaze and mouse cursor behavior (frequency and duration of visits of target areas vs. non-target areas). Performance data showed that lexical errors are easier to find than logical errors. Mouse cursor behavior was a significant indication of the level of difficulty and therefore performance. The general pattern of mouse movements was comparable with eye gaze patterns. This study indicates that mouse data does add relevant information on top of eye gaze. These results support the idea of using mouse tracking as an alternative for inferring intentions.

Keywords: eye-hand coordination, eye tracking, mouse tracking, debugging.

1 Introduction

A trend in human-computer interaction is to link eye tracking data to underlying cognitive processes. The study of eye gaze is becoming more common in HCI research. The eye tracking technique, however, is still limited to the laboratory. This study is an attempt to infer searcher's gaze position from mouse movements to see what additive information the mouse can give us. According to Chen et al. [1], the mouse can be used as an alternative for eye tracking systems. Although, the mouse is the most widely used, it is still an issue what it can tell us relatively to eye gaze for a given task. The focus of this study is to find common patterns of eye gaze and mouse cursor behavior in a debugging task. The process of debugging is very crucial in programming, a main activity when developing new technologies. To debug, a programmer has to understand the program thoroughly and be able to troubleshoot. When developing software applications, not finding bugs in early stages can be vital, since it is expensive to fix bugs in later integration or testing phases. Several issues exist with the process of debugging. First, experts often have troubles to teach beginners how to find for bugs because of the difficulty to transfer knowledge verbally. Experts seem to recognize patterns without explicit awareness [2]. Second, more training and communication occur from a distance. Therefore, there is a need to find solutions on how to improve debugging processes.

C. Stephanidis (Ed.): Posters, Part I, HCII 2013, CCIS 373, pp. 468–472, 2013.

One way for improving debugging processes is to look at differences of debugging behavior between novices and experts as they seem to differ in 1) the focus of attention, 2) the integration of multiple sources of information and 3) the use of keyboard and mouse actions [3, 4]. Debugging behavior has also been studied using eye-tracking systems to analyze individual performance of source code review [5] or to find repetitive patterns of visual attention associated with novices [6]. The use of eye tracking metrics can contribute to several software traceability tasks [7] or help another person in doing the same task [2].Beside for being restricted to the laboratory, there are reasons to question the utility of eye tracking with alternative approaches as being more effective. In a recent study done by Bieg et al. [8], users tend to minimize pointing amplitudes with little effort by carrying out approximate pointer motions in parallel to visual search when the target is unknown or initiate movements before fixating the target when the target location is known. It also seems to be possible to predict with over 70% accuracy whether gaze position and mouse position are coordinated in search tasks such as implicit feedback, query suggestion, and click prediction [9]. Furthermore, mouse movements have the potential to provide insights into users intentions behind a web page query [10. 11].Therefore, having the ability to track mouse cursor behavior that indicates users intentions would add a great value on the debugging process, which could have implications for programming instructions. Being able to infer intentions through mouse movements will also have advantages in other areas than debugging.

2 Participants, Procedure and Method

Participants consisted of 2 female and 7 male students from the University of Madeira, with the age between 21 and 35. All participants had programming experience but only 6 were doing a Computer Science related major. Figure 1 shows a source code participants were presented with containing one of the three following error types; lexical, logical or syntactic. Each considered as different levels of difficulty. The trials were presented in random order without participants' awareness on which type of error to find. A total of 27 trials, 9 for each error type, were presented. A trial ends when participants click on a chosen target. The experiment and data analysis programs were developed in C# and Java. A Tobii T60 eye-tracker was used in this experiment. Dependent variables were debugging performance (used as baseline to compare with eye and mouse data), eye gaze behavior and mouse cursor behavior. Debugging performance was measured by accuracy and duration (in seconds) of trials. Eye gaze behavior was measured by the number of eye visits inside the target area, the average number of eye visits in other areas (8 other defined non-target areas), the duration of the gaze being inside the target area and the average duration of the gaze being inside other defined non-target areas. The same data was collected to indicate mouse cursor behavior. A target area is defined as within 30 pixels on each side of the bug.

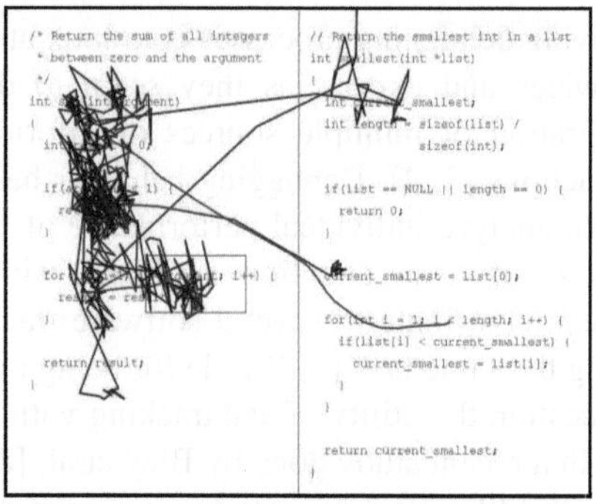

Fig. 1. The source code of one trail overlaid with eye movements (*blue*), mouse cursor traces (*red*) and a target area where the bug is (*gray rectangle*)

3 Results

3.1 Debugging Performance

To measure accuracy, a one-way repeated measure ANOVA within subject analyses was performed, showing a significant effect (F (2,240) = 9.504, p < 0.01) for error type. The Bonferroni test showed that there were significantly (p < .01) more correct answers in the lexical error type conditions (49,4%) than the logical (21,0%) and syntactic error type conditions (24,7%). These results indicate that lexical errors are the easiest to find. This same conclusion can be extracted when looking at trial duration. In the lexical error type conditions, the average duration of correct trials (M = 21,640, SE = 3,954) is much lower than the average duration of incorrect trials (M = 65,428, SE = 15,191). While for the logical and syntactic error type conditions the average duration was high for both correct and incorrect trials. This implies that when subjects are confident about their decision they tend to end the trial earlier.

3.2 Eye Gaze Behavior

For all following analyses, a 3 (error type) x 2 (accuracy) within subject repeated measures ANOVA was performed. The Bonferroni test was used to determine which, if any, of the means differed. No significant effects were found on the frequency of eye visits inside the target area or non-target areas. But there is a pattern matching performance data, as the mean frequency of eye visits during the lexical error conditions is much lower compared with the frequency of visits in the logical error type condition for correct trials. Significant main effects for correctness (F (2,240) = 30.719, p < 0.01) and interaction effects (F (2,240) = 5.710, p < 0.05) were found on the duration of the eye being inside the target area. This was significantly (p < 0.001) longer for correct trials (M = 0,167, SE = 0,022) than incorrect trials (M = 0,055, SE = 0,009). Furthermore, in lexical and logical error type conditions, the duration of the eye being inside the target area is longer for correct trials than incorrect trials

(Lexical, M = 0,210, SE = 0,037 vs. M = 0,029, SE = 0,004; Logical, M = 0,192, SE = 0,042 vs. M = 0,059, SE = 0,006). While for the syntactic error type conditions, duration seem to be comparable (M = 0,099, SE = 0,013 vs. M = 0,077, SE = 0,021). No significant main or interaction effects were found on the average duration of the eye being inside other defined non-target areas. These results implies that debugging performance cannot be extracted by looking at eye gaze duration spend in target vs. non-target areas.

3.3 Mouse Cursor Behavior

Significant main effects were found for error type ($F(2,240) = 4.455$, $p < 0.05$) and correctness ($F(2,240) = 15.557$, $p < 0.01$) on the frequency of mouse visits inside the target area. The mouse visited the target area more often in the logical error type conditions (M = 1,948, SE = 0,389) than the lexical error type conditions (M = 1,076, SE = 0,161). The mouse also visited the target area more often ($p < 0.01$) in correct trials (M = 2,033, SE = 0,288) than incorrect trials (M = 0,989, SE = 0,288). No significant main or interaction effects were found on the average frequency of mouse visits inside other defined non-target areas. These results supports performance data as the mean frequency of mouse visits during the lexical error conditions is much lower compared with the frequency of visits in the logical error type condition for correct trials. When the task is harder, in this case during the logical error type conditions, subjects visits the target area more often indicating that they are less confident. A significant main effect was found for correctness ($F(2,240) = 36.326$, $p < 0.01$) on the duration of the mouse being inside the target area. The duration was significantly ($p = < 0.001$) longer for correct trials (M = 0,198, SE = 0,024) than incorrect trials (M = 0,027, SE = 0,010). No effects were found on the average duration of the mouse being inside other defined non-target areas. These results show the same pattern as duration of eye gaze visits.

4 General Discussion and Conclusion

The aim of this study was to evaluate the relationship between eye gaze and mouse cursor movements and the additive value of mouse information to eye gaze for indicating users intentions in a debugging task. This is a step towards inferring visual attention and intentions from mouse cursor movements, which could have implications on the way we measure attention when eye tracking is not available. In this study, debugging performance was evaluated across 3 types of errors with different difficulty levels. The results for debugging performance indicated the lexical errors as easiest to find and was used as a baseline to compare with eye gaze and mouse data. In general there were no findings of eye gaze data supporting debugging performance. An explanation is because eye movements is a bottom up process while hand movements are top down processes; people control gaze movements proactively to gather visual information for guiding hand movements. Therefore, hand movements could give better information on people's real intentions [12]. This explains the findings of the current study regarding the frequency of mouse visits. Based on the collected data, the overall pattern of mouse cursor behavior for both the frequency of visits and duration of visits in target areas seem to be highly related with eye gaze behavior. This supports earlier findings [9].This study indicates that mouse data does add relevant information on top of eye gaze. These results support the idea of using mouse tracking as an alternative for inferring intentions. As a result, we argue that a mouse tracker with some cognitive inference engine built in any Integrated Development Environment could potentially enhance debugging experiences.

References

1. Chen, M., Anderson, J.R., Sohn, M.: What can a mouse cursor tell us more? Correlation of eye/mouse movements on Web browsing. In: Proceedings of CHI Extended Abstracts, USA (2001)
2. Stein, R., Brennan, S.E.: Another Person's Eye Gaze as a Cue in Solving Programming Problems. In: Proceedings of the 6th International Conference on Multimodal Interfaces, PA, USA (2004)
3. Romero, P., du Boulay, B., Cox, R., Lutz, R., Bryant, S.: Dynamic Rich-data Capture and Analyses of Debugging Processes. Proceedings of Psychology of Programming Interest Group 16, 140–150 (2004)
4. Romero, P., du Boulay, B., Cox, R., Lutz, R., Bryant, S.: Graphical Visualizations and Debugging: A Detailed Process Analyses. Proceedings of Psychology of Programming Interest Group 17, 62–76 (2005)
5. Uwano, H., Nakamura, M., Monden, A., Matsumoto, K.: Analyzing Individual Performance of Source Code Review using Reviewers Eye Movements. In: Proceedings of the Eye Tracking Research and Application Symposium, USA, March 27-29 (2005)
6. Bednarik, R., Tukiainen, M.: Temporal Eye-Tracking data; Evolution of Debugging Strategies with Multiple Representations. In: Proceedings of the Eye Tracking Research and Application Symposium, USA, March 26-28, pp. 99–102 (2008)
7. Sharif, B., Kagdi, K.: On The Use of Eye Tracking in Software Traceability. In: Proceedings of Traceability of Emerging Forms of Software Engineering, Hawaii, USA, pp. 67–70 (2011)
8. Bieg, H.J., Reiterer, H., Bülthoff, H.H.: Eye and Pointer Coordination in Search and Selection Tasks. In: Proceedings of the Eye Tracking Research and Application Symposium (2011)
9. Guo, Q., Agichtein, E.: Towards Predicting Web Searchers Gaze Position from Mouse Movements. In: Proceedings of CHI, USA, April 10-15 (2010)
10. Guo, Q., Agichtein, E.: Exploring Mouse Movements for Inferring Query Intent. In: SIGIR, Singapore, July 20-24 (2008)
11. Atterer, R., Wnuk, M., Schmidt, A.: Knowing the User's Every Move; User's Activity Tracking for Website Usability Evaluation and Implicit Interaction. In: The International WWW Conference Committee, Scotland, May 23-26 (2006)
12. Magnussen, J.S.: Moving hands reveal dynamics of thoughts. The Proceedings of National Academy of Sciences 102, 9995–9996 (2005)

Adaptive Control Elements for Navigation Systems

Benedikt Janny, Johann Winterholler, Aleko Petrov, and Thomas Maier

Institute for Engineering Design and Industrial Design
Research and Teaching Department Industrial Design Engineering
University of Stuttgart, Pfaffenwaldring 9, 70569 Stuttgart, Germany
{benedikt.janny,johann.winterholler,aleko.petrov,
thomas.maier}@iktd.uni-stuttgart.de

Abstract. An innovative navigation interface with haptic support is developed based on the idea of multimodal interaction and adaptive control elements. Thereby, for people with visual impairments interaction with the interface, e.g. indication of directions is facilitated and haptic distinction between different menus is made possible. Due to the additional haptic feedback a safe and efficient transmission of information can be ensured during use. Apart from that the use of adaptive control elements partly compensates for the lack of information based on the impaired visual channel and enables the user to experience a more immersive way of interaction.

Keywords: control elements, adaptive control elements, navigation interface, visually impaired people, user centered interface design, multimodal interaction.

1 Motivation

To improve the life of people with visual impairments a continuous development of assistive technology is essential to facilitate the mobility. Since most navigation systems only use auditory output there is a high chance that information is not being perceived properly, e.g., because of ambient noise. By adding an additional haptic output a safe and efficient interaction can be ensured.

The present paper presents the development of a navigation interface with additional haptic support. This idea was realized during the research project "Hard- and Software Interface development of map-based haptic orientation and navigation systems for people with visual impairments". The project is carried out by the University of Stuttgart in cooperation with the industrial partner Handy Tech Elektronik GmbH and funded by the German Federal Ministry of Economics and Technology. The University of Stuttgart is represented by the Institute for Visualization and Interactive Systems (VIS) and the Institute for Engineering Design and Industrial Design (IKTD), Research and Teaching Department Industrial Design Engineering. IKTD which is mainly in charge of the interface focuses on the development of ergonomic devices. VIS realizes the software of the system.

C. Stephanidis (Ed.): Posters, Part I, HCII 2013, CCIS 373, pp. 473–477, 2013.

2 State of Technology and Research

Navigation systems which help people with visual impairments have been commercialized for about four years. At this point nearly all commercialized stand-alone GPS navigation systems just use acoustic output.

This shows that there is potential for improvement. Therefore, the concept of multimodal interaction can be chosen as a basic approach to improve the usability of navigation systems. Schomaker et al. [1] define an interaction as multimodal if it is "restricted to those interactions which comprise more than one modality on either the input (perception) or the output (reaction) side". According to [2] the user's capacity of perception is enhanced through the distribution of data via multiple modalities. People with visual impairments can use two modalities (auditory and haptic). Since auditory information like a sound can be easily disturbed by ambient noise during navigation there is a high chance that information is not being perceived properly by the user. By using the somatosensory modality as an additional source of input a safe and efficient transmission of information is ensured.

An additional haptic user input for the interface of a navigation system can be made possible by the basic approach of adaptive control elements. Adaptive control elements are characterized by their ability to vary and adapt their gestalt (structure, shape) depending on the context of the human machine interaction [3]. As a consequence the user is being relieved in situations of complex information input.

3 Method

3.1 Conceptual Design

To develop the conceptual interface design, a set of essential menu functions were derived from different user questionings. Twelve control elements were defined for an ergonomic handling of the device. According to [4] control elements can be arranged based on the anticipated rate of use. Therefore those control elements were divided into a key field with three main areas, a primary, a secondary and a tertiary area. The nine keys of the primary area are expected to be used frequently and situated in direct space of reach. The two keys of the secondary area will be used less and are placed above the primary area. The last key is expected to be used least frequently and therefore located in the tertiary area. The idea of adaptive control elements was realized by two types of additional retractable and liftable tangible elements, bridge and navigation elements, permitting additional haptic information encoding. Figure 1 illustrates the final arrangement of the twelve control elements according to their absolute rate of use including the adaptive control elements.

Four movable bridge elements vary the interface gestalt of the key field and thus facilitate haptic distinction between different menus such as input / setup mode or navigation mode. By lifting all four bridge elements the key field transforms into a cross gestalt intuitively being associated with the four cardinal directions. At the same time it indicates the user that he is in navigation mode. While entering a particular destination a homogenous key field is desirable being achieved by lowering the bridge elements.

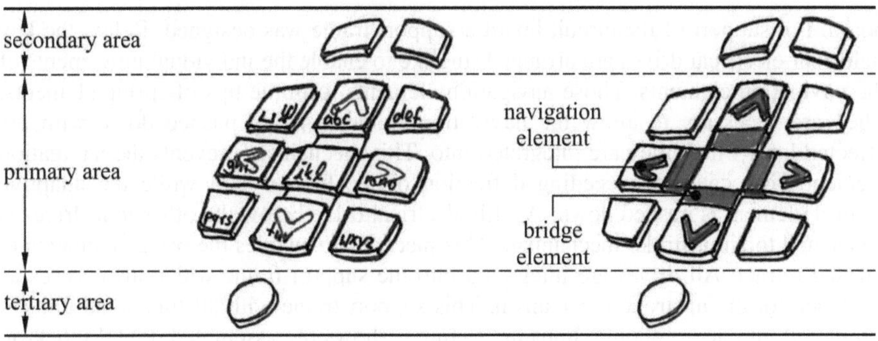

Fig. 1. Conceptual design of the interface

Four movable tangible navigation elements provide a haptic support during navigation mode. Depending on the element being lifted the aspired direction is indicated. By varying the frequency with which the elements are lifted and retracted, the distance toward the next change of direction is encoded continuously. The higher the frequency the closer the user is to the aspired waypoint.

3.2 Haptic Specifications

To develop an ergonomic device a centripetal user centered design approach is suggested. In this case the design is based on the haptic requirements of the human hand, so that the tangible feedback is well received. Especially important for proper haptic perception is the tangible height of elements which leads to deflection of the human skin during contact. According to Kaczmarek [5], the absolute threshold of haptic perception due to deflection of human skin of the fingertip is 10 µm (3.93×10^{-4} in). For the design of haptic devices Kern [6] suggests a maximum height of 1 mm (3.93×10^{-2} in). Apart from requirements concerning the haptic perception of the human skin a basic understanding of the exerted finger forces is essential for the choice of adequate drive elements. In this context measurements published in standard DIN 33411 [7] state axial forces being exerted from the index finger of 7 N maximum. Those key specifications provide a basis for the dimensions of the tangible elements.

4 Design of the Device

To enable both, the bridge and navigation elements being lifted and retracted drive elements are necessary. While all four bridge elements must be connected in parallel since they either all lift or retract together, the drive unit must enable the navigation elements to lift and retract individually. A set of electrical drives was chosen considering the necessary holding forces and lifting range. The drives must have sufficient power so that the adaptive elements remain lifted during haptic exploration by the user. The key field consisting of button caps and switches is placed on a circuit board. For support of the circuit board a support frame was designed. Below the key field four electrical drives are arranged ringlike to enable the individual movements of the navigation elements. Those navigation elements form the tips of spring elements. They are necessary to allow the navigation elements being pushed down with the affected keys which they are integrated into. This mechanism prevents the navigation element from causing exceeding deflection of the human skin while the adaptive control element is pushed down. A fifth electrical drive below the other four drives is connected to an upstroke mechanism. This mechanism enables the bridge elements to lift and retract. All drives are integrated into the support frame which also serves as guidance for the upstroke mechanism. This support frame with all functional units is integrated into an ergonomic housing. Figure 2 shows the assembled digital mock-up with the adaptively variable key field and the housing.

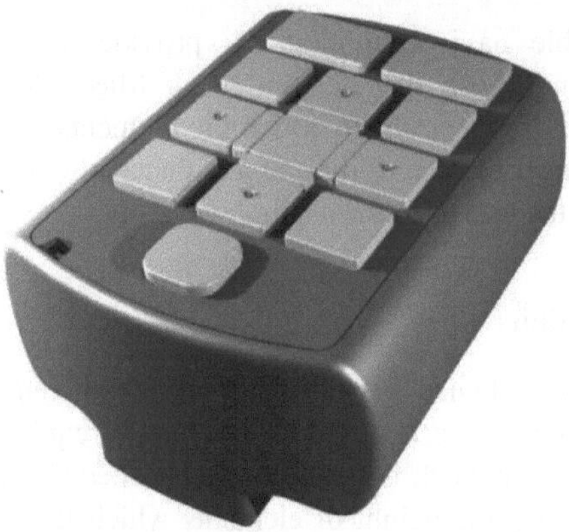

Fig. 2. Perspective view of assembled digital mock-up

5 Conclusion

An innovative navigation interface with haptic support is developed based on the idea of multimodal interaction and adaptive control elements. Thereby, for people with visual impairments interaction with the interface is facilitated and haptic distinction between different menus is made possible. Due to the additional haptic feedback a safe and efficient transmission of information can be ensured during use. Apart from that the use of adaptive control elements partly compensates for the lack of information based on the impaired visual channel. This leads to an enormous improvement of the device's usability and introduces a new kind of haptic esthetics in assistive technology. This navigation interface can be used both, for outdoor and indoor navigation even though the basic approach of adaptive control elements is not only restricted to navigation systems. It can also be adapted to other types of assistive technology.

Acknowledgements. This project is supported by the German Federal Ministry of Economics and Technology on the basis of a decision by the German Bundestag.

References

1. Schomaker, L., Nijtmans, J., Camurri, A., Lavagetto, F., Morasso, P., Benoit, C., Guiard-Marigny, T., Le Goff, B., Robert-Ribes, J., Adjoudani, A., Defée, I., Münch, S., Hartung, K., Blauert, J.: A Taxonomy of Multimodal Interaction in the Human Information Processing System. A Report of the Esprit Project 8579 MIAMI, NICI, Nijmegen (1995)
2. Schmid, M., Petrov, A., Maier, T.: HMI with Adaptive Control Elements. ATZautotechnology 8 (2008)
3. Petrov, A.: Usability-Optimierung durch adaptive Bediensysteme. Universität Stuttgart, Institut für Konstruktionstechnik und Technisches Design, Forschungs- und Lehrgebiet Technisches Design, Dissertation (2012) (in German)
4. Schmidtke, H.: Handbuch der Ergonomie. Band 4, 2 überarbeitete und erweiterte Auflage. Bundesamt für Wehrtechnik und Beschaffung, Koblenz (1989) (in German)
5. Kaczmarek, K.A., Bach-Y-Rita, P.: Tactile Displays. In: Barfield and Furness: Virtual Environments and Advanced Interface Techniques. Oxford University Press, New York (1995)
6. Kern, T.: Entwicklung Haptischer Geräte - Ein Einstieg für Ingenieur. Springer, Berlin (2009) (in German)
7. Standard DIN 33411: Körperkräfte des Menschen; Maximale statische Aktionskräfte – Teil 4 (1987) (in German)

Differences between a Young and Older Computer Users' Recognition Rate of Tactons

Ricardo Jimenez

Barry University, Math and Computer Science Department, Miami Shores, Fl. USA
rjimenez@mail.barry.edu

Abstract. Effective tacton parameters of stimuli have been identified for a young population of computer users. However, studies have shown that the detection of vibrations degrades as a natural part of the aging process. This work used stimulus parameters similar to those which have been shown to be effective in a young population, and conducted a comparison study between 40 test subjects composed of a young population of computer users between 18 and 25 years old and an older population of computer users between 55 and 75 years old. The study compared both groups' recognition rates of modulated sinusoidal waveforms and found that the older group had a significant decrease in recognition rates of modulated sinusoidal waveforms.

Keywords: Tactons, vibrotactile devices, older computer users.

1 Introduction

There is an increasing amount of research that centers on vibrotactile devices that produce vibrotactile cues known as tactons. Tactons rely on cutaneous sensation as a haptic form of output that can be used as an additional modality in Human- Computer Interaction (HCI) [1]. Tactons and vibrotactile devices can have wide-ranging potential in HCI in areas like gaming, virtual reality, navigational aids, and mobile devices. Tactons are of particular usefulness for older populations. A few examples include: supplementing visual displays, which naturally lends itself to enhancing HCI for older adult users with vision impairment. Tactons can potentially be used in multimodal design to reduce cognitive overload and as an additional sensory stimuli. Older populations are known to have additional challenges with sensory degradation and cognitive overload and thus including tactons as part of a multimodal interface could potentially be of benefit to this population [2]. The tacton works in conjunction with a vibrotactile device, which is placed on the body and mechanically produces sensations on the skin surface; these sensations can then be associated with computer functions. Defining tacton stimuli parameters and data structures as well as determining tacton recognition rates and detection thresholds, is an ongoing pursuit [5].

Studies have shown that declines can be seen in vibrotactile thresholds as well as vibrotactile recognition and discrimination with advancing age [4]. Indeed, persons over the age of 55 years old have significantly higher detection thresholds of

C. Stephanidis (Ed.): Posters, Part I, HCII 2013, CCIS 373, pp. 478–482, 2013.

sinusoidal waveforms than younger groups. In their studies, both Stuart et al. [9] and Goble et al. [7] found statistically significant differences of approximately 10 dB in actuator displacement from 10 to 400 Hz of detection thresholds of sinusoidal waveforms, between a young group under the age of 40 years old and an older group between the ages of 55 and 90 years old.

Hoggan & Brewster [8] and Brown, et al., [3] found modulated sinusodial waveforms to be effective parameters of stimuli using a C2 Tactor from EAI systems. These results were based on a young population under the age of 40 years old. Since various studies indicate that older adults over the age of 55 years old have significantly higher detection thresholds, tacton parameters that incorporate modulated sinusoidal waveforms should be tested for their effectiveness in an older population.

A comparison study was conducted between young- (18 to 25 years old) and older- (55 to 75 years old) adult computer users, using the C2 Tactor. This study used similar parameters established by Hoggan and Brewster [8] and Brown et al. [3] that used modulated sinusoidal waveforms. These parameters had recognition rates of 61% [8] and 80% [3] in a young population under the age of 40 years old.

2 Methodology

A total of 40 participants, 20 males and 20 females participated in this study. The participants belonged to one of two groups: young group (18-25) years of age and older group (55-75) years of age. There were 9 males and 11 females in the young group and 11 males and 9 females in the older group. The age of the young group was (M=22.8, SD=2.197), while the older group was (M=63.2, SD=6.725).

Participants were screened through a questionnaire to determine age and dominant hand. In addition, there were several exclusion criteria based on factors which affect vibrotactile sensation. These included: recent use of vibrating equipment, medications, and any relevant medical history. This study used the C2 Tactor vibrotactile device. The input signal to the C2 Tactor was generated by an Intel High Definition Audio sound card on a Windows based personal computer. A Crown D-75 linear amplifier was used to drive the output. The experimental interface and data collection was done on a Windows based personal computer. The signals were analyzed using a Tektronix TDS 310 oscilloscope to verify the generated parameters and output levels.

The experimental interfaces were GUI Java programs to generate the tactons, capture user responses, and write to a sequential file.

3 Experimental Protocol and Parameters

Three separate tactons consisting of three, two-second intervals of 1000 ms sinusoidal wave burst of 250 Hz, a sinusoidal wave burst of 250 Hz modulated by a sinusoidal wave of 30 Hz, and a sinusoidal wave burst of 250 Hz modulated by a sinusoidal wave of 70 Hz were generated. The modulated sinusoidal wave parameters of stimuli were similar to those used by Hoggan and Brewster [8]. The modulated sinusoidal waves were generated using Daqarta software and were produced by multiplying the base sinusoidal waveform of 250 Hz with the modulating waveform.

The baseline output amplitude for experiment 2 was determined based on an exaggerated value of threshold detection, which was done on the experimenter (49 years of age) to ensure that stimulus was felt by both experimental groups, this output was ~500 mVpp.

The chosen location for the C2 vibrotactile device was on the non-hairy portion of the volar forearm of the non-dominant hand, 5 cm from the wrist, and it was attached via a loose fitting Velcro strap. The Velcro strap was placed on the end of the wire and not the C2 Tactor itself, thus only the mass of the C2 Tactor rests on the subject's skin. This ensures uniformity of pressure for all participants as well as avoids any damping effect that woul d occur if additional pressure is applied to the C2 Tactor itself. The subject used the dominant hand to manipulate the mouse and to make selections on the experimental interface. In addition, to provide audible masking, the participants were required to wear headphones; pink noise was generated to ensure that no sound, which may have emanated from the C2 Tactor, was heard.

An initial orientation and training period was conducted, before each experiment. During this training, the participants familiarized themselves with the interface and the vibration stimuli. These are a sinusoidal wave of 250 Hz that represents an incoming "voicemail", a sinusoidal wave of 250 Hz modulated by a sinusoidal wave of 30 Hz that represents an incoming "text message", and a sinusoidal wave of 250 Hz modulated by a sinusoidal wave of 70 Hz that represents an incoming "email". When the test subject felt they could effectively discriminate each tacton the experiment began. A maximum of 30 minutes was allowed for training.

The computer testing interface presented the test subject with one of three random generated tacton cues. The subject was asked to respond which message they were receiving by selecting the appropriate response on the computer-testing interface. Test subjects were allowed only one attempt to identify a particular tacton and were asked to identify a total of 30 random generated tactons, 10 of each type.

4 Results

The level of significance for statistical tests was set at 5% ($\alpha = 0.05$). qqnorm analysis showed all data collected had normal to near normal distribution. Fisher's exact test was performed to determine if there are nonrandom associations between the test results of the two groups.

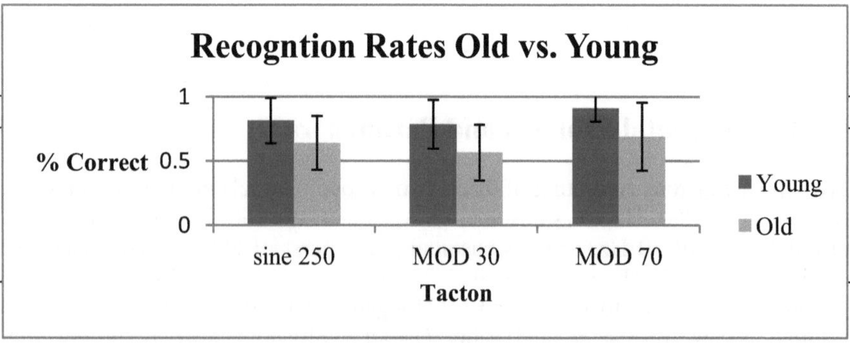

Fig. 1. Tacton recognition rates of both groups

Each waveform recognition rate was analyzed and the results are shown in table1 and figure1.

Table 1. Recognition rate results of both groups

Recognition rates		
P<=.001	**Young**	**Old**
Sinusoidal 250 Hz	**M=82%, SD=.1756**	**M=64%, SD=.2113**
MOD 30	**M=79%, SD=.1899**	**M=57%, SD=.2183**
MOD 70	**M=91%, SD=.1021**	**M=69%, SD=.2654**
Overall	**M=83%, SD=.1668**	**M=63%, SD=.2346**

5 Conclusion and Future Work

This study shows that the overall recognition rates of the younger group were consistent with those findings by

Brown et al. [3], which showed an overall recognition rate of 80%. This study confirms the findings of Brown et al. [3] that modulated waveforms with a base of 250 Hz, can serve as an effective tacton parameter in young populations. In addition, it shows that recognition rates of the same parameters are significantly lower in older adults over the age of 55 years old. The study shows that there is a statistical significance between increasing age and decreasing tacton recognition rate.

Studies have shown that persons over the age of 55 years old have significantly higher detection threshold of sinusoidal waveforms at the upper frequency range than younger groups [9]. It is also known that Pacinian receptors degrade the most with age; these receptors respond to higher frequencies, as the ones used in this study. The differences in tacton recognition rates may be a function of decreased detection thresholds at these upper frequencies.

There are also indications that non-Pacinian receptors degrade less with aging than Pacinian receptors [7], [6]. Therefore frequencies associated with these non-Pacinian receptors, those below 40 Hz may be better suited to produce more equitable results in tacton recognition and discrimination between the two groups. Furthermore, modulated waveforms may not be suitable in achieving more parity between the two groups, particularly at lower frequencies where they may be less flexible to generate and may have less effectiveness.

More studies are needed to see how effective tactons can be at this lower frequency range (10-40 Hz). If these studies show more equitable results, then tacton designers might focus on developing parameters which are most effect at these lower frequencies, and even though they are not at the optimal frequency for detection in younger groups, they may serve as a more universal parameter for detection and recognition across all age groups.

References

1. Brewster, S.A., Brown, L.M.: Tactons: Structured tactile Messages for non-visual information display. In: AUIC 2004: Proceedings of the Fifth Conference on Australasian User Interface, vol. 28, pp. 15–23. Australian Computer Society, Darlinghurst (2004)
2. Brewster, S.A., King, A.: An Investigation into the use of tactons to present progress information. Proceedings of Interact 2005 35(85), 6–17 (2005)
3. Brown, L.A., Brewster, S.A., Purchase, H.C.: A first investigation into the effectiveness of tactons. In: WHC 2005 Proceedings of the First Joint Eurohaptics Conference and Symposium on Haptic Interfaces for Virtual Environment and Teleoperator Systems, pp. 167–176. IEEE Computer Society, Washington (2005)
4. Cholewiak, R.W., Collins, A.A.: Vibrotactile localization on the arm: Effects of place, space, and age. Attention, Perception & Psychophysics 7(65), 1058–1077 (2003)
5. Craig, J.C., Rhodes, R.P., Busey, T.A., Kewley-Port, D., Humes, L.E.: Aging and tactile temporal order attention. Attention, Perception & Psychophysics 72(1), 226–235 (2010)
6. Gescheider, G.A., Valetutti, A.A., Verillo, R.T.: Vibrotactile forward masking as a function of age. Journal of Acoustical Society of Amercia 91(3), 1690–1696 (1992)
7. Goble, A.K., Collins, A.A., Cholewiak, W.: Vibrotactile threshold in young and old observers: The effects of spatial summation and the presence of a rigid surround. Journal of Acoustical Society of America 99(4), 2256–2269 (1996)
8. Hoggan, E., Brewster, S.: New parameters for tacton design. In: Proceedings of the SIGCHI 2007 Conference on Human Factors in Computing Systems, pp. 2417–2422. ACM, New York (2007)
9. Stuart, M., Turman, B.A., Shaw, J., Walsh, N., Nguyen, V.: Effects of aging on vibration detection thresholds at various body regions. BMC Geriatrics 3(1), 1–10 (2003)

Interactive Color Perspective for 3D Graphics Applications: Enhancing Depth Perception and the Understanding of Object Relations

Dietrich Kammer, Jan Wojdziak, and Rainer Groh

Technische Universität Dresden
Faculty of Computer Science, Chair of Media Design
{dietrich.kammer,jan.wojdziak}@tu-dresden.de

Abstract. Perceiving depth and spatial relations between objects in virtual environments is challenging and can be facilitated by the rendering process in 3D graphics applications. Often the perspective projection is not sufficient to visualize all necessary information because the projected image can lead to position and orientation ambiguity. Therefore, additional indicators are needed to improve the visualization of information about spatial relationships and the structure of the scene. For this purpose, we introduce a toolbox that applies color as an interactive design tool. Within this toolbox, six algorithms can be used to dynamically modulate the coloring of single objects or the scene as a whole. For evaluation, we report a study that tested whether object coloring as implemented in the toolbox can change apparent depth.

Keywords: Painting-like rendering, Non-Photorealistic Rendering, Drawing, Real-time Graphics.

1 Introduction

In computer graphics, perspective projection is used to determine spatial depth and the relations between objects, with the goal of providing a correct and natural representation of a scene. However, this projection has considerable shortcomings with regard to its visual appearance. In contrast, in the visual arts there is more to images than projection rules alone: beginning in the Renaissance, artists have developed various techniques to solve the problems associated with projecting a three-dimensional scene onto a two-dimensional surface. However, in order to communicate complex information effectively, other forms of visual abstraction are required. They should assist the viewer in directly perceiving which objects are relevant in the current context and in what relation they stand to other objects in the scene. As an overall goal, images need to be self-explanatory. A central technique is the manipulation of coloring to improve the quality of visualizations by creating depth in an image or directing the viewer to an area of interest. This paper proposes six algorithms that affect the coloring of objects based on the scene configuration and user interaction.

C. Stephanidis (Ed.): Posters, Part I, HCII 2013, CCIS 373, pp. 483–487, 2013.

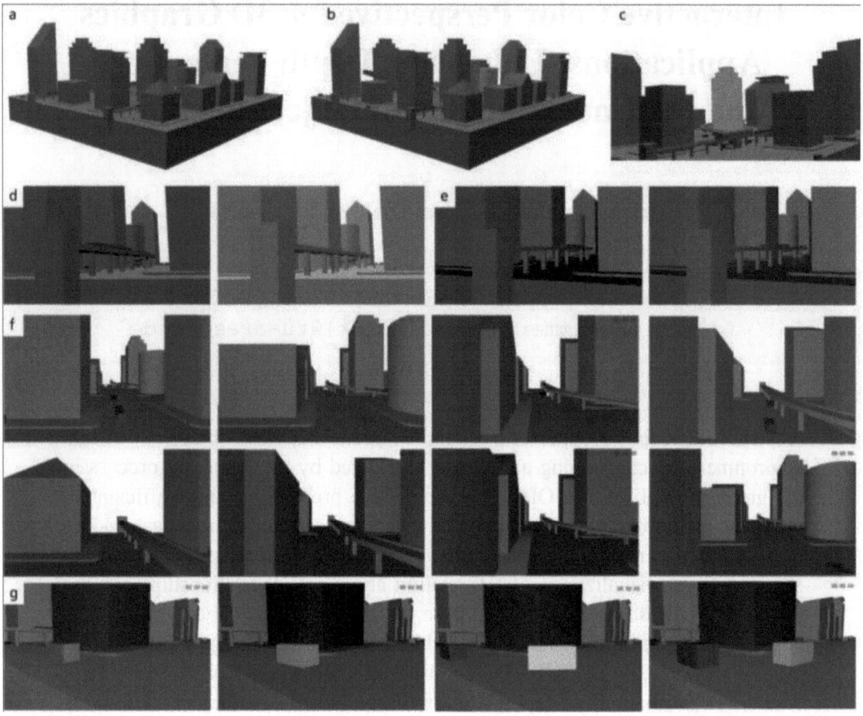

Fig. 1. Visualization results: (a) Reference scene (b) Object Identity (c) Object Interaction (d) Object Orientation (e) Spatial Depth (f) Camera Movement (g) Object Movement

2 Related Work

Two crucial aspects of the visual quality of 3D scenes are their ability to convey depth information and enable the user to understand spatial and semantic relations between scene objects. Humans consistently underestimate spatial distances in virtual environments [7]. Therefore, accurately conveying depth information poses a considerable challenge in 3D computer graphics. Beyond photorealistic imaging, artistic techniques provide other approaches to intensifying the perception of depth in a computer rendered scene [5]. For instance, Meier illustrates in [8] that depth can be implied by varying brush size. Such means for creating a depth impression are tightly coupled to the process of painting itself and thus less straightforward to apply in computer graphics. However, art provides another cue which has a high potential to inform 3D visualizations of depth: color. Until the mid 1990s computer graphics concerned with the depiction of 3D objects had widely neglected color as a depth cue [10]. Shannon argues that virtual reality is situated between science and arts, and promotes algorithmic solutions in the domain of color perspective. Empirical studies have supported the important role of color as a monocular depth cue: When judging the depth of differently colored line drawings [6], textures [3] or even 3D models of realistic objects [1], red objects are perceived to be closer than blue objects. Variations of color can serve other functions in image perception than enhancing the impression of depth. Coconu et al. [2] demonstrate that NPR is particularly efficient in conveying and transmitting selected visual information. Using Non-Photorealistic Rendering (NPR) techniques enables meaningful simplification for efficient stylization of silhouettes and realtime hatching of objects. A very effective use of color and NPR is presented by Mitchell et al. [9]. The presented methods are related to the technical illustration technique in [4] to indicate surface orientation relative to a given light source.

3 Interactive Color Perspective

Our toolbox contains six algorithms, which exploit coloring and shading in a three-dimensional scene. The properties of each algorithm can be characterized according to their global or local implementation, their application for depth perception or object relations, and their dependence on user interaction to trigger dynamic color change. With regard to user interaction, there are algorithms that vary color depending on the way the user navigates through the scene or performs explicit mouse actions. In contrast, other algorithms work independently of the user: the color overlay is fixed or dynamically changes according to the objects' own movements. Our reference scene Minitropolis depicts an abstract model of a virtual city, consisting of various buildings and moving objects like trams, cars, an airplane, and people (see Figure 1a). Despite such abstract models, further application areas are manufacturing engineering and automation or in facility and layout planning.

Object Identity. In some contexts it is necessary to highlight specific objects and distinguish them from other less relevant objects in the scene. For completeness, we provide the obvious facility of applying an individual color overlay for selected scene objects. The color overlay is achieved by adjusting the ambient material color in combination with scene related shading and illumination. Furthermore, the diffuse color component can be adjusted. Lowering the diffuse ratio reduces all lighting and shading effects, which makes it even more easy to visually extract an object from the scene context (see Figure 1b).

Object Interaction. Some tasks require an understanding of the user's actions in relation to objects in the scene. Therefore, the Object Interaction color perspective features four interaction types which can be associated with color-related effects. For instance, approach colors extract objects located on the path the user has chosen to take through the scene, while touch color is used to tag already visited objects. Hence, Object Interaction can be used to depict the navigational path through a virtual scene (see Figure 1c). Clicking arbitrary objects can result in coloring which visually extracts them from the scene context. Further interaction with objects is conceivable and can be color coded as well. For instance, introducing multi-touch interaction with objects might require additional colors. Besides a touch color, the highlighting of an object could change after a dwell time to enable hold gestures that open menus.

Object Movement. Moving objects readily attract the user's attention. However, when several objects are moving concurrently, it can be hard to distinguish relevant objects from others and overcome distraction induced by irrelevant movement. The Object Movement algorithm can be used to visually group scene objects by applying a color overlay. This overlay can be configured with colors for slow and fast movements as determined by a user defined speed threshold. Hence, a change in color emphasizes the change in speed of an object (see Figure 1g). Additionally, defining a color for Object Movement helps to distinguish it from Camera Movement.

Camera Movement. Further disambiguation of scene movement and the users' own movements is achieved by the Camera Movement algorithm. Color overlays can be defined to highlight movements of the camera (which are either induced by the user navigating through the scene or animations triggered by the system). Conversely, in achromatic mode camera movements do not lead to increased coloring but a reduction of colors in the scene by graying out pixels at the border of the screen. The achromatic approach helps to reduce color overload in a scene while still maintaining a specific coloring effect which can guide the user's perception.

Spatial Depth. As outlined before, depth information can be difficult to visually extract from virtual environments and should be emphasized. The Spatial Depth algorithm allows the definition of a differential color overlay for close-up and distant parts of the scene, respectively (see Figure 1e). Depth within the scene is calculated both in absolute and relative terms. Relative scene depth takes the position of objects relative to the camera into account, which results in a dynamic color change as the viewer navigates through the scene. In contrast, absolute scene depth is defined by the user by setting a near and far distance value, depending on the scene context. Such absolute criteria prevent undesired changes in coloring due to position changes.

Object Orientation. Based on the experiences of interior design, color can be used to influence the appearance and mood of a room. Hence, users of 3D scenes should also be able to adjust the atmosphere and impression of virtual rooms. For that purpose, the Object Orientation color algorithm allows a selective manipulation of scene elements depending on their position, visibility and orientation in relation to the camera position. Our Object Orientation algorithm provides the user with the options to configure individual colors for "walls", "ceilings", "floors" and "fronts". It then calculates the surface colors by analyzing the surface normals in relation to the viewing direction. The resulting effect is that of a consistently color-coded convex space, similar to the illusion of being inside a room.

4 Study

To evaluate the potential of our Spatial Depth algorithm to affect observers' depth perceptions, the present study applied gradual color changes to approaching objects (cp. Figure 1g). If blue makes objects appear to be further away and red makes then seem closer, the application of a congruent color perspective (blue-to-red change) should result in the perception of a faster approach. Twenty-nine participants (13 females) aged 24-55 years (M = 31.9) viewed 58 scenes of approaching spheres with a fixed or distance-dependent color overlay. Eight of them were presented in color perspective (change from blue to red with decreasing distance), eight in inverse color perspective (red to blue) and three times eight in a constant color (red, blue and grey, respectively). After each trial, participants indicated whether they had seen a constant speed, an acceleration or a deceleration. Eighteen trials contained actual speed changes and 40 did not. Only the latter were used in the analyses.

We compared the two types of errors (misperception of acceleration and deceleration) between the five color conditions. Rating frequencies for each participant were subjected to one-way repeated measures analyses of variance (ANOVAs), which revealed an effect of color for both acceleration errors, $F(4, 108) = 36.00$, $p < .001$, and deceleration errors, $F(4, 108) = 29.04$, $p < .001$ (see Figure 12). Participants wrongly perceived an acceleration more often during color perspective trials than in all other conditions (48.7 vs. < 21 %), all $p < .001$, and decelerations were perceived most often for inverse color perspective (33.6 vs. < 13 %). The results indicate that dynamic color overlays can affect speed perception in 3D scenes, presumably via their effect on perceived depth. These results are far from trivial when considering that color is a relatively weak depth cue. The fact that it nevertheless influenced the acceleration ratings clearly demonstrates its usefulness in virtual 3D scenes.

Acknowledgments. The authors received funding by the German Federal Ministry of Education and Research (Project Number: VIP 18).

References

1. Bailey, R., Grimm, C., Davoli, C.: The effect of warm and cool object colors on depth ordering. In: Proceedings of the 3rd Symposium on Applied Perception in Graphics and Visualization, APGV 2006, p. 161. ACM (2006)
2. Coconu, L., Deussen, O., Hege, H.-C.: Realtime pen-and-ink illustration of landscapes. In: Proceedings of the 4th International Symposium on Nonphotorealistic Animation and Rendering, NPAR 2006, pp. 27–35. ACM (2006)
3. Faubert, J.: Seeing depth in colour: More than just what meets the eyes. Vision Research 34(9), 1165–1186 (1994)
4. Gooch, A., Gooch, B., Shirley, P., Cohen, E.: A non-photorealistic lighting model for automatic technical illustration. In: Proceedings of the 25th Annual Conference on Computer Graphics and Interactive Techniques, SIGGRAPH 1998, pp. 447–452. ACM (1998)
5. Gooch, A.A., Gooch, B.: Enhancing perceived depth in images via artistic matting. In: Proceedings of the 1st Symposium on Applied Perception in Graphics and Visualization, APGV 2004, p. 168. ACM (2004)
6. Guibal, C.R.C., Dresp, B.: Interaction of color and geometric cues in depth perception: When does "red" mean "near". Psychological Research Psychologische Forschung 69(1-2), 30–40 (2004)
7. Loomis, J., Knapp, J.: Visual Perception of Egocentric Distance in Real and Virtual Environments, pp. 21–46. Lawrence Erlbaum Associates, Mahwah (2003)
8. Meier, B.J.: Painterly rendering for animation. In: Proceedings of the 23rd Annual Conference on Computer Graphics and Interactive Techniques, SIGGRAPH 1996, pp. 477–484. ACM (1996)
9. Mitchell, J.L., Francke, M., Eng, D.: Illustrative rendering in team fortress 2. In: ACM SIGGRAPH 2007 Courses, pp. 19–32. ACM (2007)
10. Shannon, S.: The chrome age: Dawn of virtual reality. Leonardo 28(5), 369–380 (1995)

How Humans Search Varying-Knowledge Environments: Solving Imperfect Information Mazes

Apimuk Muangkasem, Atsuo Yoshitaka, Kristian Spoerer, and Hiroyuki Iida

School of Information Science, Japan Advanced Institute of Science and Technology, Japan
{apimuk,ayoshi,kristian,iida}@jaist.ac.jp

Abstract. In our experiment, we studied the searching sequence of humans, i.e. how humans solve the game tree. We created a controlled environment of maze game to simulate the situation where the player is not allowed to observe the entire map freely. We use "fog-block" to cover the intersection of a maze. Thus, the maze becomes an "imperfect information maze." We give additional information to hint on the path that the player should choose. Then we observed the change in players' behavior. We found that hints affect searches making it best fit path towards hint.

Keywords: Knowledge, Game tree, Imperfect information, Gaze, Cognition.

1 Introduction

To solve a maze, various path-finding algorithms have been proposed [1]. In a computer, those algorithms manage sequence searches from memory. In general, the computer initially stores all the data of the maze's map which includes a path or wall or goal. The algorithm will explore mazes differently depending on search strategy. Figure 1 shows an area of search sequence between two different algorithms. 'S' is the start position and 'G' is the goal position. The colored area is the area involved in searching sequence to reach the goal position.

If the solver knows only the initial position, it evaluates neighbor nodes. Figure 1A shows how the algorithm starts searching under the given condition until the "path to goal" is found. A Dijkstra search [2] is used in this example. This algorithm repeats exploring all the unknown positions on the board, from the current position to neighbor nodes, until reaching the goal position.

If the solver knows both initial and goal position beforehand, A* algorithm is known as one of the algorithms to search more effectively [3]. Figure 1B demonstrates the A* algorithm. Search space is clearly reduced compared to Dijkstra search. Additional information enables more promising search methods as shown in our example. A question arises whether this information helps humans in searching or not.

It is known that gaze interactions can reflect human strategy [4]. It has been shown that the addition of information provided to the player affects gaze pattern [5,6,7,8,9,10]. However, in a perfect information maze, the information obtained from human eyes often involves too large area since each gaze can provide the information of several intersections and relative positions, it is difficult to tell which exact pieces of information motivate the player to search in their specific way.

C. Stephanidis (Ed.): Posters, Part I, HCII 2013, CCIS 373, pp. 488–492, 2013.

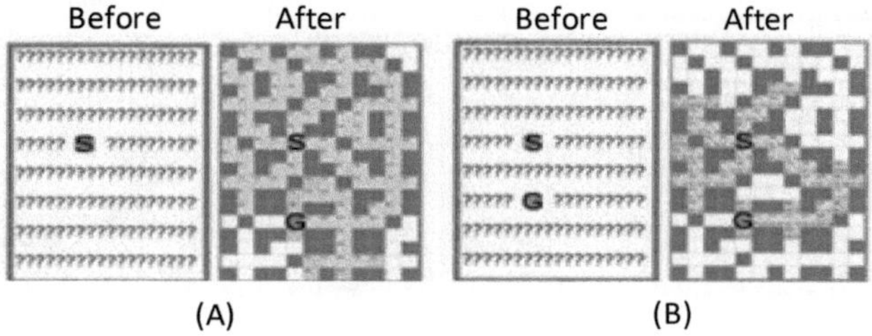

Fig. 1. Dijkstra search and A* search

2 Imperfect Information Maze

A form of game, where the player is not allowed to see the entire information provides a promising way to observe a player's thinking process, e.g. blindfold chess [11]. Figure 2 shows how a "fog-block" works in an imperfect information maze. We use the "fog-block" to cover an intersection of the maze. This environment enables to control the sequence of how a human explores the game tree.

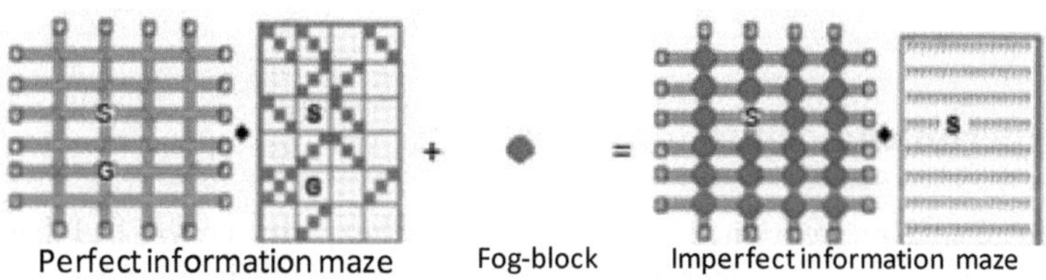

Fig. 2. Creating an imperfect information maze

We performed experiments on computer using Microsoft visual c#. Information obtained visually is limited to the interaction and interference of the "fog circle" controlled by user interface. To reveal information from under the "fog-block", user needs to move the mouse over the "fog-block" and click it. This setup reduces the ambiguity of how humans prioritize searches. Recognition process requires short-term memory [11], which affects gaze sequence due to memory capacity. In this experiment, the size of the maze problem is small and requires less memory.

3 Using Unsolvable Maze Problems for Motivation

When humans process reasoning, they need to search from the current position to each sibling position (leaf nodes) until they find a possible path to the desired outcome (winning position) in a game tree. Each maze can be modeled as a game tree because it has choices (branching nodes) and an answer (goal). Figure 3 shows how a maze can be represented in game tree format.

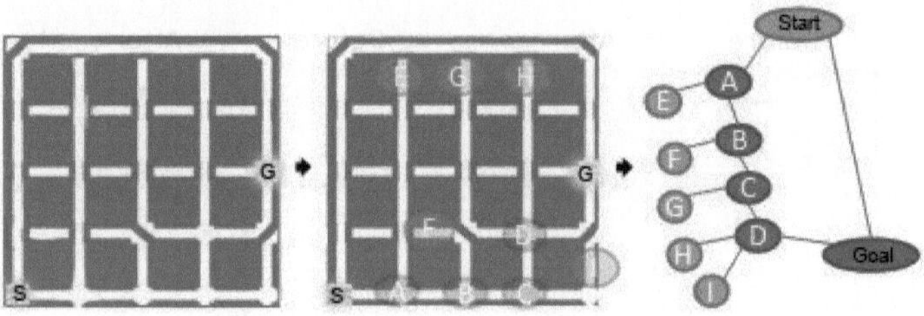

Fig. 3. Creating the game tree from a maze

There are three possibilities one can get during search through a maze, namely branching node (A,B,C,D), dead end (E,F,G,H,I) or goal position. Players will have to make a choice in the maze when they face a branching node. However, making choices in a maze problem is not as crucial of a decision as in a competitive game. Making the wrong choice in a maze will just make a player waste more time in solving it. He/she will eventually reach the goal in any maze problem. To configure the situation where the player cannot find the path to the desired outcome, we mixed a solvable maze with an unsolvable maze which includes no from start to goal. This engages the player to search through the maze like they would do in an adversarial game.

4 Experimental Setup

Two graduate students consented to participate in this experiment. We had them play 7 maze problems with a computer. During play, we captured their eye movement with using Tobii X60 & X120 Eye Trackers [8]. The objective of the maze problem is to find if there is at least one path from start to goal. We let the player play 3 different types of maze as shown in Figure 4. Figure 4A and Figure 4B are perfect information and imperfect information mazes, respectively. Figure 4C shows imperfect information with the goal position already revealed at the beginning.

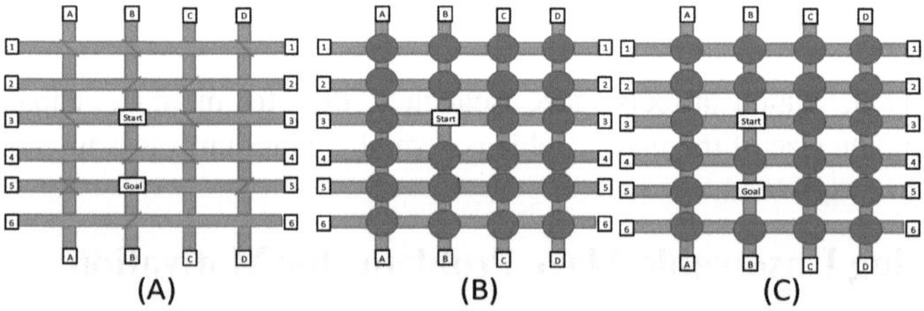

Fig. 4. Configurations in maze experiment

After playing the maze, each player was requested to answer a questionnaire. We provide the perfect information maze to the test subjects. We ask the player to pick the best intersection of the maze, considering that this hint will guide other players when they are playing the imperfect information maze with/without goal information.

5 Discussion and Concluding Remarks

We represent all maze positions as nodes in a game tree. In this way, we can recognize the position of each player's focus while solving the maze.

In a perfection information maze, the sequence of the gaze points does not fit to the exact maze position. Because it is easy to recognize obstacles in range of central vision without looking directly at them or the player simply did not pay attention to them. However, there are clear gaze patterns obtained from the player as follows:

1. The player starts looking at start and goal position as the first priority.
2. The player retrieves the straight line path from start to goal, with consideration to obstacles in each maze position as shown in Figure 5. The line represents a scan path.
3. The player attempts to construct a solution on that straight line from start to goal.

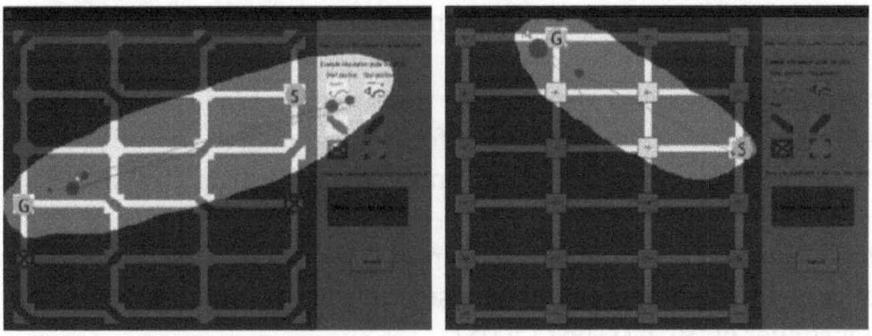

Fig. 5. Noticeable straight line, towards hint, of eye gaze sequence

In the imperfect information maze we have shown that gaze point corresponds to the cursor position. It is useful to recognize gaze point from the cursor position. In this setup, the player explores though the sibling nodes continuously. If a dead end is found, he will backtrack to the previous branching node. This search pattern is similar to Depth-First Search.

In the imperfect information maze with goal hint, the player often starts exploring the nodes from the goal position, rather than from start position. The process is similar to the perfect information maze. When the player is faced with a maze with no goal, the player tends to show less confidence when solving this problem. He/she always double-checks the path over again. The answers from the questionnaire showed that the hint guides the player to the shortest path between the start and the goal. Players comment that the straight line towards the hint guides the player when making a decision at branching nodes.

In conclusion, we found that the hint shapes the searching sequence. This straight line guides the player to make a certain decision at branching nodes. The searching sequence becomes a best fit path to the straight line toward hint.

Acknowledgement. I would like to express my greatest gratitude to the people who have helped and supported me throughout this paper. Professor. Kokolo Ikeda gave me an advice when I was having a hard time designing an experiment. Mr. Nathan Nossal helped me with English proofreading.

References

1. Kumari, S.M., Geethanjali, N.: A survey on shortest path routing algorithms for public transport travel. Global Journal of Computer Science and Technology 9(5), 73–75 (2010)
2. Dijkstra, E.W.: A note on two problems in connexion with graphs. Numerischemathematik 1(1), 269–271 (1959)
3. Dechter, R., Pearl, J.: Generalized best-first search strategies and the optimality of A*. Journal of the ACM (JACM) 32(3), 505–536 (1985)
4. Meijering, B., van Rijin, H., Taatgen, N.A., Verbrugge, R.: What eye movements can tell about theory of mind in a strategic game. PLoS one 7(9) (2012)
5. Sennersten, C.: Eye movements in am action game tutorial. Unpublished master's thesis, Lund University, Lund, Sweden (2004)
6. Gedeon, T.D., Zhu, D., Mendis, B.S.U.: Eye gaze assistance for a game-like interactive task. International Journal of Computer Games Technology 3 (2008)
7. Gowases, T., Bednarik, R., Tukiainen, M.: Gaze vs. mouse in games: The effects on user experience. In: Proceeding to International Conference on Computers in Education, pp. 773–777 (2008)
8. Sennersten, C., Alfredson, J., Castor, M., Hedström, J., Lindahl, B., Lindley, C., Svensson, E.: Verification of an Experimental Platform Integrating a Tobii Eytracking System with the Hifi Game Engine. In: Command and Control Systems, Swedish Defence Research Agency, pp. 5–15 (2007)
9. Jennett, C., Cox, A.L., Cairns, P., Dhoparee, S., Epps, A., Tijs, T., Walton, A.: Measuring and defining the experience of immersion in games. International journal of human-computer studies 66(9), 641–661 (2008)
10. Qian, Q., Shinomori, K., Song, M.: The functional role of implicit memory on gaze-evoked attention orienting. In: IEEE International Conference on Information and Automation (ICIA), pp. 148–153. IEEE (2010)
11. Campitelli, G., Gobet, F.: The mind's eye in blindfold chess. European Journal of Cognitive Psychology 17(1), 23–45 (2005)
12. Hollingworth, A., Richard, A.M., Luck, S.J.: Understanding the function of visual short-term memory: Transsaccadic memory, object correspondence, and gaze correction. Journal of Experimental Psychology: General 137(1), 163–181 (2008)

Vibration of the White Cane Causing a Hardness Sense of an Object

Kiyohiko Nunokawa[1,2], Shuichi Ino[2], and Kouki Doi[3]

[1] School of Human and Social Sciences, Tokyo International University, Kawagoe, Saitama, Japan
[2] Human Technology Research Institute, National Institute of Advanced Industrial Science and Technology, Tsukuba, Ibaraki, Japan
[3] Department of Education Information, National Institute of Special Needs Education, Yokosuka, Kanagawa, Japan
nunokawa@tiu.ac.jp, s-ino@aist.go.jp, doi@nise.go.jp

Abstract. Previously, we conducted a psychological experiment to measure sensitivity to hardness using a white cane. The Results showed that participants had higher sensitivity to hardness when using the white cane compared to when actually tapping the target with their fingertip. This suggests that the white cane acts to provide enhanced feedback on hardness. In this study, we investigated the relationship between vibration and sense of hardness using white canes. We measured frequency of vibration of the ferrule of the cane by acceleration sensor when the cane contacted with target. And using psychological experiments, we then had participants estimate their sense of hardness for each hardness degree. It was found that there is a correlation between the hardness sense and frequency of vibration.

Keywords: white cane, hardness sense, frequency of vibration.

1 Introduction

The white cane is one of the most widely used tools used by the visually impaired to support independent mobility. The white cane has a number of disadvantages. The area that users can perceive by using it is narrow, because objects can only be perceived by touching them with the cane. And it is also physically tiring to constantly swung the cane from side to side while walking. Two approaches have been making progress in addressing these issues. The first is the development of an electronic white cane that incorporates ultrasonic sensors, acceleration sensors, infrared light, lasers, etc. This electronic white cane allows people to detect and avoid obstacles from a distance, avoid hitting their head or face against objects that are above the level of the cane and there is no need to be swinging the cane. The second approach has been to make a lighter and more durable cane by improving and developing better materials. Both approach reduce fatigue. And some studies are already at the product evaluation stage. Through the developments discussed above, the convenience of the white cane has increased. To follow up on these two approaches, further developments need to

C. Stephanidis (Ed.): Posters, Part I, HCII 2013, CCIS 373, pp. 493–497, 2013.

take into account the nature of white cane use. The primary purpose of using a white cane is to be able to detect street conditions and obstacles based on the reverberations and tactile information that is gathered from the tip, not specifically what those obstacles are. But white cane users reported in interviews that in some cases they wanted to avoid directly touching a surface with their hands, and instead used their canes to distinguish between various materials or recognize certain objects. This indicates that target recognition occupies a large part of how white canes are used. Therefore, it is critical to develop a third approach that is focused on improving target recognition using the white cane. And furthermore, there are some users that imagine the cane as an extension of their hands, suggesting the possibility of somatization of tools. If the white cane were to become a part of a person's body, and could be used without discomfort, it could be considered a user-oriented tool, which is a desirable property for tools and assistive devices.

White canes are either straight and long, or collapsible. Both types consist of a grip at the top, a shaft, and a ferrule (a tip at the bottom). The grip is normally made from rubber. The shaft is crafted from materials such as aluminum, glass fiber, or carbon fiber, and the ferrule is typically made from nylon. This construction allows information, in the form of vibrations, to be transmitted to the user. Information about objects touched by the cane is transmitted to the user's palm through the structure above as vibrations. Research on the characteristics of objects, that are obtained through direct and active tactile exploration, such as texture, temperature, hardness, weight, size, shape of the whole and part of the object, has been conducted. It might be possible to obtain information about these characteristics with the white cane, by developing skills of using the cane. We conducted a psychological experiment on sensitivity to hardness [1] and [2]. Sighted university students wearing an eye mask (N=16) and blind people that usually use the white cane and walk independently (N=7) participated in the study. They were required to tap a rubber board with the tip of the forefinger of their dominant hand, and with the tip of the cane held by the dominant hand. The relationship between the actual hardness of the rubber and the sense of hardness was investigated, by using magnitude estimations. The exponents indicated by the results of the study with a standard grip were as follows: for sighted university students; 0.36 for the forefinger and 0.66 for the cane, for blind people; 0.37 for the forefinger and 0.59 for the cane. An exponent of 1 indicated that the physical and psychological values corresponded with each other. The observed exponent of less than 1 suggested that the sense of hardness did not increase significantly, even though physical hardness did increase, indicative of low sensitivity to changes in hardness. Furthermore, sensitivity to hardness when using the cane was higher than when using the forefinger, suggesting that the cane might amplify information about the hardness of a surface. In this study, we investigate the relationship between vibration and sense of hardness using white canes. We measure the frequency of vibration from the tip of the white cane at the point of contact with targets of various hardness degrees. Using psychological experiments, we then had participants estimate their sense of hardness for each hardness degree.

2 Experiment

A square rubber board 300 mm long and 12 mm thick was used to estimate hardness. Four rubber boards with the following degrees of hardness were prepared: 20, 40, 60, and 80 degrees (unit: JISA; manufactured by SHOWA RUBBER Co., Ltd, measured using Durometer Hardness Tester GS-719G type A, manufactured by TECLOCK Co., Ltd). The main body of the white cane (manufactured by G & OM Aids Inc.) was made of aluminum alloy (light metal), 1200 mm in length, including the rubber grip (260 mm) and the nylon ferrule (75 mm). The weight of the cane was approximately 200g with the inside of the shaft being hollow. Vibrations were measured using a conditioning amplifier (2-channel (single probe) Intensity Conditioning Amplifier, Type 2693-0S1, B&K Co., Ltd) , accelerometer (Miniature tear-drop CCLD accelerometer, Type 4517, B&K Co., Ltd), and an A/D converter (PowerLab/4ST , ADINSTRUMENTS, Inc.). The sensor was situated 2 cm from the tip of the ferrule (Fig.1). The floor was covered with a tile carpet during measurement and the rubber boards were placed on it.

Sighted male university students (N=3) participated in the study. They had eye masks, earplugs and year muffs, stood in front of the rubber boards (Fig.2), and held the white cane with the standard grip by stretching the forefinger along the even plane of the grip and grasping lightly with the thumb and the other three fingers (Fig.3). When the experimenter gave a sign, the participants tapped the board once to confirm the hardness of the board. Just after the tap, the magnitude was estimated and the participants were required to report the number that corresponded to the hardness. The numbers were assigned such that numbers were larger as the hardness increased. The hardness of the rubber board and the order of testing the boards were combined and randomized. The estimate of hardness was conducted five times, for each degree of hardness.

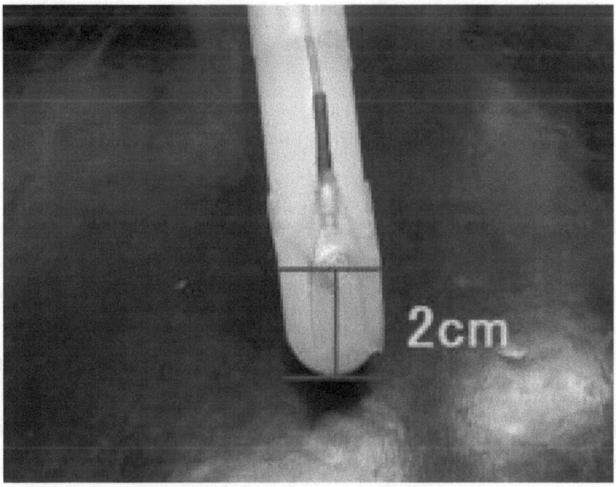

Fig. 1. Accelerometer setting

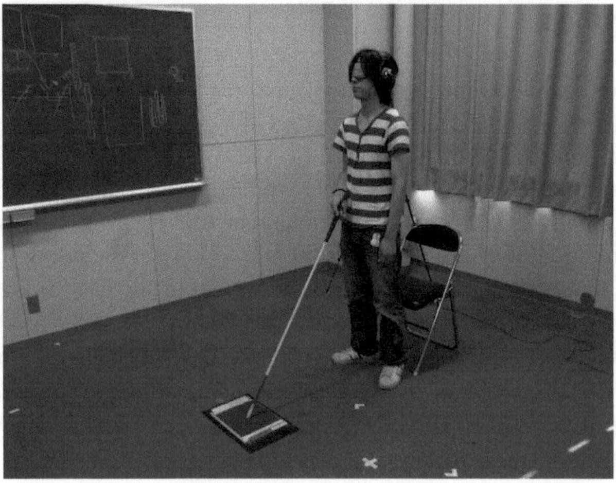

Fig. 2. Experimental setting

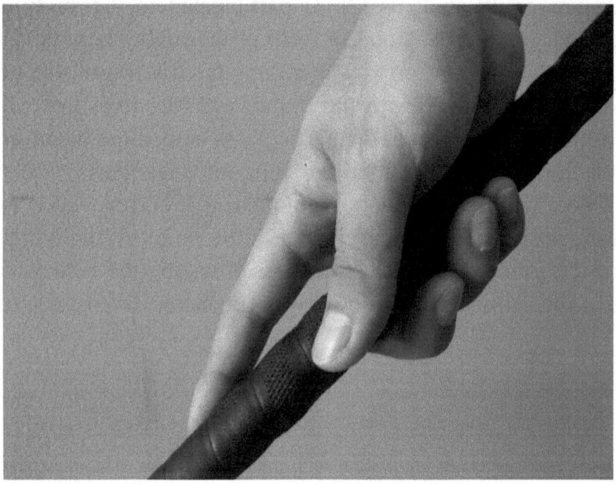

Fig. 3. Holding the white cane

3 Result

The results were processed using LabChart 7 (ADINSTRUMENTS, Inc.). Three participants indicated different frequency patterns. Moreover, each participant showed a characteristic frequency pattern to each degree of hardness. The figure shows the typical pattern indicated by subject A to each degree of hardness (Fig.4). The horizontal axis indicates the time course (sec) and the vertical axis, the frequency (Hz). This pattern was obviously different from the frequency pattern that was obtained by dropping the cane from a certain height on the rubber board, a person being involved. Furthermore, as the hardness of the board increased, the estimate given by the participants became larger.

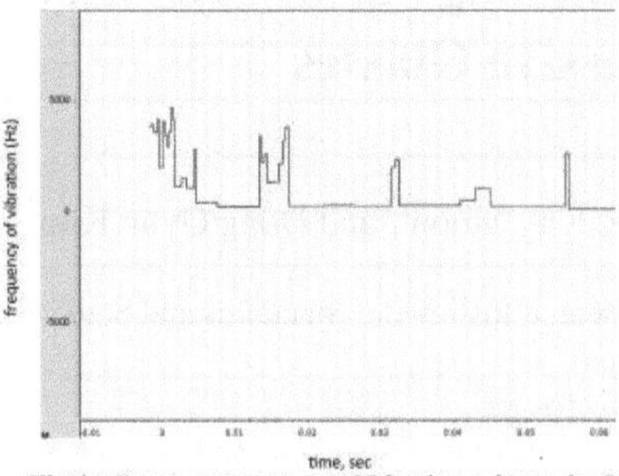

Fig.4a Frequency pattern on 20 hardness degree by Sub.A

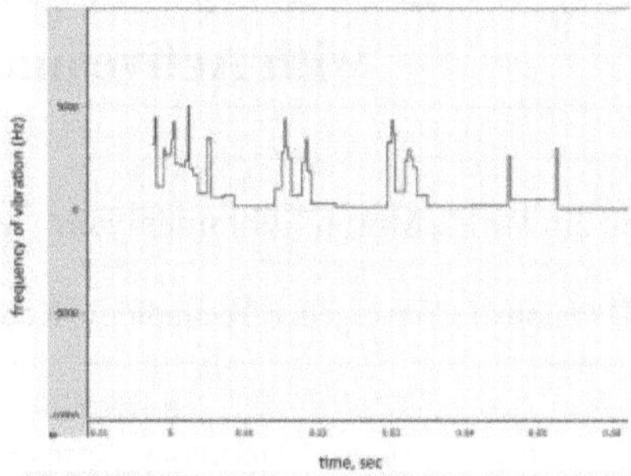

Fig.4b Frequency pattern on 40 hardness degree by Sub.A

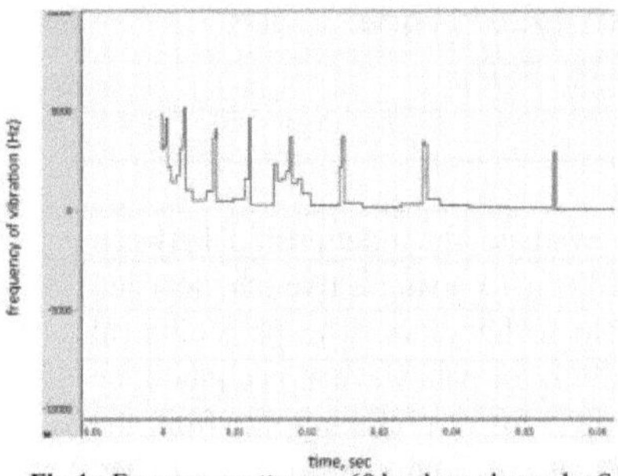

Fig.4c Frequency pattern on 60 hardness degree by Sub.A

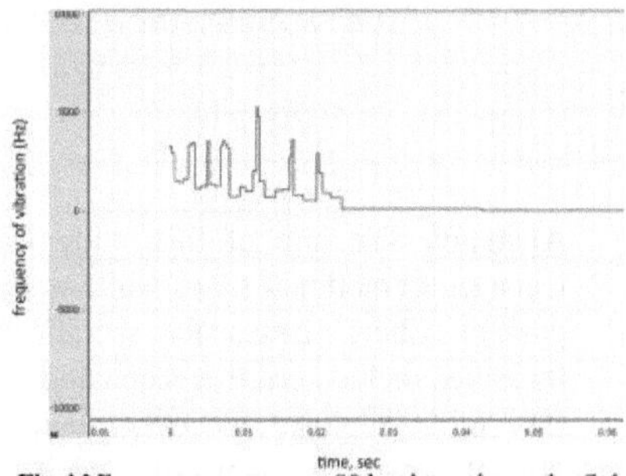

Fig.4d Frequency pattern on 80 hardness degree by Sub.A

Fig. 4. The typical Frequency pattern on each hardness degree by Sub.A

4 Discussion

It is suggested that vibrations might transmit information about the hardness of the board. Differences between the participants might have reflected differences in tapping techniques, such as the strength of the grip or the height at the position when tapping was initiated. Therefore, by investigating the relationship between tapping technique and the frequency band, and excluding the effects of the tapping technique from the resulting frequency patterns, it would be possible to identify vibration frequencies that corresponds to information about hardness of objects. And in this study, vibration at the tip of the cane, where the cane touches the object was assessed. In the next step, we should measure vibrations at participant's palm, where information is got.

References

1. Nunokawa, K., Ino, S.: A psychophysical study of indirect tactile perception on an object hardness through the white cane. In: Proc.10th SICE System Integration Division Annual Conference, pp. 147–148 (2009)
2. Nunokawa, K., Ino, S.: An Experimental Study on Target Recognition Using White Canes. In: Proceedings of IEEE EMBC 2010, pp. 6583–6586 (2010)

Physiological Responses to Watching 3D on Television with Active and Passive Glasses

Se Jin Park[1], Murali Subramaniyam[2], Myung Kug Moon[2], and Dong Gyun Kim[2]

[1] Division of Convergence Technology, Korea Research Institute of Standards and Science, South Korea
sjpark@kriss.re.kr

[2] Center for Medical Metrology, Korea Research Institute of Standards and Science, South Korea
muraliprs@yahoo.co.in, mkjy2011@gmail.com
windy6395@nate.com

Abstract. The aim of this study was to evaluate the relationship between teenager's emotional states while watching 3D on TV using active (shutter) and passive (filter) glasses and specific physiological indices. The physiological measures include electroencephalography (EEG) for beta wave at occipital lobe (O_1 and O_2 regions), electrooculography (EOG) for eye blinking rate from the dominate eye, and subjective evaluation. Eighteen healthy teenager's (9 used active glass and 9 used passive glasses) aged 18.72±0.56 years were participated. The subjects were exposed to 3D visuals for 45 min each. The relative beta band power was comparatively higher while using passive glasses. The eye blink rate was comparatively higher while using passive glasses. Subjective evaluation scores were comparatively higher while using active glasses. The contrary results between physiological responses and psychophysical were observed. Further experiments need to be performed by considering more subjects, higher viewing duration and light weight glasses.

Keywords: 3D visuals, Glass type, Subjective evaluation, Relative beta band power, Eye blinking rate.

1 Introduction

By recent advance in the multimedia processing fields, 3D TV is expected to become one of the most dominant markets in the next generation broadcasting system [1]. The basic concept of 3D TV is to provide user interactivity and 3D depth feeling. Watching 3D on TV, which involves wearing special glasses like those used for 3D movies, bombards the eyes and brain with a succession of flashing images that appear for a fraction of a second. This technology puts unusual strain on the body, especially children and teenagers may be more susceptible to health issues associated with viewing in 3D. All types of 3D glasses can be divided into two categories: passive and active. Active 3D glasses interact wirelessly with images on a screen to enhance 3D viewing, whereas passive glasses do not. Visual fatigue is a very important issue of 3D display market for implementing more comfortable display devices in terms of human

C. Stephanidis (Ed.): Posters, Part I, HCII 2013, CCIS 373, pp. 498–502, 2013.

factors. Many studies have been performed to measure the visual fatigue using objective evaluation methods namely electroencephalogram (EEG), event-related potential (ERP) signals, functional magnetic resonance imaging (fMRI), electrooculography (EOG), and electrocardiography (ECG) in 3D display environment [2-7]. The aim of this study was to evaluate the relationship between teenager's emotional states while watching 3D on TV using active (shutter) and passive (filter) glasses and specific physiological indices.

2 Materials and Methods

A total of eighteen healthy teenager's (9 used active glass and 9 used passive glasses) were participated. The average age of the participants was 18.72±0.56 years. As mentioned earlier, the goal of this study was to evaluate the relationship between teenager's emotional states while a watching 3D on TV using active and passive glasses and specific physiological indices. The physiological measures include electroencephalography (EEG) for beta wave at occipital lobe (O1 and O2 regions), electrooculography (EOG) for eye blinking rate from the dominate eye, and subjective evaluation. The subjects were exposed to 3D visuals with active and passive glasses for 45 min each. The Biopac system's Acqknowledge program was used as a physiological workstation. The physiological signals recorded while subjects were watching 3D visuals at initial, 10 min, 20 min, 30 min, 40 min and final period. To determine the optimal viewing distance, preliminary experiments were performed. The viewing distance was set at 6 times the height of the display. Subjective evaluation based on a 5 point scale includes eye pain, desire for stop watching, nausea, body pain and blurred vision. The subjective evaluation was conducted from the subjects after the experiment. Using the 10-20 international standards the EEG electrodes were placed on the O1 and O2 regions. Also, the reference electrodes were placed on the right and left ears, and a ground electrode was placed on the forehead. To measure the eye blinks count, two EOG electrodes were placed above and below the dominant eye. The sampling rate for measuring the physiological signals was set at 512 Hz. Each measurement cross resistance was less than 10 kΩ. The results were statistically analyzed in the SPSS program with 95% confidence level.

3 Results and Discussion

3.1 Relative Beta Band Power

From the EEG measurements, the percentage of relative beta band power was calculated (% relative beta band power = $\beta/\delta+\theta+\alpha+\beta)$) for O1 (Fig. 1) and O2 (Fig. 2) region, while watching 3D with active and passive glass. The relative beta band power percentage was comparatively higher while using passive glasses in both regions. The univariate ANOVA reveals that statistically significant ($p<0.05$) difference in the relative beta band power percentage between glass types was found only at the O1 region. There was not any significant difference in the relative beta band power percentage based on watching duration in both regions.

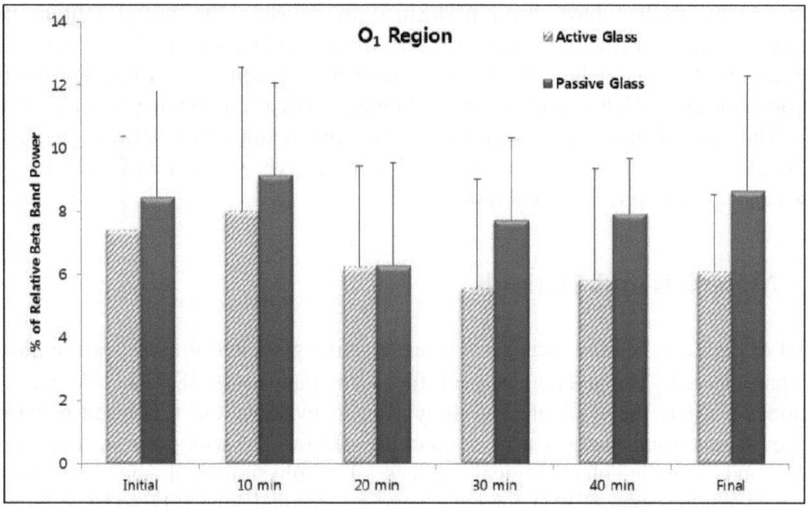

Fig. 1. O1 region relative beta band power percentage comparison (significant ($p<0.05$) difference was found between glass types)

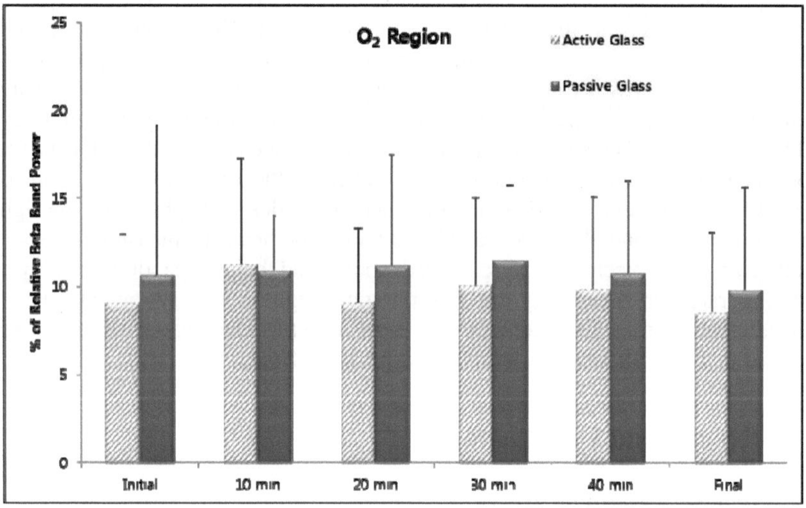

Fig. 2. O2 region relative beta band power percentage comparison

3.2 Eye Blinks Count

From the EOG measurements the eye blinks count per minute (Fig. 3) was calculated, while watching 3D with active and passive glass. The eye blink rate was comparatively higher while using passive glasses, no significant difference was found between glass types and watching duration (time).

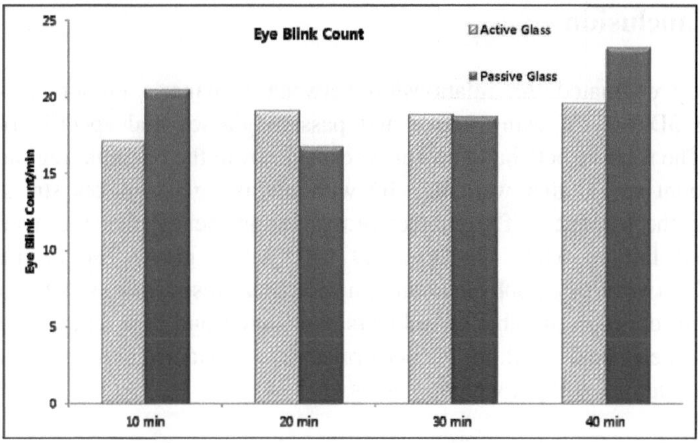

Fig. 3. Eye blinks count comparison

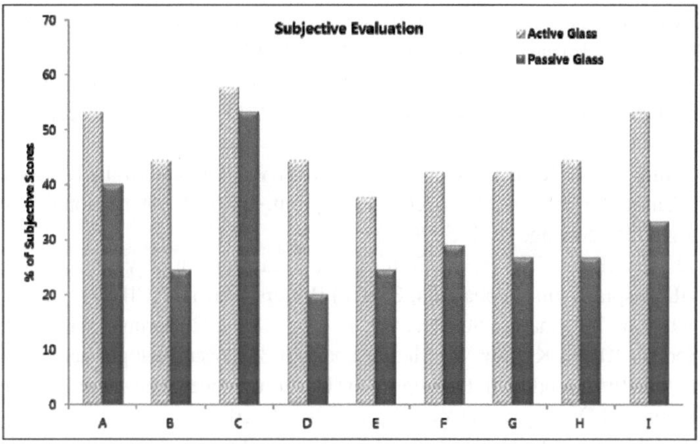

Fig. 4. Percentage of subjective evaluation scores comparison. Where: A – Eye Pain; B – Tear in the Eyes; C – Desire to Stop Watching; D – Get Stressed; E – Nausea; F – Headache; G – Stiffness in the Neck; H – Stiffness in the Shoulders; and I – Blurred Vision.

3.3 Subjective Evaluation

Subjective evaluation includes totally 28 questions and grouped based on five categories such as eye pain, desire for stop watching, nausea, body pain and blurred vision. The 5 point scores are represented as a percentage (Fig. 4) for few questions. Overall, the average scores of the subjective evaluation reveal that subjects rated high scores for watching 3D with active glass. From the figure we can see that, the percentage of subjective evaluation average scores were higher for desire to stop watching, eye pain, and blurred vision. There was no significant difference ($p<0.05$) found between the subjective scores between watching 3D using active and passive glass.

4 Conclusion

This study evaluated the relationship between teenager's emotional states while watching 3D on TV using active and passive glasses and specific physiological indices. The relative beta band power percentage from the occipital region and the eye blinks count reveal that watching 3D with passive glass makes stress and visual fatigue to the teenagers. The subjective evaluations reveal that teenagers felt stress and visual fatigue while watching 3D with active glass. The dissimilar results observed between psychophysical and physiological responses; possible reason could be viewing duration, number of subjects considered and difference in glass weight. Further experiments need to be performed by considering more subjects, higher viewing duration and light weight glasses.

References

1. Min, D., Kim, D., Yun, S., Sohn, K.: 2D/3D Freeview Video Generation for 3DTV System. Signal Processing: Image Communication 24, 31–48 (2009)
2. Kim, D., Choi, S., Choi, J., Shin, H., Sohn, K.: Visual Fatigue Monitoring System based on Eye-Movement and Eye-Blink Detection. In: Proc. SPIE 7863, Stereoscopic Displays and Applications XXII, p. 786303 (2011)
3. Kim, D., Jung, Y.J., Kim, E., Ro, Y.M., Park, H.W.: Human Brain Response to Visual Fatigue Caused by Stereoscopic Depth Perception. In: 17th International Conference on Digital Signal Processing, pp. 1–5 (2011)
4. Kim, Y.-J., Lee, E.C.: EEG Based Comparative Measurement of Visual Fatigue Caused by 2D and 3D Displays. In: Stephanidis, C. (ed.) Posters, Part II, HCII 2011. Communications in Computer and Information Science, vol. 174, pp. 289–292. Springer, Heidelberg (2011)
5. Li, H., Seo, J., Kham, K., Lee, S.: Measurement of 3D Visual Fatigue using Event-Related Potential (ERP): 3D oddball Paradigm. 3DTV conference: The True Vision - Capture, Transmission and Display of 3D Video, pp. 213–216 (2008)
6. Park, S.J., Oh, S.B., Murali, S., Lim, H.K.: Human Impact Assessment of Watching 3D Television by Electrocardiogram and Subjective Evaluation. XX IMEKO World Congress, pp. 1–4 (2012)
7. Moon, M.K., Park, S.J.: Effects of 3D Glasses on Visual Fatigue. In: Korean Society for Emotion & Sensibility Conference, pp. 10–11 (2012)
8. Park, S.J., Kim, D.K., Moon, M.K.: Research on Optimum Viewing Distance for Watching 3D TV. In: Korean Society for Emotion & Sensibility Conference, pp. 12–13 (2012)

Temporal Phase Shift: Visual Illusion by Phase-Shifted Light Projection and Its Applications

Jun Rekimoto[1,2]

[1] The University of Tokyo
7-3-1, Hongo, Bunkyo-ku, Tokyo 110-0033, Japan
rekimoto@acm.org
http://lab.rekimoto.org
[2] Sony Computer Science Laboratories, Inc.
3-14-13 Higashigotanda, Shinagawa-ku, Tokyo 141-0022, Japan

Abstract. Understanding the mechanism of human visual processing is important as a foundation for human computer interaction research, because many interactive systems are primary relying on visual information. In this paper, we report a new visual illusion caused by phased shifted light projection using our customized digital micromirror projector that appears to be related to human eyes' saccades and microsaccades. We examine the cause of this illusion, and propose possible applications using this effect.

1 Introduction

When we are looking at the fixed position, our eyes are still continuously and imperceptibly jumping and jiggling. This phenomenon is called *microsaccades*, in contrast to larger voluntary eye movements known as saccades [2,4,1]. Microsaccades are believed to be an important mechanism for visual processing, and several researches are going on to investigate its correlation to human's higher mental status such as concentration and emotion [2,4].

Meanwhile, there are a number of visual illusions are found and studied [5]. These illusions are important tools for understanding the mechanism of visual perception, and also important for creating interactive media and entertainment.

In this paper, we report a new visual illusion that occurs by using a modified DMD (digital micromirror device) projector [3] that projects images with flickering phase are slightly different. We named this effect "temporal phase shift illusion".

2 Temporal Phase Shift Illusion

Figure 1 shows a system configuration that causes this illusion. A normal projector using DMD has a configuration as shown in Figure 1 (a). A DMD device

C. Stephanidis (Ed.): Posters, Part I, HCII 2013, CCIS 373, pp. 503–506, 2013.

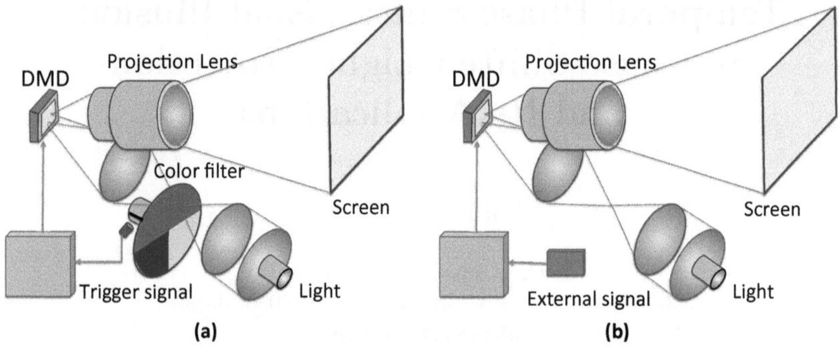

Fig. 1. Configuration of projectors: (a) normal DMD projector, (b) our customized projector to create visual illusion

has an array of micro-mirrors that control reflections of incoming light, and thus it can control projected pixel intensity. A rotating color filter is used in combination to change color from the light source. When the angle of a micro mirror is synchronously selected with color filter, it can project any selected color with selected intensity. As a result, a DMD projector can control each pixel's RGB brightness.

In contrast, our modified DMD projector, shown in Figure 1(b), has a single light source, and the color filter is removed. With this projector, light patterns those have the same brightness, the same flicker frequency, but different flicker phases can be projected.

The difference of these patterns should be imperceptible for human eyes, because the projector's flickering frequency (120Hz) is well higher than Critical Flicker Frequency (CFF, which is normally around 50Hz), at which rate our eyes are incapable of separating consecutive light stimuli. However, we found that boundaries of these patterns are still noticeable especially when our eyes' move (i.e., saccade) (Figure 2(b)). We named this effect "temporal phase shift illusion".

This effect causes when we intentionally move eyes, but it also causes (but becoming less noticeable) when we looked at one particular point on a screen. Thus we consider this effect is related to both saccades and microsaccades. Furthermore, we expect that it should be possible to measure the frequency of microsaccades occurrences by counting the noticed number of this illusion, which would be useful for knowing user status such as concentration.

Our current explanation of this effect is this. Human retina's bipolar cell has structures such as on-center or off-center so that the cell is activated when there is a difference of light stimulation at the center and the peripheral areas. This mechanism normally detects edges, but the same mechanism detects phase differences, although light stimulation's flickering frequency is much higher to be detected by photoreceptor cells (Figure 3).

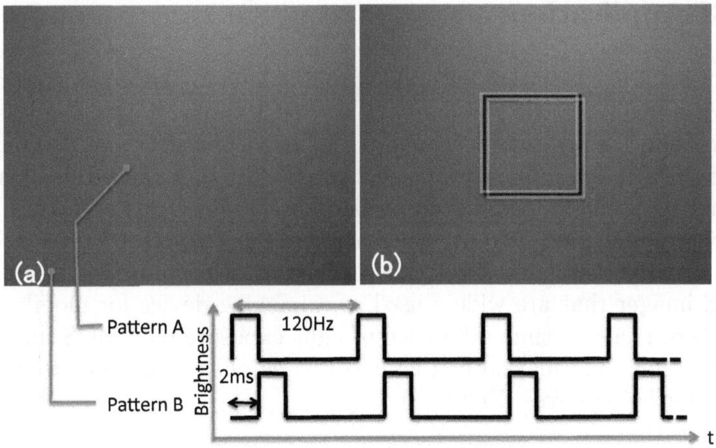

Fig. 2. Temporal Phase-Shift illusion: when flickering light patterns with the same frequency but different phases, the boundary becomes noticeable even when the frequency itself is much higher than the ability of human visual perception.((a): actual image, (b):simulation result of human visual perception)

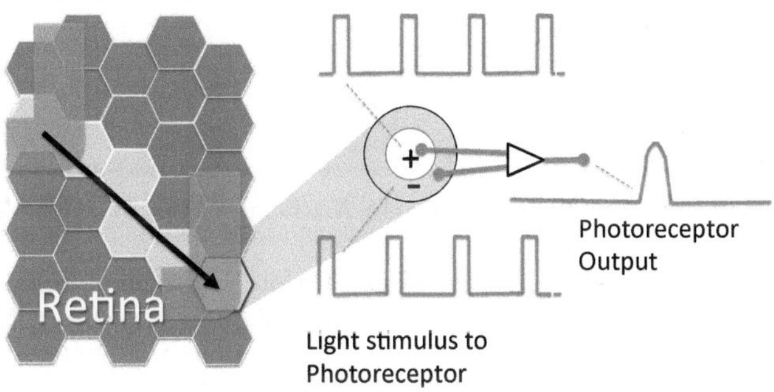

Fig. 3. A possible mechanism that causes Temporal Phase Shift Illusion: receptor detects phase difference before and after (micro-)saccades

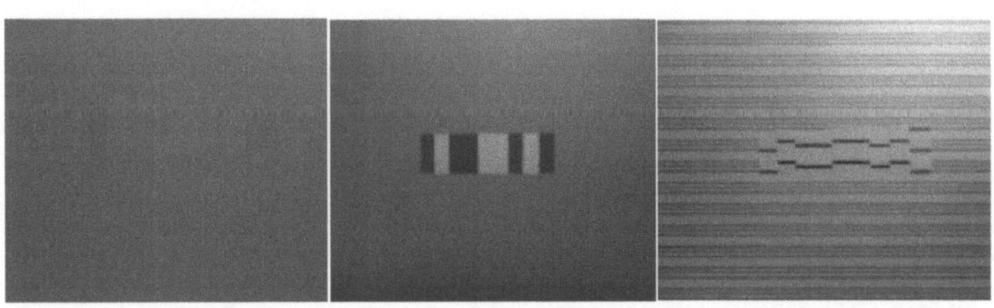

Fig. 4. Invisible barcode: left: viewed from human eyes (simulated by low-speed camera), middle: image taken by high-speed camera (1/200s), right: image taken by CMOS camera of the smartpohne

3 HCI Applications

This effect itself is interesting for understanding human visual perception mechanism. We now discuss the possibility of new HCI applications using this effect.

The first one is a measurement method for user concentration. By controlling the phase shift to determine the shortest phase shift that cause this illusion, we expect that it should be possible to measure user concentration status.

The other application is to use the feature of our customized projector itself, to create invisible barcodes. The phase difference of patterns are also detected by CMOS imager that are widely used as a imaging device for mobile phones, because there is also a time difference of light exposure on CMOS imaging device. As a result, information can be encoded as phase difference which is less noticeable for human eyes (Figure 4).

4 Conclusion

In this paper, we report our newly found visual illusion caused by phase-shifted lite projection. Although its mechanism is not perfectly explained, it should be related to our eye's saccades or microsaccades. We also reported possible HCI applications using this effect.

References

1. Bharath, A., Petrou, M.: Next Generation Artificial Vision Systems. Artech House (2008)
2. Findlay, J.M., Gilchrist, I.D.: Active Vision. Oxford University Press (2003)
3. Hornbeck, L.J., Nelson, W.E.: Bistable deformable mirror device. OSA Technical Digest Series Spatial Light Modulators and Applications 8, 107 (1988)
4. Martinez-Conde, S., Macknik, S.L.: Windows on the mind. Scientific American 297(2), 56–63 (2007)
5. Murakami, I., Cavanagh, P.: A jitter after-effect reveals motion-based stabilization of vision. Nature (395), 798–801 (1998)

Generation of the Certain Kind of Figures Using the Movement Sense of Localized Sound and Its Application

Michio Shimizu[1], Masahiko Sugimoto[2], and Kazunori Itoh[3]

[1] Nagano Prefectural College, Miwa 8-49-7
Nagano-shi, 380-8525 Japan
michio@nagano-kentan.ac.jp
[2] Takushoku University Hokkaido College, Memu 4558
Fukagawa-shi, 074-8585 Japan
sugimoto@takushoku-hc.ac.jp
[3] Faculty of Engineering, Shinshu University, Wakasato 4-17-1
Nagano-shi, 380-8553 Japan
itoh@cs.shinshu-u.ac.jp

Abstract. In this report, the easy figure which consists of a line segment and its combination is virtually expressed by the movement sense of the localized sound on a virtual sound screen. In order to create a psychological simple figure, the system which used together the movement sense of localized sound and the input tactile sense guide is proposed.

Keywords: the movement sense of the localized sound, the input tactile sense guide, a figure education.

1 Introduction

We have been examined how a visually impaired person can recognize characters or play a board game using a 2-dimensional virtual sound screen [4–8]. In this report, the easy figure which consists of a line segment and its combination is virtually expressed by the movement sense of the localized sound on a virtual sound screen. In order to create a psychological simple figure, the system which used together the movement sense of sound and the input tactile sense guide is proposed. The purpose of research is applying this system to a student's figure education in a visually impaired school.

2 Generation of Figure by the Movement Sense of Sound

The virtual sound screen is the 2-dimensional space where a vertical axis is expressed by frequency and a horizontal axis is expressed by inter aural level difference 3. Now, we realize the virtual sound screen on a PC, four localized sounds corresponding to four points A (2000Hz, -12dB), B (2000Hz, 12dB), C (400Hz, -12dB), and D (400Hz, 12dB) are specified (Fig. 1). Each of such sound is short sign waves, and output time

C. Stephanidis (Ed.): Posters, Part I, HCII 2013, CCIS 373, pp. 507–510, 2013.

is 300ms. By hearing psychology, through headphone, such sound can be heard from the upper left, the upper right, the lower left, and the lower right, respectively.

By the way, if the sound corresponding to two points on this sound screen is outputted by the suitable time lag (200ms), it is known that the interval of two points could be recognized as a line segment [5]. This psychological property is called the movement sense of the localized sound. If four points are outputted by this time lag one by one, four sides of a square and two diagonal lines will be recognized by the movement sense of sound.

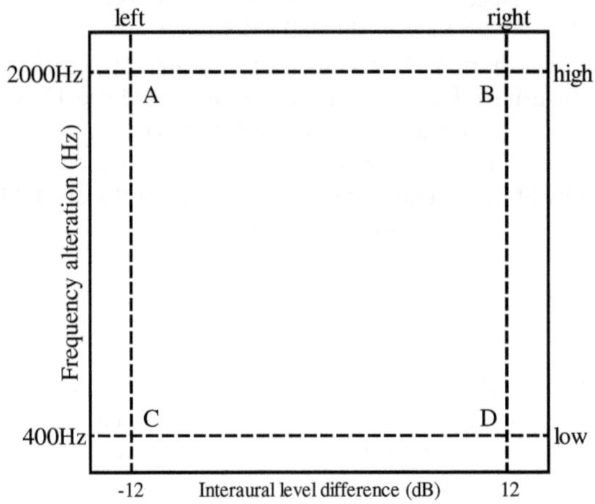

Fig. 1. Four points on a virtual sound screen

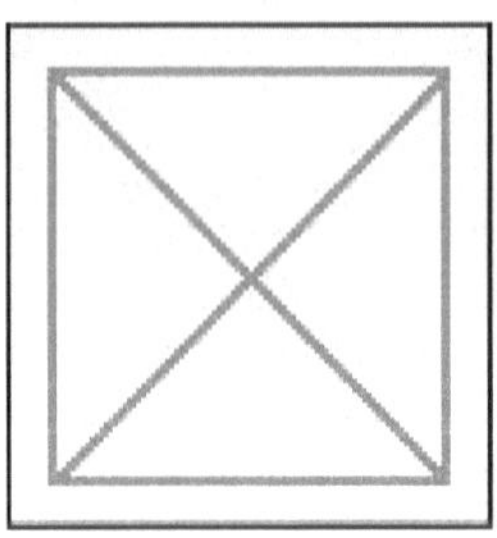

Fig. 2. Six slots on the input tactile sense guide

3 Expression of the Figure by the Input Tactile Sense Guide

On the other hand, the input tactile sense guide corresponding to the figure which consists of four slots on square and two slots on the diagonal lines is prepared (Fig. 2). This is made with the transparent plastic board of square, the size is 5cm and the thickness is 3mm. The side lines on the board are 4cm, and are made by the slot of U type with width 1.5mm and depth 0.5mm.

This input tactile sense guide is used placing on a pen tablet. If the nib of a stylus pen is placed on the slot and a side button is pushed, two sounds will be outputted in

200ms of the time lag, the movement sense of the sound corresponding to the line segment would be expressed. While continuing pushing a side button, the output of sound is repeated at intervals of 1000ms.

4 The System for Studying Fundamental Character of Figures

For visually impaired students, in order to study the fundamental character of figures, we create the PC system which consists of the localized sounds and the input tactile sense guide. In this system, the simple figures which consist of four sides and two square diagonal line segments are treated.

Depending on the fundamental character of figures, the following combinatorial figures 1 – 4 are registered into the PC. A teacher (sighted person) can take out a figure suitably using a mouse in accordance with an understanding of a student, and can show a student it. At this time, it is outputted so that the direction of movement sense of sound may become a picture drawn without lifting the brush from the paper as much as possible.

The figures that can be made using n line segments (n = 1, 2, 3, 4, 5, 6) among six line segments. The number of figures are ${}_6C_n = 6! / n!(6 - n)!$.

The figures which will overlap completely if they rotate 90 degrees, 180 degrees and 270 degrees respectively.

The point symmetrical figures (Fig.3 (a), (b)).

The figures not drawn without lifting the brush from the paper (Fig.3 (b)).

In the communication of a teacher and a student in instruction, a student with a headphone can create a figure using the input tactile sense guide, and can show a teacher it.

(a) $n = 3$ (b) $n = 2$

Fig. 3. Example of figures

5 Conclusion

We recognize that our system moves almost well. From now on, we will think that our method will be tried to students of a visually impaired school. The fundamental characters of figures that we treat in this report are the number of figures, figure rotation, point symmetry and figures not drawn without lifting the brush from the paper. We would like to examine whether this method can apply also to another fundamental characters, such as the line symmetry and the parallel movement, or it is applicable also to a little more complicated figures.

References

1. Kamel, H.M., Roth, P., Shiha, R.R.: Graphics and User's Exploration via Simple Sonics (GUESS): Providing Interrelational Representation of Objects in a Non-visual Environment. In: Proceedings of the 2001 Inter. Conf. on Auditory Display, pp. 261–266 (2001)
2. Cronly-Dillon, J., Persaud, K., Gregory, R.P.F.: The perception of visual images encoded in musical form: a study in cross-modality information transfer. In: Proceedings of The Royal Society of London Series B-Biological Sciences, pp. 2427–2433 (1999)
3. Blauert, J.: Spatial Hearing. In: The psychophysics of Human Sound Localization. MIT Press, Cambridge (1983)
4. Itoh, K., Shimizu, M., Yonezawa, Y.: A Drawing Support System for the Virtually Impaired Computer User using a Virtual Sound Screen. In: Design of Computing Systems, Elisevier, Amsterdam, pp. 401–404 (1997)
5. Shimizu, M., Itoh, K., Nakazawa, T.: Pattern Representation System using Movement Sense of Localized Sound. In: Proceedings of HCI, pp. 990–994 (1999)
6. Sugimoto, M., Itoh, K., Shimizu, M.: Simple pattern creation using a pen input guide and sound localization for the visually impaired. In: Miesenberger, K., Klaus, J., Zagler, W.L., Burger, D. (eds.) ICCHP 2004. LNCS, vol. 3118, pp. 745–752. Springer, Heidelberg (2004)
7. Shimizu, M., Sugimoto, M., Itoh, K.: Interface of Online Mini-Go-Game with Pen Input Guide for the Blind. In: Stephanidis, C. (ed.) HCI 2007. LNCS, vol. 4556, pp. 806–812. Springer, Heidelberg (2007)
8. Hamaguchi, Y., Nagasaka, D., Tamesue, T., Itoh, K., Shimizu, M., Sugimoto, M., Hashimoto, M., Kayama, M.: A Multimodal Board Game System Interface Using Finger Input for Visually Impaired Computer Users. In: Stephanidis, C. (ed.) Universal Access in HCI, Part I, HCII 2009. LNCS, vol. 5614, pp. 68–77. Springer, Heidelberg (2009)

Part VII
Ergonomic and Human Modelling Issues

The Slip-Resistance Effect Assessment of the Anti-slip Strip on Different Contaminated Floors

Ching Chung Chen[1] and Hui Chun Chen[2,*]

[1] Department of Information Management, Hsing Wu University of Science & Technology, New Taipei, Taiwan
[2] Department of Business Administration, Hsing Wu University of Science & Technology, New Taipei, Taiwan
mag@mail.hwu.edu.tw

Abstract. Anti-slip strip is one of the most popular slip-resistant products indoor and outdoor, especially on the ramp. By using anti-slip strip the roughness of floor can be increased, the COF will be increased and the risk of slips and falls will be reduced at the same time. This study wants to find out the effects of slip-resistance under different floor contamination conditions while using the emery anti-slip strip. The anti-slip strips covered by steel grit provide valid slip-resistance effect. However, the slip-resistance effect will be limited when the floor covered by oil and the grooves of footwear have been wear away. In total, to provide valid slip-resistance effect, keeping the floor dry, installing the anti-slip strips, wearing tread shoes are some useful processes to reduce the risk of falling and slipping.

Keywords: Anti-slip strip, Slip& fall, Coefficient of Friction.

1 Introduction

The fall incidences take 17% of all occupational incidences in USA and 20% of all occupational incidences in UK annually, and all those slipping and falling incidences lead huge losses on workplaces [1]. Slip and fall are more easily happened to senior people. There were 2.2 million slipping and falling cases that were sent to the emergency room due to no-fatal incidents, and more than quarter of them had to be hospitalized [2]. Therefore, slipping and falling accidents induce serious safety issues [3].

One of the most popular ways of assessing slipperiness is to measure the coefficient of friction (COF) between the shoe and floor surface [4]. The lower the COF is, the slipperier the floor will be. Due to the simplicity of measuring, the static COF (μs) has been considered as one of the major indicators of floor slipperiness. A measured static COF of 0.5 has been adopted as a safety guideline in the USA [5-6]. Prior researches have shown that falling and slipping could be affected by various factors, such as the material and the roughness of the floor; the liquid and solid contamination on the floor; the material of footwear; the groove design of shoe sole; and the gradient of ramps [7-9].

[*] Corresponding author.

C. Stephanidis (Ed.): Posters, Part I, HCII 2013, CCIS 373, pp. 513–517, 2013.

The squeeze film theory [10] is probably the most frequent adopted scientific basis describing the effects of liquid on the friction on a floor. Improving the feature of floor surface has better anti-slip effects than changing the shoe sole grooves [11-13]. In practice, the anti-slip strips are widely installed on walk ways, ramps, toilets, bathrooms and stairs to change the feature of the floor surface and prevent slipping and falling. Most of the anti-slip strips using steel grit coating to increase the floor roughness and improve the slip-resistance effects. However, the discussion about its slip-resistance effect is rare. The subject of the anti-slip strip's COF under different floor contaminations is deserved to be described. Therefore, this study wants to find out the effects of slip-resistance under different floor contamination conditions while using the emery anti-slip strip.

2 Method

The study conducted a three factors experiment. There are 4*3*2=24 combinations (4 shoe materials * 3 floor contaminations conditions * 2 floors). A total of 144 readings were collected. Four types of footwear pads were tested in this study. These included flat (no tread) and tread footwear pads made from Neolite and Rubber. For the tread footwear pad, there were grooves (1 mm wide, 3 mm deep) evenly spaced on the pad and the grooves are perpendicular to the friction measurement direction. The hardness of the Neolite and Rubber were 91±1.73 and 47±0.82 respectively.

The COF was measured under the surface conditions of dry, wet and glycerol. For the wet conditions, water was replenished in the footwear striking area during repeated strikes. The amount of water for each replenishing was 10 ml. For the glycerol conditions, glycerol was dripped evenly in the footwear striking area before each strike. The amount of glycerol replenished each time was 5 cc. There are two different terrazzo floor used in the COF measurement including regular one and the one installed 3M anti-slip strips (anti-slip floor).

The Brungraber Mark II (BM II) slipmeter was used to measure the COF. BM II has been applied to conduct friction measurement in labs and workplace [14]. The study operated BM II according to the standard test method of using the BM II published by the American Society for Testing and Materials [15]. In addition, the protocol in judging a slip or no-slip suggested by Chang [16] was used.

Finally, the study uses Paired-Samples T-test to compare the COF under different footwear materials, floor contaminates and floor.

3 Results and Discussion

The results reveal that the installing of anti-slip strips will significantly ($p<0.001$) increase the COF. Under the dry surface condition, the COF will increase 0.623、0.621、0.423 and 0.26 separately with tread Neolite、no-tread Neolite、tread Rubber、no tread Rubber shoe materials. Under the wet floor condition, with tread neolite, no tread neolite, tread rubber, no tread rubber shoe materials, the COF will increase 0.624、0.950、0.442 and 0.945 separately. Finally, under the glycerol surface condition, the COF will increase 0.799、0.068、0.572 and 0.138 separately with tread neolite, no tread neolite, tread rubber, no tread rubber shoe materials (see table 1). Therefore, as the results shown in table 1, the anti-slip strips provide better COF significantly with the floor contaminated by water. When the floor is contaminated by oil, the tread footwear pads should be used to increase the anti-slip effect.

Table 1. Mean and Standard Deviation of the COF

Footwear pads	Surface conditions	Anti-slip floor	Terrazzo floor	Friction increase	t-value	p-value
Tread Neolite	Dry	1.073 (0.008)	0.450 (0.006)	0.623	147.836	<0.001
	Wet	1.032 (0.008)	0.408 (0.008)	0.624	111.754	<0.001
	glycerol	0.827 (0.008)	0.028 (0.004)	0.799	198.894	<0.001
No-tread Neolite	Dry	1.078 (0.008)	0.457 (0.008)	0.621	154.880	<0.001
	Wet	0.990 (0.006)	0.040 (0.006)	0.950	260.168	<0.001
	glycerol	0.068 (0.008)	0.001 (0.000)	0.068	22.235	<0.001
Tread Rubber	Dry	1.100 (0.000)	0.677 (0.008)	0.423	127.000	<0.001
	Wet	1.100 (0.000)	0.658 (0.008)	0.442	143.716	<0.001
	glycerol	0.855 (0.005)	0.283 (0.008)	0.572	186.018	<0.001
No -tread Rubber	Dry	1.100 (0.000)	0.840 (0.009)	0.260	71.204	<0.001
	Wet	0.998 (0.008)	0.053 (0.005)	0.945	276.668	<0.001
	glycerol	0.138 (0.008)	0.001 (0.000)	0.138	45.013	<0.001

Only the tread rubber footwear on the wet floor and no tread footwear on the dry floor show anti-slip effects on regular terrazzo floor. The anti-slip effects are not significant when wearing no-tread footwear and walking on the floor contaminated by glycerol (see Fig.1). Therefore, adopting the tread shoes and anti-slip strips at the same time will improve the slip-resistance effect dramatically.

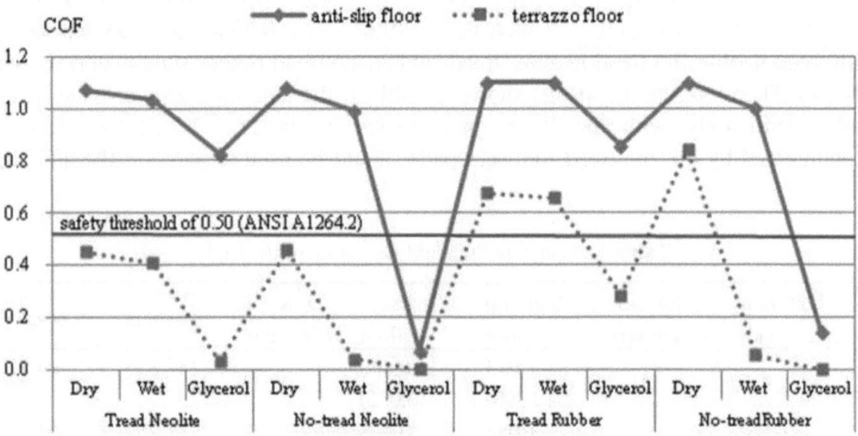

Fig. 1. The comparison of the COF under two different floors

The anti-slip strips covered by steel grit provide valid slip-resistance effect. However, the slip-resistance effect will be limited when the floor covered by oil and the grooves of footwear have been wear away. In total, to provide valid slip-resistance effect, keeping the floor dry, installing the anti-slip strips, wearing tread shoes are some useful processes to reduce the risk of falling and slipping.

4 Conclusion

Anti-slip strip is one of the most popular slip-resistant products indoor and outdoor. The study compared the effects of slip-resistant under different floor contamination conditions while using the anti-slip strip. The results demonstrated that emery anti-slip strip is really helpful on resisting slipping no matter the floor is dry or wet. However, when the floor is covered by oil, the anti-slip strips provide slip resistance effects only if the workers wear the tread shoes. Therefore, in order to perform the best ant-slip effect, the floors not only need to be kept dry, but also need to be installed with some anti-slip devices. Of course wearing the tread footwear and keeping the grooves wide & deep enough will reduces the risk of falling and slipping successfully.

Acknowledgments. This research was financially supported by the National Science Council of the Republic of China under the grant NSC 100-2221-E-266-003.

References

1. Leamon, T.B., Murphy, P.L.: Occupational slips and falls: more than a trivial problem. Ergonomics 38(3), 487–498 (1995)
2. Centers for Disease Control and Prevention, National Center for Injury Prevention and Control, Web-based Injury Statistics Query and Reporting System(WISQARS), http://www.cdc.gov/injury/wisqars/index.html (2010)

3. Grönqvist, R., Abeysekera, J., Gard, G., Hsiang, S.M., Leamon, T.B., Newman, D.J., Gielo-Perczak, K., Lockhart, T.E., Pai, Y.C.: Human-centered approaches in slipperiness measurement. Ergonomics 44, 1167–1199 (2001)
4. Chang, W.R., Matz, S.: The Slip Resistance of Common Footwear Materials Measured with Two Slipmeters. Applied Ergonomics 32(6), 549–558 (2001)
5. Li, K.W., Wu, H.H., Lin, Y.C.: The effect of shoe sole tread groove depth on the friction coefficient with different tread groove widths, floors and contaminants. Applied Ergonomics 37, 743–748 (2006a)
6. Li, K.W., Chang, W.R., Wei, J.C., Kou, C.H.: Friction Measurement on Ramps Using the Brungraber Mark II Slipmeter. Safety Science 44, 375–386 (2006b)
7. Chang, W.R., Grönqvist, R., Leclercq, S., Myung, R., Makkonen, L., Strandberg, L., Brungraber, R.J., Mattke, U., Thorpe, S.C.: The Role of Friction in the Measurement of Slipperiness, Part1; Friction Mechaniness and Definition of Test Conditions. Ergonomics 44(13), 1217–1232 (2001)
8. Miller, J.M.: "Slippery" work surface: Toward a performance definition and quantitative coefficient of friction criteria. Journal of Safety Research 14, 145–158 (1983)
9. American Society of Safety Engineers, ANSI/ASSE A1264.2, Provision of Slip Resistance on Walking/Working Surfaces, American National Standard for Construction and Demolition Operations, American National Standards Institute, Inc. (2006)
10. Moore, D.F.: The friction and lubrication of elastomers. Pergamon Press (1972)
11. Liu, L.W., Li, K.W., Lee, Y.H., Chen, C.C., Chen, C.Y.: Friction measurements on "anti-slip" floors under shoe sole, contamination, and inclination conditions. Safety Science 48(10), 1321–1326 (2010)
12. Kim, I.J., Smith, R., Nagata, H.: Microscopic observations of the progressive wear on the shoe surfaces that affect the slip resistance characteristics. International Journal of Industrial Ergonomics 28(1), 17–29 (2001)
13. Kim, I.J.: Development of a new analyzing model for quantifying pedestrian slip resistance characteristics: Part Ⅰ - Basic concepts and theories. International Journal of Industrial Ergonomics 33(5), 395 - 401 (2004a)
14. Kim, I.J.: Development of a new analyzing model for quantifying pedestrian slip resistance characteristics: Part Ⅱ - Experiments and validations. International Journal of Industrial Ergonomics 33(5), 403 - 414 (2004b)
15. American Society for Testing and Materials, F-1677-96, Standard method of test for using a portable inclinable articulated strut slip tester (PIAST), Annual Book of ASTM Standards. vol. 15.07. West Conshohochen, PA, American Society for Testing and Materials (2005)
16. Chang, W.R.: The Effect of Slip Criterion and Time on Friction Measurement. Safety Science 40(7-8), 593–611 (2002)

Analysis of Perceived Discomfort and EMG for Touch Locations of a Soft Keyboard*

Bori Choi, Sukbong Park, and Kihyo Jung**

School of Industrial Engineering, University of Ulsan, Ulsan 680-749, South Korea
bori486@hanmail.net, khaipsb2000@naver.com, kjung@ulsan.ac.kr

Abstract. With diversity of mobile services (e.g., messenger, and social network service) on smartphone, the demand of text input using a soft keyboard is increasing. However, studies on subjective and physiological responses of users for various touch locations are lacking. The present study investigated the ergonomic responses according to touch locations of a soft keyboard on smartphone. The experiment of the present study measured perceived discomfort using Borg's CR-10 scale and electromyography on forearm (abductor pollicis longus, and extensor digitorum communis) and thumb (abductor pollicis brevis, and first dorsal interossei) muscles. Perceived discomfort was significantly varied from 0.7 (extremely weak discomfort) to 2.5 (weak discomfort) depending on touch locations. %MVC at abductor pollicis brevis was significantly varied from 10% to 23% according to touch locations. The experimental results of the present study can be utilized in the ergonomic design of a soft keyboard.

Keywords: Soft Keyboard, Discomfort, EMG, Two-thumb Input, Smartphone.

1 Introduction

Recently, with diversity of the smartphone services, the frequency of text input using soft keyboard has increased. It has reported that 88% of users are using the information search, email, and web-surfing on smartphone (KISA, 2011). Furthermore, 79.6% of smartphone users have used messenger or social network services. From these reasons, the demand of the text entry with soft keyboard has been increased.

The layout of soft keyboards can be classified into 2 types: 1) 3×4 layout, 2) QWERTY layout. The 3×4 layout consists of 12 buttons and is similar to the traditional layout used in a cellular phone. On the other hands, the QWERTY layout consists of 26 buttons and is similar to the standard PC keyboard.

Various studies related to the soft keyboard have been carried out; however, they still have limits in three aspects: two-thumb entry, electromyography (EMG) analysis,

* This research was supported by Basic Science Research Program through the National Research Foundation of Korea (NRF) funded by the Ministry of Education, Science and Technology (2012-011373).

** Corresponding author.

C. Stephanidis (Ed.): Posters, Part I, HCII 2013, CCIS 373, pp. 518–522, 2013.

and grip position. First, studies on two-thumb entry are rare compared to one-thumb entry (Karlson, 2006). Second, EMG studies are few (Park, 2010; Ryu, 2011; Kim et al., 2011) because text entry on smartphone is conducted by small muscles in the thumb. Finally, most of the perceived discomfort studies for various touch locations (Park and Han, 2007) did not take account of the smartphone grip strategy for text entry.

This study analyzed perceived discomfort and EMG for touch locations of a soft keyboard. The locations of touch divided into five lows and five columns. EMG was measured on two muscles of the thumb and two muscles of the forearm by referring to Jonsson et al., 2011. The experimental results obtained in this study can be utilized to design of soft keyboard for smartphones.

2 Methods and Material

2.1 Participants

Ten male participants with smartphone usage experience were involved in this experiment. Their average age was 24.7 and their dominant hand was all right-side. The participants did not have any pain or discomfort on the thumbs and upper extremity at the experimental day.

2.2 EMG Measurement Protocol

Surface EMG system (Telemyo, Noraxon, USA) was used in this experiment. The diameter of surface electrode (Bio Protech, South Korea) was 1 cm and the centroid distance between a pair of electrodes was 2.5 cm. The MyoResearch XP Master Edition (Noraxon, USA) was used in measurement and analysis of EMG. This study used four pairs of electrodes to measure EMG signals with 1,000 Hz sampling rate on four muscles.

Four measurement muscles were selected by referring to a related study (Jonsson et al., 2011). Two muscles (abductor pollicis brevis (APB) and extrinsic muscle abductor pollicis longus (APL)) of the four were related to the movement of the thumb. APB and APL identically relate to thumb abduction motion; however, they are intrinsic muscle and extrinsic muscle, respectively. The rest of two muscles (first dorsal interossei, (FDI), extensor digitorum communis (EDC)) were related to the movement of the fingers (index, middle, ring, and little fingers). FDI and EDC relate to flexion and extension motions, respectively. They are intrinsic and extrinsic muscles.

2.3 Experimental Design

One factor (touch location) within-subject design was applied in the experiment. Touch location consisted of 5 rows and 5 columns as illustrated in Fig 1. The touch thumb was designated to each of the column based on users' touch behavior. For the left 2 columns, the buttons were touched by the left thumb; for the right 2 columns, the buttons were touched by the right thumb; lastly, for the middle column, the buttons were touched by both the left and right thumbs.

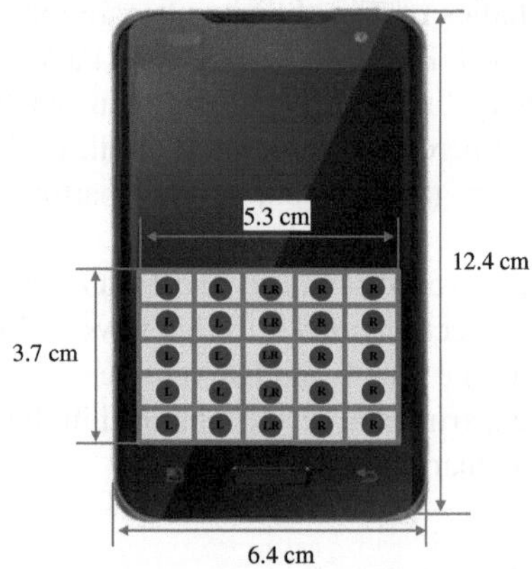

Fig. 1. Touch locations (L: left thumb, R: right thumb, LR: left and right thumb)

Dependent variables were two (rating of perceived discomfort and percent of maximum voluntary contraction (%MVC)). Perceived discomfort was measured by Borg's CR-10 scale (Kwon et al., 2009; Borg, 1998). %MVC was calculated by dividing measured voltage with MVC of each participant. MVC of the present study was measured by applying the Caldwell protocol (Chaffin et al., 1999).

The experiment of this study was conducted by 6 stages (introduction, electrode attachment, MVC measurement, practice, main experiment, and debriefing). First, we explained research purpose and experimental methods to each participant and obtained informed consent. Second, the electrodes were attached on the muscles of participants. Third, MVC of each participant was measured by applying the Caldwell protocol. Fourth, enough practice was allowed participants to accustom the experiment method and procedure. Fifth, the main experiment was conducted which presses the button of soft keyboard in random order. Finally, a brief debriefing was carried out.

2.4 Analysis Protocol

EMG data was analyzed in 4 stages (rectification, smoothing, RMS calculation, %MVC calculation). First, EMG data was rectified. Second, rectified data was smoothed (RMS window = 100 ms) in order to eliminate noise. Third, root mean square (RMS) for the smoothed data was calculated. Finally, %MVC was calculated by dividing RMS with MVC.

The statistical analysis of the present study was conducted using MINITAB 16.0 (Minitab Inc., USA) with significance level (α) 0.05. One-factor within subject ANOVA was carried out for each of touch location (25 levels), touch row (5 levels), and touch column (5 levels). As post-hoc analysis, Bonferroni test was applied.

3 Results

The perceived discomforts for each touch location were significantly different ($F(24, 215) = 7.38$, $p < 0.001$). Maximum value (2.5: weak) of the perceived discomforts was 3.5 times greater than the minimum value (0.7: very weak). On the other hand, the perceived discomforts between the left and right thumbs were not significant ($F(1, 238) = 0.04$, $p = 0.84$).

The perceived discomforts of 2nd and 4th columns were significantly lower than those of other columns ($F(4, 235) = 2.99$, $p = 0.02$; Fig 2.a). The perceived discomforts were divided into two: 1) small discomfort group: 2nd column ($\bar{x} \pm SE$; 1.19 ± 0.13) and 4th column (1.21 ± 0.13), 2) large discomfort group: 1st column (1.45 ± 0.13), 5th column (1.54 ± 1.13), and 3rd column (1.55 ± 1.60). This tendency seems to be caused because the initial locations of the left thumb and right thumb were located around 2nd and 4th columns, respectively.

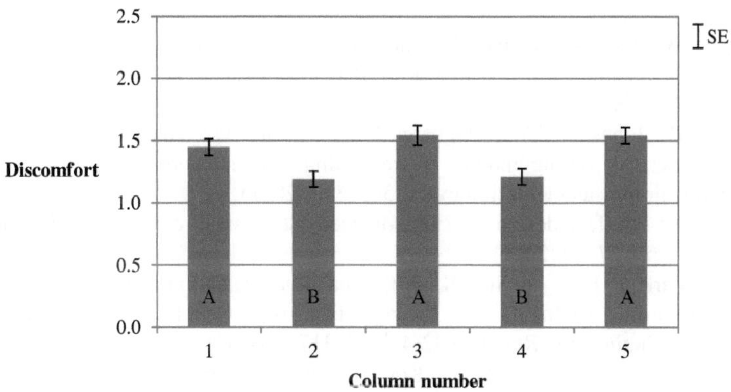

(a) Touch column

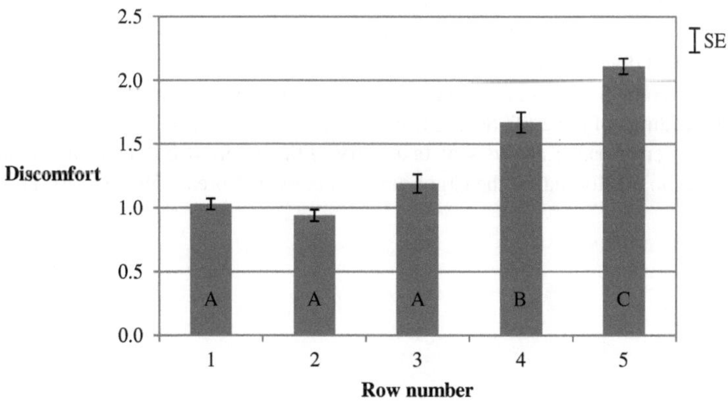

(b) Touch row

Fig. 2. Perceived discomfort for touch columns and rows

The perceived discomforts of upper rows (1st - 3rd) were significantly lower than those of lower rows (4th and 5th) ($F(4, 235) = 36.37$, $p < 0.001$; Fig 2.b). The perceived discomforts for rows were divided into two: 1) small discomfort group: 2nd row (0.94 ± 0.09), 1st row (1.03 ± 0.09), 3rd row (1.03 ± 0.09), 2) large discomfort group: 4th row (1.67 ± 0.16) and 5th row (2.11 ± 0.12). This tendency seems to be explained by the initial location of the thumbs, which located around 2nd row.

%MVC for APB was only significant across touch rows ($F(24, 216) = 3.55$, $p< 0.001$) and columns ($F(24, 216) = 3.55$, $p< 0.001$). %MVC for the left thumb's APB increased 1st (10 ± 0.9), 2^{nd}(13 ± 1.2), and 3rd (23 ± 1.8) columns in ascending order. Similarly, %MVC for the right thumb's APB increased 5th (16 ± 1.8), 4th (18 ± 1.5), and 3rd (23 ± 1.8) columns in ascending order. In addition, %MVC for APB significantly increased from 1st row (13 ± 1.4) to 5th row (20 ± 1.8). This trend was occurred because APB muscle is contracted while the thumb is abducted.

References

1. Borg, G.: Borg's Perceived Exertion and Pain Scales. Human Kinetics, Champaign (1998)
2. Chaffin, D.B., Andersson, G.B.J., Martin, B.J.: Occupational Biomechanics, 3rd edn. John Wiley & Sons, New York (1999)
3. Jonsson, P., Johnson, P.W., Hagberg, M., Forsman, M.: Thumb joint movement and muscular activity during mobile phone texting – A methodological study. Journal of Electromyography and Kinesiology 21, 363–370 (2011)
4. Karlson, A.: Interface design for single-handed use of small devices. UIST 2006 Adjunct Proceeding, pp. 27–30 (2006)
5. Kim, K., Park, J., Kim, G., Son, K.: A Comparative evaluation about force and fatigue on thumb according to input type for repetitive use of mobile phone. Journal of the Biomedical Engineering Research 32(4), 312–317 (2011)
6. KISA, Smartphone Usage Statistics. Korea Internet and Security Agency (2011)
7. Kwon, O., You, H., Jung, K.: Identification of the maximum acceptable frequencies of upper-extremity motions in the sagittal plane. Human Factors and Ergonomics in Manufacturing 19(3), 212–222 (2009)
8. Park, Y.: User Interface Design for One-handed Touch Interaction with Mobile Devices. Unpublished doctorial dissertation. POSTECH, Pohang (2010)
9. Park, Y., Han, S.: Effects of touch key location and size on one-handed thumb input. In: Proceedings of the 2007 Spring Conference of Ergonomics Society of Korea (2007)
10. Ryu, T.: Performance analysis of text entry with preferred one hand using smart phone touch-keyboard. Journal of the Ergonomics Society of Korea, 259–264 (2011)

Servo-actuated Stylus for Post Stroke Arm and Fore Arm Rehabilitation

Mario Covarrubias, Monica Bordegoni, and Umberto Cugini

Politecnico di Milano, Dipartimento di Meccanica
via G. La Masa, 1, 20146 Milano, Italy
{mario.covarrubias,monica.bordegoni,umberto.cugini}@polimi.it
www.kaemart.it

Abstract. This paper describes the design and implementation of a 1-DOF servo-actuated stylus, which is used as an end effector in a desktop haptic device. The desktop haptic device is part of a multimodal system aimed for the assessment, training and rehabilitation of the arm, forearm and hand while the user perform several tasks. Patients will use the haptic device which carries out the servo-actuated stylus in order to draw simple and complex sketches, in this way, the patient is able to feel the virtual sketch by using the haptic device, which acts as a virtual guide taking advantages of its force feedback capabilities. The therapist is able to control the 1-DOF-stylus rotation according to the requirements of the patient.

Keywords: Haptic Guidance, Sketching task, Stroke patient, Multimodal system.

1 Introduction

Rehabilitation after a stroke is a long process and usually the therapist guides the patient verbally as well as physically. For example, if the patient needs to perform a 2D rectangular sketch motion, the therapist will say now, lets draw a rectangle as she or he begins guiding the patients hand. A sketch is a rapidly executed freehand drawing that is not intended as a finished work. Sketching is one of the most important and complex human activities in which the hand movements are controlled by the central nervous system, which regulates the activity of the hand and arm muscles to act in synergy. The central nervous system receives dynamic feedback information from visual sensors and from other body sensors located on the skin, muscles and joints while regulating the motor output. In case of rehabilitation after a stroke, one important factor is motivation [1]. The guidance haptic device concept has been described in [2], while the multimodal system has been described in [3] which consisting in a combination of visual, haptic and sound technologies, aims to be a step forward in the field of multimodal devices for supporting unskilled people to improve their skills and in the assessment of manual activities. Sketching, hatching and cutting tasks are assisted through the haptic guidance device. The drawn shape can also be physically produced as a piece of polystyrene foam as shown in Figure 1.

C. Stephanidis (Ed.): Posters, Part I, HCII 2013, CCIS 373, pp. 523–527, 2013.

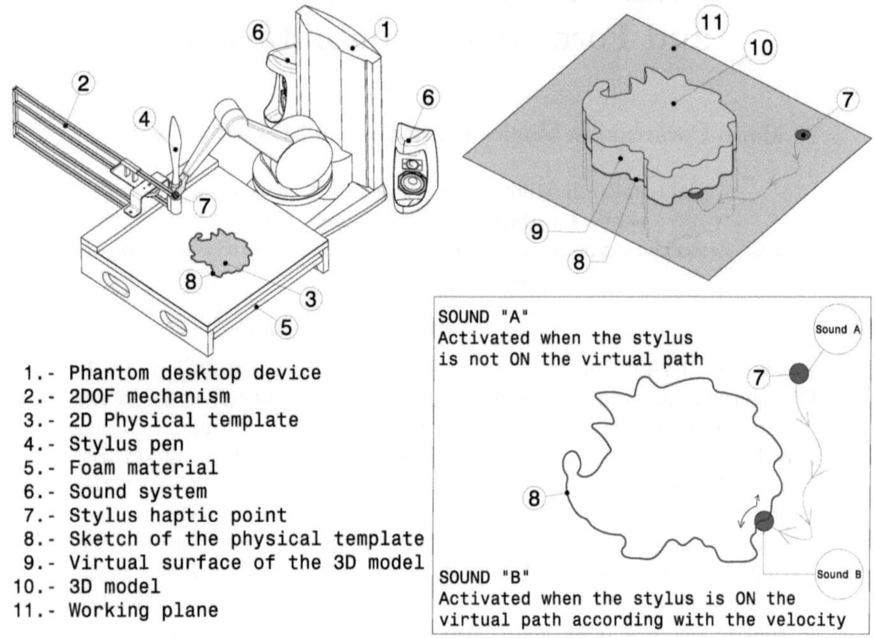

Fig. 1. Concept of the Multimodal System

The user is sitting in front of the haptic guidance device in a comfortable way, and then by handling the stylus (4) tries to follow the sketch (8) from the physical template (3) in order to perform the 2D tasks. These tasks are driven by the operators movement and assisted by the Magnetic Geometry Effect (MGE). The MGE constraint is linked to the external surface (9) of the virtual object that has been previously created by using a CAD software and the stylus haptic point (7). When this option is activated, a spring force tries to pull the sphere of the stylus (7) of the haptic device towards the virtual surface (9) of the 3D model (10). In fact, this effect is used to assist the users hand movements. In the cutting modality, while user follows the 2D template (8) by using the MGS, the wire tool, which is carried out by the 2DOF mechanism (2) cuts the polystyrene foam (5). The polystyrene foam is an interchangeable element. Note that in the intersection between the external surface (9) and the stylus haptic point (7), there is a working plane (11). In fact, this working plane is a physical constraint created by the 2DOF mechanism linked to the Phantom device (1). Figure 1 also shows in detail the sound strategy that has been adopted. In the multimodal system, the stylus (4) can freely rotate according to the hand movement.

2 Servo-controlled Stylus

According to preliminary test with stroke patients using our system, in which the therapist was involved in order to run a therapy session, we have noted the necessity to provide an additional degree of freedom to the stylus (4). Figure 2-a shows the patient's hand while tries to grasp the stylus. Figures 2-b and Figure 2-c show the therapist hand while guiding the patients hand in order to perform the sketching test. Figures 2-d and Figure 2-e show the patient performing the test without the therapist help. The patient is not able to control the radial deviation, flexion and extension of the hand as a result of the stroke and is not able to correct positioning the stylus in order to perform the sketching test.

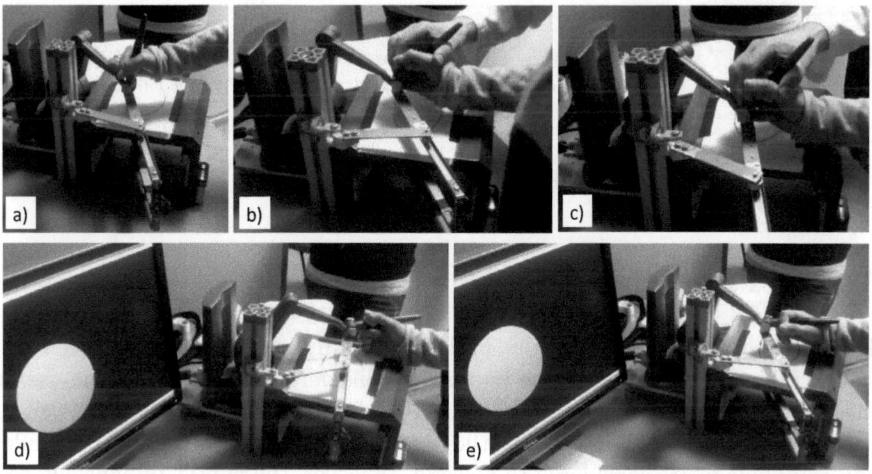

Fig. 2. Therapist guiding the user's hand

2.1 Biomechanics of Human Arm

The human arm has seven degrees of freedom: Abduction/adduction and flexion/extension of the shoulder; rotation of the upper arm; flexion/extension of the elbow; rotation of the forearm; and radial/ulnar deviation and flexion/extension of the wrist.

This paper presents the design and implementation of a 1-DOF servo-actuated stylus, which is driven by the therapist in order to allow the patient to correct handle the stylus according to the rehabilitation task. Figure 3-a shows the ideal position for the users hand while Figures 3-b and Figure 3-c show several problems in reaching the stylus. Figure 3-d shows the concept of our approach in which the stylus is driven by a servo-actuator. This servo-actuator is driven by the therapist in order to rotate the stylus according to the specific needs required in the rehabilitation task. In this way, once the user is able to correct handle the stylus, then is able to perform the sketch operation by using the multimodal system.

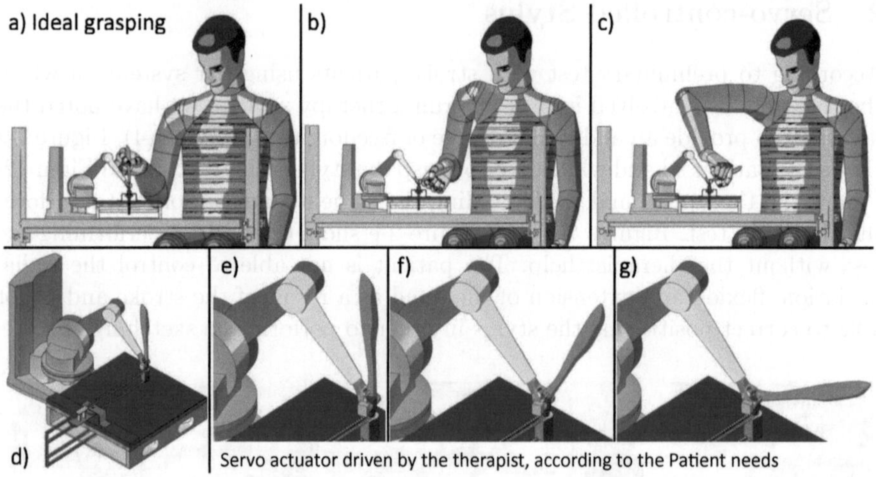

Fig. 3. Postural position problems

3 The Prototype

The main structure used for the Multimodal Guidance System has been designed taking into account some important considerations related to the use of sheet metal and aluminum components that implies: low inertia, light weight parts and low friction. Regarding the static and dynamic modeling, the links and components are considered to be rigid. However, the haptic guidance device is not a rigid structure. To provide this stiffness, the links have been designed as beams or shell structures. Also, the mounting arrangement of the main structure has been designed to accommodate manufacturing tolerances. Figure 4-a shows the prototype of the device and Figures 4-b and Figure 4-c show two different positions on the stylus while the user sketching a circle in a therapy session. A force and torque analysis have been performed in Visual Nastran 4D.The results of these analysis have been used to select the actuators. In fact, the servo drives have been selected so as to guarantee high reliability: the servo motor with titanium gears provides up to 2.35 Nm of continuous torque. The servo drives are HS-5955TG manufactured by HITEC [4]. This allows us to get high stiffness and load capacity.

The therapist is able to control the rotation of the stylus from -75 to 0 degrees through a computer interface which allow the signal communication between the computer and the DMX Servo-12 controller board.

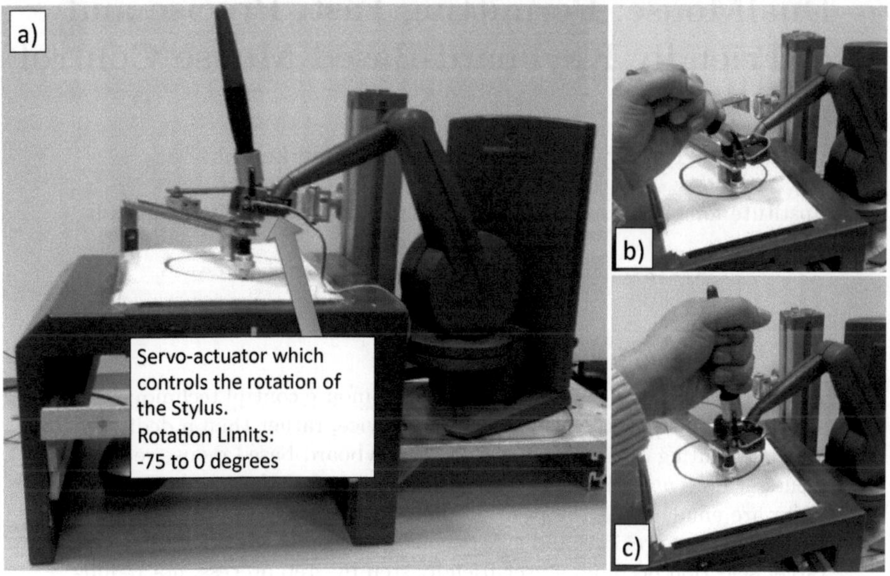

Fig. 4. The prototype

References

1. Mihelj, M., Novak, D., Milavec, M., Ziherl, J., Olenšek, A., Munih, M.: Virtual rehabilitation environment using principles of intrinsic motivation and game design. Presence: Teleoperators and Virtual Environments 21(1), 1–15 (2012) ISBN 1054-7460, http://www.mitpressjournals.org/doi/abs/10.1162/PRES_a_00078 (April 05, 2013)
2. Covarrubias, M., Bordegoni, M., Cugini, U.: Sketching haptic system based on point-based approach for assisting people with down syndrome. In: Stephanidis, C. (ed.) Posters, Part I, HCII 2011. CCIS, vol. 173, pp. 378–382. Springer, Heidelberg (2011)
3. Covarrubias, M., Gatti, E., Mansutti, A., Bordegoni, M., Cugini, U.: Multimodal guidance system for improving manual skills in disabled people. In: Miesenberger, K., Karshmer, A., Penaz, P., Zagler, W. (eds.) ICCHP 2012, Part I. LNCS, vol. 7382, pp. 227–234. Springer, Heidelberg (2012)
4. HITEC servos, http://www.hitecrcd.com/ (accessed January 25, 2013)

DualMouse: Permitting Fast, Precise and User-Friendly Keyboard-Based Mouse Control

Torsten Felzer and Stephan Rinderknecht

Institute for Mechatronic Systems, Technische Universität Darmstadt,
Darmstadt, Germany
{felzer,rinderknecht}@ims.tu-darmstadt.de

Abstract. This paper presents an unusual mouse control technique, designed to be used with a keyboard-type device, rather than a dedicated manual pointing device. Unlike ordinary keyboard-based mouse replacements, it does not rely on pointer movements across the screen. Instead, clicks are emulated at the position directly chosen by the user (who recursively selects regions and sub-regions to do that). As a consequence, target selection becomes a user-friendly step-by-step process, not requiring any time-critical interaction.

Keywords: human-computer interaction, keyboard replacement, word completion, ambiguous keyboards, mouse emulator, neuromuscular diseases, Friedreich's Ataxia.

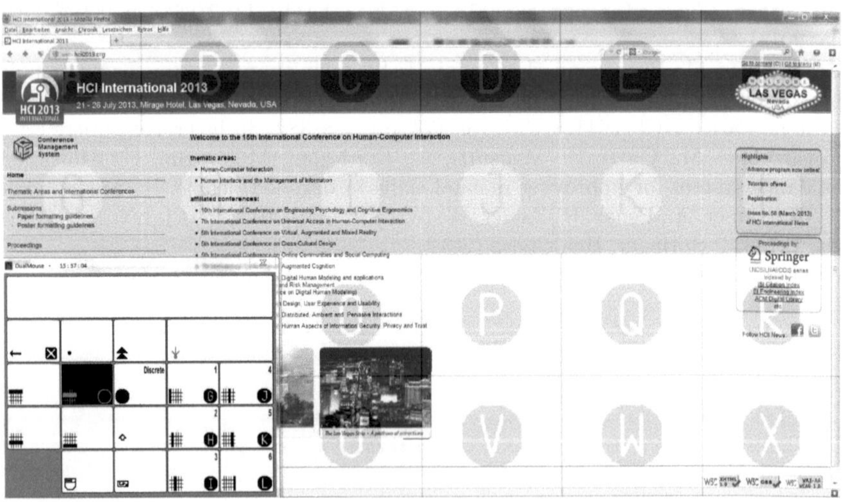

Fig. 1. Initial target acquisition step in *DualMouse* when issuing a click on the HCI International 2013 website

C. Stephanidis (Ed.): Posters, Part I, HCII 2013, CCIS 373, pp. 528–532, 2013.

1 Introduction

Persons with neuromuscular diseases – who usually have specific problems with fine motor control – regularly struggle with the standard input device when operating a computer: a large manual keyboard. As typing can often only be done with few fingers and with a limited individual range, "traveling" from one key to the next generally requires constant lifting and repositioning of the hands. This makes keyboard usage a very slow and cumbersome task, involving a lot of erroneous keystrokes.

To facilitate computer operation for the mentioned population, we developed the asistive tool *OnScreenDualScribe* [2], which is based on the modified numerical keypad depicted in fig. 2. The tool is a replacement of the full-size keyboard and as such primarily optimized for text entry (offering word completion and an ambiguous keyboard [4] – both using a 100,000 word dictionary based on [1]). However, it depends on an internal mouse mode for efficient operation (since using a second manual device for pointing operations – to switch windows, for example – would be very uneconomical).

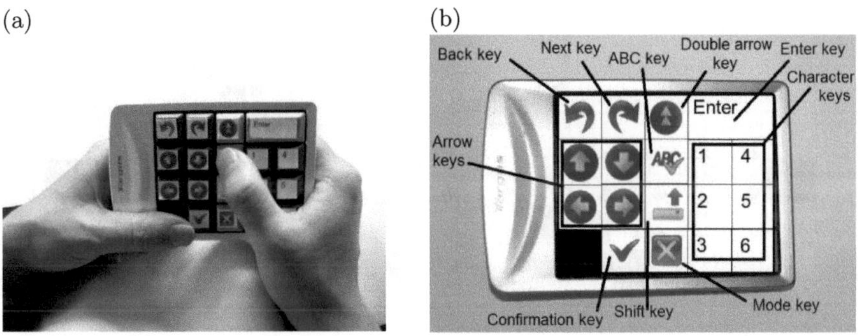

Fig. 2. Input device used in *OnScreenDualScribe*; (a) user can reach every key with either thumb without repositioning the hands; left and right edges serve as tactile guide when aiming at the keys; (b) key layout

The current implementation of this mouse mode poses a problem for many of the intended users. An alternative technique, called *DualMouse*, eliminates these shortcomings. Currently implemented as an own application (supporting the same input device), the technique suggests itself to be included in a new version of *OnScreenDualScribe*.

2 Keyboard-Based Mouse Control

When designing a mouse control that depends on keystrokes only (as opposed to two-dimensional displacements with – or on – a dedicated pointing device), the challenge is to allow for quickly bridging large distances on the screen, while simultaneously fostering a high precision near the target area. In an ordinary keyboard mouse (e.g., [5]), some keys allow moving the mouse pointer in a cardinal direction, while others trigger clicks of various types at the current pointer position. Pointer movement can either be active (meaning that the pointer moves in one direction for as long as the corresponding key is held down) or passive (where the user starts a movement in one direction, which continues until a particular input event).

In this sense, the currently implemented mouse mode of *OnScreenDualScribe* is a passive keyboard mouse. Using the terminology of fig. 2, the mouse pointer begins moving up, down, to the left, or to the right, in response to pressing one of the four Arrow keys. This movement is repeated until the user either selects a different direction or presses one of the six Character keys (each generating a different type of click – single, double, left, right, drag – at the current position). To make it possible to pinpoint a single pixel, the movement is initially very slow. By pressing the Arrow key belonging to the selected direction again, the movement speed can gradually be increased (to coarsely slide over the screen). Unfortunately, this is a pitfall for the target population of *OnScreenDualScribe*: persons with neuromuscular diseases. Due to a longer reaction time, they often fail to stop a movement early enough (once accelerated), potentially resulting in repeated overshooting.

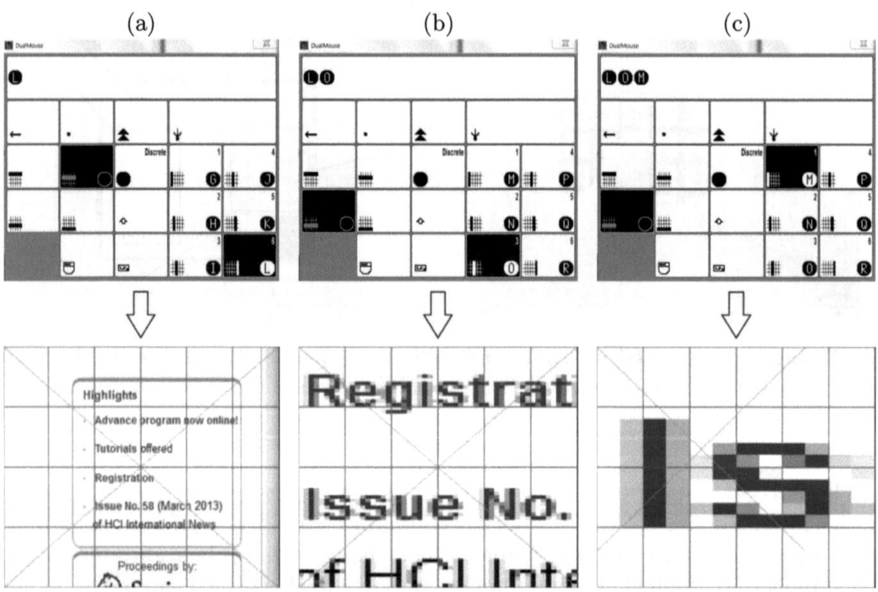

Fig. 3. Using the *DualMouse* technique, the link to HCI International News (being an example click target) is reached with six keystrokes: ↓, 6, ←, 3, ←, 1

3 *DualMouse* Approach

DualMouse does not rely on the mouse pointer traveling across the screen. Rather, the user directly determines where to issue a click, and the software emulates necessary input events. To realize that, the screen is split into 24 rectangular regions, arranged in four rows and six columns (as in fig. 1).

Let's say, we want to click on the link to HCI International News on the HCI International 2013 website. By successively pressing the second Arrow key (↓) and the sixth Character key (6), the user selects the region that contains the desired click target (region L). The selected region is then split into 24 sub-regions, and the selection process is recursively repeated until the target is narrowed down (see fig. 3). Pressing the Enter key evokes the emulation of a click in the center of the sub-region selected at that instant (as shown in fig. 4).

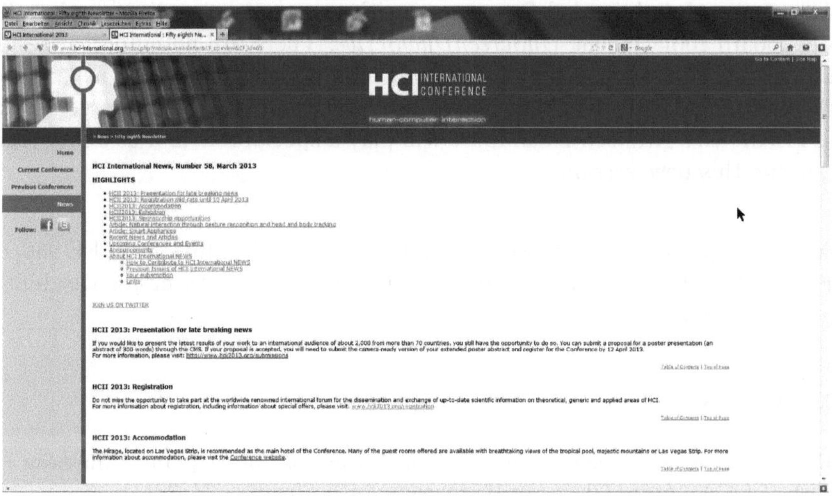

Fig. 4. Result after finally pressing the Enter key

The type of that click event can be selected any time prior to the final trigger signal, that is, before, during, or after target selection. Since also dragging is supported (by prompting for start and endpoint one after another), the idea can be used to replace a two-button mouse device almost completely. Only hovering does not work: of course, it is possible to set the pointer to a new position without actually performing a click in the initial implementation of the approach, but that only approximates the true functionality of hovering.

Target acquisition is rather efficient. Suppose, for example, the user's computer has a screen resolution of 1600×900 (or less). Since $6^5 \geq 1600$ *and* $4^5 \geq 900$, at most 5 recursive steps (or – including Enter at the end – at most 11 keystrokes) are needed to perform a single left click (the default) on any arbitrary pixel. To facilitate precise clicking, sub-regions along the way are visually enlarged (as in [3]) – pressing the Back key at any point takes back the last recursive step and, thus, zooms out. Most importantly, the user can apply the technique at his or her own pace, and is not forced to make an input at a split second dictated by the software.

4 Conclusion

DualMouse, an alternative interaction technique allowing to perform pointing operations with the help of a keyboard-type device, has been described. What makes the approach different from other mouse replacements is that the mouse pointer does not steadily move to a target position, but it "jumps" to the point specified by the user. Choosing the click target is done in a recursive process involving zooming in on rectangular portions of the screen. The method is very user-friendly since it does not require producing particular input signals within a certain time frame.

The approach is intended for persons with neuromuscular diseases, just like the keyboard replacement *OnScreenDualScribe*. There are no empirical results available yet. However, it is planned to include the technique in a new version of the aforementioned tool (which is in use – on a daily basis – by a gentleman with Friedreich's Ataxia). *DualMouse* will play a special role in a usability study evaluating this new version.

Acknowledgments. This work is partially supported by DFG grant FE 936/6-1 "EFFENDI – EFficient and Fast text ENtry for persons with motor Disabilities of neuromuscular orIgin".

References

1. Davies, M.: Word frequency data from the Corpus of Contemporary American English (COCA), `http://www.wordfrequency.info` (January 27, 2011)
2. Felzer, T., MacKenzie, I.S., Rinderknecht, S.: OnScreenDualScribe: A computer operation tool for users with a neuromuscular disease. In: Stephanidis, C., Antona, M. (eds.) UAHCI/HCII 2013, Part I. LNCS, vol. 8009, pp. 474–483. Springer, Heidelberg (2013)
3. Grossman, T., Balakrishnan, R.: The bubble cursor: Enhancing target acquisition by dynamic resizing of the cursor's activation area. In: Proc. CHI 2005, pp. 281–290. ACM Press (2005)
4. MacKenzie, I.S., Felzer, T.: SAK: Scanning Ambiguous Keyboard for efficient one-key text entry. ACM Transactions on Computer-Human Interaction (TOCHI) 17(3), 11:1–11:39 (2010)
5. RH Designs: Mouse emulator, `http://rhdesigns.browseto.org/mouseemulator.html` (accessed on April 3, 2013)

Comparisons of Computer Exposure and Forearm Musculoskeletal Symptoms among Three Computer Groups-The Application of an External Logger

Wei-Hsien Hong[1], Hsieh-Ching Chen[2], Ya-Hsiu Hsu[3], and Hsin-Chieh Wu[3]

[1] Department of Sports Medicine, China Medical University, Taiwan
[2] Department of Industrial Engineering and Management, National Taipei University of Technology, Taiwan
[3] Department of Industrial Engineering and Management, Chaoyang University of Technology, Taiwan
whhong@mail.cmu.edu.tw

Abstract. This study aim was to compare the computer exposure and forearm musculoskeletal symptoms among three computer use groups by an external logger. 30 participants were recruited in this study and divided into three groups: 10 computer-document (CD) processors, 10 computer-aided design (CAD) draftsmen, and 10 online gamers. Computer use of each participant was recorded for 10 consecutive days. Questionnaire survey was conducted to collect musculoskeletal complaints in participants' upper limbs right after data collection period. Quantitative parameters computed using recorded data were daily keystrokes, mouse clicks, wheel scrolling counts, mouse movement and dragged distance. Experimental results showed that the online gamers had the significantly higher keyboard activities than typical keyboard users, CD processors. Also, it had the higher mouse activities than the typical mouse users, CAD draftsmen. However, musculoskeletal complaint in their upper limbs was not greater than that of CD processors and CAD draftsmen. There existed a complicate relationship between cumulative hazards and computer uses. Experimental results indicated that computer use duration alone could not accurately represent the workloads of various computer tasks. Adequate tools are needed for quantifying user computer exposure and providing detailed information for various computer tasks.

Keywords: Computer exposure, Online game, Computer input, External logger.

1 Introduction

Previous studies showed that prolonged computer use was positive correlation with work-related upper extremity disorders. Study investigation pointed out that the hand, wrist, and arm pain of computer operators exceeded other body parts [1,2]. Szabo (1998) study showed that 21% of work-related carpal tunnel symptoms (CTS) cases were engaged in the repeated data entry [3]. Recently, the musculoskeletal injury problems of young people caused by using computer had drawn a lot of scholars'

C. Stephanidis (Ed.): Posters, Part I, HCII 2013, CCIS 373, pp. 533–537, 2013.

attention [4-5]. To date, many studies determined computer exposures based on computer use time, and a strong relationship existed between computer use time and risk of musculoskeletal symptoms [3,6]. However, different computer tasks might have different times spent typing, mouse clicking, and mouse dragging. Determining computer exposure by total computer use time might be insufficient for discovering differences in physical workload. Therefore, the purpose of this study was to explore computer exposure and forearm musculoskeletal symptoms among three computer groups. The computer groups included computer-document (CD) processors, computer-aided design (CAD) draftsmen, and online gamers.

2 Material and Method

Subjects. Ten CD processors (aged 33.4±4.8 years), 10 CAD draftsmen (aged 31.8±5.2 years), and 10 online gamers (aged 23.5±1.5 years) were recruited in this study. Each subject self-reported used only the test PC during work and had a regular work-rest schedule and consistent work content (i.e., routine or similar computer tasks). Table 1 showed the demographic data of each group.

Table 1. Demographic data (mean ± SD)

Groups	Sex	Age (year)	Height (cm)	Weight (kg)	Seniority (year)
CD processors (n=10)	F: n=8 M: n=2	33.4±4.8	167.2±5.0	64.6±5.5	9.5±6.4
CAD draftsmen (n=10)	F: n=3 M: n=7	31.8±5.2	166.6±4.8	65.4±7.2	6.8±5.8
Online gamers (n=10)	M: n=10	22.5±1.5	170.5±6.8	70.6±5.8	5.6±1.7

CD computer-document; *CAD* computer-aided design.

Equipment and Test Procedure. Three sets of logger systems which were developed by Chen et al. (2009) were utilized to record subject computer activities [7]. The system consisted of a hardware logger and KMlog analytical software. The computer activities of each subject were recorded for 10 consecutive days. Participants provided informed consent before participating in the study. Demographic data were collected, included personal characteristics, computer use, and subjective feelings about regional pain during the past year. Pain in the neck, shoulders, arms, wrists, and upper and lower back areas were recorded. Response categories were scored on a scale from 0 to 4. Each test run was started on a weekday by an investigator who installed and initiated the hardware logger on each subject's computer at 8:00 a.m. Data recording continued for 10 consecutive days and was stopped by the investigator on day 10 at 6:30 p.m. During each test, the same keyboard, mouse set and gain settings were applied to each test PC. Each participant then performed regular work-rest activities during the test period.

Data Processing and Statistical Analysis. Parameters derived by KMlog software from recorded computer activities consisted of the number of workdays, total keystrokes, mouse click counts, wheel scrolling counts, mouse movement and distance dragged (in 1000*mickeys). The time intervals (pause definitions) were set to 5 seconds and 30 seconds to categorize computer use time as dynamic (<5s), static or resting (>30 s) durations [7]. Average daily exposures were computed by dividing the above PC usage parameters by the number of workdays measured during the 10-day survey period. Statistical analysis used SYSTAT 12.0. Group differences for all daily exposure parameters were performed by a one-way analysis of variance (ANOVA). Post hoc Bonferroni tests were conducted for multiple comparisons. Group differences and side differences (dominant vs. non-dominant) for musculoskeletal complaints in each body part were tested using the Kruskal-Wallis test and Wilcoxon signed rank test, respectively, an analytical result was considered significant at $p< 0.005$.

3 Results

Table 2 showed that computer exposure differences (operating period, speed and number of keystroke, speed and number of mouse button clicks, and mouse move No) in three groups differed significantly ($p<0.005$). Post hoc results showed that online gamers had significantly higher operating period than CD processors and CAD draftsmen ($p<0.001$). The stroke speed was higher in online gamers than in CD processors and CAD draftsmen ($p<0.001$). The keystroke number was higher in online gamers than in CAD draftsmen ($p<0.001$). In mouse use, results showed click speed was higher in CAD draftsmen than in CD processors ($p=0.003$). The click number and move distances were higher in online gamers than in CD processors ($p=0.002$). But there was no difference in mouse use between online gamers and CAD draftsmen (Table 2). In regional pains, no significant group difference existed in musculoskeletal complaints of any body part, but the shoulder and arm of dominant side had higher tendency in CAD draftsmen than in online gamers ($p=0.028\sim0.047$). However, subjects had a significantly higher number of complaints in the shoulder, arm and wrist of dominant than in those of non-dominant ($p<0.002$) (Table 3).

4 Discussion

The results showed the computer average exposure (operating time) were high within three groups; further, the exposure amount of daily operating period were more than 3 hours that the scholars have suggested [3]. Among three groups, the average daily operating period was over 8.2 hours for online gamers. Many studies determined that increased duration of computer use was positively associated with increased risk of musculoskeletal symptoms [3]. However, previous study suggested that computer exposure of different tasks would not be based solely on duration of computer use [8]. Village et al. (2005) concluded that the risk of CTS increased as computer use increased, especially when used a mouse for more than 20 hours per week [9].

Previous study suggested high typing speed and force caused significant musculoskeletal discomforts [10]. This study found that online gamers had the fastest stroke speed of keyboard, and lowest CAD draftsmen. In addition, the keyboard use

Table 2. Average daily computer exposures of document processors, draftsmen, and online gamers

Parameters / Groups	Total operation period (hr/day)	Keyboard: Stroke speed (counts /min)	Keyboard: Keystroke (counts /day)	Mouse: Click speed (times /min)	Mouse: Click (times /day)	Mouse: Scroll (counts /day)	Mouse: Move (k mickey /day)	Mouse: Drag (k mickey /day)
CD processors (n=12)	3.8 (0.9)	34.8 (13.5)	7785.5 (3598.2)	14.3 (2.9)	3224.2 (1250.3)	4085.2 (1525.4)	885.2 (304.6)	48.9 (26.3)
CAD Draftsmen (n=12)	4.8 (0.8)	7.5 (3.6)	2024.0 (816.0)	23.4 (3.7)	6594.0 (1672.6)	8531.6 (4410.5)	1743.0 (538.5)	152.0 (112.2)
Online gamers (n=14)	8.2 (2.6)	38.8 (25.2)	20250.0 (15834.5)	17.8 (8.8)	9136.4 (5940.2)	5982.5 (5292.3)	2466.0 (1580.5)	452.2 (512.4)
p_{abc}	<0.000**	<0.000**	<0.000**	0.005*	0.003*	0.043	0.003*	0.07
p_{ab}	n.s.	0.003*	n.s.	0.003*	n.s.	n.s.	n.s.	n.s.
p_{bc}	<0.000**	<0.000**	<0.000**	n.s.	n.s.	n.s.	n.s.	n.s.
p_{ac}	<0.000**	n.s.	n.s.	n.s.	0.002*	n.s.	0.002*	n.s.

$^*p<0.01$, $^{**}p<0.001$; p_{abc}: difference among three groups; p_{ab}: difference between CD processors and CAD draftsmen; p_{bc}: difference between CAD draftsmen and online gamers; p_{ac}: difference between CD processors and online gamers; *CD* computer-document; *CAD* computer-aided design.

Table 3. Subjective regional pains and related response score among three groups

Groups	Neck	Dominant side: Shoulder	Dominant side: Arm	Dominant side: wrist	Non-dominant side: Shoulder	Non-dominant side: Arm	Non-dominant side: wrist	Upper back	Lower back
CD processors (n=12)	1.83 (0.83)	1.50 (0.80)	1.25 (0.62)	1.58 (0.79)	1.25 (0.62)	1.08 (0.29)	1.25 (0.62)	1.42 (0.67)	1.08 (0.29)
CAD draftsmen (n=12)	1.83 (0.94)	2.25 (0.87)	1.75 (0.87)	2.25 (0.97)	1.33 (0.49)	1.25 (0.45)	1.42 (0.51)	1.33 (0.65)	1.25 (0.62)
Online gamers (n=14)	1.79 (0.80)	1.50 (0.65)	1.07 (0.27)	2.21 (0.97)	1.14 (0.36)	1.00 (0.00)	1.07 (0.27)	1.21 (0.43)	1.43 (0.76)
p_{abc}	n.s.	0.033	0.026	n.s.	n.s.	n.s.	n.s.	n.s.	n.s.
p_{ab}	n.s.	n.s.	n.s.	n.s.	n.s.	n.s.	n.s.	n.s.	n.s.
p_{bc}	n.s.	0.047	0.028	n.s.	n.s.	n.s.	n.s.	n.s.	n.s.
p_{ac}	n.s.	n.s.	n.s.	n.s.	n.s.	n.s.	n.s.	n.s.	n.s.

p_{abc}: difference among three groups; p_{ab}: difference between CD processors and CAD draftsmen; p_{bc}: difference between CAD draftsmen and online gamers; p_{ac}: difference between CD processors and online gamers; *CD* computer-document; *CAD* computer-aided design.

of online gamers excessively concentrated on some specific keys, results in causing pressure load to concentrate in few small muscle groups. This study speculated that people addicted to online game should have a high risk of musculoskeletal injury.

The online gamers may have a higher risk of musculoskeletal injuries, but are not the most serious in musculoskeletal complaints of the upper extremity in this study. The results were consistent with the previous findings [11]. Even the young people frequently used computers due to computer games, but upper extremity pain were not significantly higher than in other computer users [11]. This observation shows upper extremity musculoskeletal symptoms should be complex cumulative damage. Both the quantitative records by short-term few days and questionnaire data collection may not be sufficient on behalf of actual exposure by operating keyboard and mouse for a long time.

5 Conclusions

The computer average exposure (operating time) are high within three groups. The online gamers had significantly higher keyboard and mouse exposures than other groups, but not greater musculoskeletal complaint of upper extremity than CAD draftsmen. Experimental results derived from onsite measurements indicated that computer use duration alone could not accurately represent the workloads of various computer tasks. Adequate tools are needed for quantifying user computer exposure and providing detailed information for these computer tasks. To better understand computer-associated risk of musculoskeletal disorders, future study should further collect long-term data of computer exposure.

References

1. Sauter, S.L., Schleifer, M., Knutson, S.: Work posture, work station design, and musculoskeletal discomfort in a VDT data entry task. Human Factors 33, 151–167 (1991)
2. Rempel, D.R., Tittiranonda, P., Burasteno, S., Hudes, M.: Effect of keyboard key switch design on hand pain. J. Occup. Environ. Med. 41, 111–119 (1999)
3. Szabo, R.M.: Carpal tunnel syndrome as a repetitive motion disorder. Clin. Orthop. Relat. Res. 351, 78–89 (1998)
4. Szeto, G.P.U., Lau, J.C.C., Siu, A.Y.K.: A study of physical discomfort associated with computer use in secondary school students. In: Proceedings of CybErg (2002)
5. Paula, T.H., Rimpela, A.H., Saarni, L.A., Salminen, J.J.: Frequent computer-related activities increase the risk of neck–shoulder and low back pain in adolescents. Eur. J. Publ. Health 16(5), 536–541 (2006)
6. Chang, C.H., Amick III, B.C., Menendez, C.C., et al.: Daily computer usage correlated with undergraduate students' musculoskeletal symptoms. Am. J. Ind. Med. 50, 481–488 (2007)
7. Chen, H.C., Wu, H.C., Liu, Y.P.: Design and functional evaluation of a novel external logger for computer input activities. Int. J. Ind. Ergon. 39(5), 790–797 (2009)
8. Wu, H.C., Liu, Y.P., Chen, H.C.: Differences in computer exposure between university administrators and CAD draftsmen. Draft submitted for publication (2009)
9. Village, J., Rempel, D., Teschke, K.: Musculoskeletal disorders of the upper extremity associated with computer work: a systematic review. Occup. Ergon. 5, 205–218 (2005)
10. Szeto, G.P.Y., Straker, L.M., O'Sullivan, P.B.: The effect of typing speed and force on motor control in symptomatic and asymptomatic office workers. Int. J. Ind. Ergon. 35, 779–795 (2005)
11. Zapata', A.L., Moraes, A.J.P., Leone, C., Doria-Filho, U., Silva, C.A.A.: Pain and musculoskeletal pain syndromes related to computer and video game use in adolescents. Eur. J. Pediatr. 165, 408–414 (2006)

Laser Pointer Interaction and Its Properties in Pointing Performance

Makio Ishihara[1] and Takuya Nakashima[2]

[1] Fukuoka Institute of Technology, 3-30-1 Wajiro-higashi, Higashi-ku, Fukuoka, 811-0295 Japan
m-ishihara@fit.ac.jp
http://www.fit.ac.jp/~m-ishihara/Lab/

[2] Graduate School of Computer Science and Engineering, Fukuoka Institute of Technology, 3-30-1 Wajiro-higashi, Higashi-ku, Fukuoka, 811-0295 Japan

Abstract. This manuscript conducts an experiment in properties of pointing performance for laser pointer interaction. Fitts's Law is used to evaluate pointing performance of traditional pointing devices like mouses and touchpads but it is not suitable to evaluate it for laser pointer interaction. This manuscript introduces a model function to express and parameterize pointing performance of a Nintendo Wii-based pointing device. The result shows that the obtained model function can express it by the error ratio of about 3%.

Keywords: pointing performance, Nintendo Wii, laser pointer interaction, ISO9241-9.

1 Introduction

Laser pointers are common tools for presentations. They are simple devices that emit a light ray for a projection screen and used to draw the audience attention to the laser spot.

Laser pointer interaction uses laser pointers for interaction between presenters and computers. It allows presenters to move the laser spot in a specific pattern on the projection screen in order to manipulate a mouse cursor, click on contents, or forward/backward PowerPoint slides in the distance. Shizuki, B. et al. [1] build a protopype of laser pointer interaction using peripheral areas of the projection screen. The laser spot is captured by a USB camera and the movement of the laser spot crossing the boundary of the projection area is interpreted into commands to the computer. Presenters, for example, move the laser spot into the projection area in order to forward PowerPoint slides. In a commercial field, Nintendo Wii and Sony Move are good examples of laser pointer interaction.

There are several ways to design laser pointer interaction. The first one is to capture the laser spot by a camera and locate it on the projection screen. Shizuki, B. et al. take this way. The second one is to use a handheld camera to capture the quadrilateral of the entire projection screen so that the center of the camera performs the laser spot. Nintendo Wii and Sony Move take this way.

C. Stephanidis (Ed.): Posters, Part I, HCII 2013, CCIS 373, pp. 538–542, 2013.

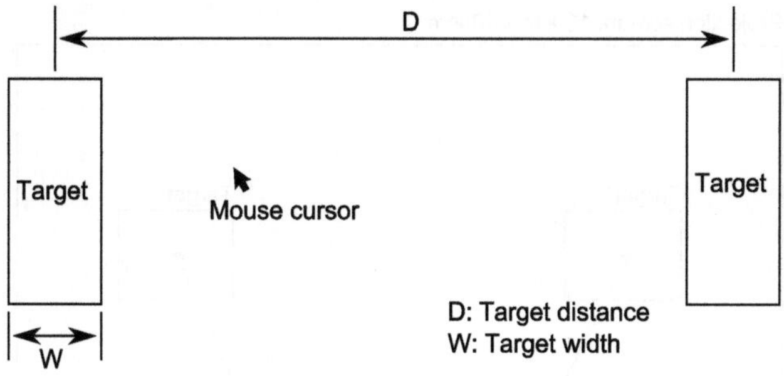

Fig. 1. Parameters for Fitts's Law

The third one is to use invisible gray-code for the camera to capture not the entire screen but a position on the screen to locate it. Gray-code binary patterns appear on the screen in order then the temporal pattern at a position of the screen uniquely represents its own position.

One of the key issues around laser pointer interaction is how to evaluate usability of their various designs. Each design should vary in pointing performance such as accuracy and time. This manuscript conducts an experiment in properties of pointing performance of a Nintendo Wii-based pointing device.

2 Fitts's Law

Fitts's Law [2] is used to evaluate the usability of traditional pointing devices like mouses and touchpads. It says, pointing performance $T_{(sec.)}$, which is the elapsed time to point, depends on the target width $W_{(cm)}$ and the target distance $D_{(cm)}$. Fig. 1 shows a schematic diagram of the target's parameters. Mackenzie, I.S. et al. [3] expresses the pointing performance T as a function of W and D:

$$T = a + b \log_2 \left(\frac{W + D}{W} \right) \tag{1}$$

Constants of a and b are specific to a given pointing device. a represents the start/stop time in seconds for the device and b represents the inherent speed of the device. The smaller the constants of a and b are, the better the pointing device is.

Graham, E. et al. [4], meanwhile, suggest that considering the behavior of the hand, rather than the mouse cursor, will lead to more effective modeling of human performance with certain types of pointing devices. At this point, we confirmed that Fitts's Law is not suitable to express pointing performance for laser pointer interaction in our previous work.

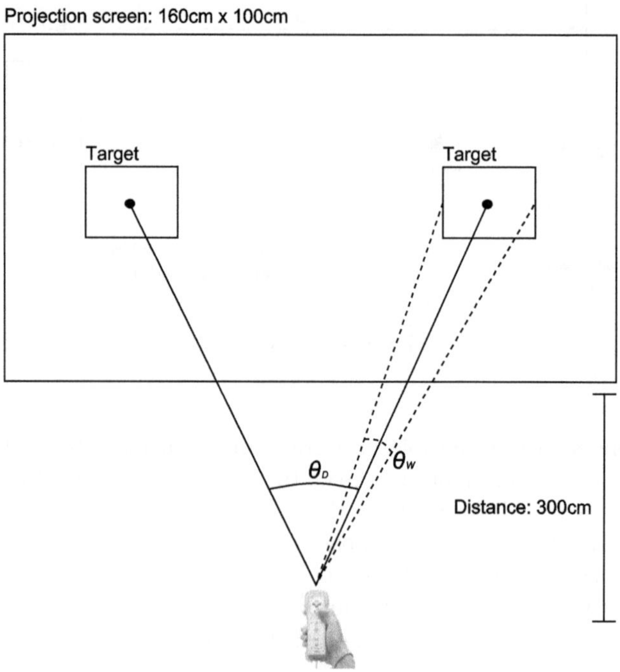

Fig. 2. Parameters for the behavior of the hand

3 Wii-Based Laser Pointer Interaction

3.1 Samples of Pointing Performance

An experimental pointing device with Nintendo Wii is built to see properties of its pointing performance. As regards Graham's suggestion, the pointing performance is supposed to depend on the behavior of the hand. Fig. 2 shows parameters for the behavior of the hand: θ_D represents the angular distance between two targets and θ_W represents the angular distance of the target width.

The one-directional tapping test (ISO9241-9)[5] is conducted to obtain 6,250 samples of the pointing performance T under 25 conditions varying in θ_W and θ_D. There are 5 subjects between the ages of 22 and 23. All are right-handed. They stand 300cm to the projection screen which is 150cm wide and 100cm high. Each subject is asked to point and click alternately on two targets 25 clicks each, resulting in 50 clicks.

$$25(conditions) \times 5(subjects) \times 50(clicks) = 6,250(samples) \quad (2)$$

The elapsed time (sec.) to point and click on a target is measured. Table 1 shows the elapsed time on average.

Table 1. Pointing performance T of the Wii-based pointing device

Elapsed time (sec.)		$\theta_W(deg.)$				
		0.71	1.25	1.79	2.32	2.86
$\theta_D(deg.)$	5.72	0.80	0.67	0.46	0.41	0.36
	9.94	0.99	0.72	0.61	0.53	0.44
	14.17	1.15	0.85	0.67	0.63	0.51
	18.39	1.27	0.94	0.77	0.70	0.59
	22.61	1.46	1.07	0.80	0.79	0.64

3.2 Approximate Expression

A new function F is proposed to express properly the pointing performance T of the Wii-based pointing device, taking into account the behavior of the hand:

$$T = F(\theta_W, \theta_D). \tag{3}$$

The function F can be used to optimize the design of user interface such as the size of buttons or check boxes, and their layout. Referring to the samples, this manuscript supposes the following model function.

$$F(\theta_W, \theta_D) = a * b^{-\theta_W} * \theta_D + c \tag{4}$$

Using the model function, the least squares method acquires an approximate expression to the samples as follows.

$$F(\theta_W, \theta_D) = 0.0899 * 2.41^{-\theta_W} * \theta_D + 0.428. \tag{5}$$

Fig. 3 shows the approximate expression together with the samples. The solid graph indicates the samples and the dotted one does the approximate expression.

3.3 Accuracy

A further experiment of the one-directional tapping test is conducted to see error ratio of the approximate expression to measured values. In this experiment, three pairs of θ_W and θ_D are randomly selected: (θ_W, θ_D)=$(0.9, 7)$, $(1.9, 16)$, $(1.4, 19)$. There are other 3 subjects between the ages of 22 and 23. All are right-handed. Any other settings are the same with the previous one in **3.1**.

$$3(conditions) \times 3(subjects) \times 50(clicks) = 450(samples) \tag{6}$$

Table 2 shows the measured values on average and their expression values. The error ratio is the ratio of the difference between the two values to the expression value. It is about 3%.

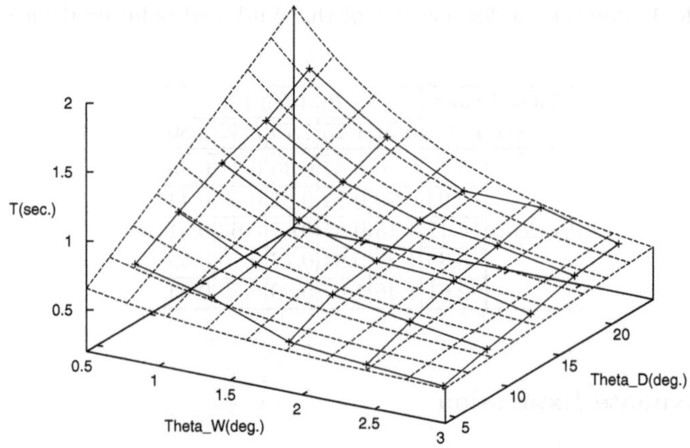

Fig. 3. Approximate expression to the samples

Table 2. Accuracy of the approximate expression

Elapsed time (sec.)	$\theta_W(deg.)/\theta_D(deg.)$		
	0.9/7	1.9/16	1.4/19
Measured values	0.69	0.71	0.89
Expression values	0.71	0.69	0.92
Error ratio	2.54%	2.02%	3.26%

4 Conclusions

This manuscript conducted an experiment in pointing performance of a Nintendo Wii-based pointing device and introduced a model function to express it. In the future work, we are going to examine generalization of the model function by including more samples from various designs of laser pointer interaction.

References

1. Shizuki, B., et al.: Laser pointer interaction techniques using peripheral areas of screens. In: Proc. of the Working Conf. on Advanced Visual Interfaces, pp. 95–98 (2006)
2. Fitts, P.M.: The information capacity of the human motor system in controlling the amplitude of movement. Journal of Experimental Psychology: General 121(3), 262–269 (1992)
3. Mackenzie, I.S., Buxton, W.: Extending Fitts's Law to two-dimensional tasks. In: Proc. of the SIGCHI Conf. on Human Factors in Comp. Sys., pp. 219–226 (1992)
4. Graham, E., MacKenzie, C.L.: Pointing on a computer display. In: Conf. Companion on Human Factors in Comp. Sys., pp. 314–315 (1995)
5. International standard: Ergonomic requirements for office work with visual display terminals - Part 9: Requirements for non-keyboard input devices, ISO 9241-9 (2000)

Relationship between Surface Property and Operability of Tablet Terminal with Touch-Sensitive Screen

Takahiro Nishimura[1], Kouki Doi[2], and Hiroshi Fujimoto[3]

[1] Graduate School of Human Sciences, Waseda University, Tokorozawa, Saitama, Japan
[2] Department of Education Information, National Institute of Special Needs Education, Yokosuka, Kanagawa, Japan
[3] Faculty of Human Sciences, Waseda University, Tokorozawa, Saitama, Japan
t.nishimura@akane.waseda.jp, doi@nise.go.jp, fujimoto@waseda.jp

Abstract. Intuitively operated touch-sensitive screens are becoming more prevalent in our daily lives. Particularly, the rapidly growing demand for tablets, which are beginning to be used in the educational and medical environments, is said to be leading the market. However, it has been pointed out that it is hard to slide a finger easily on the tablet screen when operating the device, making it difficult to use the device. The present study investigates the relationship between the surface property of a tablet touch-sensitive screen and the easiness of sliding a finger on the screen, and evaluates the influence of the surface property on the operability based on the experimental results.

Keywords: Touch-sensitive screen, tablet, surface property, operability.

1 Introduction

Touch-sensitive screens that serve as displays and input devices have been adopted mainly in smartphones and slate PCs, and their market has been greatly expanded. Particularly, the rapidly growing demand for tablets is said to be leading the touch-sensitive screen market. The touch-sensitive screen tablets are used in a variety of situations, from educational to medical environments.

Although the touch-sensitive screens are being applied in many fields, some operability problems arose concerning difficulty in sliding a finger easily on the screen to operate the device. These problems are specific to touch-sensitive screens where the "touching" action itself serves as an interface, but the quantitative data on the relationship between the easiness of sliding a finger on the screen surface and the operability have not been available. Furthermore, although screen protection films having the surface property that enables easy sliding of a finger are commercially available, the ease of sliding a finger is evaluated subjectively based on experience. Therefore, quantitative operability data in humans that can be used as the reference in designing the screens are required. In view of these facts, it is likely that a design guideline based on the operating characteristics in humans can be obtained by evaluating the influence of the ease of sliding a finger on the screen surface on the operability of the touch-sensitive screen tablet.

C. Stephanidis (Ed.): Posters, Part I, HCII 2013, CCIS 373, pp. 543–547, 2013.

Accordingly, the present study aims to investigate the relationship between the screen surface properties of a touch-sensitive screen tablet, the ease of sliding a finger, and explain the influence of the surface property on operability. Specifically, films with quantitatively different finger-sliding ease were selected to reproduce the display surfaces with different finger-sliding ease. Then, using the selected films, an experiment for evaluating the touch-sensitive screen tablet operability was conducted to evaluate the relationship between the display surface property and operability.

2 Relationship between the Screen Surface Property and the Ease of Sliding a Finger

This chapter describes the quantitative evaluation of the ease of sliding a finger on films performed to select the films used for the operability evaluation experiment of a touch-sensitive screen tablet. Specifically, four films on which the ease of sliding a finger is subjectively different (films A to D) were prepared in cooperation with a film manufacturer. The selected films were quantitatively evaluated for their ease of sliding a finger using two parameters—roughness average [1] and coefficient of kinetic friction—which are to be used as the experimental factors in the operability evaluation experiment described in the next chapter.

2.1 Measurement of the Roughness Average

The roughness average was measured using a non-contact surface texture measuring device (Mitaka Kohki Co., Ltd., PF-60). The measured range was 1000 μm in vertical direction by 1000 μm in the horizontal direction. The roughness average was measured 10 μm apart in the vertical direction along the horizontal measurement axis. After the measurement, the values for five measurement targets were randomly extracted, and their mean value was used as the roughness average value for evaluation.

Figure 1 shows the measurement results. As a result of the variance analysis for the factor "film", the main effect by the film was revealed [$F(3, 12) = 1125.04$, $p < 0.001$]. By reviewing the significant difference between the levels based on the Bonferroni multiple comparison correction, it was also revealed that the roughness average became significantly smaller in the order films A, B, C, and D.

2.2 Measurement of the Coefficient of Kinetic Friction

It is known that the friction acting between two objects generally follows the Amontons-Coulomb law of friction expressed by the formula (1):

$$F = \mu' \cdot N \tag{1}$$

where F [N] is the kinetic friction, μ' is the coefficient of kinetic friction, and N [N] is the normal component of reaction. By measuring the kinetic friction F and the normal

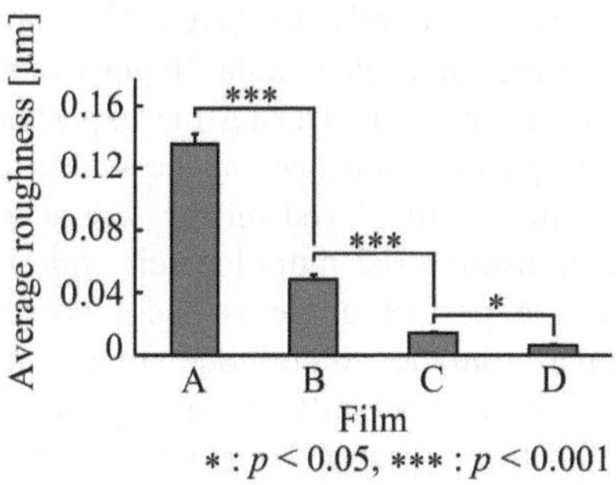

Fig. 1. Results of the average roughness

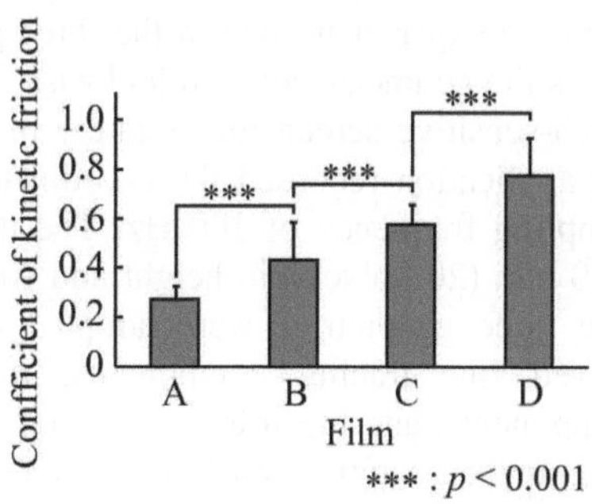

Fig. 2. Results of the coefficient of kinetic friction

component of reaction *N*, the coefficient of kinetic friction μ' can be calculated by the formula (1). Therefore, the kinetic frictions *F* and the normal components of reaction *N* while sliding a finger on the films were measured using a three-component load cell (Kyowa Electronic Instruments Co., Ltd., LSM-B-50NSA1) to calculate the coefficients of kinetic friction based on the measured data. The sliding speed of the finger and the normal component of reaction during measurement were 50 mm/s and 1.0 N, respectively, which were determined based on the values obtained from several subjects while they are operating on a touch-sensitive screen display naturally. The total number of trials was 48 (4 film conditions × 4 friction directions × 3-time trials under each condition). The time required for measurement was approximately 1 hour.

In the measurement, three adult subjects (aged 23.0 ± 2.0 in average) without injury in the fingertip skin or related past history participated and cooperated. To control the perspiration and sebum conditions of the finger during the experiment, the finger was wiped clean with ethanol and dried in the air immediately before each measurement. For information, the experiment was conducted after being approved by the Ethics Committee on Human Research of Waseda University.

Figure 2 shows the results of the coefficient of kinetic friction. As a result of the variance analysis for the factor "film", the main effect by the film was revealed [$F(3, 140) = 92.77$, $p < 0.001$]. The Bonferroni multiple comparison correction also revealed that the coefficient of kinetic friction became significantly larger in the order films A, B, C, and D, and that the coefficient of kinetic friction for the anti-glare film (film A) was one third of that for the hard coat film (film D).

3 Evaluation of the Touch-Sensitive Screen Tablet Operability

3.1 Experimental Task

As an experimental task, an original application software for tracing simple geometries (perfect circle, regular triangle, and square) using the index finger of the dominant hand was prepared, and executed on a capacitive touch-sensitive screen tablet (Apple Inc., USA, iPad 2).

In the experiment, one of the three geometries is randomly displayed. The subject traces the geometry counterclockwise for three times and releases the finger from the touch-sensitive screen immediately on completing the task. During the experiment, the application recorded the coordinates of the position touched on the screen at a sampling frequency of 100 Hz. The three geometries displayed on the screen were 40.0 mm (208 pixels) in height and were drawn using a 0.2 mm (1 pixel) wide line. The three geometries were adopted because the perfect circle is decomposed to curved line tracing components, the regular triangle to oblique line tracing components, and the square to straight line tracing components. In writing letters or dragging on a touch-sensitive screen tablet, the finger draws straight lines, oblique lines, curves, and multi-segment lines in different directions by dragging the finger while keeping the finger in contact with the screen. Therefore, by using the three geometries that contain these operation components in the evaluation, the basic data on the relationship between the ease of sliding a finger and the usability are likely to be obtained. Also, the tracing path on the screen by the finger was displayed as a 0.2 mm wide black line to provide visual feedback of the operation.

3.2 Procedure

Each subject sat on a chair with adjustable height, rested his/her arms on a desk, and operated the tablet using the index finger of a dominant hand. The touch-sensitive screen tablet used in the experiment was fixed horizontally to the desk. The total number of trials was 36 (4 film conditions × 3 geometry conditions × 3-time trials under each condition). To control the perspiration and sebum conditions of the finger during the experiment, the finger was wiped clean with ethanol and dried in the air immediately before operating the tablet. To let the subjects become accustomed to the experimental procedure and the experimental task, the subjects had sufficient practice before they start the actual trials. The experiment was conducted taking intermittent rest breaks as required, and the time for the experiment was approximately 2 hours.

In evaluating the experimental results, "deviation" was adopted as the operability evaluation parameters to evaluate how correctly the experimental task is performed. Specifically, the deviation was evaluated using the deviation between the traced path and the displayed geometry.

3.3 Results and Discussion

For the results regarding deviation, a variance analysis for the factor "film" was conducted. Where the main effect by the film was significant, the significant difference between the levels was tested by the Bonferroni multiple comparison correction.

Regarding the deviation observed with the curved line in the circle shown in Figure 3 (a), the main effect by the film was significant [$F(3, 33) = 7.91$, $p < 0.001$]. As a result of the multiple comparison, it was revealed that the deviation in tracing curves on films A and D is increased. As to film A, the deviation may have been increased because the finger was slippery on the film and it was difficult to control the slipping of the finger. As to film D, on the other hand, the deviation may have been increased

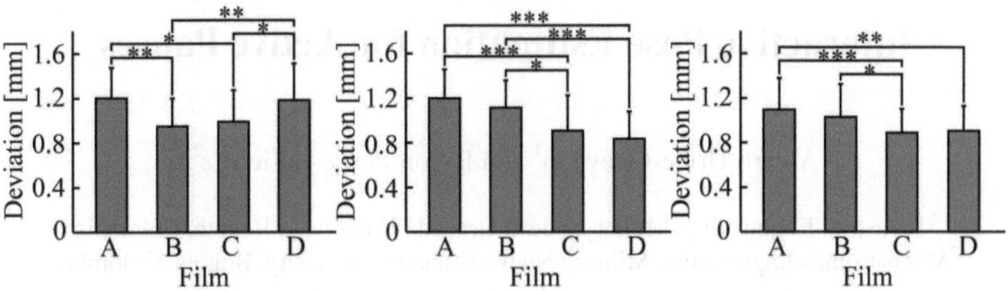

Fig. 3. Results of the deviation

because the finger was caught by the film and it was difficult to control the fine movement of the finger. Regarding the deviation observed with the oblique line in the triangle shown in Figure 3 (b), the main effect by the film was observed [F(3, 33) = 14.75, p < 0.001]. Regarding the deviation observed with the straight line in the square shown in Figure 3 (c), the main effect by the film was significant [F(3, 33) = 8.89, p < 0.001]. As to oblique and straight lines, it was revealed that the deviation was reduced in films C and D that have great coefficients of kinetic friction. In these films, a certain degree of difficulty in sliding a finger may have suppressed slipping of the finger and the deviation was reduced as a result. The reason the deviation did not increase in the films with small coefficients of kinetic friction as it did when tracing curves may be because tracing of curves required more skillful maneuvering than tracing oblique and straight lines.

4 Conclusion

In the present study, the relationship between the surface property of a touch-sensitive screen tablet and the ease of sliding a finger was investigated, and the experiment was conducted to demonstrate the effect of the surface property on the operability. As a result, we obtained the following information.

1. The greater the roughness average of the film surface, the smaller the coefficient of kinetic friction becomes, and the coefficient of kinetic friction of the anti-glare films is approximately one third of that of the hard coat films.
2. In tracing curves, the correctness of the operation is improved by providing an appropriate range of frictional resistance on the surface
3. In tracing oblique and straight lines, the correctness of the operation is improved by increasing the surface frictional resistance.

Reference

1. International Organization for Standardization: ISO 4287, Geometrical Product Specifications (GPS) – Surface Texture: Profile Method – Terms, Definitions and Surface Texture Parameters (1997)

Interactive Pose Estimation for Active Pauses

Alvaro Uribe-Quevedo[1] and Byron Perez-Gutierrez[2]

[1] Industrial Engineering, Military Nueva Granada University, Bogota, Colombia
[2]Mechatronics Engineering, Military Nueva Granada University, Bogota, Colombia
{alvaro.j.uribe,byron.perez}@ieee.org

Abstract. Occupational health affections related to ergonomics result in musculoskeletal problems that affect the locomotion apparatus through the muscles, tendons, ligaments and nerves, yielding to numerous cases of work absence. The World Health Organization (WHO) has acknowledged occupational health problems associated with excessive computer work resulting in the execution of repetitive tasks and sedentary cycles. With increased use of mobile electronic devices (laptops, smartphones and tablets) and initiatives as bring your own device, work time has increased recently and users do not take care of their posture or joints during usage of these devices. Recommendations on taking active pauses and do exercises for avoiding occupational health problems are promoted with videos, animations, reminders, guides and surveys, however use of this tools or taking time for active pauses is not done by several users. This project addresses the problem through an application for reminding the pause and monitor user exercises using Kinect.

Keywords: Active pause, Interaction, Motion tracking, Occupational health.

1 Introduction

Occupational health affections related to ergonomics result in musculoskeletal problems that affect the locomotion apparatus through the muscles, tendons, ligaments and nerves, yielding to numerous cases of work absence [1]. Solutions for tackling the occupational health problem regarding sedentary are based on surveys for monitoring user's health while at work [2], consulting enterprises [3], reminding active pause software [4], and reports such as the one presented by the World Health Organization in [5], that aims to raise awareness about this problem for avoiding occupational health risks, recommending active pauses, changing routines, and exercising among others according to different working scenarios. The growth information and technology indexes is the result of current technological trends [6], where computers and mobile devices have become widely used tools for developing daily tasks whether, for studying, working, procrastinating, entertainment or reading among many other activities.

At Military Nueva Granada University the office of Preventive Medicine and Occupational Health uses an active pause flash-based multimedia application with

C. Stephanidis (Ed.): Posters, Part I, HCII 2013, CCIS 373, pp. 548–551, 2013.

still images and animations along with information for users to download and follow on their own. Research on this area have presented studies showing that software assisted breaks leads to an increased execution of exercises, while others state that passive pauses make little difference in decreasing the overall loading produced while working seated, and suggests that pauses should introduce more physical activity [7]. An approach to raise awareness used eLearning as a tool for improving and understanding computer ergonomics which resulted in better work habits for their users.

This work presents the development of a prototype tool for increasing computer workers interest in taking active pauses based on motion tracking and data monitoring. The application aims not only to remind the user of taking the active pause, but also to improve exercise accuracy by presenting a visual feedback of how each motion sequence is performed while tracking the user within each taken pause.

This paper is organized as follows, in Section 2 the methods are presented; in Section 3 the results and findings are documented; finally, in Section 4 the conclusions are discussed.

2 Methods

For developing the application, the occupational health guidelines for our university were taken as design parameters. Active pauses are to be perform from one to two minutes for every 45 minutes of work, additionally, exercises are presented for lower member, back, neck and hands (each series to be performed for 10 s) [8]. The first active pause sequence begins with neck rotation from either side; shoulder rotation backward and forward; alternate arm rising by arm abduction, elbow extension, elbow flexion and arm adduction; torso flexion and extension; and finally, knee flexion and extension while standing. It is worth noting that each of the previous exercises is recommended to be executed for a period of 15 seconds, for achieving the time frame of 1 to 2 minutes.

For tracking the user, the Kinect sensor was chosen as it allows body tracking from a range of 1 m (using a magnifying lens) to 3 m. The sensor uses depth maps and tracks joint's positions and orientation in 3D, however, only frontal tracking is recognizable and environmental characteristics as light and clothing color may affect the tracking [9]. For the proposed prototype only upper member active pause exercise was chosen as it can be performed while standing up or seated within 2 m from the sensor and it is successfully recognized by the sensor.

The upper member exercises consist on alternating arm motion going from sideways of the body to fully extend arose above the head by combining flexion/extension and adduction/abduction, this sequence is presented in Fig.1.

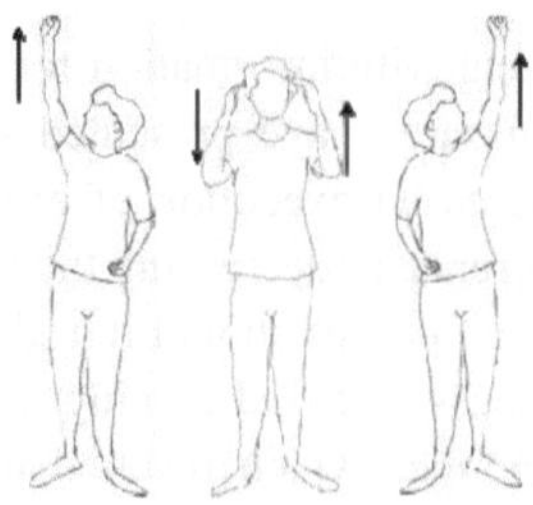

Fig. 1. Upper member sequence

The application development was achieved using the Kinect SDK and XNA for the graphics user interface. This combination allowed creating an interface were the user follows the respective sequences and executes it, an image was inserted to inform if the posture was successfully achieved or not. The application was programmed to emit an alert after 45 minutes of being launched, then instructs the user to step away from the sensor in a standing position and executes the programmed sequence. Additionally, while the user is performing the sequence, a plain text file is created with spatial data of each joint's motion for monitoring and further analysis.

3 Results

After testing the application, results showed that while the Kinect tracked each user, lights and clothing color were only affected in overexposed spaces. Tracking motion and having visual feedback proved to increase accuracy in exercise execution as presented in Fig.2. A survey was applied to 15 computer users whose time in front of the device is around 8 hours a day, this included students, teachers and laboratory assistants. The goal was to check if a tool for active pauses would encourage them for improving their occupational health through motion tracking and monitoring.

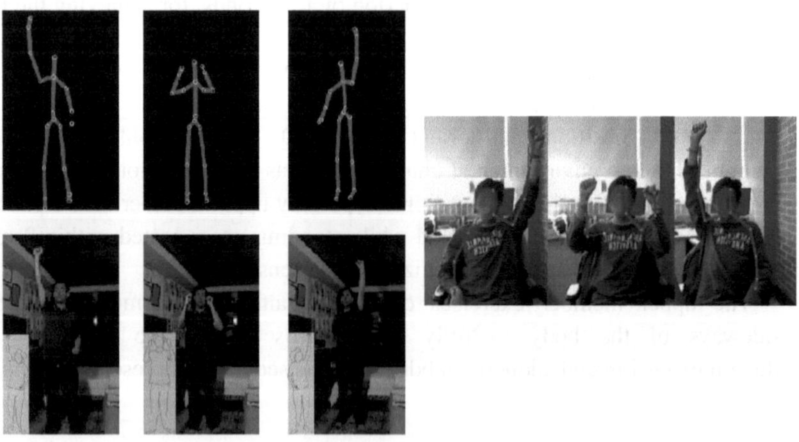

Fig. 2. Standup and seated results

The survey results showed that all participants do not practice active pauses; they are aware of the consequences of occupational health risks, 79% would be interested in using passive active software and considers it an useful tool.

4 Conclusions

The sequence information offered enough information for defining the inputs and outputs of the application, postures and motion for each exercise are programmed considering each joint relation to another, so the application can be used by several users without needing personalized configuration. With the previous information user motion is captured through skeletal tracking implemented with Microsoft ® Kinect, whose three-dimensional information for each joint allows comparing user the motion to the programmed exercises. The outputs are entirely visual, as the sequence is presented for the user to follow, while a tracked body is also visualized for the user to check how he or she is doing, also, time and numbers of exercises are displayed for user information.

Further improvements to the application will consider more exercise sequences, the ability to choose independent exercises and data exportation and statistics for further analysis by a specialist.

Acknowledgements. The Authors would like to thank the Military Nueva Granada University for their support.

References

1. World Health Organization WHO, Occupational and work related diseases (January 2013), http://www.who.int/occupational_health/activities/occupational_work_diseases/en/index.html
2. Stanford, Computer Workstation Ergonomic Evaluation (2013), http://www.stanford.edu/dept/EHS/prod/general/ergo/PDFs/self_evaluation.pdf
3. The Human Solution, Ergonomic Office Desk, Chair and Keyboard Height Calculator (2013), http://www.thehumansolution.com/ergonomic-office-desk-chair-keyboard-height-calculator.html
4. Philip Worthington, Posture minder (2013), http://www.postureminder.co.uk/
5. Luttman, A., Jager, M., Griefahn, B., Caffer, G., Liebers, F.: Prevención de trastornos musculoesquéleticos en el lugar de trabajo: World Health Organization (2004)
6. World Economic Forum, The Global Information Technological Report 2012, World Economic Forum, Insight report 2012 (2012)
7. Richter, J.M., Smeets, J.B., Frens, M.A., Slijper, H.P.: The effects of pause software on the temporal characteristics of computer use. Ergonomics 50(2), 178–191 (2007)
8. Universidad Militar Nueva Granada, Salud Ocupacional y Gestión Ambiental (2013), http://www.umng.edu.co/web/guest/la-universidad/gestion-ambiental-y-salud-ocupacional
9. Microsoft, Kinect gallery (2013), http://www.microsoft.com/en-us/kinectforwindows/discover/gallery.aspx

One Possibility for Computer Syndrome: Rethinking Computer Break Software Program

Sy-Chyi Kiky Wang[1,*], Jin-Yuan Chern[2], and Wei-Hsin Teng[3]

[1] Dept. of E-learning Design and Management, National Chiayi University, Chiayi, Taiwan
[2] Dept. of Healthcare Administration, Chang Jung Christian University, Tainan, Taiwan
[3] Dept. of Visual Communication Design, Kun Shan University
kiky@mail.ncyu.edu.tw, chern@mail.cjcu.edu.tw,
Jeffteng3d@yahoo.com.tw

Abstract. This paper first explored the possibilities of redefining computer break software for advanced function and redesigning the interface for more proper and effective delivery of the informed message, and then discussed the potentiality of drawing the targeted health information online for advanced uses on updated information. It presents an example of how we can create an interactive interface to better motivate users to adopt the program, and how we can fetch online the targeted health information and then present it in a local computer via break software.

Keywords: ergonomics, computer syndrome, interface design, computer break software, stretch exercise.

1 Introduction

Several ergonomics training programs provide ergonomics software packages, designed to prompt computer users to take a break and guide them toward regular exercise. However, most of the software packages either contain only limited information or are not very user friendly. Most of the functions of the ergonomics programs focus only on a lower level of commitment such as reminding computer users to take a break or do some stretches. The content design of the programs alike usually aims on providing "take a break" text and/or office stretches. There were not many content or interface design concerns for the program design. Besides, all of the ready-to-be-delivered information, such as stretch animation, is supposed to be downloaded to local computers at one time as a package. There is no further information or updated data available for advanced uses. This study tries to rethink and redefine computer break software for advanced function and commitment, and to redesign the interface for more effective delivery of the informed massages.

The computer and Internet use has increased substantially and is becoming increasingly commonplace at home, in school, and at work nowadays. The Workplace Employee Relations Survey (WERS) reported that 75% of all workers in the US used

---

[*] Corresponding author.

C. Stephanidis (Ed.): Posters, Part I, HCII 2013, CCIS 373, pp. 552–556, 2013.

computers at work in 2004; the US Census Bureau reported that 68.7% of the households (78.2% of the population) had access to the Internet at home and on average the Internet users spent more than three hours a day online (United States Census Bureau, 2009). A population-based prevalence study showed that on average children and adults in the US spent 54.9% of their waking time, or 7 hours 42 minutes per day, in sedentary behaviors, or leading a sedentary lifestyle (Matthews et al., 2008). Stanford University annual Student Computing Survey (2010-2011) reported that almost 100% of undergraduate students have their own computers and most of them use their computers between 4 and 8 hours a day, with 32% using them between 4 and 6 hours a day, 32% between 6 and 8 hours a day, and 18% more than 8 hours a day (Stanford University, 2010-2011).

The benefits of increased convenience, connectivity, and flexibility that the computer and Internet has brought to us are tremendous. However, these new technologies also add more stress and new demands to our lives. It has been shown that extended computer use may contribute to symptoms of visual impairment (commonly dry eyes), musculoskeletal injuries (e.g., neck, shoulder, and low back pain), skin problems, and even emotional disorders (Hayes et al., 2007). Among the many possible causes of injuries, not taking regular breaks from computer work has been acknowledged as an important factor (Broughton, 2008).

With increasing interest in how to help prolonged sitting computer users avoid computer syndrome, there are studies investigating the effects of computer break programs. Although the relevant programs showed positive effects on health behaviors and conditions (Marangoni, 2010; Van den Heuvel et al., 2003; Wang et al., 2012), in practical, there are still not many people adopt the programs while they worked with computer. Although most of the participants were aware of the benefits of the program to their health and reach the agreement on the necessaries of the programs alike, they still hesitated on the adoption of the interventions. Therefore, more efforts on how to motivate potential users for long-term use of the programs alike are needed in this tech-savvy generation.

2 Method

With a focus on the media and interface design of the program, this study interviewed 30 college students for their perspectives on the user experiences of the programs. The users raised three main concerns. First, for the media design, a 3D (compared to 2D) character design with poor body shape image (compared to perfect body figure) was more welcomed by the participants. Second, for the interface design, animation pop-up windows should be more user friendly; for example, animations pop-up timing should follow users' computer activities on demand (based on keyboard and mouse idle time), and the sound should fade in after the image (to avoid startles), etc. Third, for the sake of long-term users, the content of the program carrying should be further updated from time to time.

3 Result

The project first worked on the 3D character design, which started with an image about some negative effects of extended computer use, such as big belly and weak vision. Please see Figure 1 for the screen shots.

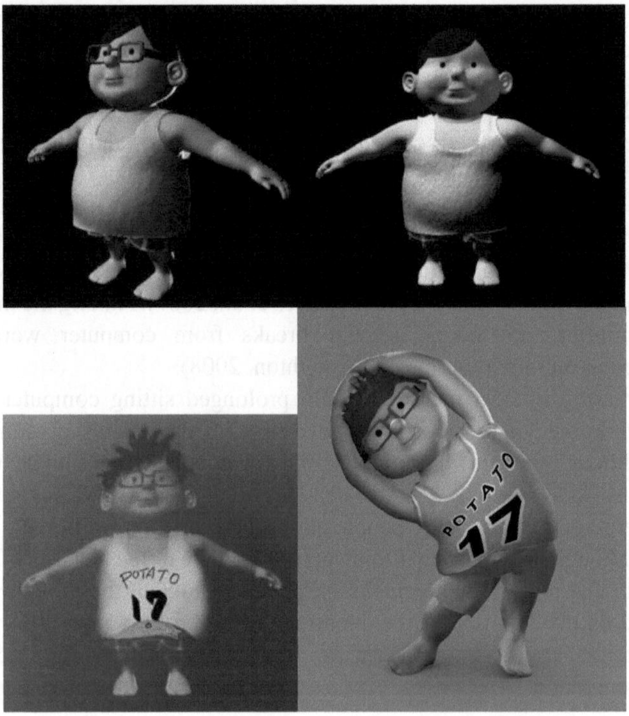

Fig. 1. The screen shots on the 3D character design for the computer break software

For the interface design, this study has the designed character wave his hand at the lower right corner of the computer window whenever the user has worked for a certain period of time. The figure will initially show up as a tiny one at the corner. The user can choose to ignore or cancel it. However, the figure will become a bigger size after a certain period of time which can be preset. If the user clicks on it, the animation will start to show the designed stretch content. Besides, the designed character will reveal itself on the screen without a window frame. Please see Figure 2 for the screen shots.

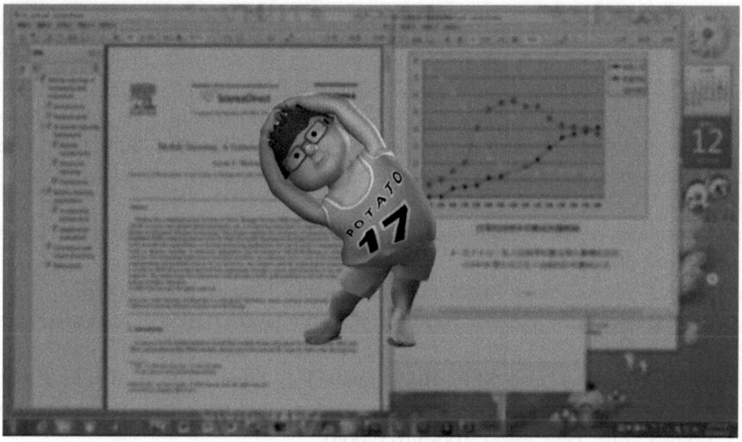

Fig. 2. The screen shots of the interface design demonstrations

For now, we are working on the online system to allow the users to access the server for informed information for updating. We also conducted an investigation on the program experiment with college students. Please see Figure 3 for the visual concept presentation of the implementation.

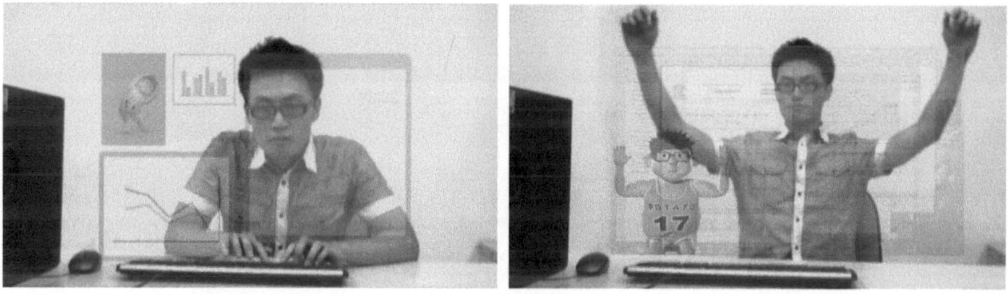

Fig. 3. The visual concept presentation of the program implementation

This study tries to call for attention to the negative effects of extended computer use and to advocate a better content and interface design for computer break/stretch software programs. In addition to the proposed ideas, more solutions to the more and more severe problems of computer syndromes in the field are expected.

References

1. Broughton, A.: Eurofound: Place of work and working conditions (2008), `http://www.eurofound.europa.eu/ewco/studies/tn0701029s/tn0701029s_4.htm` (accessed January 14, 2012)
2. Hayes, J.R., Sheedy, J.E., Stelmack, J.A., et al.: Computer use, symptoms, and quality of life. Optometry Vision Sci. 84(8), E738–E755 (2007), doi:10.1097/OPX.0b013e31812f7546

3. Marangoni, A.H.: Effects of intermittent stretching exercises at work on musculoskeletal pain associated with the use of a personal computer and the influence of media on outcomes. Work 36(1), 27–37 (2010)
4. Matthews, C.E., Chen, K.Y., Freedson, P.S., et al.: Amount of time spent in sedentary behaviors in the United States. Am. J. Epidemiol. 167(7), 875–881 (2003-2004, 2008)
5. Stanford University: Student Computing Survey 2010-2011: Undergraduate Results (2010-2011), `http://acomp.stanford.edu/surveys/2010_2011_undergraduate` (accessed April 20, 2012)
6. United States Census Bureau: Internet use in the United States: 2009 (2009), `http://www.census.gov/hhes/computer/index.html` (accessed December 22, 2011)
7. Van den Heuvel, S.G., Looze, M.P., Hildebrandt, V.H., et al.: Effects of software programs stimulating regular breaks and exercises on work-related neck and upper limb disorders. Scand. J. Work. Env. Hea. 29(2), 106–116 (2003)
8. Wang, S.C., Jiang, C., Chern, J.Y.: Promoting healthy computer use: timing-informed computer health animations for prolonged sitting computer users. Journal: Behaviour & Information Technology - Behaviour & IT ahead-of-p(ahead-of-p), 1--7 (2012)

Lower Limb Musculoskeletal Model Validation during One Legged Forward Hopping and Side Jumping in Healthy Subjects Using EMG

Adhi D. Wibawa[1,2], Nico Verdonschot[6,7], Jan P.K. Halbertsma[3], J.G.M. Burgerhof[5], Ron L. Diercks[4], and G.J. Verkerke[3,7]

[1] Department of Electrical Engineering, Institute of Technology Sepuluh Nopember, Surabaya, Indonesia
[2] Department of Biomedical Engineering
[3] Rehabilitation Medicine
[4] Orthopaedics
[5] Epidemiology, University of Groningen, University Medical Center Groningen, The Netherlands
[6] Orthopaedics Research Laboratory, Radboud Nijmegen University Medical Center, Nijmegen, The Netherlands
[7] Department of Biomechanical Engineering, University of Twente, Enschede, The Netherlands

{wibawa.a.d,j.p.k.halbertsma,j.g.m.burgerhof, r.l.diercks}@umcg.nl, n.verdonschot@orthop.umcn.nl

Abstract. Musculoskeletal modeling is a powerful tool for analyzing human biomechanics during active movement. It has the ability to determine important kinetic data during motion such as muscle force, muscle activity and knee joint force. However, validation of these models need further study to determine the quality of their predictions. In the past, we validated the GaitLowerExtremity model (GLEM) of the AnyBody modeling system (AMS) by a series of experiments, where subjects walked normally, while their movements and EMG were measured. The movements were used by AMS to predict muscle activity, and these predictions were then compared by EMG activities. Although visual inspection showed a good comparison, quantitative comparison results were rather disappointing. We think that a more prescribed movement could result in a better comparison such as during one legged forward hopping (FH) and side jumping (SJ). In this study two variables were used to quantify muscle activity, number of onsets and offsets. The Kappa value (K) was calculated to determine the level of agreement. During FH, for all variables, 7 muscles showed a positive agreement and only one muscle showed a negative agreement. During SJ, for all variables, all muscles showed a positive agreement. This result demonstrates that during more prescribed movements, AMS predicts muscle activity much better than compared to our previous validation study during normal walking, even though some differences between AMS and EMG still did existed.

Keywords: one legged forward hopping, side jumping, EMG, AnyBody Musculoskeletal System, Inverse dynamics analysis.

C. Stephanidis (Ed.): Posters, Part I, HCII 2013, CCIS 373, pp. 557–560, 2013.

1 Introduction

Numerical modeling such as AnyBody Modeling System (AMS) can be a breakthrough of many complexities of studying human biomechanics, since measuring them in vivo is still challenging nowadays [Delp. et al 2007; Komistek., et al 2005]. The GaitLowerExtremity model (GLEM) of the AnyBody modeling system (AMS) is capable to predict muscle forces and muscle activity by a series of assumptions. The influence of these assumptions is never determined, so the accuracy of these models is not known. We did a first attempt in determining the accuracy of GLEM by performing a walking test. In that study we compared the number of onset and offset between the predicted muscle activity by AMS with EMG. Visual inspection showed a reasonable match for most muscles, but after quantifying the results were disappointing. The main reasons for this were the type of movement [Wibawa, et al 2013], besides the assumptions and simplifications of the modeling process. To our opinion, a better way to compare predicted and measured muscle activity is to use a more prescribed movement like one legged forward hopping (FH) and side jumping (SJ). These movements have more defined moments in which muscles are active. So a better comparison between predicted and measured muscle activity could be possible.

The main goal of this study was to validate quantitatively muscle activity predicted by AMS with EMG measurements during FH and SJ in eight lower limb muscles by calculating the level of agreement in number of onset and offset variable using kappa analysis. The novelty of this study is, proving our hypotheses that during more prescribed movement like FH and SJ, the validation result is better when compared to a walking test.

2 Materials and Methods

Ten healthy subjects participated in this experiment (age> 18 years). The characteristics of the subjects (6 males and 4 females) were: mean age of 29.8 ± 6.6 years, mean body weight 67.7 ± 8.18 kg, mean body height 168 ± 4.6 cm. This study was approved by the Medical Ethical Committee of the University Medical Center Groningen (UMCG). Every subject signed an inform consent before performing the trials in the gait lab.

2.1 Test Set-up

This experiment was performed at a Gaitlab with a 9.0 m long walkway for performing FH and SJ, two force plates (BP400600-1000, AMTI, Watertown) with a sampling frequency of 1000 Hz and two video cameras (Basler A602 FC, DE). Recording, synchronising and analysis were performed with a motion system (Vicon Motion System, Oxford, UK). Sixteen reflective markers were attached to bony landmarks on both lower limbs [Davis et al 1991].

Non-invasive sEMG Zerowire electrodes (ConMedCleartrode ref. 1720-003, Aurion SRL, Milan, Italy) were used to record the activity of: Rectus Femoris (RF), Vasti Medialis (VM) and lateralis (VL), Semitendinosis (ST), Bicep femoris (BF), Gastrocnemius Medialis (GM) and lateralis (GL) and Tibialis anterior (TA). The EMG electrodes placement was based on the Seniam standard placement [Hermens et al 2000].

2.2 AnyBody Modeling System (AMS)

GLEM from AMS version 5.0 (AMMR.1.3.1) was used to model FH and SJ activity. EMG data was filtered using a Butterworth band pass filter with a frequency range of 30-200 Hz and 6 Hz Low pass filter [Carlo J. De Luca et al 2010].

2.3 Comparison Strategy

Before quantifying the number of onset/offset, EMG data were threshold two times. The first was min/max threshold to crop the graph. The second was the duration threshold. This threshold was defined as a position where the EMG signal has the same duration as AMS. For AMS graphs, there was only one threshold level (value of 10^{-7}) applied in order to define the zero level. Kappa analysis was used to calculate the level of agreement in both variables, number of onset and offset.

3 Result

During FH activity, from the 10 healthy subjects, two were excluded due to errors in marker trajectory data. Since every subject performed 3 good hopping trials, in total 24 models of FH activity were analyzed, while in SJ the total model was 27 (obtained from 9 subjects). Results are shown in Fig. 1.

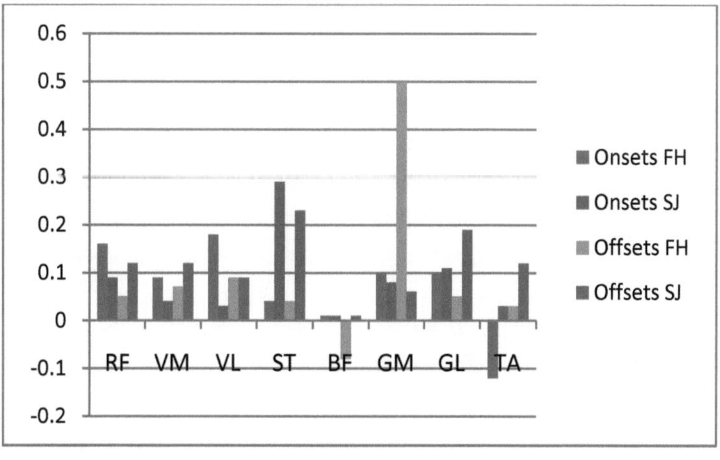

Fig. 1. Kappa value of variable number of onset and offset during FH and SJ

4 Discussion and Conclusion

When compared to the results of our previous study on walking, FH and SJ showed much better validation results. When we consider the kappa value (K), for walking there were only 3 muscles that showed a positive agreement in onset variable (VM, BF and TA), 4 muscles in offset variable (VM, VL, BF and TA). In this study for FH there were 7 muscles that showed a positive agreement (only TA did not). During SJ all 8 muscles showed a positive agreement, in all variables. So indeed a more prescribed motion improves the validation results.

Despite the better agreement results, some differences are still present, mainly due to AMS-simplifications, like a fixed hinge as knee model. In general the GLEM-AMS predicts muscle activity during FH and SJ very well. Suggestions for improvement of AMS are inclusion of time delay between predicted muscle activity and EMG and improving the knee joint from a single hinge one to the one that mimics the anatomical movements.

References

1. Delp, et al.: OpenSim: Open-source Software to Create and Analyze Dynamic Simulations of Movement, TBME-00014-2007 & 00592-2006
2. Komistek, et al.: Knee mechanics: a review of past and present techniques to determine in vivo loads. Journal of Biomechanics 38, 215–228 (2005)
3. Wibawa, et al.: Simulating muscle activity using the AnyBody Modeling System (AMS): Comparison of measured EMG and predicted muscle activity patterns during normal walking (2013)
4. Davis, et al.: A gait data collection and reduction technique. Human Movement Sciences 10, 575–587 (1991)
5. Hermens, et al.: Development of recommendations for SEMG sensors and sensorplacement procedures. Journal of Electromyography and Kinesiology 10, 361–374 (2000)

Research on Two Dimensional Touched Position Distributions of the Touch Screen QWERTY Keyboard

Yuma Yanai[1] and Mitsuhiko Karashima[2]

[1] Tokai University, Graduate School of Information and Telecommunication Engineering, Japan
2bjnm024@mail.tokai-u.jp
[2] Tokai University, School of Information and Telecommunication Engineering, Japan
mitsuk@keyaki.cc.u-tokai.ac.jp

Abstract. This research explored the characteristics on two dimensional touched position distributions in each key of a touch screen QWERTY keyboard through the experiment. The results of the experiment revealed that the mistyping ratio was more than 5% and it suggested the necessity of an approach for key input performance improvement. The results also revealed that the center of distribution of the key touched position tended to be positioned in the low part of the key regardless of keys and the mistyping concentrated under the bottom of the key area. A new approach that the key input performance could be improved by using these characteristics of key touched position and mistyping was proposed.

Keywords: Software keyboard, Touch panel, Touch Screens.

1 Introduction

Recently iPad, android based tablet PC, and Windows based tablet PC have been developed and the touch screen input devices have been increasingly used. The user can input a long sentence by using the touch screen QWERTY keyboard (the virtual keyboard). However the software keyboard brings the disadvantages that the typing speed is slower and the typing accuracy is lower than the hardware keyboard (Andrew(1992)). This disadvantage is caused by the lack of the physical feedbacks. Many kinds of tools for inputting the text from the virtual keyboard were proposed in order to improve the performance of inputting the text from the virtual keyboard (Altinsoy (2009), Go(2007, 2010), Jeong(2012)). However few literatures discussed the characteristics on two dimensional touched position distributions of the virtual keyboard (Leah(2011)). The characteristics on two dimensional touched position distributions could be expected to be the significant information in order to propose the new tool for the virtual keyboard.

This research explored the characteristics on two dimensional touched position distributions in each key of a touch screen QWERTY keyboard through the experiment in order to propose a new approach that the key-input performance could be improved.

C. Stephanidis (Ed.): Posters, Part I, HCII 2013, CCIS 373, pp. 561–565, 2013.

2 Methods

2.1 Participants

12 right-handed university students ranging in age from 19 to 24 (M=21.9) participated in the experiment. All subjects regularly use the hardware QWERTY keyboard but they cannot use blind touch perfectly. They also have experience of the usage of the virtual keyboard but they don't regularly use it.

2.2 Experimental Task

In the experiment 12 participants were required respectively to input five sets of meaningless text strings via the virtual keyboard on the tablet PC without blind touching. The participants were also required to neglect the mistyping and input the next character when they recognized their own mistyping.

Each set of the strings consisted of 156 characters, 26 alphabetical characters times 6, and were displayed on the same tablet PC.

2.3 Apparatus

Participants sat at the desk and the tablet (Iconia Tab A500) was tilted five degrees to the desk as well as the normal hardware keyboard. The tablet had the capacitive sensing touch screen and the screen size was 10.1 inches wide (1280×800 resolution).

The strings of the task were displayed at the top of the screen. The virtual keyboard was displayed at the bottom of the screen, and every key size was set 1.35cm square. As the visual feedback, a character was painted out with white in each touch.

The original application, which was made in Java, displayed the keyboard and the strings, controlled the visual feedback to each touch, and acquired the two dimensional position of each touch.

2.4 Experimental Procedure

In order to understand the experiment task clearly and be acclimated to the experimental environment, the participants were required to input a set of meaningless text strings before the experiment. After that, the participants were required to input five sets of meaningless text strings. The participants were required to take one minute break between each set.

3 Results

In this experiment, if the touched key was more than 2 keys away from the target key, this touch was regarded as the irregular such as the touch by the other parts of the body because the participants input the characters without blind touching. So this kind of the touched key was excluded from the data. In Figure 1, 3σ limits of the two dimensional touched position of each key were shown by the circles. As shown in Figure 1, the center of 3σ limits circle tended to be positioned in the low and slightly right part of the key regardless of keys. A one-way ANOVA within keys was conducted to compare the position between the center of keys and the center of circles and the results confirmed the tendencies statistically ($F(1,25)= 1673.53$, $p<0.01$, $F(1,25)=10.21$, $p<0.01$).

As shown Figure 1, the sizes of 3σ limits circle tended to be different between keys in both vertical and horizontal directions. A one-way ANOVA was conducted to compare the effect of keys on the square deviation of each touched position from the center of circle and the results confirmed the tendencies statistically ($F(25,8309)=1.74$, $p<0.05$, $F(25,8309)=1.65$, $p<0.05$)..

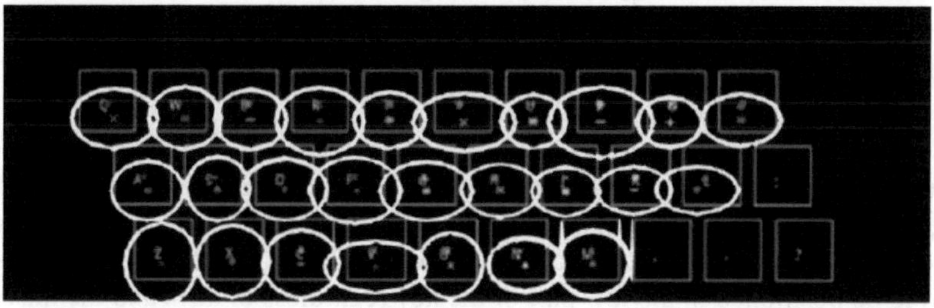

Fig. 1. The virtual keyboard and 3σ limits circles of the two dimensional touched position

4 Discussions

The experimental results showed that the center of distribution of the key touched position tended to be positioned in the low and slightly right part of the key regardless of keys, the same as tendency in the virtual QWERTY keyboard of the mobile phone for one-hand typing (Niels(2012)).

4.1 Mistyping Characteristics

The averaged mistyping ratio was 6% even though the participants input characters without blind touching and a part of a 3σ limits circle was not included within the key area regardless of keys as shown in Figure 1. In order to clarify the characteristics of the mistyping, a one-way ANOVA within keys and the Bonferroni's multiple comparison was conducted to compare the effect of the eight mistyping areas which were out of the key area, as Figure 2 shows, on the ratio of the whole mistypes. The results of the ANOVA revealed that the ratio of the whole mistypes was significantly different between the areas ($F(7,175)=51.05$, $p<0.01$), and the results of the multiple comparison revealed that the ratio in the area "B" was significantly higher than all the others and the ratio in the area "R" was significantly higher than "LT", "T", "RT", and "RB" as shown in Figure 2. These results revealed that the mistypes concentrated under the bottom of key area.

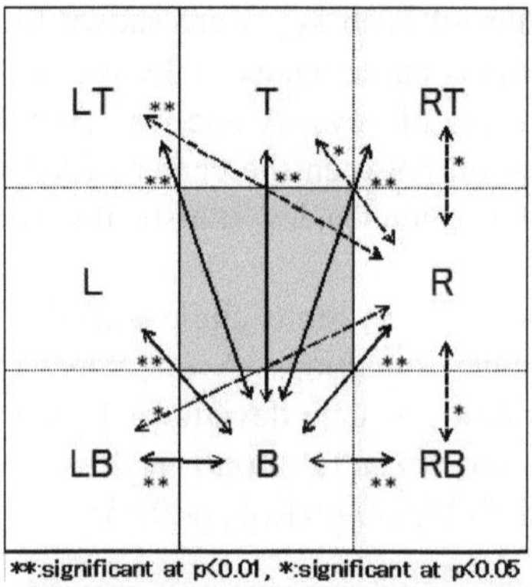

Fig. 2. The eight mistyping areas and the results of the multiple comparison

4.2 New Approach for Key Input Performance Improvement

The results of the experiment revealed that the mistyping ratio was more than 5% and it suggested the necessity of an approach for key input performance improvement. The results also revealed that the center of distribution of the key touched position tended to be positioned in the low part of the key regardless of keys and the mistyping concentrated under the bottom of the key area. We proposed a new approach that the key input performance could be improved by using these characteristics of key touched position and mistyping. The new approach was named the Pop-Up Key system that the users could chose the second possible key by the flick input if the users touched the area within a 3σ limits circle of a certain key but on the visual surface of another key or the overlapped area of 3σ limits circles of two keys. In this system if the users didn't use the flick input and release the finger from the screen, the first possible key was chosen automatically. The priority for the possible characters was according to the rules as follows.

1. In case that the users touch the area within a 3σ limits circle of a certain key but on the visual surface of another key, the first possible key is the corresponding key to the circle and the second possible key is the touched key.
2. In case that the users touch the overlapped area of 3σ limits circles of two keys, the first key is the key of which Mahalanobis distance from the center of the circle is shorter and the second key is the longer one.

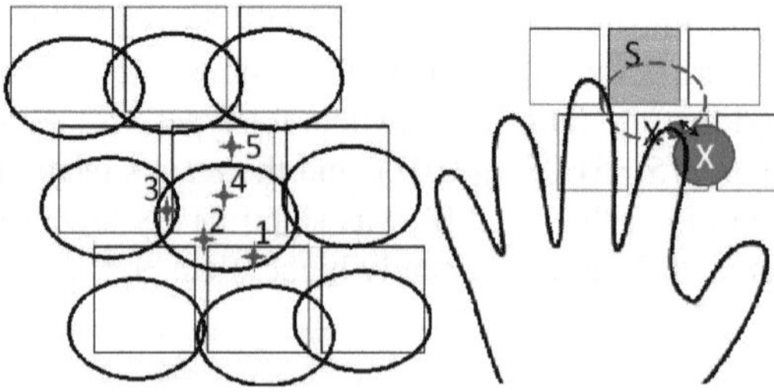

Fig. 3. The rule's number and the touched area and the example of the Pop-Up Key system

Figure 3 shows the relationship between the rule's number and the touched area and the example of the Pop-Up Key system.

This system had also the other rules as follows.

3. If the users touch the area within a 3σ limits circle of a certain key and on the visual surface of the key, only the touched key is chosen automatically.
4. If the users touch the area within a 3σ limits circle of a certain key but not on any key, only the corresponding key to the circle is chosen automatically.
5. If the users touch the area in a certain key which does not belong to any circle, only the touched key is chosen automatically.

5 Conclusion

This research explored the characteristics on two dimensional touched position distributions in each key of a touch screen QWERTY keyboard through the experiment. The results of the experiment revealed that the mistyping ratio was more than 5% and it suggested the necessity of an approach for key input performance improvement. The results also revealed that the center of distribution of the key touched position tended to be positioned in the low part of the key regardless of keys and the mistyping concentrated under the bottom of the key area. A new approach that the key input performance could be improved by using these characteristics of key touched position and mistyping was proposed. Further researches will be held in order to exam the effectiveness of the proposed Pop-Up Key system through experiments.

References

1. Sears, A., Revis, D., Swatski, J., Crittenden, R., Shneiderman, B.: Investigating Touchscreen Typing: The effect of Keyboard size on typing speed. Behaviour & Information Technology 12(1), 17–22 (1993)
2. Ercan Altinsoy, M., Merchel, S.: Audiotactile Feedback Design for Touch Screens. In: Altinsoy, M.E., Jekosch, U., Brewster, S. (eds.) HAID 2009. LNCS, vol. 5763, pp. 136–144. Springer, Heidelberg (2009)
3. Go, K., Endo, Y.: CATKey: Customizable and Adaptable Touchscreen Keyboard with Bubble Cursor-Like Visual Feedback. In: Baranauskas, C., Abascal, J., Barbosa, S.D.J. (eds.) INTERACT 2007. LNCS, vol. 4662, pp. 493–496. Springer, Heidelberg (2007)
4. Go, K., Tsurumi, L.: Arranging Touch Screen Software Keyboard Split-keys based on Contact Surface. In: CHI 2010, Work-in-Progress, Atlanta, GA, USA, pp. 3805–3810 (2010)
5. Kim, J.M., Ishibashi, K., Iwanaga, K.: The effect of invisible touch sensitive area on target acquisition. The Japanese Journal of Ergonomics 48(suppl.), 188–189 (2012)
6. Findlater, L., Wobbrock, J.O., Daniel, W.: Typing on Flat Glass: Examining Ten-Finger Expert Typing Patterns on Touch Surfaces. In: CHI 2011 Session: Text Entry &Typing, Vancouver, BC, Canada, pp. 2453–2461 (2011)
7. Henze, N., Rukzio, E., Boll, S.: Observational and Experimental Investigation of Typing Behaviour using Virtual Keyboards on Mobile Devices. In: CHI 2012 Session: Touch Text Entry, Austin, Texas, USA, pp. 2659–2462 (2012)

Part VIII
Capturing Gaze, Biosignals and Brainwaves

Brainwave Typing: Comparative Study of P300 and Motor Imagery for Typing Using Dry-Electrode EEG Devices

Hadeel Al-Negheimish[1], Lama Al-Andas[1], Latifah Al-Mofeez[1], Aljawharah Al-Abdullatif[1], Nuha Al-Khalifa[1], and Areej Al-Wabil[2]

[1] Information Technology Dept.
College of Computer and Information Sciences, King Saud University
Riyadh, Saudi Arabia
[2] Software Engineering Dept.
College of Computer and Information Sciences, King Saud University
Riyadh, Saudi Arabia
halnegheimish@acm.org, aalwabil@ksu.edu.sa

Abstract. This paper presents the findings of an exploratory study comparing two of Brain-Computer Interface approaches, P300 and Motor Imagery, with EEG signals acquired using the Emotiv Neuroheadset. It was conducted to determine the most suitable approach for typing applications based on BCI. Results show that while selection accuracy is similar for both, with mean of 50%, the speed varies greatly, with the former approach being approximately 2 times more efficient in typing. Implications presented in this document are useful for BCI researchers who seek to build brain-controlled Augmentative and Alternative Communication technologies.

Keywords: BCI, Brain Computer Interface, P300, Motor Imagery, Brain Machine Interface, BMI, Augmentative and Alternative Communication, AAC, EEG.

1 Introduction

Brain-Computer Interface has engendered much research in recent years, with focus on providing people with severe motor disabilities, such as amyotrophic lateral sclerosis or spinal cord injury, with an alternative means of control [1]. This research, however, is mostly based on Gel-based signal acquisition devices that are too expensive for the average user. This experiment explores EEG BCI with consumer-market headset, the Emotiv EEG headset [2]. It is part of on-going research aimed to build a BCI typing applications for Arabic-speaking users. Non-invasive electroencephalography (EEG), where EEG signals are recorded from the surface of the scalp, is one of the popular ways to implement BCI. In fact, it has already been used to develop communication systems, where users can spell words via brain activity, and control systems, where they can drive a simulated wheelchair, for example [3].

There are two main approaches for EEG-BCI. First, Evoked Potential; methods of this kind depend on EEG components (features) evoked and time-locked to a specific

C. Stephanidis (Ed.): Posters, Part I, HCII 2013, CCIS 373, pp. 569–573, 2013.

sensory stimuli, which are also called cue-guided [4]. The most widely used example of this approach is P300 method [5]. Second, Motor Imagery; Methods of this kind use features that are processed in the frequency domain instead of the time domain, as it depends on recording rhythmic activities over the sensorimotor cortex [5]. In this type, instead of needing an external stimulus to generate a command, a user can voluntarily issue a command by controlling his brain activity, by imagining moving a virtual object in a certain direction, for example [4].

Visual representation of the physical and virtual interface for mind-typing.	**Descriptive representation of the functionality of navigation and selection in the typing program.**
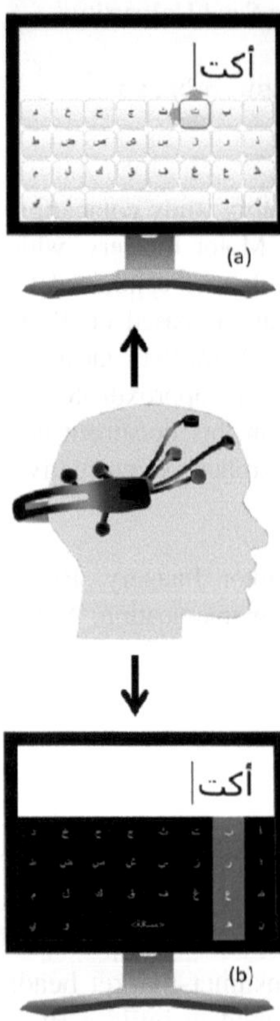	Mind-typing with Motor Imagery: Navigation on the virtual keypad is conducted with imagery movements in the horizontal and vertical directions. Navigating in the top-down direction rotates vertically when then top of the column of virtual keys is reached. Navigating in the right-left direction rotates horizontally when the left-most virtual key on a row is reached.
	Electrical activity of the brain is recorded by 14-channels on the surface of the scalp.
	Mind-typing with Evoked-Responses: The rows and columns in the matrix display Arabic alphabet and numbers. These flash successively and randomly at a rapid rate, and users select a character by directing and sustaining their attention on the Arabic character when it flashes. The row or column that contains this character evoke a P300 response, whereas all others do not. The system determines the desired row and column which exhibited the highest P300 amplitude to select the desired character for the typing task.

Fig. 1. Conceptual design of a typing application with the two approaches: (a) With Motor Imagery, keyboard is navigated in two directions, plus selection. (b) A traditional P300 matrix with Arabic letters.

P300 is characterized by a positive peak 300ms after the presentation of a stimuli, and is most prominent across the area between the two hemispheres [5]. This method is reportedly most suitable for applications where there is a finite number of options [6].

In an effort towards designing an affordable BCI application, Emotiv's EEG Neuroheadset is used for signal acquisition. This, however, introduces the challenge of limited electrode positions, and low signal-to-noise ratio [7]. Thus, this means that eliciting P300 responses for control may not be the best option. The Emotiv headset is shipped with a Cognitiv Suite that discerns a user's intended action on a physical or virtual object, such as pushing or rotating it. This is done by asking the user to imagine moving the object in the desired way while signals are recorded. Before this can be done, the system must be trained to detect an action, the more actions that are trained, the more difficult it is to control them [8].

This study provides an evaluation of the two Brain-Computer-Interface (BCI) approaches; P300 and Motor Imagery, for typing applications using a dry electrode signal acquisition device, the Emotiv Neuroheadset. The P300 approach is evaluated with P3Speller task provided in the BCI2000 [9] distribution, while the latter is done with the Cognitiv Suite in Emotiv's Control panel. To the best of our knowledge, there is no published work that provides such a comparison.

2 Method

To evaluate both approaches, we measured the dependent variables: accuracy and approximated speed of typing with each value of the independent variable, the approach: P300 and Motor Imagery, using a within-subjects design on 5 subjects. Equipment used comprised of the 14-channel Emotiv EEG headset, and a laptop to run the software for each approach. For the Motor Imagery we used the Cognitiv Suite included with Emotiv's Control panel. As for P300, we used P3Speller module included with the BCI2000 platform. The experiment was divided to three parts, the first two parts were to evaluate motor imagery. With motor imagery, three actions are needed to navigate a virtual keyboard; one for moving across the vertical axis, the other for moving across the horizontal axis, and finally, the third for selecting the desired button. These actions were mapped in the Control Panel to Lift, Left and Push respectively. To evaluate the P300, we used the P3Speller included with BCI2000, adjusting the parameters to make up for the relatively noisy signals produced by the headset. We set the number of sequences in a set of row/column intensifications to 15, the stimulus duration to 125ms, and duration of inter-stimulus interval to 250ms, with a 1.5s pause between each sequence.

3 Results and Discussion

The measures we are interested in are the accuracy and speed of typing for each of the two EEG-BCI approaches. With P300, we calculated accuracy by finding the percentage of the correctly typed letters to the total number of letters in the testing session, where the subjects were asked to spell "COOKIE". Speed was calculated directly by multiplying the stimulus and inter-stimulus duration by the number of flashes in a given sequence.

In Motor Imagery's testing sessions, subjects were given commands to move the virtual box in a random order to control for order effects, whether or not they have managed to move it in the specified direction was recorded. Each testing session contained commands testing each of the actions approximately 4 times. In addition to the time that was needed to complete that session. Each subject has completed at least 10 testing sessions. Accuracy for each subject was found by averaging the accuracies of all testing sessions for that subject. In a traditional 6x6 keyboard, same size as P300's, to navigate from one letter to another we need on average 5 movements, and one more action for selection. Thus, to approximate the speed of selecting a certain letter, we multiplied the average duration of an action (movement) by 6. The average accuracy for all subjects is somewhat similar, but P300 has generally higher values with 40% of the subjects achieving more than 80% accuracy. Variations in typing efficiency were found between the two approaches; P300 can provide typing speed more than twice that of Motor Imagery. Both are far too slow and are in need of improvement.

Preliminary investigations with the Emotiv headset for the two EEG-BCI approaches showed that both achieve more or less the same accuracy, but P300 was more efficient than Motor Imagery. Since the incorrect letters in the former approach resulted from letters adjacent to the target letter distracting the user, it can be argued that using the checkerboard paradigm, where no adjacent locations can flash concurrently, would improve accuracy. Additionally, Motor Imagery is an approach that depends on the adaption of both the user and the system; the user must train himself or herself to control their brain activity to type, much like learning to walk or write for the first time. Results that were found by this study did not allow the subjects to gain sufficient experience to control the virtual box, which can take a substantial amount of time. Hopefully, this would reduce the generation of false positives, whose presence significantly decreases the usability of keyboards using Motor Imagery.

There remains an issue of how to balance between system and user training in Motor Imagery, increasing the number of system training sessions can lead to distorting the signature of a certain action [8], but improvements in user control should also be propogated to the system. Further investigation is required to establish some threshold.

Additional work is needed to examine the usability of these applications with people with severe motor disabilities. It remains unknown whether they can control an application with Motor Imagery if they had lost control of their limbs prior to learning how to use it [10]. Hence, it is important to find out if our target population would achieve the same results.

4 Conclusion

This document describes an evaluation of a dry-electrode EEG acquisition device with P300 and Motor Imagery for typing applications. The former approach was deemed more suitable because of its relative efficiency. The document also presented changes that can be introduced to improve accuracy and speed. Further investigation is needed to validate the results for our target population, people with severe motor disabilities.

References

1. Vaughan, T.M., Wolpaw, J.R.: Special issue containing contributions from the Fourth International Brain–Computer Interface Meeting. Journal of Neural Engineering 8(2), 020201 (2011)
2. Emotiv SDK Research Edition Specifications. Emotiv (2010)
3. McFarland, D.J., Wolpaw, J.R.: Brain-computer interfaces for communication and control. Communications of the ACM 54(5), 60 (2011)
4. Rao, R., Scherer, R.: Brain-Computer Interfacing (In the Spotlight). IEEE Signal Processing Magazine 27(4), 152–150 (2010)
5. Wolpaw, J., Wolpaw, E.W. (eds.): Brain-Computer Interfaces: Principles and Practice, 1st edn. Oxford University Press, USA (2012)
6. Fazel-Rezai, R., Allison, B.Z., Guger, C., Sellers, E.W., Kleih, S.C., Kübler, A.: P300 brain computer interface: current challenges and emerging trends. Front. Neuroeng. 5, 14 (2012)
7. Duvinage, M., Castermans, T., Dutoit, T., Petieau, M., Hoellinger, T., De Saedeleer, C., Seetharaman, K., Cheron, G.: A P300-based Quantitive Comparison between the Emotiv Epoc Headset and a Medical EEG Device. Biomedical Engineering / 765: Telehealth / 766: Assistive Technologies 764 (2012)
8. Emotiv Software Development Kit User Manual for Release 1.0.0.3. Emotiv
9. Schalk, G., McFarland, D.J., Hinterberger, T., Birbaumer, N., Wolpaw, J.R.: BCI2000: a general-purpose brain-computer interface (BCI) system. IEEE Trans. Biomed. Eng. 51(6), 1034–1043 (2004)
10. Kübler, A., Nijboer, F., Mellinger, J., Vaughan, T.M., Pawelzik, H., Schalk, G., McFarland, D.J., Birbaumer, N., Wolpaw, J.R.: Patients with ALS can use sensorimotor rhythms to operate a brain-computer interface. Neurology 64(10), 1775–1777 (2005)

Eye-Controlled Games for Behavioral Therapy of Attention Deficit Disorders

Ashwag Al-Shathri[1], Areej Al-Wabil[2], and Yousef Al-Ohali[1]

[1] Computer Science Department
College of Computer and Information Sciences, King Saud University, Saudi Arabia
[2] Software Engineering Department
College of Computer and Information Sciences, King Saud University, Saudi Arabia
ashwag.alshathri@gmail.com, {aalwabil,Yousef}@ksu.edu.sa

Abstract. This paper describes an eye-controlled game designed for behavioral therapy of ADHD. A user-centered design approach was adopted in the development cycle of these games in close collaboration with domain experts and target user populations. The games have an Arabic language interface and include multimodal interaction. Game scenarios were designed with increasing complexity depicted in visual design, dwell time for controlling elements within the games, and combinations of key presses with eye-control at higher levels of attention training. The visual design, interaction design and the system's conceptual designs are discussed.

Keywords: Eye tracking, Serious Games, Attention Deficit, ADD, ADHD.

1 Introduction

The proliferation of computer usage in medicine and rehabilitation has changed the way health care is delivered. Attention Deficit Hyperactivity Disorder (ADHD) is a neurobehavioral developmental disorder and is one of the most common disorders of childhood, with a reported prevalence of approximately 3–9% [1]. It is characterized by hyperactivity, short attention span, and impulsiveness, which is thought to contribute to learning disabilities and many behavioral problems. This consequently affects all areas of an individual's life. ADHD is a persistent and chronic condition, however behavioral modification strategies have been shown to be effective in remedial interventions with individuals. ADHD can be challenging for a parent or caregiver with an individual who has this disorder. Interventions often include medications for individuals with ADHD to control the neurotransmitter imbalance that has an impact on brainwave activation patterns. However, these medications only work a relatively short period of time and often cause unwanted side effects. A number of systems have been developed to improve the attention span of children and adolescents with cognitive or behavioral problems and help them to increase the focus and concentrate on some tasks for long periods of time. These projects offer patients the behavioral intervention treatment which when combined with other therapies can provide improvements in the specific deficits associated with ADHD for these patients.

C. Stephanidis (Ed.): Posters, Part I, HCII 2013, CCIS 373, pp. 574–578, 2013.

Tarkeezy 'تركيزي' is a game focusing on exploiting existing eye tracking technologies to leverage the potential of creating engaging behavioral therapy programs. Tarkeezy's design is based on incorporating unobtrusive stand-alone eye tracking devices that capture eye gaze of individuals and using that to control objects embedded in interactive computer games. The objective of the proposed behavioral intervention program with games that can be controlled solely through movement of the eyes is to help individuals with ADHD to improve focus, visual and auditory attention, and concentration and learn to ignore distractions.

2 Attention Deficit Disorders

Attention Deficit Hyperactivity Disorder (ADHD) is the most common neurobehavioral disorder of childhood that affects neurobehavioral functioning and development. ADHD is a life-long chronic problem. It is believed that up to 50% of children who were diagnosed with ADHD continue to have symptoms into adulthood. This disorder is characterized by inattention, hyperactivity and impulsivity and associated with impairment affecting various aspects of an individual's life [2]. Considerable evidence has accumulated showing that ADHD is linked to impairment in working memory capacity, which refers to the ability to hold goal-relevant information and skip goal-irrelevant for brief periods of time. Individuals with ADHD often seem immature for their age and unable to control their impulsiveness and hyperactivity. They have difficulty forming friendships with others and may have difficulty understanding the social consequences of their actions [3].

Although ADHD is considered a relatively mild disorder, the negative effects of untreated ADHD can have very serious and long-lasting consequences. People with ADHD often feel depressed or anxious. They often have substance abuse problems. Since they have problems forming friendships, it follows that adults with ADHD may have marital issues as well. People who have ADHD easily feel overwhelmed and have low motivation. In addition to these issues, children and adults with ADHD often have problematic employment histories. Difficulties in school are also common among teens and adults with ADHD. Hence, early diagnosis and treatment is essential for people with this disorder to minimize the risk of such serious impacts upon all aspects of life [4]. A range of interventions and therapies for individuals with mental health problems have been explored to develop appropriate behavior and adequate social skills according to rules and societal norms. Some commonly used remedial programs for individuals with ADHD include interventions such as pharmacological, behavior, cognitive behavior, neural-based, and play. Each one has its own merits and demerits and quite often a combination of two or more interventions are sought by the clinicians in treating individuals with ADHD. Some individuals with ADHD take stimulant medications to correct the neurotransmitter imbalance that affects their brainwave activation patterns. However, medications only work for a short period of time and often cause unwanted side effects. In recent years, interventions for ADHD often consider treatment plans that involve behavioral interventions, neurofeedback, non-invasive, drug-free approach to rehabilitating brain function and overcoming ADHD [5,6].

Play is an important part of childhood development and the natural context within which children develop complex social behaviors and competence. The use of play as an intervention plan to treat individuals with cognitive difficulties and mental health disorders may bridge the gap between the exceptional individual's mental health needs and the available services. Play acts as a medium to help therapists interact with individuals and help them express their feelings and emotions [7]. Play therapy is widely used as an intervention for individual's behavioral, cognitive and emotional disorders because it's focus on the developmental needs. As noted by the Association for Play Therapy [8], play therapy is "a systematic use of a theoretical model to establish an interpersonal process in which trained play therapists use the therapeutic powers of play to help clients prevent or resolve psychosocial difficulties and achieve optimal growth and development". It is an intervention based on the cognitive, social, and emotional development. Evidence suggests that play therapy is effective with individuals who experience social, emotional, behavioral, and learning problems.

In recent years, research studies have also demonstrated that play therapy is effective with individuals with ADHD in particular, and that it has a positive impact on self-concept, self-efficacy, depression, anxiety, general behavioral problems, and treatment compliance. The individuals participating in play therapy have been shown to be less stressful, emotional distress and difficulties with withdrawal [9].

3 Eye Tracking: Diagnostic and Interactive

Eye tracking is a technique that allows users to determine where individuals are focusing their visual attention at a given time. The point being focused upon in an inter-face is called a gaze point. Tracking eye gaze of users has been used in the design and development of assistive technologies and in diagnostic contexts of HCI research. The direction of gaze indicates the direction of attention. In this way we can gain insight into what the observers looked at, what they might have perceived, and what object drew their attention [10]. Eye tracking is a computerized remote video-based corneal reflection device that captures individual's gaze without being attached to them [11]. Gaze control is a feasible alternative to hand-based interaction that gives users the ability to control the computer in situations when hands-off control is desired. It has recently become of central concern in several application domains of disciplines such as biology, medicine, psychology, and neurology [12]. Recently, two lines of research have emerged that involve eye tracking. The first one is diagnostic eye tracking which examines human cognition and perception through experimentation; application domains for this type of research are HCI, psychology, medicine, and neurosciences. The second line is interactive eye tracking which integrates gaze within applications to use the eyes as a control mechanism; application domains for this type of research are gaze-controlled games, biometrics, and assistive technology [11]. Recent discoveries in the field have led to an abundance of new applications. New improvements in interactive methods of using gaze control and eye movement have the potential to make human-computer interfaces faster and more efficient. This potential could benefit users with and without disabilities.

4 Tarkeezy

The Tarkeezy program is a behavioral intervention serious game designed to be controlled solely through movement of the eyes using eye tracking technology to help individuals with ADHD to improve attention, concentration and learn to ignore distractions. This program depends on objective gaze metrics gathered by corneal-reflection eye trackers (e.g. gaze coordinates, fixation duration, and the number of fixations) for the purpose of controlling objects embedded in the games. The system is comprised of a pre analysis stage in which the specialist selects and configures the games with the suitable dwell time and size of area of interest (AOI) according to the subject's disorder severity. This step includes: design sessions' procedures according to the subject's needs, select the game, the level, and set the dwell time and the size of AOI. The system also includes a playing and data analysis component which processes the gaze measurements that are read from the eye tracker's live stream to control the game such as the gaze coordinates after mapping game window's coordinates to the eye tracker coordinates, fixation duration, and the number of fixations. The final component of the system is the reporting component which analyzes the data derived from the sessions to produce progress charts for the specialist, and to print reports. Before the session, the specialist will register the subject and enters their demographic data. After logging in to the system, several tasks can be performed to manage the subject. Calibration follows before launching the games as depicted in Fig 1.

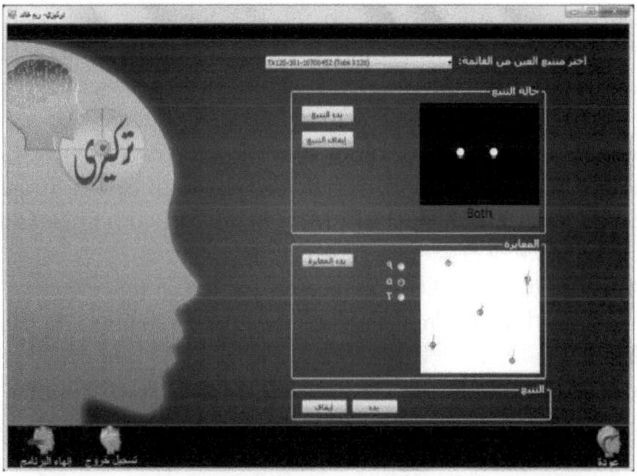

Fig. 1. Calibration of the eyes in the Tarkeezy games

The specialist will select the game and appropriate level for the subject. Then, the user starts using the system. After starting the game, the system will read the data from the stream of gaze captured with the eye tracker to facilitate gaze interaction with controlling objects within the game. The specialist can show data in a graph format to monitor the individual's progress across game sessions. Games were designed with increasing complexity to introduce challenge at progressive levels in the games. Complexity factors include increasing distraction with background images, manipulating dwell time to increase the difficulty of controlling objects or avatars within the games, and adding elements of control to increase the complexity (e.g. combining a key press with visual attention on objects to manipulate them within the game scenario).

5 Conclusion

This paper described the design of eye-controlled games for behavioral therapy of attention deficit disorders. The system was designed in UCD design cycles and underwent initial user-acceptance testing. Preliminary evaluations demonstrated good usability measures by heuristic evaluations of specialists and target user populations. The testing phase is underway. Future work involves conducting user evaluations of the effectiveness of these games in the context of behavioral therapy for ADHD.

Acknowledgement. This project was supported in part by Research Group Grant RGP-VPP-157 from the Deanship of Scientific Research in King Saud University.

References

1. Greydanus, D.E.: Attention Deficit Hyperactivity Disorder. In: Patel, D.R., Greydanus, D.E., Omar, H.A., Merrick, J. (eds.) Neurodevelopmental Disabilities, pp. 111–140. Springer, Heidelberg (2011)
2. Goldstein, M.L., Morewitz, S.: Attention-Deficit Hyperactivity Disorder. Chronic Disorders in Children and Adolescents, pp. 99–123. Springer, New York (2011)
3. Tannock, R.: A meta-analysis of working memory impairments in children with attention-deficit/hyperactivity disorder. J. Am. Acad. Child Adolesc. Psychiatry 44, 377 (2005)
4. Resnick, R.J.: Attention deficit hyperactivity disorder in teens and adults: They don't all outgrow it. Journal of Clinical Psychology 61, 529–533 (2005)
5. Ravichandran, S., Qunfang Jacklyn, H.: Behavior Modification Strategy for Motivating Children with Attention Deficiency Disorder. Journal of Abnormal Child Psychology 34, 584–601 (2009)
6. Goh, D.H., Ang, R.P., Tan, H.C.: Strategies for designing effective psychotherapeutic gaming interventions for children and adolescents. Computers in Human Behavior 24, 2217–2235 (2008)
7. Wilkes, S., Cordier, R., Bundy, A., Docking, K., Munro, N.: A play-based intervention for children with ADHD: A pilot study. Australian Occupational Therapy Journal 58, 231–240 (2011)
8. Association for Play Therapy – Home, `http://www.a4pt.org/ps.index.cfm`
9. Leblanc, M., Ritchie, M.: A meta-analysis of play therapy outcomes. Counselling Psychology Quarterly 14, 149–163 (2001)
10. Corno, F., Farinetti, L., Signorile, I.: A cost-effective solution for eye-gaze assistive technology. Multimedia and Expo, 2002. In: Proceedings of the IEEE International Conference on ICME 2002, pp. 433–436 (2002)
11. Duchowski, A.T.: Eye tracking methodology: Theory and practice. Springer (2007)
12. Drewes, H.: Eye gaze tracking for human computer interaction (2010), `http://edoc.ub.uni-muenchen.de/11591/`

Towards an Emergent and Autopoietic Approach to Adaptative Chord Generation through Human Interaction

Francisco de Paula Barretto[1], Suzete Venturelli[1], and Gabriel Gaudencio do Rego[2]

[1] Computer Art Research Lab, University of Brasilia, Brasilia, Federal District, Brazil
{kikobarretto,suzeteventurelli}@gmail.com
[2] Laboratory of Cognitive and Social Neuroscience, Mackenzie Presbyterian University, So Paulo, Brazil
gabrielgaudenciorego@gmail.com

Abstract. This poster describes a transdisciplinary practical-theoretical on-going research, which address on the discussion about the possible applications of Artificial Intelligence (AI) techniques, such as genetic algorithms, which underlie the Maturana and Varela's autopoietic concept considering the achievement of emergent results as heuristic to creativity. Through human interaction using neuronal bio-feedback it is possible to provide more natural fitness function to such algorithms.

Keywords: autopoiesis, emergence, bio-feedback, creativity, genetic algorithms.

1 Theoretical Framework

1.1 Autopoiesis

The concept of autopoiesis, as the organization of the living, originated in the work of Chilean biologists Humberto Maturana and Francisco Varela in the 1970s [1] . This idea was developed in the context of theoretical biology and was early associated with the artificial life simulation long before the term "artificial life" have been introduced in the late 1980s in [2] .

Autopoiesis (from the Greek auto which means itself and poiesis which means creation) describes the autonomous systems, able to self-reproduce and self-regulate, while iterating with the environment. This environment iteration might unroll, only in an indirect way, changes on the autopoietic systems internal processes and structures that might lead to a deterministic-emergent transition.

Today the concept of autopoiesis continues to have a significant impact in the field of artificial life computing. Pier Luisi presents a good review in [3]. Furthermore, there was also an effort to integrate the notion of autopoiesis to the field of cognitive sciences.

C. Stephanidis (Ed.): Posters, Part I, HCII 2013, CCIS 373, pp. 579–583, 2013.

To be more precise, an autopoietic system is organized as a production processes network of components (synthesis and destruction) which: (i) continuously regenerate themselves in order to form a network able to reproduce components and (ii) this network constitutes the system as a distinct unit in the domain in which it exists. In addition to these two explicit criteria for autopoiesis, we can add another important point: that identity self-constitution implies on the creation of a relational domain between the system and its environment. Froese and Ziemke describes this relational domain in [4]. This emergent domain is not predetermined but possibly co-determined by the system and environments organization. Any system that meets the criteria for autopoiesis also generates its own domain of interactions while its identity emerges.

The concept of self-organization can be interpreted in many different ways, but in terms of autopoietic is worthy of being presented by two aspects: (i) determining local-to-global, so that the process has its emerging identity global constituted and constrained as a result of local interactions and (ii) determining global-to-local and global identity where its ongoing contextual interaction constrain local interactions [5].

Finally, autopoietic systems are also autonomous systems since they are characterized by such a dynamic co-emergence but are specified within a specific domain. It is important for the creativity of a system that it's changes and adaptations of the internal mechanisms are not performed directly by an external agent, but through an internal self-regulation mechanism.

1.2 Emergency

The emergent behavior can be defined, according to Peter Cariani [6] , as something fundamentally new, that could not be predicted before it happened, such as natural evolution. This characteristic might be seen as a useful heuristic towards achievement of creative behavior. Being the human not only a part of the autopoietic system's environment, but also an active agent, the interaction occurs in a higher cognitive level, influencing the artificial agent cognitive construction.

In general, emergence designates a behavior that has not been explicitly programmed in a system or agent. Pfeifer and Bongard [5] point out three kinds of emergence: (i) a global phenomenon arising from a collective behavior, (ii) individual behavior as the result of an interaction between the agent and the environment and (iii) emergence behavioral from a time scale to another.

The artistic installation named La Funambule Virtuelle [7], from Marie-Hlne Tramus and Michel Bret, where a virtual acrobat evolves to keep up on a tightrope, reacting to the movements of the public. The character tries to reproduce the position of the iterator while trying to stay on the rope. In this installation, through a ANN, the balancer is able to learn to remain on the rope during the user interaction. From the learned gesture, a new behavior emerges through movements that were not taught, endowing the character of what the artist calls the ability to improvise. This is a nice example of the individual behavior as the result of an interaction with the environment.

A deeper level of emergence called epistemic emergence involves, of course, the emergence of new perspectives intrinsically linked to the sensorial changes. The improvement or development of new sensorial organs allows an organism to evolve into another lineage, along with new world perspectives. This kind of development also occurs in our technological evolution as we build artifacts such as thermometers, clocks, telescopes, and that extend our senses or reactions as an extension of our natural biological functions.

2 The Evolutionary Chord Generation Case

Genetic algorithms are an Artificial Intelligence technique proposed by John Holland [8] and uses a metaphor based on the theory of natural evolution. In the genetic algorithms, the solutions for the problem are evolved through multiple generations, improving the solutions prior to each new iteration. Just like in natural evolution, genetic operators such as mutation and recombination allow each new generation of individuals to improve the previous generated potential solutions. This evolution towards the "best" solution is given by a fitness function that calculates the degree of adaptation of the individual and its neighbors, inferring the most likely to reproduce and therefore which variations are more able to extinction.

These populations of individuals composed by a genotype and a phenotype. The genotype is the individual coded information, like our chromosomes and is composed by some alleles. The information coded in the individual genotype is represented by the phenotype. For example, the color of our eyes (phenotype) are coded into our DNA (genotype).

For example, in one possible approach to chord formation, we must consider that there are many standards and rules that define various categories of chords as major, minor, diminished or increased and that these patterns are usually represented by intervals between notes, expressed in semitones, and we can, from a note, build several different chords using other notes at specific intervals. So,as a first experiment there was implemented a Genetic Algorithm (GA) chord generator.

In this experiment the individuals chromosome are formed by 4 alleles and each one of these alleles contains a musical note. Groups of 4 notes forms a chord. The fitness function, in this case evaluates the distance between chromosomes, considering the notes contained in alleles in relation to the notes required for formation of a major chord, classifying individuals with interpolated values between 0 and 100 (maximum fitness).

Once an initial population randomly generated containing 10 individuals were performed 100 rounds using two genetic operators with different rates probability for this population: crossover and mutation. For the crossover operator there was applied a percentage rate of 80

At each round played the individual sound (phenotype) with the highest fitness. This mapped chromosome (genotype) evolution allowed us to realize that, while not struck a major chord, all the other types of chord system emerged.

Even with a fixed and hard fitness function, the application of recombination and mutation operator has enabled the emergence of chords not provided as minors diminished and augmented, for example, suggests an emergent behavior of the autopoietic system.

3 A Human-Guided Evolutionary Chord Generation Experiment

It is possible to use human bodys physiological signals as a fitness function, which could indicate cognitive and affective processes relevant for the implemetation of a human-computer interface (HCI). In the specific case of a musical experiment, two classes of physiological signals could be used to assign: (1) affective processes, like emotional states [9]; or (2) cognitive processes, like error detection in the harmonic field expectation [10]. The first proposed class is being subject of intensive research since the last decade, resulting in systems with acceptable accurate rates that can identify and classificate a subjects emotion only using his physiological responses [11]. In the other hand, the second proposed class got less attention from researchers, mainly because the subjacent complexity in tracking and using its signals in accurate online systems for HCI. Only in the last few years some papers proposed online systems based in error detection signals, but yet with low accuracy rate or with better accuracy rates, but limited by the kind of the task [12], that is different from the experiment proposed in this research.

However, the use of cognitive process like error detection (which represents a biological feedback system) opens a broad branch of HCI possibilities and, in this particular experiment, it serves as an innovating way in creative interaction, where the fitness function is not oriented by a determined function leading to a final state, but it develops to a endless state oriented by a constant homeostasis process.

As said before, there are some eletrophysiological potential related to cognitive processing of music in human beings, like the Early Right Auditory Negativity (ERAN) detected by Electroencephalography (EEG). The ERAN is related to the detection of violations in the harmonic patterns, taking in count some harmonic scale which a person has familiarity (such as Western music) [10]. The problem is that ERAN potential is well detected by offline (post-analysis) and multi-trial processing, such as ERP experiments. But, by this moment, the literature lack conclusive studies about the use of ERAN in a online (real-time) system. There are studies with similar potentials, like ERN (Error-related Negativity) [12], which behaves in a similar way of ERAN and are detected in similar spacial distribution of electrodes (frontal lobe).

4 Conclusion

In the research, we propose a system that could integrate the musical genetic algorithm with a HCI based on a feedback detection using error signals, like

ERAN. To potentialize the signal detection, the analysis process will be designed to a user-dependent system, which requires training of the user to optimize the algorithm detection of the system according to individuals error signal characteristics. There are also the possibility to integrate different physiological signals, like pupillometry, skin conductance or electromyography that could be involved with error and feedback detection (yet this assumption still lack conclusive studies), or affective responses (like tension, arousal or unpleasantness) that could compound a integrative system for the HCI system proposed in this study.

This approach might seem simple at first sight but opens several doors to the development of adaptative interfaces based on bio-feedback, for exemple. In the other hand it can provide to natural-based artificial intelligence techniques evaluation functions more natural than the rigid ones used today.

References

1. Maturana, F., Varela, H.: De Máquinas y Seres Vivos. 3rd edn. Editorial Universitaria (1972)
2. Langton, C.: Artificial life. In: Artificial Life: Proceedings of an Interdisciplinary Workshop on Synthesis and Simulation of Living Systems, vol. 4, pp. 1–47 (1989)
3. Luisi, P.: Autopoiesis: a review and a reappraisal. Naturwissenschaften 90(2), 49–59 (2003)
4. Froese, T., Ziemke, T.: Enactive artificial intelligence: investigating the systemic organization of life and mind. Artificial Intelligence 173(4-3), 446–500 (2009)
5. Pfeifer, R., Bongard, J.: How The Body Shapes The Way We Think: a new view on intelligence. The MIT Press (2007)
6. Cariani, P.: Emergence and creativity. Emoção Artificial 4.0, 21–41 (2009)
7. Tramus, M.H., Chen, C.Y.: La funambule virtuelle et quorum sensing, deux installations interactives s'inspirant du connexionnisme et de l'évolutionnisme. La création artistique face aux nouvelles technologies (2005)
8. Holland, J.H.: Adaptation In Natural and Artificial Systems. The University of Michigan Press (1975)
9. Sourina, O., Liu, Y., Nguyen, M.: Real-time eeg-based emotion recognition for music therapy. Journal of Multimodal User Interfaces 5(1-2), 27–35 (2012)
10. Steinbeis, N., Koelsch, S., Sloboda, J.: The role of harmonic expectancy violations in musical emotions: Evidence from subjective, physiological, and neural responses. Journal of Cognitive Neuroscience 18(8), 1380–1393 (2006)
11. Liu, Y., Sourina, O.: Eeg based dominance level recognition for emotion-enabled interaction. In: IEEE International Conference on Multimedia and Expo (2012)
12. Vi, C.T., Subramanian, S.: Detecting error-related negativity for interaction design. In: 30th Conference on Human Factors in Computing Systems, pp. 493–502 (2012)

Stress Resilience Training System (SRTS)

Joseph V. Cohn[1,*], Theodore Morrison[2,**], Gershon Weltman[3,**], Donald Chartrand[4,**], Rollin McCraty[5,**], David J. Combs[6,*], Antonio Anglero Jr.[7,***], Brian R. Johnson[8,*], David Rozovski[9,*], Stephen Eggan[10,*], Brennan Cox[9,*], Kirsten Carlson[11,*], and Elizabeth O'Neill[12]

[1] Office of Naval Research
[2] Naval Center for Combat and Operational Stress Control
[3] Perceptronics Solutions, Inc.
[4] Ease Interactive, Inc.
[5] Institute of HeartMath
[6] Naval Research Laboratory
[7] Naval Safety Center
[8] United States Air Force Academy
[9] Naval Aerospace Medical Institute, Pensacola, FL
[10] Naval Medical Research Unit–Dayton
[11] Naval Air Warfare Center Aircraft Division
[12] Strategic Analysis, Inc.
eoneill@sainc.com

Abstract. The SRTS is an eLearning iPad app that incorporates both cognitive knowledge and proven neurological biofeedback based on Heart Rate Variability (HRV) Coherence. SRTS uses HRV-controlled games as a way of motivating today's young soldiers and sailors. The objective is both to minimize the adverse effects of stress and enhance its productive effects in order to help improve immediate performance as well as help prevent the occurrence of future problems such as post-traumatic stress disorder (PTSD). The initial phase of the research resulted in a PC-based SRTS demonstration system, as well as positive responses to formal and informal usability and utility studies. The current phase of the project has involved the complete development of the iPad version of the SRTS, and also its operational evaluation for efficacy by the Naval Center for Combat and Operational Stress Control (NCCOSC), US Navy Bureau of Medicine and Surgery (BUMED). Many potential customers for SRTS in the Navy, Marine Corps, Air Force and Army are waiting completion of the NCCOSC efficacy evaluation.

Keywords: Stress resilience training, eLearning, Heart Rate Variability, PTSD.

1 Introduction

Stress resilience is an important issue in the military today. The negative effects of stress can be evident before, during and after exposure; they include decrements

* Ph.D., Medical Service Corps, United States Navy.
** Ph.D.
*** Psy.D., Medical Service Corps, United States Navy.

C. Stephanidis (Ed.): Posters, Part I, HCII 2013, CCIS 373, pp. 584–588, 2013.

in performance both on and off the battlefield, psychological injuries leading to high-risk behaviors such as alcohol and drug use, and in extreme cases, PTSD and suicide.

At the same time, there are positive aspects to stress as well. It has long been recognized that warfighters adapt to combat stress after the first few experiences and that training can help duplicate this process [1], with recent studies showing that experienced military personnel are able to control and even utilize stress productively [2]. An important part of what experienced personnel learn is self-awareness of their stress state and self-regulation of stress energy. Accordingly, the current DOD definition of stress resilience is: The ability to withstand, recover, and grow in the face of stressors and changing demands.

Our Stress Resilience Training System (SRTS) is completely consistent with current DOD resilience doctrine and objectives in that it aims both to minimize adverse effects of stress and enhance its productive effects in order to improve immediate performance and prevent the occurrence of future problems such as PTSD. In fact, the SRTS emphasizes the performance-improving aspects of stress resilience. This differentiates it from the great majority of other stress resilience programs and methodologies, which tend to be more focused on stress pathology and therapy.

2 Hypotheses

The key hypotheses upon which we have based the development of SRTS are:

- Incorporating both *Cognitive Learning* and *Evidence-Based Biofeedback* in a scientifically-designed system to enhance stress resilience can minimize the adverse effects of stress.
- Minimizing the adverse effects of stress *and enhancing its productive effects* at exposure will_improve immediate performance and will also help prevent the occurrence of longer term psychological injuries such as PTSD.
- A state-of-the art mobile device such as the *iPad* will greatly improve training effectiveness by enabling individualized, on-the-spot refreshment training and practice before, during and after deployment.
- Embedding the Neurological Biofeedback methods in a set of *Casual and Serious Games* will help motivate today's young military population [3].

3 Technical Description

The initial phase of the research resulted in an end-to-end PC-based SRTS demonstration system that contained most of the key features of the final product. Formal and informal studies showed that the SRTS interface, training modules and practice games were easy to understand and enjoyable as well, and yielded very positive comments [4]. As a result, the research progressed to development of the originally-planned complete iPad-based mobile stress resilience training course. SRTS is now available as an iPad app that provides access to four main training components:

- **KNOW HOW:** Provides a set of short narrated video modules that include: an introduction to SRTS; general information about stress effects, stress resilience and putting stress in perspective; and also specific instructions on preparing for, performing in, and recovering from stressful situations or operations.

- **TECHNIQUES:** Teaches the HeartMath Coherence Advantage technique, which includes self-regulation of Heart Rate Variability (HRV) and shifting from negative to positive emotions.
- **GAMES:** Provides a set of entertaining HRV-controlled games in which the trainee can practice maintaining HRV Coherence while performing under increasingly absorbing and challenging conditions.
- **REVIEW**: Allows the user to review his or her progress in learning the cognitive material and in the acquisition of Coherence Advantage skills.

In addition, there is a built-in Adaptive Coach that monitors the trainee's progress and self-test results, and provides recommendations on how best to progress through the training program. Each component has been human factored for ease of use, and professionally designed and produced to the highest standards of iPad apps. The current iPad SRTS has a Navy orientation because it fit the Navy's Operational Stress Control Program so well [5], but the framework is applicable to many different users.

An important part of SRTS is Coherence Advantage training using methods developed and validated by our team member the Institute of HeartMath. Coherence Advantage employs Heart Rate Variability biofeedback to control the neuropsychological responses associated with counter-productive emotional states. Heart Rate Variability (HRV) is a measure of the strength and regularity of the changes in the heart's beat-to-beat interval, sometimes called Heart Rhythm. The intervals between heart beats vary, and can be expressed as a variation in Heart Rate with time. A strong and regular Heart Rate Variability is called Coherence; it is when the sympathetic and parasympathetic nervous systems are in synch, and is associated with good neurophysiological function and stress resilience. A weak and irregular variability is called Incoherence, and is associated with poor neurophysiological function and stress. The top graph in Figure 1 shows the edgy, jerky HRV pattern associated with Incoherence. The bottom graph shows the more even HRV pattern associated with Coherence. Coherence represents the neurophysiology of optimal function, when everything seems easy and cognitive performance is high. Athletes call this *THE ZONE*.

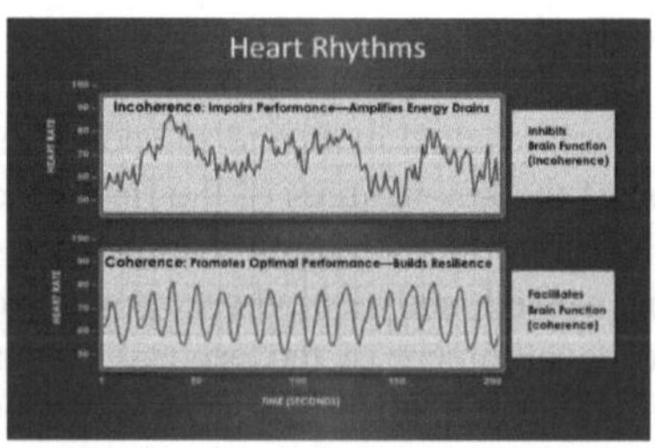

Fig. 1. Heart Rate Variability (HRV) in Incoherence and Coherence

In SRTS the heart beat is detected with an ear pulse sensor. The HRV value goes from 0 to 100, and is calculated using an algorithm developed by Institute of Heartmath that uses power spectral analysis. A low HRV number is associated with Incoherence, a high number with Coherence. Using biofeedback techniques coupled with voluntary shifts in emotion, individuals can learn to increase their HRV value, thus improving their immediate performance and enhancing their stress resilience.

Figure 2 shows how Coherence feedback is included in a typical HRV-controlled SRTS game. This game, Slingshot Racer, is the most challenging and requires the trainee to increase the speed of the jet racer while avoiding various obstacles. A breath pacer time-graph helps the trainee regulate his or her breathing rhythm, while HRV is shown in three ways: one, as a Heart Rate time-graph above the breath pacer; and two, as a slider on a red-to-green Coherence bar; and three, as a numerical Coherence value. The trainee can use the feedback mode or combination of modes that best helps him or her to achieve and maintain higher Coherence in the game.

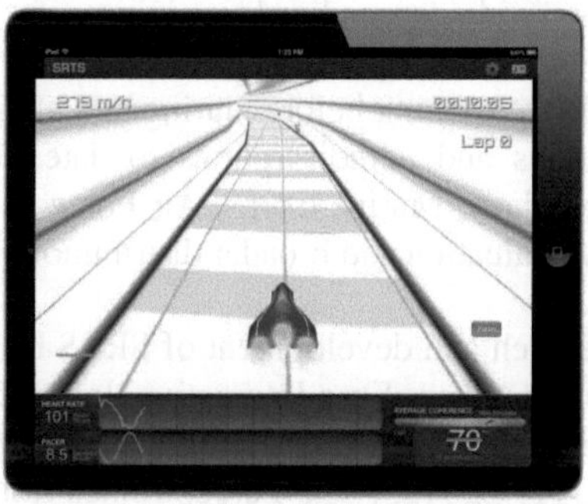

Fig. 2. HRV-Controlled Slingshot Racer Game

4 Efficacy Evaluation

Usability of the initial PC-based SRTS and current iPad SRTS app has been validated by several experimental studies at the George Mason University Psychology Dept. The first usability study was done in 2011with the PC-based SRTS version using questionnaires, observations and interviews. The results showed that the interface, modules and games were easy to understand, fast to learn, and enjoyable. The second study was done in 2012 with the iPad SRTS app and also produced very positive results on measures of usability and stress control potential [6].

The military utility of SRTS has been initially established in a series of trial evaluations by military groups such as Navy Operational Stress Control (OSC) Program Office, the Navy Special Warfare Group 1, Naval Air Station Lemoore, the Army Family Advocacy Program at Ft. Sam Houston, the Army CSF-PREP Program at Ft. Hood, and others. Typical comments included, "…it's great; very engaging. Would give it to our guys." And "Catches my attention all the time. Will work with adolescents."

SRTS' operational efficacy is being tested in a large-scale, formal evaluation study now under way at the Naval Center for Combat and Operational Stress Control (NCCOSC), San Diego. The NCCOSC evaluation study will provide groups of about

35 subjects with SRTS units for several weeks. It will base efficacy on pre- and post-trial stress and resilience questionnaires (and potentially other available performance measures) as compared with two other groups: one group will receive an iPad app on Progressive Muscle Relaxation (PMR) and the other group will receive no training for the period. The total study will involve about 200 volunteer subjects from two Navy commands in the San Diego area; the study protocols have received IRB approval and the experimental portion of the study is scheduled to begin in early May, 2013.

5 Conclusions

Two major problems have precluded effective stress control in the military: the stigma of weakness prevents personnel from seeking psychological help; and existing soft programs do not build transferable skills. SRTS addresses both of these problems by its "de-stigmatizing" emphasis on performance over pathology, and by its combination of instruction about stress with specialized training in how to build actual neurophysiological resilience. Its mobile iPad format allows personnel to obtain individualized stress resilience training before, during and after deployment. As a result of the successful evaluations and demonstrations to date, there are many potential customers for SRTS in the Navy, Marine Corps, Air Force and Army who are waiting completion of the efficacy evaluation and broader distribution of the SRTS product.

Acknowledgements. Research and development of SRTS by Perceptronics Solutions, Inc., with the help of team members Ease Interactive, Inc. and Institute of HeartMath, has been supported by DARPA through SBIR Phase I contract N10PC20058 and SBIR Phase II contract D11PC20125. The Perceptronics Solutions team's support of the efficacy evaluation at the Naval Center for Combat and Operational Stress Control has been funded by ONR BAA contracts N0001412M0198 and N0001412M0408.

References

1. Fenz, W.D., Jones, G.B.: Individual Differences in Physiologic Arousal and Performance in Sport Parachutists. Psychosomatic Medicine 34, 1–8 (1972)
2. McCraty, R.: Psychophysiological Coherence: A Link between Positive Emotions, Stress Reduction, Performance and Health. In: Proceedings of the Eleventh International Congress on Stress, Mauna Lani Bay, HI (2001)
3. Fletcher, J.D., Tobias, S.: Using Computer Games and Simulations for Instruction: A Research Review. In: Proceedings of the Society forApplied Learning Technology (SALT) Meeting, Orlando, FL (February 2006)
4. Cohn, J., Weltman, G., Chartrand, D.: Stress Inoculation through Cognitive and Biofeedback Training. In: Proceedings of Interservice/Industry Training, Simulation, and Education Conference, I/ITSEC (November 2010)
5. US Navy. Operational Stress Control. All Hands Magazine of the U.S. Navy (March 2010)
6. Smith, M.A., Woo, H.J., Parker, J.P., Youmans, R.J., LeGoullon, M., Weltman, G., de Visser, E.J.: Using Iterative Design and Testing Towards the Development of SRTS: A Mobile, Game-Based Stress Resilience Training System. In: Proceedings of the Human Factors and Ergonomics Society, Annual Meeting. Vol. 57 (in press, 2013)

Proposal of PC Input Method by Combination of Gaze Detection and Head Movement Detection

Yoshinobu Ebisawa, Hayato Hakamada, and Kiyotaka Fukumoto

Graduate School of Engineering, Shizuoka University, Hamamatsu, 432-8561 Japan
ebisawa@sys.eng.shizuoka.ac.jp

Abstract. We propose a PC input methodology combining the gaze detection technology and the PupilMouse technology (head movement detection). Both technologies are based on the remote pupil detection technique using video cameras with near-infrared light sources. In the PupilMouse method, a user can move the cursor on the PC display screen smoothly and accurately, based on the movements of the user's two pupils in the camera image caused by the user's smooth head movement. The biggest advantage of PupilMouse is to be able to point a very small area without a scattering of the cursor. However, in order to move the cursor largely on the screen, the user must move the head largely. This is a burden for the user. In contrast, the gaze point moves quickly and largely by just looking. However, at present, there is no remote gaze detection system that can detect the gaze point on the PC screen accurately, as a replacement for computer mouse. Moreover, as the ability of the user, it might be very difficult to continue to direct the line of sight exactly to small areas. In the experiment that subjects type twelve Japanese letter string using a software keyboard, the input speed, number of typing mistakes, and the usability were investigated. The results show that the proposed method is comprehensively superior to both the gaze detection method and the PupilMouse method.

Keywords: Gaze detection, Head movement detection, pupil detection.

1 Introduction

The remote video-based gaze detection system is considered to be useful as a PC input device. One of the reasons is that the gaze shift is very quick. So far, however, there is no gaze detection system having high accuracy enough to able to choose a small menu option in the GUI environments. Even if the system has enough high accuracy, it is may be difficult to continue to direct the line of sight within the small area due to a limit of human eye-movement control system. On the other hand, we had developed the system where a user can move a mouse cursor very precisely by the head movement [1]. We named the system PupilMouse because the cursor moves according to the movement of the pupils detected by a video camera. However, when the user wants to move the cursor largely, it takes a long time compared to the gaze detection method. According to our consideration, the gaze detection and PupilMouse have the opposite properties. The present paper proposes a novel method using only the advantages of both methods. We experimentally shows that the proposed method is comprehensively superior to both the gaze detection method and the PupilMouse method.

C. Stephanidis (Ed.): Posters, Part I, HCII 2013, CCIS 373, pp. 589–593, 2013.

2 Gaze Detection System and Method

Our gaze detection system used in the present experiment is described elsewhere [2]. The system uses two optical devices (Fig. 1(a)). Each of the optical devices consists of a camera and a two concentric near-infrared LED ring light source attached to the camera (Fig. 2(b)). The inner and outer LED rings generate bright and dark pupil images, respectively. The pupils are detected from the difference image created by subtracting the bright and dark pupil images. Basically, the line of sight is determined by the difference of the pupil center from the corneal reflection in each of the camera images. Here, the corneal reflection is the reflection image of the light source. The gaze point is determined as an intersection between the line of sight and the PC screen plane. By camera calibration of the optical devices, the 3D coordinates of the pupils are determined by the stereo matching. This enables to allow the user's head movements. Owing to our gaze detection theory, gaze detection with accuracy of less than one degree becomes possible by looking at only one point whose coordinates is known [2].

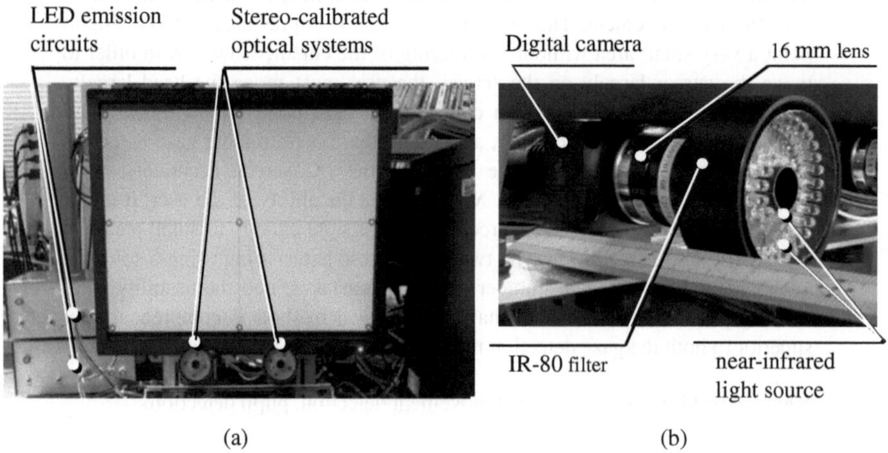

Fig. 1. (a) Gaze detection system and (b) optical device for pupil detection including camera and near-infrared light source

3 Cursor Control by Head Movement (PupilMouse)

The algorithm of the PupilMouse method can be implemented in the same hardware system as the gaze detection system. In the PupilMouse method, the cursor on the PC screen is moved basically by the averaged displacement of the two pupils in the images obtained from the two cameras [3]. The horizontal and vertical components of the cursor movement on the screen are related to the respective components of the pupil movements in the images. Here, the dead zones have been provided so that the cursor does not move by a little pupil movement due to an oscillation of the user's head. Also the cursor does not move very little by eye movement (eye rotation). The user can even stop the cursor completely.

4 Proposed Method and System

The displacement of the detected gaze point is calculated every frame as a gaze shift amount. We assumed that a saccadic eye movement is occurring when the amount is exceeding an empirically determined threshold. While the user stops the gaze and fixates something, the gaze shift becomes less than the threshold. In the proposed algorithm, according to the assumption, the gaze detection mode and the PupilMouse mode are switched by always monitoring the gaze shift amount. The PupilMouse mode works when the amount is not more than the threshold. The gaze detection mode works when the amount is more than the threshold. In the gaze detection mode, the cursor is presented at the coordinates of the detected gaze point. When it is switched from the gaze detection mode to PupilMouse mode, the last gaze position of the gaze detection mode is handed over as the first cursor position of the PupilMouse mode. In the PupilMouse mode, note that the cursor is not presented where the user is looking.

5 Experiments

Four university students participated in the experiment. They were explained about the mechanisms of the gaze detection and PupilMouse methods. The subject was seated approximately 80 cm from the 19 inch PC display (Fig. 2(a)). Near the bottom of the display screen, a software keyboard (26 mm by 60 mm) is presented (Fig. 2(b)). In each key area of the keyboard, the respective letter is displayed.

Three experimental conditions were given to the subjects: the gaze detection condition, the PupilMouse condition, and the combination of both conditions (the proposed method). In all experimental conditions, the subject was asked to type a twelve Japanese Hiragana letter string that means 'Shizuoka University'. The same procedure was repeated ten times for each of the three conditions. In order to type the letter string, the subject was asked to move the cursor into within the respective key area one by one. When the cursor stopped to some period of time at almost the same position, the letter indicated in the key area where the cursor has existed was automatically typed. Even if there were typing mistakes, the subject was asked not to correct the mistake but to proceed to type the next letter. Time necessary for typing all of the letter string and the number of typing mistakes were measured. After the experiment, a questionnaire about the usability was taken.

The experimental results showed that the PupilMouse condition significantly took more time than the gaze detection conditions or the combination of both conditions although there was no significant difference between the latter two conditions (Fig. 3). However, the number of typing mistakes in the gaze detection condition was much more than the other two conditions (Table 1). Concerning the usability, the proposed method was most excellent (Table 2). These results indicate that the proposed method is comprehensively more excellent than both the gaze detection method and PupilMouse.

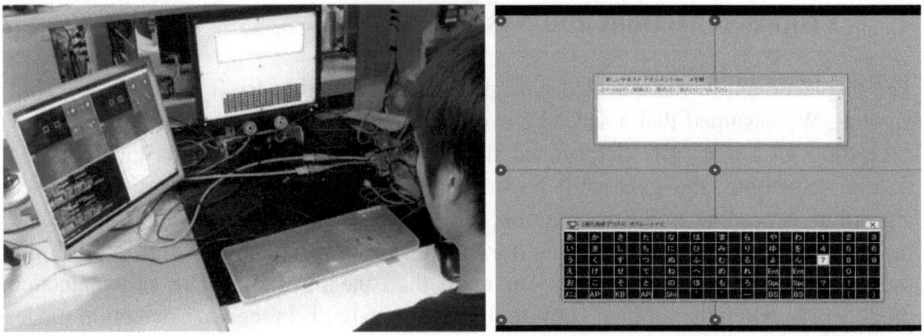
(a) (b)

Fig. 2. (a) View of the experiment and (b) software keyboard presented on the PC screen

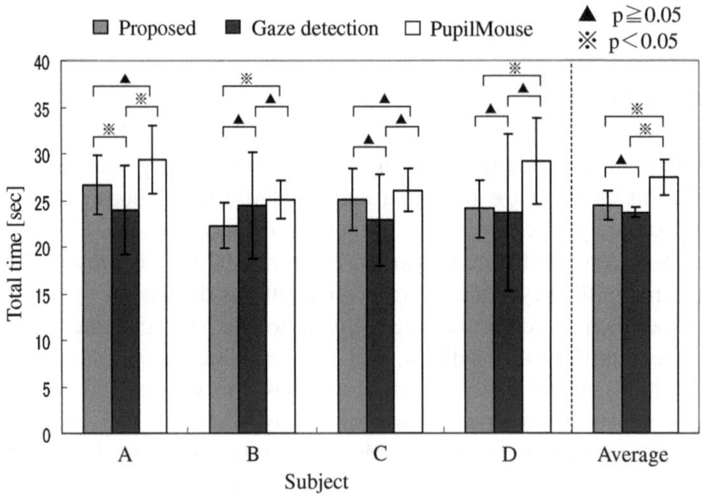

Fig. 3. Comparison of total typing times in the three conditions

Table 1. Average typing mistake number among the three conditions

Subject	Proposed	Gaze detection	PupilMouse
A	0.7	2.4	0.3
B	0.2	1.7	0.1
C	0.7	1.2	0.5
D	0.6	2.3	0.5
Average	0.55	1.90	0.35

Table 2. Questionnaire result concering usability of three methods

Subject	Proposed	Gaze detection	PupilMouse
A	3	1	4
B	5	2	4
C	5	3	3
D	4	2	3
Average	4.3	2.0	3.5

6 Conclusion

In the present paper, we proposed a PC input methodology combining the gaze detection technology and PupilMouse technology (head movement detection). The proposed method employs only the advantages of both methods. In the experiment, the subject was asked to type the twelve Japanese Hiragana letter string using the software keyboard. The total time for input, the number of typing mistakes, and the usability were investigated. These results showed that the proposed method is comprehensively superior to both the gaze detection method and the PupilMouse method.

References

1. Ebisawa, Y., Ishima, D., Inoue, S., Murayama, Y.: PupilMouse: Cursor Control by Head Rotation Using Pupil Detection Technique. In: Proceedings of International Conference on Computing, Communications and Control Technologies (CCCT 2004), pp. 209–214 (2004)
2. Ebisawa, Y., Fukumoto, K.: Head-Free, Remote Gaze Detection System Based on Pupil-Corneal Reflection Method with Using Two Video Cameras – One-Point and Nonlinear Calibrations –. In: Proceeding of 15th International Conference, HCI International 2013 (2013)
3. Ebisawa, Y.: PupilMouse having two optical systems. In: Proceedings of The 3rd International Symposium on Nanovision Science and The 9th Joint International Conference on Advanced Science and Technology, JICAS 2007, pp. 13–18 (2007)

Pupil Detection Using Stereo-Matching Method and a Constant Interpupillary Distance Condition for a Solution of Glasses Reflection Problem in the Video-Based Gaze Detection System

Yoshinobu Ebisawa, Kiyotaka Fukumoto, and Hiroki Yamaguchi

Graduate School of Engineering, Shizuoka University, Hamamatsu, 432-8561 Japan
ebisawa@sys.eng.shizuoka.ac.jp

Abstract. In the pupil-corneal reflection detection-based eye-gaze detection method, glasses reflection of near-infrared LED light sources for producing the corneal reflection is misdetected as the pupil when a user wears eyeglasses. To improve the robustness of the pupil detection, we propose novel pupil searching and tracking methods in the gaze detection system using two stereo-calibrated cameras. The pupil searching method first chooses the true pupils from all stereo-matched pupil candidates using the suitable depth range condition, and second chooses the true pair of the right and left pupils under the constraint of the suitable 3-D interpupillary distance. Even if one pupil is not detected in the image of either camera owing to the glasses reflections, the pupil tracking method estimates the 3-D coordinates of the undetected pupil by using the constant interpupillary distance and the temporal continuity of the 3-D coordinates of the moving pupil. The experimental results show that the accuracy of pupil searching and tracking was better than that of the conventional one-camera method.

Keywords: Pupil detection, Gaze detection, Head movement, Glasses reflection.

1 Introduction

Most of the remote video-based gaze detection systems basically determine the gaze position from the relative position between the center of the pupil image and the corneal reflection image of near-infrared light source(s), which usually produce a bright pupil or a dark pupil. However, the light source causes reflection images from eyeglasses. In the gaze detection system which we have been developed, the pupils are detected from the difference image made of the bright and dark pupil images. Even if using this image difference method, the glasses reflection image remains due to the positional difference of the two light sources for generating bright and dark pupil images. Sometimes the wreck of the glasses reflection image is misdetected as the pupil because of the similarity of their images. This is a problem for general purposes of the gaze detection system. Fortunately, our gaze detection system detects the 3-D pupil position. In the present paper, we propose the pupil detection method

C. Stephanidis (Ed.): Posters, Part I, HCII 2013, CCIS 373, pp. 594–598, 2013.

using an interpupillary distance as a constraint condition in order to distinguish the pupils from the glasses reflections. The effectiveness of the proposed method is shown experimentally.

2 Our Gaze Detection System

We have been developed a pupil-corneal reflection method-based gaze detection system, which allows head movements and achieves easy gaze calibration [1]. The system includes two stereo-calibrated cameras and two light sources attached to each of the cameras, etc. as shown in Fig. 1. They were arranged under a PC display. The light source has near-infrared LEDs arranged in two concentric rings (inner: 850 nm, outer: 940 nm). The inner ring generates a bright pupil image and the outer ring generates a dark pupil image. The pupils are detected from their difference image. The image difference method is very useful for robust pupil detection because the image except the pupils is cancelled out. However, when a user wears eyeglasses, the glasses reflection images remain and sometimes are misdetected as the pupil.

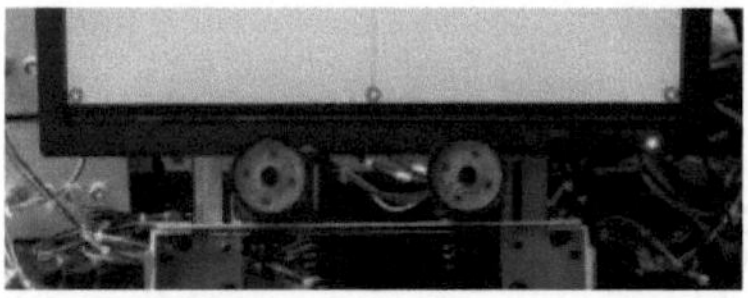

Fig. 1. Overview of two stereo-calibrated optical systems in our gaze detection system

3 Proposed Pupil Detection Method

The proposed method first detects several 2-D pupil candidates (up to 5) from the difference image for each of the two cameras. Next, the positions of 3-D pupil candidates (up to 25) are obtained by stereo-matching all 2-D candidates obtained from both cameras. If stereo-matching is wrong, the depth of the 3-D candidates is out of user's working space. So such a 3-D candidate is excluded. Furthermore, the distances between all pairs of the remaining 3-D candidates are calculated. When the distance is within the predetermined range suitable for an interpupillary distance, the corresponding pupil candidate pair is determined as the final pupil pair.

The above-mentioned processing (searching mode) is used to search the 3-D pupil pair. Once the 3-D pupil pair is found, tracking of the pupil pair (tracking mode) begins. By assuming that the midpoint of the paired pupils and the directional vector passing through them vary at a constant velocity, the 3-D positions of the pupils in the next frame are estimated. The 3-D positions are transformed into the 2-D positions in each camera. The small windows are applied to the 2-D positions. The window serves to prevent to detect the glasses reflection instead of the pupil. When the user's head moves, the effectiveness of the image difference method decreases due to the positional discrepancy between the bright and dark pupil images. During the tracking mode, the positional compensation by the corneal reflection for differentiation is performed [2].

In general, as shown in Fig. 2, there is a case when one camera cannot detect one of the two pupils (e.g., P_R) owing to overlying of the glass reflection while another camera detects the two pupils. In such a case, the 3-D position of the one pupil (P_R) is not obtained. The proposed method estimates the 3-D position of the pupil using the interpupillary distance as follows. Assume a spherical surface where the center is the pupil detected by both cameras (P_L) and the radius is the interpupillary distance. The 3-D position of the undetermined pupil (P_R) is estimated as an intersection between the spherical surface and the line determined by the direction vector (u_{L1}) and the position of the camera (O_L) that has detected the pupil (P_R). Here, when two intersections are obtained, the intersection close to the 3-D pupil position in the previous frame is chosen. Finally, the 3-D position is transformed into the 2-D position in the image of the camera (O_R) that has not been able to detect the pupil (P_R). As a result, the small window is applied around the pupil in the image of the camera. Previously, in our study, the small window was released when the pupil was not detected owing to glasses reflection overlying. The release sometimes leads to tracking the glasses reflection instead of the pupil. The proposed method (tracking mode) would make it possible to continue tracking the pupil without releasing the window even when the glasses reflection image moves across the pupil image.

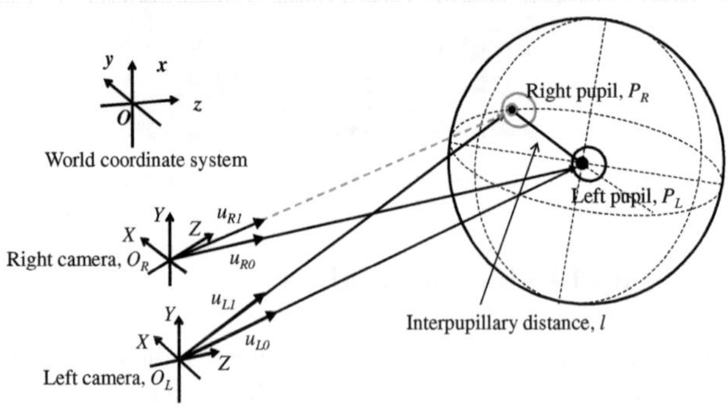

Fig. 2. Pupil tracking method using interpupillary distance as constraint condition

4 Experimental Methods and Results

Five university students wearing eyeglasses participated in two experiments: searching and tracking experiments. The position of the user's head was approximately 80 cm from the PC screen. In the searching experiment, the subject was asked to blink a few times and not to move the head during 10 sec. In the tracking experiment, the subject was asked to rotate the head from side to side during 10 sec so that the glasses reflections crosses the pupils. The same program was used for both experiments. The depth of the working space of the subject was set between 70 cm and 90 cm. The interpupillary distance was predetermined set between 63 mm and 70 mm.

Fig. 3(a) shows the sample images indicating the pupil detection results when eyes were closed in the conventional and proposed methods. Here, the conventional method is a method relying on the image processing by one camera. The conventional

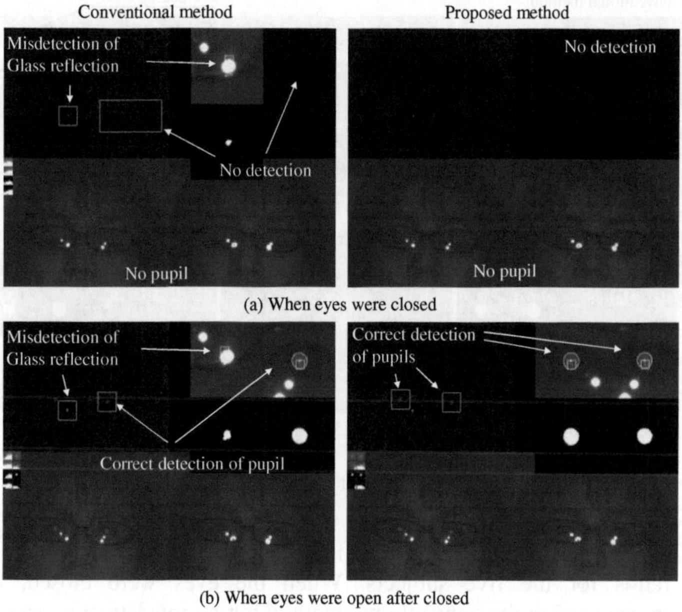

Fig. 3. Resultant samples of pupil detection when the subject blinks. In each panel, lower right and left segments indicate bright and dark pupil images. Several glasses reflection spots are seen diagonally downwards from the pupils. Squares in the difference image (upper left segment) show the small windows. Upper right segment shows the magnified images around the detected objects and shows that it detects glasses reflection or pupil, or nothing.

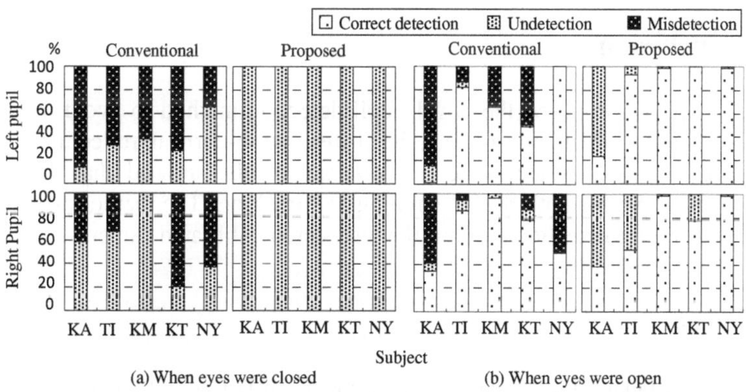

Fig. 4. Pupil detection ratios for five subjects when eyes were (a) closed and (b) open

method misdetected the glasses reflection as the pupil. However, the proposed method did not misdetect: no pupil was surely detected. Fig. 3(b) shows the results when eyes were open after closed. The conventional method continued the right pupil misdetection by the window tracking process. However, the proposed method surely

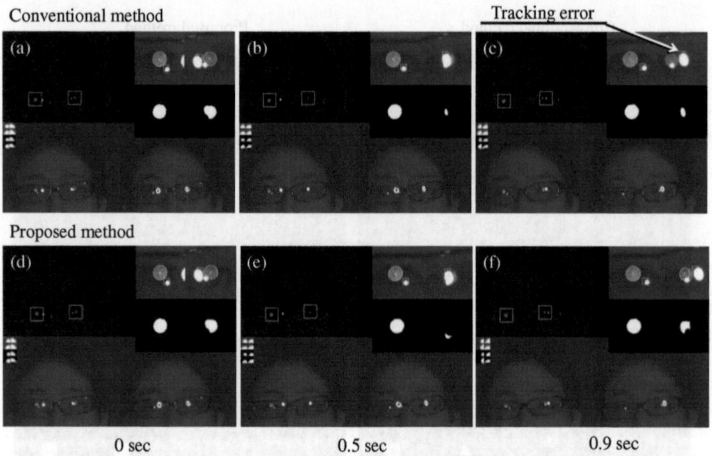

Fig. 5. Pupil detection when subject rotated his head to the right and left

detected the pupils by the proposed tracking method. Fig. 4(a) and (b) compare the detection ratios for the five subjects. When the eyes were closed, high ratio misdetection occurred in the conventional method but no misdetection occurred in the proposed method. When the eyes were open, there was no misdetection.

Fig. 4(a) and (b) show the samples of pupil detection when the subject rotates his head to the right and left in the conventional and proposed methods. The glasses reflection overlay the left pupil at 0.5 sec. After this time, glasses reflection tracking started in the conventional method but pupil tracking was kept in the proposed method.

5 Conclusion

The present paper proposed the novel pupil detection method to avoid misdetecting the glasses reflection in our remote, head-free, pupil-corneal reflection detection-based gaze detection system. The experimental results showed that the proposed method is effective for both pupil searching and tracking. The method would be also useful in other gaze detection systems that use stereo-calibrated cameras.

References

1. Ebisawa, Y., Fukumoto, K.: Head-Free, Remote Gaze Detection System Based on Pupil-Corneal Reflection Method with Using Two Video Cameras – One-Point and Nonlinear Calibrations –. In: Proceeding of 15th International Conference, HCI International (to appear, 2013)
2. Ebisawa, Y., Nakashima, A.: Increasing Precision of Pupil Position Detection Using the Corneal Reflection. The Institute of Image Information and Television Engineers 62(7), 1122–1126 (2008)

Rules of Engagement: Brain-Computer Interfaces for Military Training

Cali M. Fidopiastis[1] and Tami Griffith[2]

[1] University of Alabama at Birmingham, School of Health Professions, Birmingham, AL, USA
[2] U.S. Army Research Laboratory, Human Research and Engineering Directorate, Simulation and Training Technology Center, Orlando, FL USA
cfidopia@uab.edu, Tami.Griffith@us.army.mil

Abstract. Simulation based training systems execute our 'intention to perform' an action in computer space by means of intermediary physical manipulations, such as pressing keys or directing a joystick. Transferring actions through these traditional input devices place an intermediary between the human operator and the simulation that can negatively affect user performance. To eliminate some of these bottlenecks, we explore the use of brain-computer interface techniques to improve the naturalistic interactivity within a military gaming environment using Second Life. We used a P300 speller approach to map action codes of the game to user actions (e.g., walk or run) within the environment. We report on the results of the study as well as discuss implications for future use of hybrid brain-computer interfaces as part of naturalistic interaction schemas for military training.

Keywords: Simulation Based Training, Serious Games, P300, Active BCI, Reactive BCI, brain states.

1 Introduction

Brain Computer Interfaces (BCIs) afford the possibility of removing the computer interface-as-middleman in both gaming and virtual reality contexts [1]. A typical BCI system consists of three processing modules: 1) a brain activity-monitoring device (EEG or fNIRs) that records brain activity, 2) a signal-processing module that identifies specific brain patterns or features related to a person's intention to initiate action, 3) and a translator that converts these brain features into meaningful control commands [2]. Electrophysiological sources of control (ESC) are the mental activities and their associated EEG measures that become the control mechanism that perform actions within a given application. ESC are currently elicited in an active (user conscious control without external stimulation), a reactive (external stimuli elicits user brain response), or a passive (brain activity associate with a cognitive state drives system change) manner. The feature vector represents the ESC and once translated into commands becomes the trigger for action in the application.

For use within military applications, each module of the BCI processing loop needs modification. For example, neurosensing devices should be lightweight, portable,

C. Stephanidis (Ed.): Posters, Part I, HCII 2013, CCIS 373, pp. 599–602, 2013.

ruggedized, and wireless with low battery requirements. Signal processing methods should account for motion artifacts and identify more robust brain signatures that are not solely motor cortex dependent. Additionally, translating neural commands into action within the simulator should be direct and not require traditional interaction schemas (e.g., emulating button presses).

Low cost BCI solutions are making their way to the consumer through the gamming community. Products such as the Emotiv EPOC (http://www.emotiv.com) and NeuroSky Mindset (http://www.neurosky.com) sell for less than 300 US dollars and provide a wireless lightweight BCI solution for gaming platforms. While inexpensive and wireless, these BCI systems limit the user's capability of creating new EEG channel configurations and translation algorithms, which in turn affects the generalizability and extensibility of the interface when moving from pre-defined gaming interaction schemas to non-linear simulations that models real life [3]. As well, researchers estimate that 50% of the end user populations will not be able to use such devices without taking into account individual differences [4].

Pfurtscheller and fellow BCI researchers suggest that a hybrid approach to BCIs using two different brain signals (e.g. EEG and fNIR) or one brain signal in combination with other physiological signals (e.g., heart rate or eyegaze) should address the issues of generalizability and individual differences [5]. This convergent approach of using multiple sensors to detect a user's intention to act is consistent with the adaptive training systems literature where EEG and other psychophysiological measures such as heart rate improve cognitive state detection [6]. In an effort to explore hybrid BCI solutions for military serious training games, we used a P300 speller approach to map the gaming action codes to the ESCs within the 3D virtual world Second Life.

2 Materials and Methods

The 3D virtual world Second Life provided the testing environment for this phase of the research. We implemented a P300 speller paradigm using BCI2000 software to map Second Life interaction codes for moving an avatar forward and backward while walking or running. We acquired brain activity data needed for extracting relevant BCI features using a 10 channel EEG with EKG system made by Advanced Brain Monitoring (ABM, advancedbrainmonitoring.com) for a sample of 15 participants. In addition, we collected eye-tracking data for later data fusion with the BCI P300 data stream.

Participants performed tasks that required movement through the environment and interaction with other avatars and objects as related to a military task scenario. Figure 1 displays one task that required participants to walk to a helicopter, enter the aircraft, and then assume the role of pilot. The main advantage of the BCI approach was that only a single controller was necessary to switch tasks. For example, the same button commands could map from controlling the avatar to controlling the aircraft.

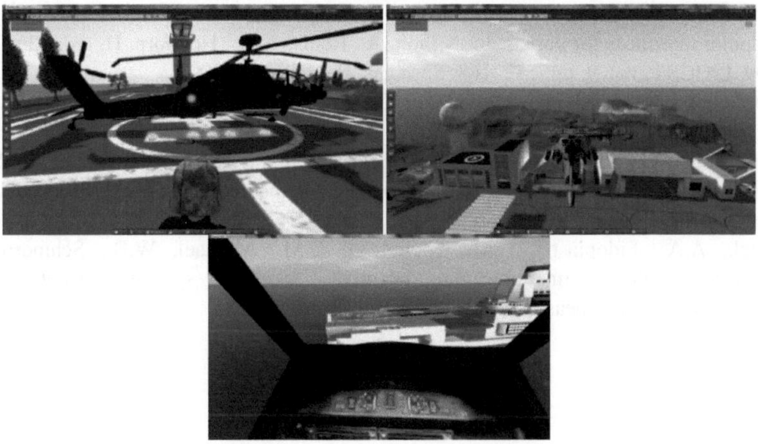

Fig. 1. Second Life user testing tasks for the prototype BCI

3 Results

All participants were able to navigate the 3D environment once they completed training. However, once engaged in an action (e.g., walking), participants had difficulty stopping that action to switch to a new action or task. Despite the frustration, participants reported that the use of BCI augmented their user engagement in the task and felt that the technique would be acceptable to end-users once the technique became more reliable.

4 Discussion

While the goal of this work was to assess the capability of a P300 approach as a means to more naturally interact within a 3D gaming environment. We found that there were several barriers to successful implementation. For example, very few open source BCI software integrate with all EEG manufacturers. While the ABM EEG integrates with BCI2000, there were issues in setup that would preclude a novice who would like to explore the potential use of BCI in their applied work. Once the system reliably performed, tasking issues emerged that highlight the need for improved action code mapping to ESCs for more flexible and fluid interaction within these dynamically changing training environments. Regardless of the current issues, participants reported that they would use this type of system if it became more reliable.

References

1. Lalor, E.C., Kelly, S.P., Finucane, C., Burke, R., Smith, R., Reilly, R.B., McDarby, G.: Steady-state VEP-based brain-computer interface control in an immersive 3D gaming environment. EURASIP J. Appl. Signal Processing 19, 3156–3164 (2005)
2. Wolpaw, J.R., Birbaumer, N., McFarland, D.J., Pfurtschellere, G., Vaughan, T.M.: Brain-computer interfaces for communication and control. Clinl. Neurophy. 113(6), 767–791 (2002)

3. Nijholt, A., Reuderink, B., Bos, D.O.: Turning shortcomings into challenges: Brain-computer interfaces for games. In: Nijholt, A., Reidsma, D., Hondorp, H. (eds.) INTETAIN 2009. LNICST, vol. 9, pp. 153–168. Springer, Heidelberg (2009)
4. Popescu, F., Blankertz, B., Müller, K.: Computational challenges for noninvasive brain computer interfaces. IEEE Intelligent Systems, 78–79 (2008)
5. Pfurtscheller, G., Allison, B.Z., Brunner, C., Bauernfeind, G., Solis-Escalante, T., Scherer, R., Zander, T.O., Mueller-Putz, G., Neuper, C., Birbaumer, N.: The hybrid BCI. Front. Neurosci. 4, 42 (2010)
6. Vartak, A.A., Fidopiastis, C.M., Nicholson, D.M., Mikhael, W.B., Schmorrow, D.: Cognitive state estimation for adaptive learning systems using wearable psychophysiological measures. Biosignals 2, 147–152 (2008)

A Novel Approach for Adaptive EEG Artefact Rejection and EOG Gaze Estimation

Mohammad Reza Haji Samadi and Neil Cooke

School of Electronic, Electrical & Computer Engineering, University of Birmingham, UK
{mrh833,n.j.cooke}@bham.ac.uk

Abstract. An adaptive system for Electroencephalography (EEG) artefact rejection and Electrooculogrum (EOG) gaze estimation is proposed. The system inputs optical gaze information, and accuracy of the EOG gaze classification into an adaptive Independent Component Analysis (ICA) algorithm, for improving EEG source separation. Finally two evaluation methods based on EOG gaze estimation are suggested to assess the performance of the proposed system. The work will be of use to researchers considering using BCI and eye-tracking paradigms in real life applications.

Keywords: EEG, Artefact, Adaptive ICA, BCI, Gaze.

1 Introduction

In recent years, there has been a significant increase in the development of assistive technologies and innovative interfaces based on human modalities eye (gaze), touch, speech and brain. This way, traditional computer inputs are supplemented or replaced with others that promise richer and more realistic human computer interaction schemes, for both normal people and people with severe disabilities.

Among the new interaction methods, eye-tracking systems and Electroencephalography-based (EEG-based) Brain-Computer Interfaces (BCI) can be considered as the final frontiers for Human-Computer Interactions (HCI), which are gaining more interests in recent HCI research [1]. This is due to minimum motor control requirement of BCI and eye tracking systems, which makes the interaction possible for both normal people and people with limited motor control or severe disabilities.

The brain is the centre of human's nervous system and exerts control over the other organs of the body and controls all of human actions and cognitive states [2]. Humans use their eyes to gain information about their environment. As a result, the underlying patterns in both the brain activity and eye movement can distinguish between activities. For example they can be used to reflect the cognitive states of users [3], estimate users' intentions [4], moving a cursor across the screen [5, 6], monitoring visual attention of the drivers [7] and providing an interface for disabled people [8].

One of the main sources of biological artefacts (noise) which contaminate EEG signals is eye related artefact (Electrooculogrum). EEG artefact identification and removal and developing low-cost, consumer grade eye-tracking apparatus for daily life applications are still active topics of the researches [9-12].

C. Stephanidis (Ed.): Posters, Part I, HCII 2013, CCIS 373, pp. 603–607, 2013.

To reap the potential benefits of the BCIs and eye-tracking systems in daily human-computer interactions, the development of a signal processing method for removing artefacts from EEG signals, and development of affordable and robust eye-tracking systems are necessary. Additionally, fusion of brain signals and eye movements has the potential to a more robust method for human activity detection and human intention and/or attention detection.

Here, we proposed an adaptive artefact rejection system, which utilises time-variant optical gaze tracking information to accurately identify Electrooculogrum (EOG) signals from EEG. The aim of this work is to build a system which outputs artefact free EEG and EOG signals, for BCI and gaze-tracking applications, respectively. Moreover it will assess the feasibility of incorporating brain and eye movement signals for human activity and attention detection.

1.1 Independent Component Analysis-ICA

Independent Component Analysis (ICA) is the most widely used method for separating biological artefacts from EEG signals, and cleaning the EEG recordings [10]. ICA assumes that the observed EEG signals from electrodes $X(t)$, are linear mixture of independent source signals (components) $S(t)$, that build them.

$$X(t)= AS(t) \tag{1}$$

where A is the mixing matrix, and source signals $S(t)$, are assumed to be independent, non-Gaussian and stationary. The objective is to estimate a time-invariant invertible mixing matrix A in order to reconstruct original source signals $S(t)$, from only the observations $X(t)$.

Before obtaining the independent sources, first the "unmixing" matrix W should be obtained, so that:

$$S(t) = WX(t) \tag{2}$$

where, $W = A^{-1}$. After obtaining the independent sources, those sources which are attributed to artefact can be identified; therefore EEG signals can be reconstructed without the identified artefact components.

2 Method

2.1 Proposed System

EEG recordings are a mixture of cognitive signals originating from cerebral sources, and artefact signals originating from non-cerebral sources (e.g. EOG artefacts). To recover cognitive signals, the measured voltages $X(t)$ at time t have to be filtered, to remove artefacts which are originated from non-cerebral sources. The prevalent environmental artefact is power line noise (50 Hz Mains hum); and prevalent biological artefacts are EOG and EMG, which have higher amplitude than EEG signals. The primary objective of this work is to propose an adaptive ICA method, for improving the EOG and EEG signal separation, by incorporating time-variant optical gaze information. The idea is to simultaneously record EEG signals and point of gaze, using an EEG headset and an optical eye-tracker, respectively. Therefore, efficiently employing the optical gaze information, $I(t)$, to optimise the estimation of the mixing matrix in the ICA algorithm.

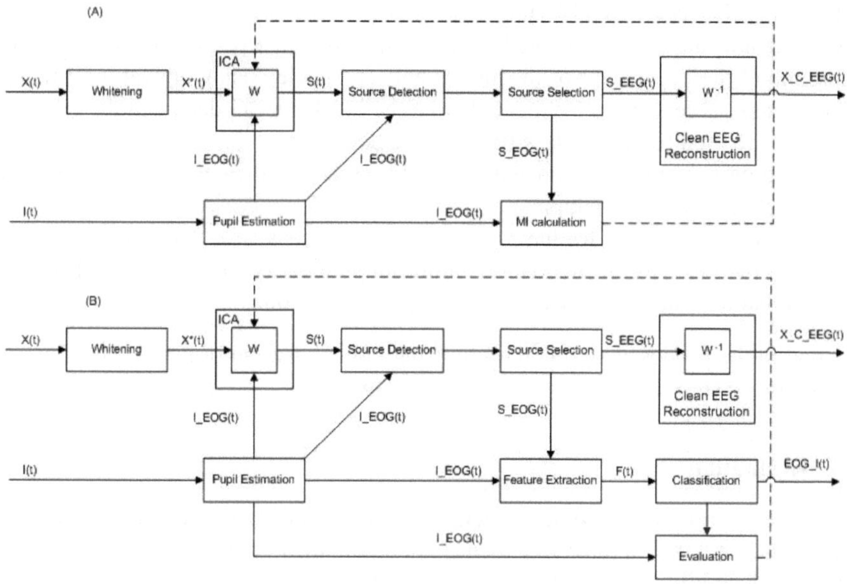

Fig. 1. (A) Proposed system for artefact rejection; use of Mutual Information for evaluation. (B) Proposed system for artefact rejection and gaze estimation; use of classification accuracy for evaluation

The proposed system consists of seven stages (Figure 1.B):

1. Whitening the observation signals $X(t)$, in which, mean values are subtracted from the recorded signals and the covariance matrix of $X(t)$ transforms to an identity matrix (i.e. decorrelation and normalisation to unit variance). This step is undertaken for de-correlating the sources and improving the convergence speed.
2. Exploiting the optical gaze information $I(t)$, for estimating optimal mixing matrix A, in order to recover linear mixture of sources $S(t)$, from the recorded EEG observation $X(t)$at time t.
3. Identifying and labeling eye-related sources $S_{EOG}(t)$, using optical gaze information.
4. Reconstructing cleaned EEG signals for use in BCI. To reconstruct cleaned EEG, the weights of the artefactual sources in the mixing matrix W^{-1} are set to zero. Finally, multiplication of the sources to the unmixing matrix leads to back-projection of the cleaned EEG.

From equation (1) we have:

$$X(t) = AS(t)$$

hence,

$$S_{EEG}(t)W^{-1} = X_{C_{EEG}}(t) \tag{3}$$

where, $S_{EEG}(t)$ is matrix of the sources which are labeled as cerebral activities, and $X_{C_{EEG}}(t)$ is cleaned EEG.

5. After identifying sources related to different types of eye-movements, time and duration of the occurrence of the movements are labeled using optical information. Then temporal features are extracted from the labeled EOG data, and the extracted features are used to train a classifier for gaze detection.
6. Detected movements are validated, and the accuracy of the detections is evaluated, using optical gaze information.
7. An additional step is to feedback the obtained accuracy of EOG gaze detection to the step (2); and use a raw vector optimisation strategy to estimate such mixing matrix that maximises the accuracy of the gaze detection.

Note that in the proposed system, before using optical gaze information; they have to be transformed (modeled) into synthetic EOG data.

2.2 Evaluation

To validate the proposed artefact detection/rejection and gaze estimation approach, it is also demanded to undertake an existing evaluation method or propose an evaluation approach. Generally, there can be two types of evaluation methods; cerebral-based and ocular-based. In the cerebral-based method, the performance of the proposed system can be evaluated using the changes in the accuracy of EEG signal classification during a real BCI paradigm, or changes of the signal to noise ratio on the simulated data. In the ocular-based evaluation method, the performance of the system can be measured using the accuracy of the gaze estimation on the real data or measuring the signal to noise ratio on the simulated data. Due to lack of information about the actual sources of the brain signals, and since, there is available optical gaze information which can be transformed to synthetic EOG data; it is more desired to use the ocular-based method of evaluation. Consequently in the evaluation method the optical information can be considered as the gold standard, and its synthetic EOG information can be used for measuring the performance of the proposed system. Following are two methods that can be employed for evaluating the proposed artefact rejection and gaze detection system.

Method1 (Figure 1.B): Taking the accuracy of EOG gaze classification (which has been measured using optical gaze information) as the performance measure; higher accuracy of EOG signal classification represents higher performance.

Method2 (Figure 1.A): Comparing the Mutual Information (MI) between the synthetic EOG data obtained from optical eyetracker, and EOG data obtained from ICA algorithm. In this method, higher mutual information between optical data and EOG data shows better performance of the system (see Figure 1.A).

3 Conclusion

In this paper, we provided an adaptive EEG artefact rejection and EOG gaze estimation system. The system is based on an adaptive ICA algorithm which uses information coming from an optical gaze tracker for better estimation of EOG sources (eye-related artefacts). The proposed system is not yet applied on real or simulated data. A further study could assess the performance of the proposed system through a real life BCI paradigm.

References

1. Graimann, B., Allison, B., Pfurtscheller, G.: Brain–computer interfaces: A gentle introduction. Brain-Computer Interfaces, 1–27 (2010)
2. Levenson, R.W.: The intrapersonal functions of emotion. Cognition & Emotion 13(5), 481–504 (1999)
3. Marshall, S.P.: Identifying cognitive state from eye metrics. Aviation, Space, and Environmental Medicine 78(suppl. 1), B165–B175 (2007)
4. Asteriadis, S., et al.: Estimation of behavioral user state based on eye gaze and head pose—application in an e-learning environment. Multimedia Tools and Applications 41(3), 469–493 (2009)
5. Pan, S.: Method and apparatus for controlling cursor movement. Google Patents (1994)
6. Wolpaw, J.R., McFarland, D.J.: Control of a two-dimensional movement signal by a noninvasive brain-computer interface in humans. Proceedings of the National Academy of Sciences of the United States of America 101(51), 17849–17854 (2004)
7. Ji, Q., Yang, X.: Real time visual cues extraction for monitoring driver vigilance. Computer Vision Systems, 107–124 (2001)
8. De Santis, A., Iacoviello, D.: Robust real time eye tracking for computer interface for disabled people. Computer Methods and Programs in Biomedicine 96(1), 1–11 (2009)
9. Croft, R.J., Barry, R.: Removal of ocular artifact from the EEG: a review. Neurophysiologie Clinique/Clinical Neurophysiology 30(1), 5–19 (2000)
10. Vigário, R.N.: Extraction of ocular artefacts from EEG using independent component analysis. Electroencephalography and Clinical Neurophysiology 103(3), 395–404 (1997)
11. Kenemans, J.L., et al.: Removal of the ocular artifact from the EEG: a comparison of time and frequency domain methods with simulated and real data. Psychophysiology 28(1), 114–121 (2007)
12. Topal, C., Dogan, A., Gerek, O.: A wearable head-mounted sensor-based apparatus for eye tracking applications. In: IEEE Conference on Virtual Environments, Human-Computer Interfaces and Measurement Systems, VECIMS 2008. IEEE (2008)

Point-and-Click Interface Based on Parameter-Free Eye Tracking Technique Using a Single Camera

Shinichi Hikita and Yasuhiro Seto

Graduate School of Information Sciences, Hiroshima City University, 3-4-1 Ozuka-Higashi, Asa-Minami-Ku, Hiroshima, 731-3194, Japan
hikita@hiroshima-cu.ac.jp, seto@ics.info.hiroshima-cu.ac.jp

Abstract. We propose a method for the estimation of point of gaze with neither user- nor environment-dependent parameters. The gaze direction is calculated from the centers of both the pupil and the eye rotation. The center of the eye rotation is determined using the centers of both the pupil and the iris and the edge of the iris when at least four calibration targets, for which only the distances between them are known, are fixated on the screen. The mean horizontal and vertical errors for seven subjects were 0.91 deg and 0.77 deg, respectively. Next, a point-and-click interface, in which a user can move a cursor by a gaze shift and click a computer mouse by a voluntary eye blink or short fixation, was developed. On average, it took 1.2, 0.9, and 0.8 sec to point and click for each target with eye blink, short fixation, and normal hand manipulation, respectively.

Keywords: Eye-gaze estimation, Pupil, Iris, Center of eye rotation.

1 Introduction

An eye tracking technique using a single camera could be a key for an eye-gaze input interface of a wearable head-mounted computer. However, previous methods with a single camera require user parameters that depend on the shape of the eyeball and/or environmental parameters such as distances between the eye and the camera or the screen to calculate gaze direction from the pupil and corneal reflections of near-infrared lights in the eye image [1, 2]. The cumbersome calibration procedures that determine these parameters would reduce the convenience of using a wearable computer with an eye-gaze input interface.

In this paper, we propose a method for the estimation of point of gaze with neither user- nor environment-dependent parameters and introduce a point-and-click interface as an example of an implementation of the proposed technique. Just looking at a few calibration targets makes it possible to calculate gaze direction and point of gaze on the screen. Pupil and iris detection are described in Section 2. The parameter-free eye tracking technique and estimation of point of gaze are described in Section 3. The accuracy of the estimated point of gaze is shown in Section 4. The point-and-click interface is described in Section 5. Finally, the conclusion is given in Section 6.

C. Stephanidis (Ed.): Posters, Part I, HCII 2013, CCIS 373, pp. 608–612, 2013.

2 Pupil and Iris Detection

Fig. 1 shows eye images under near-infrared light after the detection of the pupil and iris. First, the pupil area is extracted from the segmented images. Next, the center of the pupil is computed from an ellipse fitted to the edge of the pupil after removal of outliers. An algorithm based on the Taubin method [3, 4] is employed to fit the ellipse. The ellipse parameter $\boldsymbol{u}$ is obtained by solving a generalized eigenvalue problem, shown in equation 3.

$$Ax^2 + Bxy + Cy^2 + Dx + Ey + F = 0 \tag{1}$$

$$\boldsymbol{u} = (A\ B\ C\ D\ E\ F)^T \tag{2}$$

$$\boldsymbol{Vu} = \lambda \boldsymbol{Wu} \tag{3}$$

where $\boldsymbol{V}$ is a 6×6 matrix obtained from the data of the pupil $(x_i\ y_i)$ and $\boldsymbol{W}$ is a 6×6 weighting matrix. The edge of the iris is detected using a differential filter. An ellipse is fitted to the edge to obtain the center of the iris and feature points that are two intersection points of the fitting ellipse and the horizontal axis of the ellipse.

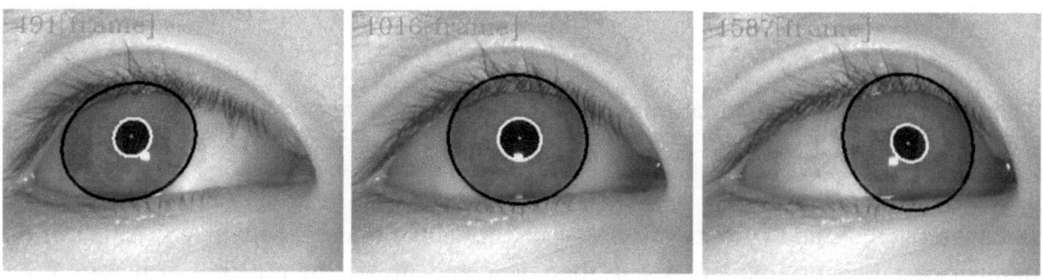

Fig. 1. Ellipses fitted to the pupil and iris

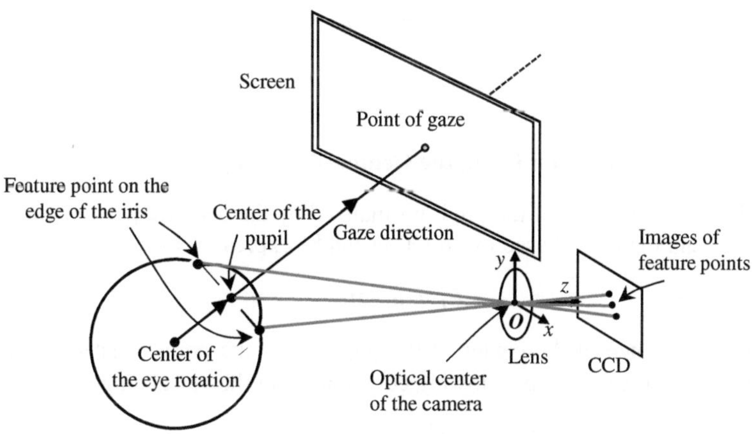

Fig. 2. Schematic view of the eye, a camera, and point of gaze on the screen

3 Parameter-Free Eye Tracking Technique

Fig. 2 shows the camera coordinate system when a user fixates on a point on a screen. The center of the eye rotation and position of the screen are determined based on *N*-point calibration when at least four targets are sequentially fixated. The eyeball is assumed to be a sphere and to rotate around a fixed point relative to the camera.

3.1 Estimation of Visual Angles Using Feature Points of the Iris

When a user fixates on the calibration target, the normalized position of a feature point on the edge of the iris $\boldsymbol{Q}_{ij}$ $(i = 1, \ldots, N,\ \ j = 1,2)$ divided by the distance between the centers of both the iris and the iris-based eye rotation can be expressed as the following equation with unknown parameters α_{ij} and an image of the feature point $\boldsymbol{q}_{ij}$:

$$\boldsymbol{Q}_{ij} = \alpha_{ij} \cdot \boldsymbol{q}_{ij} \tag{4}$$

Next, the feature point $\boldsymbol{Q}_{ij}$ is located on the surface of a sphere with a radius of one from the center of the eye rotation $\boldsymbol{E}_I$.

$$|\, \boldsymbol{Q}_{ij} - \boldsymbol{E}_I \,|^2 = 1 \tag{5}$$

The distance between the feature points on the iris is expressed as:

$$|\, \boldsymbol{Q}_{i1} - \boldsymbol{Q}_{i2} \,|^2 = D^2 \tag{6}$$

In equations 4, 5, and 6, there are *2N+4* unknown parameters and *3N* equations. If the number of calibration targets $N \geq 4$, then we can estimate the position of feature point $\boldsymbol{Q}_{ij}$ and the center of the eye rotation $\boldsymbol{E}_I$. The iris-based direction vector $\boldsymbol{g}_I$ between the centers of both the iris $\boldsymbol{Q}_C$ and the eye rotation $\boldsymbol{E}_I$ is given by:

$$\boldsymbol{g}_I = \boldsymbol{Q}_C - \boldsymbol{E}_I \tag{7}$$

The visual angles between calibration targets can be obtained from the above vectors.

3.2 Eye-gaze Estimation Using the Center of the Pupil

The position of the center of the pupil normalized by the distance between the centers of the pupil and the pupil-based eye rotation can be expressed by:

$$\boldsymbol{P}_i = \beta_i \cdot \boldsymbol{p}_i \tag{8}$$

The moving distance of the center of the pupil when the point of gaze moves from one to another is given by the following equation using the visual angle θ.

$$\left|\boldsymbol{P}_i - \boldsymbol{P}_j\right|^2 = \{2\sin\left(\tfrac{\theta_l}{2}\right)\}^2 \tag{9}$$

where $i = 1, \ldots, N-1, j = 2, \ldots, N$ $(i<j)$, $l = 1, \ldots, {}_N\mathrm{C}_2$

The position of $\boldsymbol{P_i}$ is determined by solving the above equations for β_i. The center of the pupil-based eye rotation $\boldsymbol{E_P}$ can be obtained from the following equations.

$$|\boldsymbol{P_i} - \boldsymbol{E_P}|^2 = 1 \tag{10}$$

The center of the pupil in any gaze direction can be obtained from the above equation using $\boldsymbol{E_P}$. The eye-gaze vector is determined by the following equation:

$$\boldsymbol{g_P} = \boldsymbol{P} - \boldsymbol{E_P} \tag{11}$$

The parameters of a screen plane can be estimated using the eye-gaze vector and the distances between the calibration targets by the least squares method. Finally, the point of gaze on the screen is determined as an intersection point of the line through the eye-gaze vector and the screen plane.

4 Accuracy of Estimated Point of Gaze

An experiment was performed to evaluate the accuracy of the proposed method. The subject, with the head fixed by a chin rest and a bit bar, was instructed to fixate on a target on the screen 580 mm away from the right eye. The target sequentially appeared for three seconds on one of 21 grid points shown in Fig. 3. Five calibration targets, located at (0mm, 0mm), (0mm, ±150mm), and (±200mm, 0mm), were used to estimate parameters. Images of the eye were captured in 320×240 size at 30 frames per second by a CCD camera. Fig. 3 shows the accuracy of the estimated point of gaze. The mean horizontal and vertical errors for seven subjects were 0.91 deg and 0.77 deg, respectively.

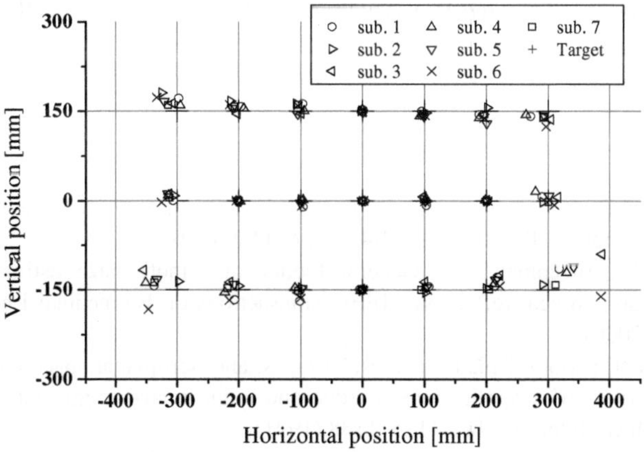

Fig. 3. Accuracy of the estimated point of gaze on the screen 580mm away from the eye

5 Application

A point-and-click interface was developed as an example of an implementation of the proposed method. A user can move a cursor presented on a point of gaze on the screen and click a computer mouse by a voluntary eye blink or short fixation. Duration of eye blink was computed using the derivative of the horizontal to the vertical ratio of the pupil. An eye blink longer than 0.33 sec (10 frames) was detected as a voluntary eye blink for a mouse click. Short fixation was detected using the variance in the position of the center of the pupil in a time window of 0.5 sec (15 frames). A usability test was conducted for a subject familiar with the system in the same environmental condition as in Section 4. The subject was instructed to point and click a 50×50mm-sized target, which was selected from among 15 grid points in the horizontal range of ±200mm, appeared in a pseudo-random order immediately after five-point calibration for approximately 5 sec. Another target appeared after the click within the current target area. Each trial consisted of 45 targets. On average, for five trials, it took 1.2, 0.9, and 0.8 sec to point and click per target with eye blink, short fixation, and normal hand manipulation, respectively.

6 Conclusion

In this paper, we proposed a method for the estimation of point of gaze with neither user- nor environment-dependent parameters using a single camera. A point-and-click interface that implemented the proposed technique made it possible to utilize an eye-gaze input with less calibration effort. This method would be more useful for a mobile computer with a wearable display and an eye camera.

Acknowledgements. This work was supported by JSPS KAKENHI Grant Number 23700670.

References

1. Ohno, T., Mukawa, N., Yoshikawa, A.: Just Look at Two Points: A Gaze Tracking System with Easy Calibration. IPSJ Journal 44(4), 1136–1149 (2003)
2. Guestrin, E.D., Eizenman, M.: General theory of remote gaze estimation using the pupil center and corneal reflections. IEEE Transactions on Biomedical Engineering 53(6), 1124–1133 (2006)
3. Taubin, G.: Estimation of planar curves, surfaces, and non-planar space curves defined by implicit equations with applications to edge and range image segmentation. IEEE Trans. Patt. Anal. Mach. Intell. 13(11), 1115–1138 (1991)
4. Sugaya, Y., Kanatani, K.: Optimization computation for 3-D understanding of image [II]: ellipse fitting. The Journal of the Institute of Electronics, Information and Communication Engineers 92(4), 301–306 (2009)

Automatic Sleep Stage Classification GUI with a Portable EEG Device

Chih-Sheng Huang[1,2], Chun-Ling Lin[1], Li-Wei Ko[1,3,*], Yu-Kai Wang[1,4], Jyun-Wei Liang[1], and Chin-Teng Lin[1,2,4,*]

[1] Brain Research Center, University System of Taiwan, Hsinchu, Taiwan
[2] Institute of Electrical Control Engineering, National Chiao-Tung University, Hsinchu, Taiwan
[3] Department of Biological Science and Technology, National Chiao-Tung University, Hsinchu, Taiwan
[4] Department of Computer Science, National Chiao-Tung University, Hsinchu, Taiwan
{chih.sheng.huang821,sean7558}@gmail.com, gera-late.ece95g@nctu.edu.tw, {lwko,ctlin}@mail.nctu.edu.tw, yukai-wang@cs.nctu.edu.tw

Abstract. In this study, a developed automatic sleep stage classification system with a portable EEG recording device, (Mindo-4s) is implemented by JAVA-based sleep graphical user interface (GUI) in android platform. First, the parameters of the developed sleep stage classification system, including extracting effective sleep features and a hierarchical classification structure consisting of preliminary wake detection rule, adaptive adjustment scheme, and support vector machine, were trained by our existing sleep database, which collected using polysomnogram (PSG), in MATLAB program. Finally, this classification system would be reedited by JAVA language, and the corresponding JAVA-based sleep GUI software was working in android platform and Mindo-4s. The connection between JAVA-based sleep GUI software and the portable Mindo-4s was through Bluetooth communication. The performance of this JAVA-based sleep GUI can reach 72.43% average accuracy comparing to the result from manual scoring. This JAVA-based sleep GUI can on-line display, record and analyze the forehead EEG signals simultaneously. After sleep, the user can received a complete sleep report, including sleep efficiency, sleep stage distribution, from JAVA-based sleep GUI. Thus, this system can provide a preliminary result in sleep quality estimation, and help the sleep doctor to decide someone needs to have a complete PSG testing in hospital. Using this system is more convenient for long–term and home-based daily caring than traditional PSG measurement.

Keywords: Sleep stage classification, Polysomnogram, JAVA-based sleep graphical user interface.

1 Introduction

Having a good sleep was proved that related with our physiological and psychological healthy [1]. Long time monitoring the sleep quality is a hard and difficult task in our

* Corresponding author.

C. Stephanidis (Ed.): Posters, Part I, HCII 2013, CCIS 373, pp. 613–617, 2013.

daily life, and many choices can be used, such as sleep questionnaires, polysomnography (PSG) measurement. In the real environment, adopting sleep questionnaire were a general choice to monitor the sleep quality usually. However, adopting sleep questionnaire is not possible to measure the sleep quality and physiological state directly and objectively. The most effective way to measure the physiological state is to make a clinical and complete PSG in sleep laboratory of hospital. PSG is a system measures including electroencephalography (EEG), electrocardiography (ECG), electromyography (EMG), electrooculography (EOG) and oxygen saturation (SpO2) et al, and the sleep technologist would assistant to score these physiological signals to a sleep stage by the manual of American Academy of Sleep Medicine (AASM) [2]. The distribution of sleep stage and the physiological state will be estimated by visual scoring from the sleep technologist. In the AASM scoring manual, five sleep stages, 1) Wake stage, 2) Rapid eye movement stage (REM) , 3) Non-REM stage 1 (N1) , 4) Non-REM stage 2 (N2) , 5) Non-REM stage 3 (N3), are recommended for the stages of sleep. Although using PSG to measure the sleep quality is the most direct and objective way, the process for a diagnostic sleep test by PSG is complication and time-consuming, in the other points of view, the PSG system is also not possible to use in the daily life for long time monitoring.

In order to overcome the hair problems in EEG measurement, the study of automatic sleep classification was developed to classify the sleep stages by only forehead EEG channels, such as FP1 and FP2 [3]. In this study, we adopted the developed sleep classification system [3] to develop a JAVA-based sleep GUI software. In addition, we use a portable EEG recording device (Mindo-4s) with foam sensors to record the FP1 and FP2 EEG signals for overcoming the conductive adhesive of EEG [4, 5]. For evaluating the performance of the JAVA-based sleep GUI software with Mindo-4s, we took the sleep experiment with recording the full montage PSG data and the Mindo-4s data simultaneously. All PSG data would be manual scoring with manual rules of AASM by an experienced sleep clinician to obtain the ground truth of the sleep distribution in the sleep experiment.

2 Materials and Methods

2.1 Subjects

Five healthy voluntary subjects participate in the sleep experiment to evaluate the performance of JAVA-based GUI software with the Mindo-4s. All subjects were required to complete the experiment in the night (10:00 pm- 08:00 am). Experiment protocol was approved by the Institutional Review Broad of Taipei Veterans General Hospital, Taiwan. Subjects were informed of the experimental procedure and written consent was obtained from each subject prior to the experiment.

2.2 Data Acquisition

The PSG signals were measured and recorded with a sampling rate of 128 Hz using Sandman Elite (PSG, Nellcor Puritan Bennett), and the additional forehead EEG (FP1 and FP2) recording was recorded by the Mindo-4s with sampling rate of 128 Hz simultaneously. The full PSG recording contained six channels EEG, two channels EOG, one channel EMG, one channel ECG and many other physiological signals, such as Airflow, and SpO2 et al., see as Fig. 1. Figure 2 shows the photograph of Mindo-4s and the real situation the Mindo-4s recording. The Mindo-4s includes the development of wearable, wireless EEG device with the dry foam sensors (Figure 2B) that allows high temporal resolution EEG monitoring in realistic operational environments.

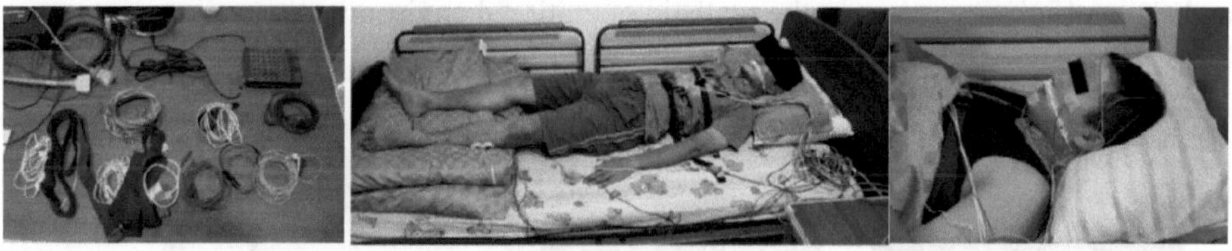

Fig. 1. Real situation of PSG recording

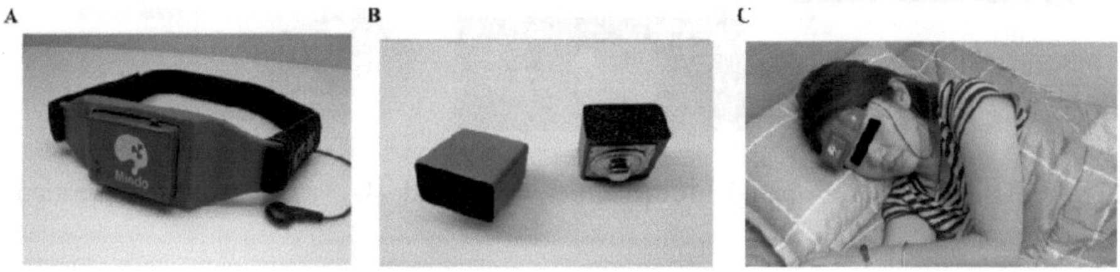

Fig. 2. Mindo-4s with the dry foam sensors

2.3 Data Analysis

Sleep physiological signals of five subjects were visual scored from an experienced sleep clinician who works on identifying different sleep stages by AASM scoring manual in hospital. In this study, the sleep stages scoring by experienced sleep clinician were redefined as follow: Wake, Light sleep (Stage N1 and N2), Deep sleep (Stage N3) and REM. The distribution of sleep epochs belonging to five subjects is shown in Table 1.

Table 1. The distribution of sleep stages of five subjects

	Wake	Light sleep	Deep sleep	REM
S01	14	522	97	122
S02	102	127	182	91
S03	116	337	47	176
S04	254	227	35	98
S05	106	308	156	117

2.4 JAVA-Based Sleep GUI Software

The developed sleep classification system [3] is implemented using JAVA application. This JAVA-based sleep GUI application included the displaying, recording and online analysis function. The prediction of the sleep stages and the prediction of subject's sleep efficiency would be shown in the immediate sleep report after finishing the whole night sleep recording. Raw data and sleep report were stored to the hard disk by JAVA-based sleep GUI program. Fig. 3 shows the way to record forehead EEG signal using Mindo-4s, and JAVA-based sleep GUI and the sleep stage and sleep efficiency report in the realistic operational environment.

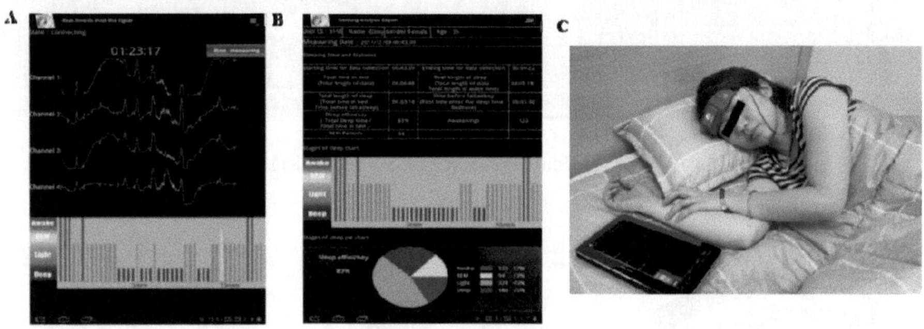

Fig. 3. Using the JAVA-based sleep GUI with Mindo-4s in the realistic operational environment

3 Evaluation of the JAVA-Based Sleep GUI with Mindo-4s

The results shows in Table 2, the performance of this Java-based sleep GUI with Mindo-4s can reach 72.43% of average accuracy, and 0.60 of kappa coefficient. The sensitivity of deep sleep stage can reach 96.92%.

Table 2. The classification performance of the JAVA-based sleep GUI. ACC. is accuracy, and κ is kappa coefficient.

	Sensitivity (%)				Acc.	κ
	W	Light	Deep	REM		
Average	75.78%	71.35%	96.92%	46.30%	72.43%	0. 60

4 Discussion

The JAVA-based sleep GUI, working in the android platform, with a portable EEG recording device, Mindo-4s, is proposed in this study. The Mindo-4s with dry foam sensors can overcome the hair and conductive adhesive problems of traditional EEG recording. In the classification performance of this GUI aspect, the sensitivity of REM stage is only 46.30%. Classifying the REM stage very well is difficult if we just apply only FP1 and FP2 EEG channel without EOG and EMG, so it still has a great improvement in classifying the REM stage by only forehead EEG. This JAVA-based sleep GUI can reach 72.43% average accuracy, and it's enough to provide a preliminary result for long-term monitoring and estimating the sleep quality at the home.

Acknowledgments. This work was supported in part by the UST-UCSD International Center of Excellence in Advanced Bio-engineering sponsored by the Taiwan National Science Council I-RiCE Program under Grant Number: NSC-101-2911-I-009-101, in part by the Aiming for the Top University Plan of National Chiao Tung University, the Ministry of Education, Taiwan, under Contract 102W963, and in part by the National Science Council, Taiwan, under Contract 100-2628-E-009-027-MY3. Research was also sponsored in part by the Army Research Laboratory and was accomplished under Cooperative Agreement Number W911NF-10-2-0022. The U.S. Government is authorized to reproduce and distribute reprints for Government purposes notwithstanding any copyright notation heron.

References

[1] Gallagher, S., Phillips, A.C., Carroll, D.: Parental stress is associated with poor sleep quality in parents caring for children with developmental disabilities. Journal of Pediatric Psychology 35(7), 728–737 (2010)

[2] Iber, C., American Academy, M.: of Sleep, The AASM manual for the scoring of sleep and associated events: rules, terminology and technical specifications. American Academy of Sleep Medicine (2007)

[3] Huang, C.S., Lin, C.L., Ko, L.W., Liu, S.Y., Su, T.P., Lin, C.T.: A Hierarchical Classification System for Sleep Stage Scoring via Forehead EEG Signals. In: 2013 IEEE Symposium Series on Computational Intelligence (2013)

[4] Lin, C.-T., Ko, L.-W., Chiou, J.-C., Duann, J.-R., Huang, R.-S., Chiu, T.-W., Liang, S.-F., Jung, T.-P.: Noninvasive neural prostheses using mobile and wireless EEG. Proceedings of the IEEE 96, 1167–1183 (2008)

[5] Lin, C.-T., Liao, L.-D., Liu, Y.-H., Wang, I.-J., Lin, B. S., Chang, J.-Y.: Novel dry polymer foam electrodes for long-term EEG measurement. IEEE Transactions on Biomedical Engineering 58, 1200–1207 (2011)

Intelligent Workload Control for Exercise Game

Changhoon Park

Dept. of Game Engineering, Hoseo University,
165 Sechul-ri, Baebang-myun, Asan, Chungnam 336-795, Korea
chpark@hoseo.edu

Abstract. Regular physical activity is associated with enhance health and reduced risk of all-cause mortality. But, most people who repeat the exercise easily feel the boredom and tend to give up. And, there are real risks of injuries or side effects of exercise. We introduce a video game for exercise motivation and aerobics with providing a modified fitness bike as a special controller. This paper aims to make exercise games personalized for safe and effective exercise by introducing intelligent workload control. Intelligent workload control is implemented to customize exercise time and intensity based on exercise prescription. Exercise game will be personalized according to individual physical abilities. And, experimental results will be presented to illustrate the effect of our personalized exercise game.

Keywords: exercise game, workload control, racing track, feedback, smartphone, intensity.

1 Introduction

It is increasingly desirable to have good health. And, regular exercise is the most effective way to improve fitness. But, most people who repeat the exercise easily feel the boredom and tend to give up. And, there are real risks of injuries or side effects of exercise. We introduce a video game for exercise motivation and aerobics with providing a modified fitness bike as a special controller. This paper aims to make exercise games personalized for safe and effective exercise by introducing racing track based on exercise prescription. And, exercise game will be personalized in order to customize exercise time and intensity according to individual heart rate.

This game is intended to support aerobic exercise to improve heart and lung function has a strong organization, has the effect of the blood vessels. And we believe that it is important to ensure exercise safety and effectiveness. So, we apply exercise prescription to game mechanics. Then, game can adjust exercise intensity and time for a player based on their heart rate.

2 Intelligent Exercise Game

This game system is consisted of a modified exercise bike and wireless heart rate monitor. Our exercise bike has rotation sensors connected to the handlebar and pedals. This enables to exercise and play video game at the same time with pedaling and steering. And, the level of resistance in the pedal can be controlled by PC. And, wireless heart monitor is used to estimate calorie expenditure and exercise stress.

C. Stephanidis (Ed.): Posters, Part I, HCII 2013, CCIS 373, pp. 618–622, 2013.

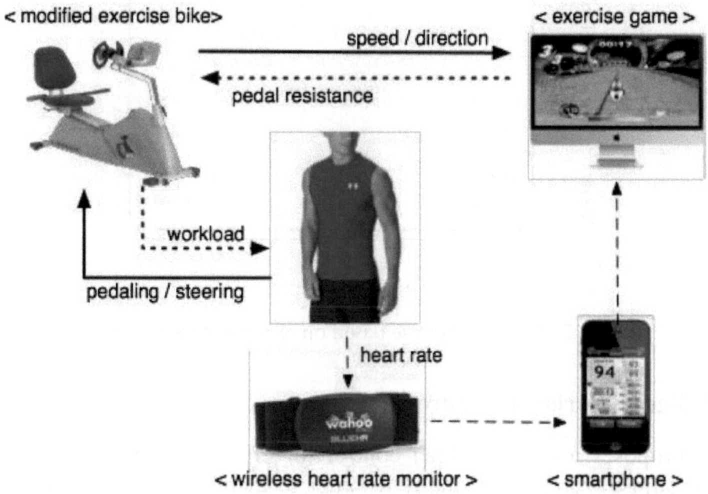

Fig. 1. System overview

2.1 Virtual Racing Track

In this game, virtual racing track is closely related to the intensity and time of aerobic exercise. The exercise intensity increase in proposition to the resistance of the bike pedals. And the level of resistance in the pedal is controlled by means of slope of the track in the game. The higher slope of virtual world is, the more the pedal resistance increase. At this moment, player can experience virtually uphill and downhill while watching the game screen. And, the total exercise time is depends on the overall length of virtual track and the speed of virtual avatar. This means that aerobic exercise program can be designed by the virtual racing track in the game.

First, the length of virtual track is designed to guarantee at least of the 20 minutes exercise per session with considering the maximum speed of virtual avatar. Second, there is a zone named A for warm-up at the beginning of the track. For cool-down, there is a zone named B at the ending of the track. These zones are designed to take about 3 minutes and the slope of zone A and B is designed at an easier pace to let player's legs warm up and cool down. Third, there are two different zones named B1 and B2 for main exercise. Each zone takes about 7 minutes equally. But, the slope of B1 is relatively higher than B2. This means that the exercise intensity of B1 is harder than B2. In the game, we will control the path of main exercise depending on the player's physical status. After all, player will race B1-B1, B2-B2, B1-B2, or B2-B1 in order to perform 14 minutes of main exercise.

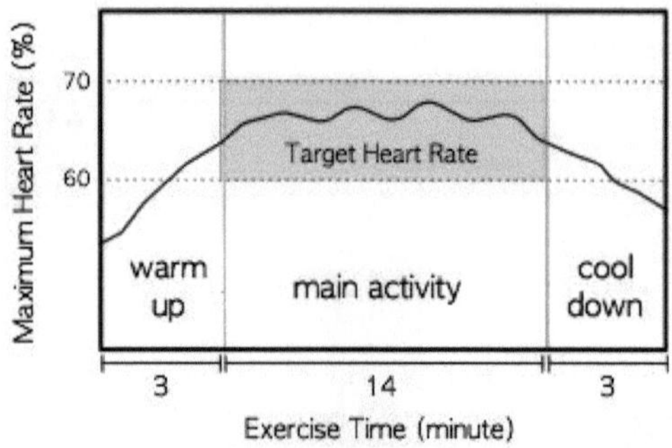

Fig. 2. Aerobic exercise based on exercise prescription

2.2 Intelligent Workload Control

This game proposes a dynamic load control for effective and safe exercise. This control will adjust exercise personally in order to maintain heart rate to target heart rate zone. it's important to work at a certain level of intensity during cardio exercise.

First, we will control the path of zone B1 and B2 for main exercise. Zone A and C will be provided to all players statically. In the other hand, B1 or B2 will be provided dynamically depending on their heart rate. Because the average slope of B1 and B2 is different each other, the intensity of exercise will be also different. In the game, there are two times of path control for main exercise. Depending of the average heart rate of previous zone, B1 or B2 will be provided as shown in Table 1. This aims to maintain In the game, These controls will be adjusted by means of the average heart rate of previous zone. If the average heard rate is low, B1 will be provided. Otherwise, B2 will be provided.

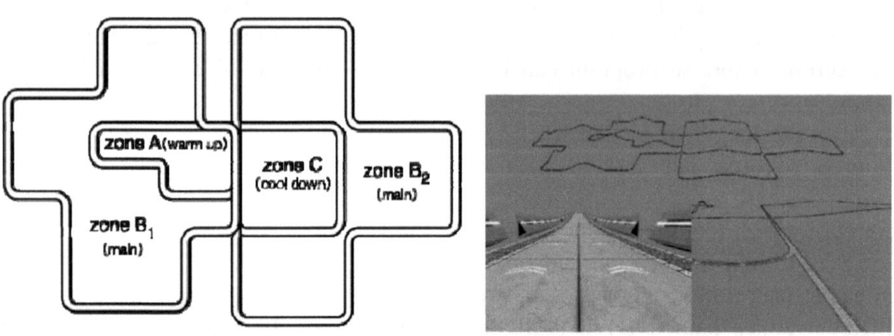

Fig. 3. Design of racing track and 3d model for aerobic exercise

Second, game feedback is used to control the workload for the player's safety during exercise. Feedback is provided in order to reduce the intensity of exercise. When the player's heart rate is grater than 68% of maximum heart rate, the resistance of pedal will be decrease . In spite of this control, if player's heart rate is grater than 80% of maximum heart rate, the exercise game will be paused until player's heart rate become less than 70% of maximum heart rate.

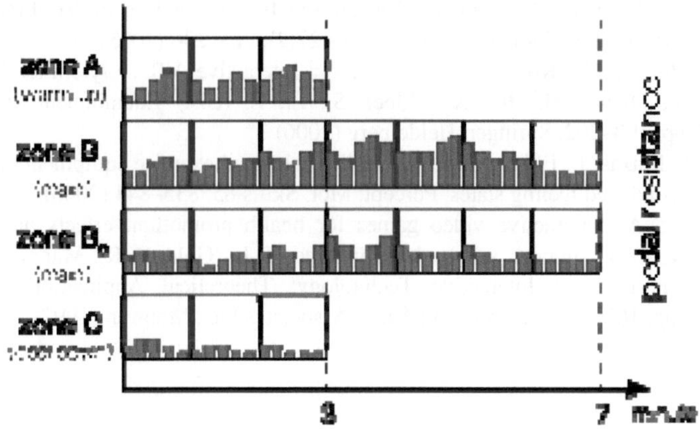

Fig. 4. Pedal intensity design for racing track

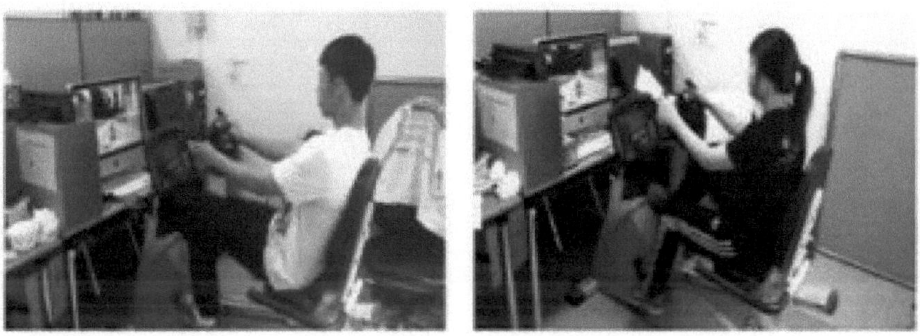

Fig. 5. Experiments of exercise

3 Conclusion

This project has been executed with 20 students for a period of 2 months. This game aims to support exercise safety and effectiveness. To achieve this goal, we applied exercise prescription to virtual racing track and game feedback. Then, the game provide intelligent workload control in order to adjust exercise intensity and time for a player based on his or her heart rate. We. expect this game will help people increase their interest and motivation, so exercise can be a part of their daily routine.

Acknowledgement. This research was supported by the Academic Research fund of Hoseo University in 2012 (2012-0134).

References

1. Mokka, S., Vaatanen, A., Heinila, J., Valkkynen, P.: Fitness computer game with a bodily user interface. In: Proc. of the 2th Intl. Conference on Entertainment Computing, vol. 38 (2003)
2. Van Dan, N., Kameyama, M.: Bayesian-networks-based motion estimation for a highly-safe intelligent vehicle. In: SICE-ICASE International Joint Conference, pp. 6023–6026 (2006)

3. Park, C., Ko, H., Kim, T.: NAVER: Design and Implementation of VR Framework for Gyeongju VR Theater. Computer and Graphics 27(2), 223–236 (2003)
4. Park, C., Hirose, M., Ko, H.: A platform for interactive VR storytelling. In: Pan, Z., Aylett, R.S., Diener, H., Jin, X., Göbel, S., Li, L. (eds.) Edutainment 2006. LNCS, vol. 3942, pp. 193–202. Springer, Heidelberg (2006)
5. Annesi, J.J., Mazas, J.: Effects of virtual reality-enhanced exercise equipment on adherence and exercise-induced feeling states. Percept. Mot. Skills 85, 835–844 (2006)
6. Lieberman, D.A.: Interactive video games for health promotion: effects on knowledge, self-efficacy, social support, and health. In: Street, R.L., Gold, W.R., Mannings, T. (eds.) Health Promotion and Interactive Technology: Theoretical Applications and Future Directions, pp. 103–120. Lawrence Erlbaum Associates Inc., Mahwah (1997)

Measurement of the Characteristics for BCI by SSVEP

Hisaya Tanaka and Hiromi Sakata

Department of Information Design Kogakuin University, 1-24-2 Nishi Shinjuku, Shinjuku-ku, Tokyo 163-8677, Japan
hisaya@cc.kogakuin.ac.jp, j209055@ns.kogakuin.ac.jp

Abstract. This paper describes the fundamental study for the research and development of SSVEP-BCI. Experiments were carried out with flash and pattern reversal stimulation. A stimulus size of 4.6x4.6cm/40x40cm, time-frequency characteristics from 5 to 20Hz, and three types of stimulus patterns were investigated. As the result, the condition where SSVEP strongly appeared was the flash stimulation of a 4.6x4.6cm square. Moreover, the frequency band was 7 to 17Hz. SSVEP-BCI which transmits at least five intentions may be able to be developed from this experiment.

Keywords: Electroencephalogram (EEG), Brain-Computer Interface (BCI), Steady-State Visual Evoked Potential (SSVEP).

1 Introduction

Attempts to create intuitive input interfaces have been made in many fields in recent years by utilizing interaction between biological signals and computers. One interface utilizing brainwaves is known as a Brain-Computer Interface (BCI).This study aims to develop a communication tool with less mental burdens from attention concentration on the assumption that BCI is utilized by physically handicapped people represented by those with ALS (amyotrophic lateral sclerosis). It is believed that the body of a person with ALS continues to have normal central nerves in the process of weakening of motor neurons in peripheral nerves. For this reason, brainwaves can be utilized for a long time even during the progress of symptoms; therefore are used to measure various characteristics for utilization of steady-state visual evoked potential (SSVEP) as one component of brainwaves. We have researched and developed BCI with P300 event-related potential [1], which had a problem of mental burdens imposed on users due to attention concentration. On the other hand, the SSVEP is neural response that induces brainwaves near the vision field only by casting a glance at the flickering light source. We noted it, therefore, expecting the possibility to reduce mental burdens in comparison with P300. With SSVEP, Fast Fourier Transform (FFT) is applied to brainwaves, based on which frequency at the time of gaze is determined from the power spectrum analyzed. If a spectrum corresponding to the flickering cycle presented is obtained from the brainwaves measured, it is possible to design a BCI that can transmit multiple intentions. If we know the method of stimulation that gives less visual fatigue and can observe and determine multiple spectra, it will be useful to design a BCI with SSVEP; therefore we researched the size, type, presentation time, and frequency band of stimuli.

C. Stephanidis (Ed.): Posters, Part I, HCII 2013, CCIS 373, pp. 623–627, 2013.

2 Measurement of Various Characteristics

Five items were established to investigate the size, type, presentation time, and frequency band of stimuli as follows, to conduct experiments and spectrum analyses. For size of stimuli, two types of stimulus display (large and small) are prepared. For Frequency of stimuli, seven types are prepared within the range of 5-20Hz in reference to previous studies [2] and [3]. In regards to Type of stimuli, two types including pattern reversal stimulation (pattern reversal: reverse stimulation) and flash stimulation (flash: flickering stimulation) are prepared in reference to previous studies [2] and [3]. FFT is applied to each power spectrum 5, 10, 15 and 20 seconds after commencement of stimulus presentation, respectively. For Subjective assessment of stimuli, a four-stage questionnaire survey on subjective assessment is conducted in regards to stimulus displays. Stimuli to be presented are prepared with the evoked response testing device (Neuropack8: MEB-4204 manufactured by Nihon Koden Corporation) and displayed on a 20" CRT display with the size of 40cm x 30cm (SONY, PUM-20420). The stimulus size indicated on this overall display is set as a "large size" (Figure 1).

Fig. 1. Stimulus display - large size (40cm×30cm)

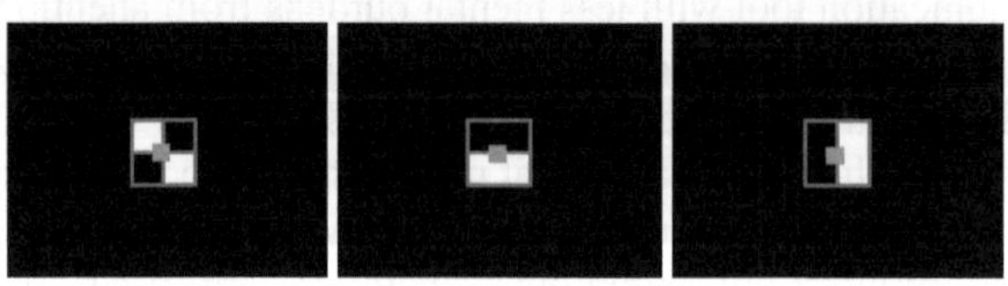

Fig. 2. Stimulus display - small size (4.6cm×4.6cm)

The stimulus display with a 4.6cm square indicated with 2x2 black and white checked squares is set as a "small size" (Figure 2). There are seven types of stimulus frequency presented in the actual experiment: 5, 7, 9, 13, 15, 17 and 20Hz. For the stimulus type, three types of images with pattern reversal where black and white flip (CHECK, H-BAR, V-BAR) and one type of image where the image itself flickers (CHECK) are used.

3 Experiment

Subjects are asked to sit 75cm away from a display placed on an 81cm high desk. The viewing angle is 15 degrees in the case of a large-size stimulus display and 1.7 degrees in the case of a small-size display. Brainwaves are measured with the unipolar derivation method and electrodes are placed at positions A1, A2, O1 and O2 and attached to the electrode box (JE-311B manufactured by Nihon Koden Corporation), beyond which the bio-amplifier (Neurotop: MME-3132 manufactured by Nihon Koden Corporation) is connected. The low-pass filter of the bio-amplifier is set at 30Hz, the high-pass filter at 1.6Hz, and sensitivity at $15\mu V/V$. Furthermore, amplified output from the bio-amplifier is incorporated into a personal computer (Lenovo; ThinkPad X61 7673-A98) using the measurement system, through the BNC terminal box. This experiment has been approved by the Research Ethical Review (H22-2) of Kogakuin University.

SSVEP's power spectra for the subject A are indicated in Figure 3. (a) and (b) show the results when pattern reversal and flash were presented, respectively. The small-size CHECK is used for both stimulus displays. ▼ marks are used at the locations of spectrum with the same frequency as the stimulus presented. Since the spectrum for flash tends to be larger in comparison with pattern reversal, the values on the vertical axis are different.The condition where the power spectrum can be clearly observed includes (a) 9Hz and (b) 15Hz in Figure 4. The condition where the power spectrum cannot be observed includes the case when the size is $1.0\mu V^2/Hz$ or less such as Figure 4(a) 17Hz or the case when a spectrum equivalent to or higher

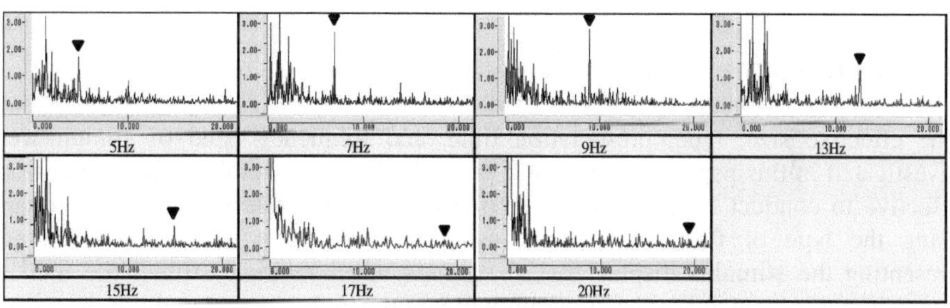

(a) Pattern Reversal

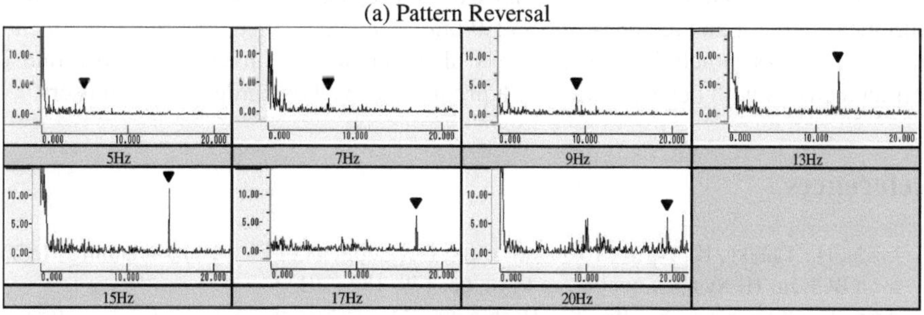

(b) FLASH

Fig. 3. Spectra of SSVEP (Subject A)

than the frequency near ▼ appears like Figure 3(b) 20Hz. The power spectrum up to 5-13Hz can be confirmed in the case of pattern reversal in Figure 3. The power spectrum up to 7-17Hz can be confirmed in the case of flash. This is the result of subject A, while the power spectra were obtained for other subjects in the same way.

4 Discussion

It is considered from the results that the SSVEP's power spectrum appears the most often with the method of using small stimulus size with a 4.6cm square and the stimulus type of flash and presenting the stimulus display for 20 seconds at the frequency band of 7-17Hz. Discussion is as follows. Presentation of a smaller stimulus size can be considered; however since the power spectrum was known to be smaller in proportion to the size, determination might become difficult. By using the stimulus style of flash, the frequency band up to 7-17Hz becomes available. In other words, transmission of at least five-choice intentions is possible when multiple stimuli are used with SSVEP-type BCI. This is more useful than pattern reversal that can only determine up to 5-13Hz. However, 4/6 answers related to "felt slightly difficult to see/felt sick" in the case of small size of flash in the results of questionnaire in Table 1. Thus, utilization for long hours or continuous presentation might cause burdens on users. It was found from Figure 6 that SSVEP's power spectrum increases in proportion to the presentation time. Based on the results of all subjects, the determination rate increases when the spectrum exceeds $2.0\mu V^2/Hz$ in general; therefore it is considered to be desirable to present the stimulus display for 20 seconds.

5 Summary

The effective size, type, presentation time, and frequency band of stimuli were investigated in this paper to design BCI with SSVEP. As a result, it was found to be effective to conduct experiments by setting the stimulus size with a 4.6cm square, using the type of flash stimulation, using the frequency band of 7-17Hz and presenting the stimulus display for 20 seconds when multiple stimuli are used to transmit multiple intentions. A program will be prepared to detect multiple intentions with measurement and analysis of SSVEP online in accordance with this fundamental study. Study for practical application is also planned by investigating the rate of correct answers with determination by a program as well as burdens, etc. on users.

References

1. Inada, H., Tanaka, H.: Need Investigation and Development of Pictogram-Scanning Method for a BCI. In: HI Symposium Proceedings, pp. 179–182 (2011)
2. Arai, Y., Yonezawa, Y., Ito, K., Hashimoto, M., Ushiyama, Y.: Basic Characteristics of VEP and Application to its Input System, Technical Research Report by the Institute of Electronics, Information and Communication Engineers. MBE, ME and Bio Cybernetics 96(257), 13–18 (1996)

3. Ando, J., Toyama, J., Shigemasu, H., Matsuzaki, N.: Quantitative Steering of a Driving Simulator by Steady-State Visual Evoked Potentials. Journal of the Virtual Reality Society of Japan 15(1), 33–40 (2010)
4. Cheng, M., Gao, X., Gao, S., Xu, D.: Design and Implementation of a Brain-Computer Interface with High Transfer Rates. IEEE Transactions on Biomedical Engineering 49(10) (October 2002)
5. VitalRecorder2, BIMUTAS, http://www.kicnet.co.jp/bimutas-video/index.html

Evaluation of Independent Component Analysis Algorithms for Electroencephalography Source Separation

Masoud Zakeri and Zohreh Zakeri

School of Electronic, Electrical & Computer Engineering, University of Birmingham, UK
{mxz848,zxz849}@bham.ac.uk

Abstract. Since each ICA algorithm employs a different approach for source estimation, the result of the estimated sources could be changed. The proposed evaluation method applies three different ICA algorithms on EEG datasets including FastICA, Infomax and Extended-Infomax algorithms. The analysis demonstrates that different ICA algorithms do not have a significant effect on the accuracy of the Support Vector Machine (SVM) classifier in detecting right and left hand imagery movements.

Keywords: Independent Component Analysis, EEG, Artefact rejection.

1 Introduction

Electroencephalography (EEG) is a measure of the brain's electrical activity that can be recorded by placing electrodes on the scalp [1]. It can explore brain function, which is useful for cognitive processing in clinical applications. The EEG brain signals are linearly mixed with non-brain signals due to volume conduction [2]. In order to study brain function, it is desired to remove non-brain signals from the EEG data such as eye movement artefacts.

Among EEG artefact rejection methods, Independent Component Analysis (ICA) is the most commonly used method for EEG source separation and artefact rejection. ICA is a statistical method that is able to separate the brain and non-brain signals from the observed EEG data [3]. It belongs to Blind Source Separation (BSS) methods and can estimate underlying sources of EEG data, which are temporally independent. Several ICA algorithms exist to decompose EEG data into independent components such as FastICA, Infomax and Extended-Infomax. The approach of each ICA algorithm is different in estimating independent components; hence the results of decompositions and artifacts by each ICA algorithm may be different. FastICA is based on a fixed-point iteration scheme that attempts to maximize non-Gaussian properties of the recovered components' distributions. Negentropy is employed to measure the non-Gaussianity and independence of components. Infomax and Extended-Infomax are natural gradient-based algorithms that minimise the mutual information of the component probability distributions. The difference between Info-max and Extended-Infomax is the type of the component distribution that can be estimated by each of them. Infomax is able to separate source signal with

C. Stephanidis (Ed.): Posters, Part I, HCII 2013, CCIS 373, pp. 628–631, 2013.

super-Gaussian distribution (positive kurtosis), while Extended-Infomax can separate sources with both sub-Gaussian (negative kurtosis) and super-Gaussian distributions.

In the scope of this research, the performance of three common ICA algorithms, FastICA [4], Infomax [5], and Extended-Infomax [6], in terms of increasing the accuracy of the Support Vector machine (SVM) classifier [7] for motor imagery task detection will be analysed.

2 Method

2.1 EEG Data

The raw EEG dataset has been provided by 2008 BCI competition IV, Data set II [8]. The data was recorded from 9 subjects while executing four motor imagery tasks: left and right hand imagined movements. The EEG signals were sampled at 250 Hz and filtered by a 0.5-100 Hz band-pass filter with and a 50 Hz notch filter. C3, Cz and C4 are three EEG electrodes that are used to record the data according to the 10-20 international electrodes position [9]. At the beginning of the trials, subjects were shown a fixation cross on the computer screen. Subsequently, different of eye movements of blinking, rolling, up-down or left-right movements were instructed to the subjects. Subjects have to imagine the corresponding hand movements over a period of 4 seconds. A short break was considered between each trial.

2.2 Data Analysis

Three selected ICA algorithms including FastICA, Infomax and Extended-Infomax have been applied to the data to separate EEG brain and non-brain sources from the EEG mixture. The patterns of EEG signal artefacts associated to the different eye movements including blinks, vertical and horizontal eye movements have been obtained by ICA decompositions and removed from the recordings.

The EEG data channels have been split into epochs of 1 second with 90% overlap. Fast Fourier Transform (FFT) is used to extract features of delta, theta, alpha and beta frequency bands of 1-4 Hz, 4-8 Hz, 8-13 Hz and 13-20 Hz, respectively. Then, other features including Root Mean Square (RMS) amplitude, kurtosis, skewness, average power, minimum amplitude, variance and peak to peak values of the signal are extracted. Also, Principal Component Analysis (PCA) [10] has been used to reduce the dimension of the feature vector for avoiding the effect of noise and outliers in to the classifier.

2.3 Classifier

SVM classifier is applied to distinguish the left and right hand imagery movements. The SVM classifier is trained on a sub-space of the data using a set of extracted features. In order to evaluate the performance of the trained SVM classifier, a 10-fold cross validation method is employed.

3 Results and Discussion

The effect of the FastICA, Infomax and Extended-Infomax algorithms on the accuracy of SVM classifier for motor imagery task detection is shown in Figure 1. On one hand, the accuracy of the SVM classifier is different for each individual EEG data. The between subject difference can be due to the distinctness of subjects from whom EEG data was collected and different conditions of each individual. On the other hand, the variability of the SVM classifier's accuracy is small across ICA algorithms for each individual EEG data.

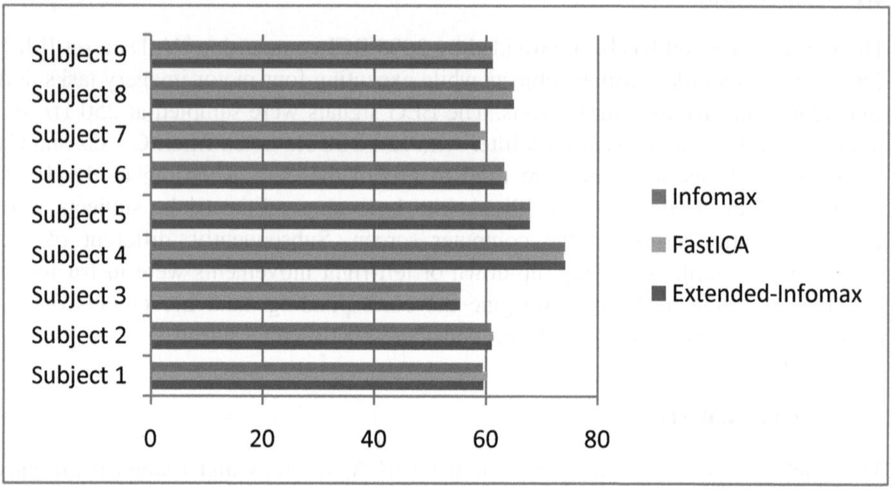

Fig. 1. The performance of SVM classifier method using three different ICA algorithms of FastICA, Infomax and Extended-Infoamx

The Analysis of Variance (ANOVA) test at 5% significance level represents no significant different between ICA algorithms' effect on the accuracy of SVM classifier performance. Although the selected ICA algorithms employ different approaches of source estimation, they are able to estimate and separate eye related components from EEG data. The eye movement components can be detected and separated as single individual sources and removed from the EEG mixture. The difference between ICA algorithms implementations does not affect the performance of SVM classifier to classify right and left imagery movements.

4 Conclusion

In this study, the accuracy of the SVM classifier to distinguish the left and right hand imagery movements are assessed. The imagery movements are distinguished by SVM with no significant difference in the accuracy of the classifier regardless of using different ICA algorithms in the EEG data pre-processing. Different ICA algorithms are applied to pre-process the EEG data and eye movement artifact rejection has no significant effect on the performance on SVM classifier. They all can detect and separate bran non-brain sources from EEG mixture and clean the data to be given to the classifier method. Further studies can be done on the comparison of the effect of ICA algorithms and other artifact rejection methods on classification method's accuracy.

References

1. Berger, H.: Über das elektrenkephalogramm des menschen. European Archives of Psychiatry and Clinical Neuroscience 87(1), 527–570 (1929)
2. Sanei, S., Chambers, J.A.: EEG signal processing. Wiley-Interscience (2008)
3. Comon, P.: Independent component analysis, a new concept? Signal Processing 36(3), 287–314 (1994)
4. Hyvarinen, A.: Fast and robust fixed-point algorithms for independent component analysis. IEEE Transactions on Neural Networks 10(3), 626–634 (1999)
5. Cardoso, J.-F.: Infomax and maximum likelihood for blind source separation. IEEE Signal Processing Letters 4(4), 112–114 (1997)
6. Lee, T.-W., et al.: A unifying information-theoretic framework for independent component analysis. Computers & Mathematics with Applications 39(11), 1–21 (2000)
7. Suykens, J.A., Vandewalle, J.: Least squares support vector machine classifiers. Neural Processing Letters 9(3), 293–300 (1999)
8. Leeb, R., et al.: BCI Competition 2008–Graz data set B. Graz University of Technology, Austria (2008)
9. Homan, R.W., Herman, J., Purdy, P.: Cerebral location of international 10–20 system electrode placement. Electroencephalography and Clinical Neurophysiology 66(4), 376–382 (1987)
10. Jolliffe, I.T.: Principal component analysis, vol. 487. Springer, New York (1986)

Part IX
Development Environments

Ants Can Schedule Software Projects

Broderick Crawford[1,2], Ricardo Soto[1,3], Franklin Johnson[4], and Eric Monfroy[5]

[1] Pontificia Universidad Católica de Valparaíso, Chile
FirstName.Name@ucv.cl
[2] Universidad Finis Terrae, Chile
[3] Universidad Autónoma de Chile, Chile
[4] Universidad de Playa Ancha, Chile
FirstName.Name@upla.cl
[5] LINA, Université de Nantes, France
FirstName.Name@univ-nantes.fr

Abstract. This paper presents the design of an algorithm based on Ant Colony Optimization paradigm to solve the Software Project Scheduling Problem. This problem consists in deciding who does what during the software project development, finding an optimal schedule for a project so that the precedence and resource constraints are satisfied and the final project cost and its duration are minimized. We present the design of an general ant algorithm to solve it.

Keywords: Software Engineering, Software Project Scheduling Problem, Project Management, Ant Colony Optimization.

1 Introduction

We present the design of an algorithm based on Ant Colony Optimization (ACO) paradigm to solve the Software Project Scheduling Problem (SPSP). The SPSP is related to the Resource-Constrained Project Scheduling (RCPS), an existing problem very popular in the literature. It is a problem of finding an optimal schedule for a project so that the precedence and resource constraints are satisfied and the final project cost consisting of personal salaries and project duration is minimized. The RCPS is known to be a NP-hard optimization problem. That means that is not possible to find an efficient algorithm to optimally solve large-size instances in reasonable computational time. Most of the methods used for solving the problem belong to the class of priority-rule-based-methods or to the class of metaheuristic. The first kind of methods starts with none of the jobs being scheduled. Subsequently, a single schedule is constructed by selecting a subset of jobs in each step and assigning starting times to these jobs until all jobs have been considered. By other side, metaheuristics improve an initial solution executing operations which transform one or several solutions into others. ACO has demonstrated to solve several NP-hard combinatorial problems effectively [5]. We believe that the constructive nature of ACO is effective attacking this problem.

C. Stephanidis (Ed.): Posters, Part I, HCII 2013, CCIS 373, pp. 635–639, 2013.

Table 1. SPSP Model

Item	Description
$S = \{s_1, ..., s_{sk}\}$	set of skills associated with software projects
$T = \{t_1, ..., t_T\}$	set of tasks necessary for the project
$G(V, A)$	precedence graph defined in the project's Gantt
$V = \{t_1, t_2, ..., t_T\}$	is a vertex set consisted of all tasks
$A = \{(t_i, t_j), ..., (t_n, t_T)\}$	is an arc set, the task t_i must be done before t_j
t_j^{skills}	is a set of skills for the task j. It is a subset of S
t_j^{effors}	is a effort person-months to complete the task t_j
$EM = \{e_1, ..., e_E\}$	is a set of employees
e_i^{skills}	is the set of skills of e_i. It is a subset of S
e_i^{maxded}	is the maximum degree of dedication of e_i, $e_i \in (0, 1)$
e_i^{salary}	is the monthly salary of e_i

2 The Software Project Scheduling Problem

SPSP is one of the most common problems in managing software engineering projects [12]. It consists in deciding who does what during the software project lifetime. SPSP should consider salaries and employee skills which must be assigned to project tasks according to the requirements of these tasks [14,2]. We describe the model in Table 1:

The SPSP solution can be represented as a matrix $M = [E \times T]$ and $m_{ij} \in [0, 1]$ which represents the degree of dedication of employee e_i to task t_j. If $m_{ij} = 0$ the employee e_i is not assigned to task t_j, if $m_{ij} = 1$ the employee e_i work all day in task t_j. We define some constraints to be feasible solutions from the matrix M, first, all tasks are assigned at least one employee:

$$\sum_{i=1}^{E} m_{ij} > 0 \; \forall j \in \{1, ..., T\} \tag{1}$$

Second, the employees assigned have all the necessary skills to carry out the task. for this all $m_{ij} > 0$, t_j^{skills} is a subset of the union $e_{i \in \{1,...,E\}}^{skills}$ for $\forall j \in \{1, ..., T\}$. It follows that the skills needed for the task t_j are a subset of the union of the skills the employees assigned to the task. To evaluate the quality of the solutions should be evaluated the feasibility of the solution, the whole project cost and duration of the project. We calculate the duration t_j^{dur}, $j \in \{1, ..., T\}$ for each task according to the solution matrix as the following formula:

$$t_j^{dur} = \frac{t_j^{effort}}{\sum_{i=1}^{E} m_{ij}} \tag{2}$$

Now we can calculate the start time t_j^{start} and the end time t_j^{end} for task j. We must consider tasks without precedence, in this case the start time $t_j^{start} = 0$, and the end time is $t_j^{end} = t_j^{start} + t_j^{dur}$. To calculate the start time of tasks with precedence, must be calculated first the end time for all previous tasks. In this case t_j^{start} is defined as $t_j^{start} = max\{t_i^{end} | (t_i, t_j) \in A\}$ else 0. For the total duration of a project p_{dur} just need the end time of task that ends later. We can calculate as $p_{dur} = max\{t_j^{end} | \forall k \neq j (t_j, t_k) \notin A\}$. For the total cost of the software project we need to calculate the cost of each task and then the total cost is the sum of costs according to the following formulas:

$$t_j^{cost} = \sum_{i=1}^{E} e_i^{salary} m_{ij} t_j^{dur} \quad (3) \qquad p_{cost} = \sum_{j=1}^{T} t_j^{cost} \quad (4)$$

The target is minimize the project duration p_{dur} and the total cost p_{cost} of project. Therefore a fitness function is used, where w_{cost} and w_{dur} are values weighting the relative importance of the total cost and duration of the whole project. Then, the fitness fuction to minimize is given by:

$$f(x) = (w_{cost} p_{cost} + w_{dur} p_{dur}) \quad (5)$$

3 ACO for Schedule Software Project

Ant Colony Optimization (ACO) is a Swarm Intelligence technique which inspired from the foraging behavior of real ant colonies. The artificial ants seek the solutions according to a constructive procedure as described in [9,6]. This ACO exploits an optimization mechanism for solving discrete optimization problems in various engineering domain [7,11]. To adapt SPSP to ACO using a Hyper-Cube Framework (ACO-HC) [10] must establish an appropriate construction graph and define the use of pheromone and heuristic information associated with the specified problem [4,1].

The construction graph structure and pheromone matrix, with the respective ACO-HC algorithm is presented in the following subsections. This algorithm makes the association of employees to tasks according to the needs of the tasks, evaluating the quality of the solution [13].

3.1 Construction Graph

The ants travel through the construction graph starting from an initial point and select the nodes which travel according to a probability function that is given by the pheromone and heuristic information of the problem, their relative influence is given by α and β respectively[3,8]. The proposed construction graph makes the association of employees for each task. The construction graph consists of each employee and the ratio of dedication contributions of employees for the task defined as *ded* $\in [0, 1]$ This structure is presented in Fig 1.

The ants travel through the construction graph selecting ways of probabilistically way. Using the following function:

$$p_{ij}^t = \frac{[\tau_{ij}]^\alpha [\eta_{ij}]^\beta}{\sum_{l=0}^{ded} [\tau_{il}]^\alpha [\eta_{il}]^\beta}, j \in \{1, ..., ded\} \quad (6)$$

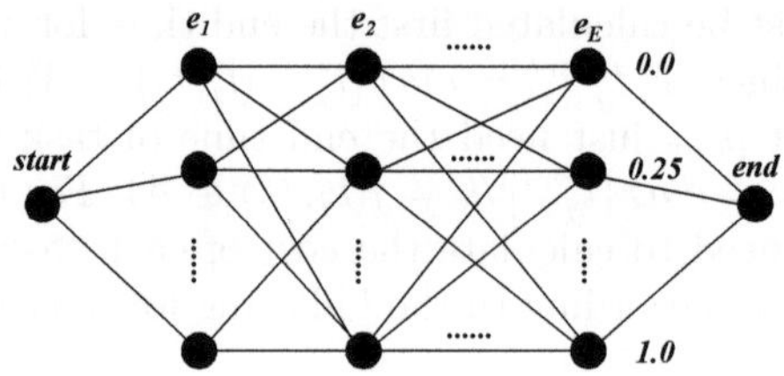

Fig. 1. Construction Graph, $CG = [ded \times E]$

Where τ_{ij} is the pheromone and η_{ij} is the heuristic information of the problem on the path between node i to j in the graph CG for de t task. The heuristic information can be defined according to the importance of the task.

3.2 Pheromone

In the hyper-cube framework the pheromone trails are forced to stay in the interval $[0, 1]$.We represent computationally the evaporation of pheromone and in addition the amount of pheromone in the ant path through the graph, once is completed a tour using the following formula:

$$\tau_{ij} = (1 - \rho)\tau_{ij} + \rho \Delta\tau^k \tag{7}$$

Where ρ is a rate of evaporation $\rho \in \ ]0, 1]$. And $\Delta\tau$ it is associated with quality of the current solution of ant k. We can use a updating pheromone strategy considering the cost and duration of the whole project as follows [10]:

$$\Delta\tau^k = \frac{((w_{cost}p_{cost} + w_{dur}p_{dur})^{-1})^k}{\sum_{h=1}^{m}((w_{cost}p_{cost} + w_{dur}p_{dur})^{-1})^h} \tag{8}$$

3.3 Algorithm Description

ACO-HC algorithm to solve the software project scheduling problem can be briefly described as follow:

Step 1: to initialize the pheromone values and splitting tasks.
Step 2: to allocate first ant in the initial node.
Step 3: each ant travels on the graph choosing nodes (it is to fix the dedication degree of one employee in the task).
Step 4: when the tours are finished, a solution matrix is determined per each ant.
Step 5: to evaluate the quality of the solutions.
Step 6: to calculate the duration and cost of the whole software project and to evaluate its feasibility.
Step 7: to select the best solution and update the pheromone values.
Step 8: to repeat the steps (3-7) until the termination condition is satisfied (iterations).
Step 9: to obtain the best solution according to the fitness.

4 Conclusion

We presented an overview to the resolution of the SPSP using an ACO-HC framework. We design a representation of the problem in order to ACO algorithm can solve it, proposing a construction graph and a pertinent heuristic information. Furthermore, we defined a fitness function able to allow optimization of the generated solutions.

References

1. Abdallah, H., Emara, H.M., Dorrah, H.T., Bahgat, A.: Using ant colony optimization algorithm for solving project management problems. Expert Systems with Applications 36(6), 10004–10015 (2009)
2. Barreto, A., de Oliveira Barros, M., Werner, C.M.L.: Staffing a software project: A constraint satisfaction and optimization-based approach. Comput. Oper. Res. 35(10), 3073–3089 (2008)
3. Berrichi, A., Yalaoui, F., Amodeo, L., Mezghiche, M.: Bi-objective ant colony optimization approach to optimize production and maintenance scheduling. Computers and Operations Research 37(9), 1584–1596 (2010)
4. Chen, W., Zhang, J.: Ant colony optimization for software project scheduling and staffing with an event-based scheduler. IEEE Transactions on Software Engineering 39(1), 1–17 (2013)
5. Crawford, B., Castro, C.: Integrating lookahead and post processing procedures with ACO for solving set partitioning and covering problems. In: Rutkowski, L., Tadeusiewicz, R., Zadeh, L.A., Żurada, J.M. (eds.) ICAISC 2006. LNCS (LNAI), vol. 4029, pp. 1082–1090. Springer, Heidelberg (2006)
6. Dorigo, M., Di Caro, G.: Ant colony optimization: a new meta-heuristic. In: Proceedings of the 1999 Congress on Evolutionary Computation, CEC 1999, vol. 2, p. 1477 (1999)
7. Dorigo, M., Gambardella, L.M.: Ant colony system: A cooperative learning approach to the traveling salesman problem. IEEE Transactions on Evolutionary Computation (1997)
8. Dorigo, M., Maniezzo, V., Colorni, A.: The ant System: Optimization by a colony of cooperating agents. IEEE Transactions on Systems, Man, and Cybernetics Part B: Cybernetics 26(1), 29–41 (1996)
9. Dorigo, M., Stutzle, T.: Ant Colony Optimization. MIT Press, USA (2004)
10. Johnson, F., Crawford, B., Palma, W.: Hypercube framework for aco applied to timetabling. In: Bramer, M. (ed.) Artificial Intelligence in Theory and Practice. IFIP, vol. 217, pp. 237–246. Springer, Boston (2006)
11. Liao, T.W., Egbelu, P., Sarker, B., Leu, S.: Metaheuristics for project and construction management a state-of-the-art review. Automation in Construction 20(5), 491–505 (2011)
12. Ozdamar, L., Ulusoy, G.: A survey on the resource-constrained project scheduling problem. IIE Transactions 27(5), 574–586 (1995)
13. Rubio, J.M., Crawford, B., Johnson, F.: Solving the university course timetabling problem by hypercube framework for aco. In: Cordeiro, J., Filipe, J. (eds.) ICEIS (2), pp. 531–534 (2008)
14. Xiao, J., Ao, X.-T., Tang, Y.: Solving software project scheduling problems with ant colony optimization. Computers and Operations Research 40(1), 33–46 (2013)

Visualizing Software Ecosystems as Living Cities

Clinton Jeffery

University of Idaho, Moscow ID 83844, USA
jeffery@uidaho.edu
http://www2.cs.uidaho.edu/~jeffery/personal.html

Abstract. Several groups visualize software systems using "city" metaphors, mapping software onto features such as buildings and roads. This abstract introduces a "living city" metaphor, where programs are visualized as a city populated by users, data structures, threads of execution, and bugs. A living city is a 3D, multi-user virtual world in which the visible artifacts are software and data.

Keywords: software visualization, virtual environments.

1 Introduction

Software visualization includes static views such as UML Class Diagrams, as well as animated program execution behavior.

1.1 Visualizing Software as Cities

Wettel and Lanza [1] developed CodeCity to visualize software as a city. Classes are buildings, whose height indicates the number of methods. Width and length depict the number of attributes. CodeCity depicts large software systems, such as this 8,000 class program.

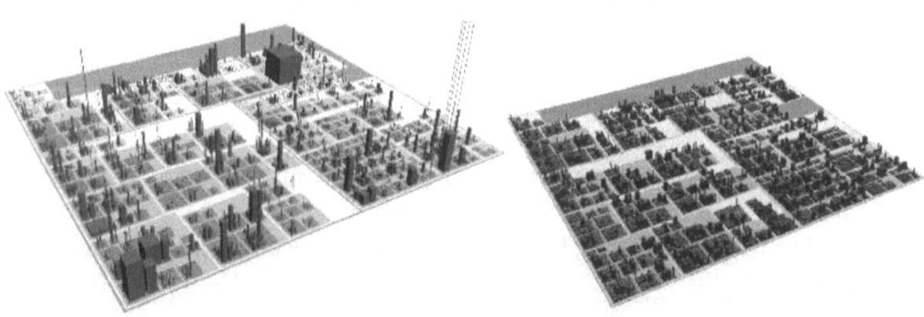

Fig. 1. CodeCity buildings are classes. Height gives the number of methods.

In CodeCity, topography depicts package structure. Layout groups classes in the same package together, and then uses a modified treemap algorithm [2]. CodeCity's static views show how software systems evolve over time. Their metaphor provides the backdrop for the visualization of dynamic program behavior proposed in this paper.

C. Stephanidis (Ed.): Posters, Part I, HCII 2013, CCIS 373, pp. 640–644, 2013.

1.2 Related Work

Knight and Munro [5] developed a tool in which a program is a virtual world, a directory is a country, each file is a city, each class is a district, and each method is a building. They do not map the building interiors, but exterior characteristics show size, parameters, and so on. Kuhn et al [3] developed topological software maps, with island chains depicting relationships of software components.

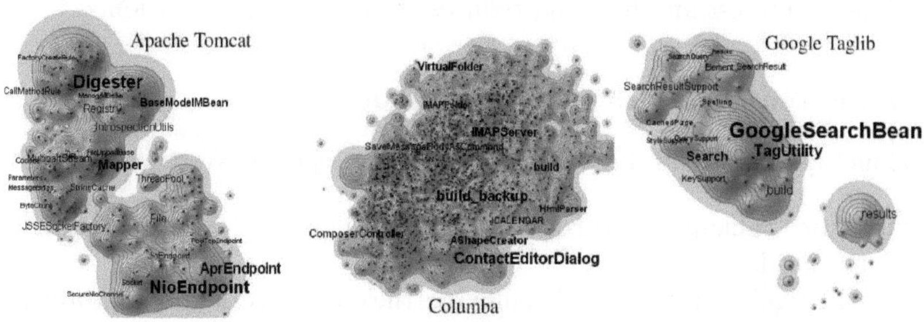

Fig. 2. Topological software maps constructed from component relationships

In CrocoCosmos, [4] a primary model depicts the software system; secondary and tertiary models depict details. Subsystems are streets, with contained classes as buildings. Age is depicted by centrality and elevation.

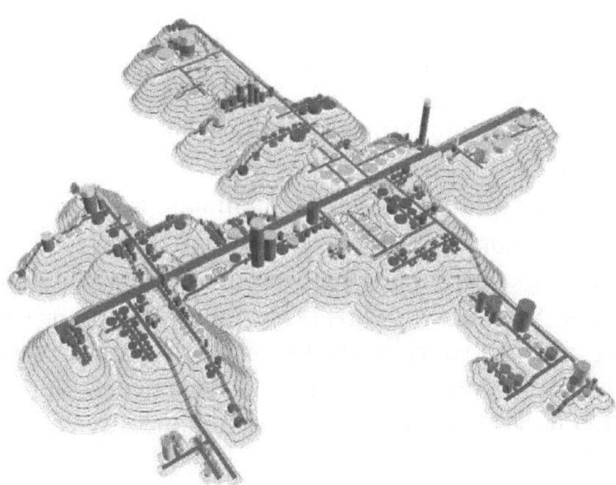

Fig. 3. CrocoCosmos

2 The Living City Metaphor

The "city" metaphor enables sharing, interacting, and debugging collective software development efforts. Extensions to the static software city metaphor are required. The primary extensions introduce dynamic entities.

2.1 Visualizing a Software Ecosystem

Besides peer assistance and review, working in a software city on a set of related programs injects interest and fun, and reduces the cost of collaboration.

2.2 Static Extensions to the City Metaphor

Additional metaphors extend the static backdrop developed by Wettel and Lanza.

directories and packages are roads sizes equivalent to street, arterial, and freeway are needed.

classes' buildings' dimensions height gives the number of methods (storeys). The width is the number of variables. The length is log(| longest method in C|).

Building exterior appearance A texture shows class age and a blended color suggests last commit time. Some old programs are maintained, while others are in ruins.

Class internals Inside a class building is an informative layout for users to walk around in. Starting from ground floor constructors and a directory, one accesses methods via elevator.

Method body details building interiors contain dynamic information: number of activation records live, threads executing there, etc.

Time model Unlike wall-clock time, CPU time may be frozen, or go backwards, a la the Dagger of Time.

Processes and threads Tasks appear as "weeping angels": frozen when seen; moving when unseen.

Functions Functions are singletons containing one public method. A function library resembles a village.

Representing heap Applications are humanoids. Libraries are robots.

Garbage Unused memory lies on the ground.

Atoms data appears as books (string), hammers (int) and saws (real).

External entities Networks are airports, databases are sea ports, local files are mines. Handles are runtime entities such as aircraft or ships.

Associations Class references add connectivity, beyond the street system.

Inheritance Subclasses have a physical resemblance, such as copied buildings with extra floors.

Aggregation Part-of relationships are physical adjacency or containment.

The call stack A beam-of-light model points backwards from callee to caller.

Bugs and warnings A bug report is a spawn-point that emits monsters that attack executions. Killing the bug in-game is temporary; until the bug is fixed, the spawn-point remains.

Building layout After placing the largest buildings first, and placing others around them, and placing associated or coupled classes together, Loretan [6] suggests associating classes by their lexical vocabulary.

Ghosts The city contains remembrances of fixed bugs and deleted code

2.3 Dynamic Extensions

A software city is changed by the software developers that write the code.

Users End users are depicted by computer controlled avatars (NPC's). Users work on use cases, suspend, log out, or crash due to bug attacks.

Developers Developers are NPC's when not present.

Processes and threads The software code forms buildings, but executions are NPC's that move around in a building. A thread standing still is blocked or thrashing and needs help.

3 Case Study: Unicon

This section explores living cities by proposing one for the Unicon programming language, called Unicon City. The case study considers the code that is bundled with the language distribution. The Unicon source code includes 195K lines of C code in the language implementation.

About 350K lines of Unicon code in the distribution was written by 60+ authors. Unicon City has a horizontal axis street (`unicon`), sized so that a person can walk across. The length of the axis street is proportional to the number of lines of code. A street 1cm/LOC long would be 5.7km. The width of this primary arterial is scaled ln(LOC) meters (13.2m).

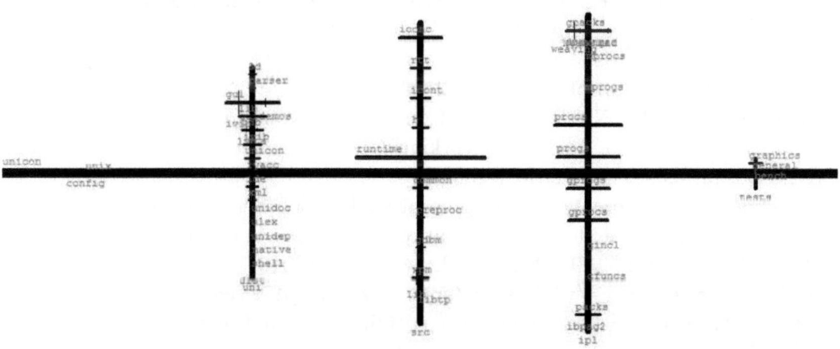

Fig. 4. First street layout for Unicon City

This first street layout for Unicon City is based on the Unicon directory hierarchy. The "CodeCity" treemap algorithm has more crossroads, laying out disconnected parts of the tree adjacently. The "CrocoCosmos" street-based layout is closer to Unicon City. An automatic city layout algorithm might generate a software city atop a map of a real city to increase the aesthetics of the result.

4 Implementation

These tools under construction are needed to complete the living city:

collaborative virtual environment CVE (cve.org) is one.
world generation from a software codebase generate street layouts and buildings from code.
incremental algorithms for code updates update data models from repository commits
high performance dynamic data Unicon reports ~120 types of events such as control flow, calls, returns, data structures, and garbage collection. Dynamic program behavior events will be used to animate the software city.
NPC AI NPC's need "intelligent" behavior.
early adopter user base Some of the Unicon language community might use this project, but others will prefer or require more privacy than it affords.

5 Conclusions and Future Work

The Living Cities metaphor is a vision of the future of software development: an IDE, visualization tool, and MMO. Although this vision requires substantial time and effort to achieve, the enabling technologies are all in place.

References

1. Wettel, R., Lanza, M.: Visualizing Software Systems as Cities. In: Proceedings of VISSOFT 2007 (4th IEEE International Workshop on Visualizing Software For Understanding and Analysis), pp. 92–99. IEEE Computer Society Press (2007)
2. Shneiderman, B.: Tree visualization with Treemaps: a 2-D Space-filling Approach. ACM Transactions on Graphics 11(1), 92–99 (1992)
3. Kuhn, A., Loretan, P., Nierstrasz, O.: Consistent Layout for Thematic Software Maps. In: Proceedings of the 15th Working Conference on Reverse Engineering, WCRE 2008, pp. 209–218 (October 2008)
4. Steinbruckner, F., Lewerentz, C.: Representing Development History in Software Cities. In: Proceedings of the 5th International Symposium on Software Visualization, SOFTVIZ 2010, pp. 193–202. ACM, New York (2010), `http://csbob.swan.ac.uk/visWeek10/softvis/docs/p193.pdf`
5. Knight, C., Munro, M.: Comprehension with[in] Virtual Environment Visualizations. In: Proceedings of the Seventh International Workshop on Program Comprehension, Pittsburgh, PA, May 5-7, pp. 4–11.
6. Loretan, P.: Software Cartography. M.S. Thesis, University of Bern (2011)

Modeling the Portfolio Selection Problem with Constraint Programming

Claudio León de la Barra[1], Ricardo Soto[1,2], Broderick Crawford[1,3], Camila Allendes[1], Hans Berendsen[1], and Eric Monfroy[4]

[1] Pontificia Universidad Católica de Valparaíso, Chile
[2] Universidad Autónoma de Chile, Chile
[3] Universidad Finis Terrae, Chile
[4] CNRS, LINA, Université de Nantes, France
{claudio.leondelabarra,ricardo.soto,broderick.crawford}@ucv.cl,
{camila.allendes.f,hans.berendsen.m}@mail.ucv.cl,
eric.monfroy@univ-nantes.fr

Abstract. Portfolio selection is a relevant problem in finance and economics. It consists in selecting a portfolio of assets considering a given expected return such that the risk of the portfolio is minimized. Several approaches have been proposed to tackle this problem, which are mainly based on mathematical programming techniques and metaheuristics. In this paper we illustrate how this problem can easily be modeled and solved by a relatively modern and declarative programming paradigm called constraint programming.

Keywords: Constraint Modeling, Portfolio Selection Problem, Constraint Satisfacion.

1 Introduction

Portfolio selection is a relevant problem in finance and economics. It consists in selecting a portfolio of assets considering a given expected return such that the risk of the portfolio –measured in terms of variance– is minimized. This problem can be modeled as an optimization problem over real domains with a quadratic objective function and linear constraints.

Several approaches have been proposed to solve portfolio selection problems. Earlier techniques were based on mathematical programming. For instance, traditional methods such as linear and quadratic programming were employed to solve the problem [1,12]. Metaheuristics have also been involved in this context, some examples are simulated annealing [4], genetic algorithms [15], particle swarm optimization [9,8], local search [14,7] as well as hybrid approaches [6,10].

In this paper, we focus on solving the portfolio selection problem (PSP) by using Constraint Programming (CP). CP is a programming paradigm for the efficient solving of constraint-based and optimization problems, which has been successfully employed in several application domains [5]. In CP, a problem is modeled in terms of variables and relations among these variables, namely the

C. Stephanidis (Ed.): Posters, Part I, HCII 2013, CCIS 373, pp. 645–649, 2013.

constraints. Then, the model representing the problem is launched in a search engine, which is commonly called solver.

From a user standpoint, the CP paradigm has a main advantage with respect to metaheuristics: there is no need to design a specific algorithm to solve the problem, the user only models the problem and the solver autonomously search for a solution. This paper focuses on illustrating how this problem can easily be modeled by using CP via the MiniZinc modeling language [13].

2 The PSP Model

In this paper, we use the classic portfolio selection problem introduced by Markowitz in [11]. The corresponding mathematical model is described as follows:

$$\texttt{minimize} \ f(x) = \sum_{i=1}^{n} \sum_{j=1}^{n} \delta_{i,j} x_i x_j \tag{1}$$

$$\texttt{subject to} \ \sum_{i=1}^{n} r_i x_i \geq R \tag{2}$$

$$\sum_{i=1}^{n} x_i = 1 \tag{3}$$

$$0 \leq x_i \leq 1, for \ i \in \{1, \ldots, n\} \tag{4}$$

where n is the number of assets, r_i is the expected return of asset i, $\delta_{i,j}$ is the covariance between assets i and j, R is the expected return, and x_i corresponds to the percentage of the budget invested in asset i. The first equation is the cost function that aims at minimizing the total variance associated to the portfolio. Equation 2 is a constraint that guarantees a given expected return and equation 3 defines that the 100% of the budget must be invested.

3 Modeling the PSP in MiniZinc

As previously mentioned, the CP paradigm has a main advantage with respect to metaheuristics: there is no need to design a specific algorithm to solve the problem, the user only models the problem and the solver autonomously search for a solution. In practice, when problems are solved using metaheuristics a specific algorithm must be designed and implemented according to some pre-established patterns. In CP, it suffices to encode the mathematical model in the language of the solving engine as illustrated in Figure 1.

The model begins by including the `globals.mzn` library. This is necessary to use some specific predicates of the MiniZinc Language. Then, a constant defining the number of assets and three arrays are defined: `r_i` holds the expected return of assets, `covariance` stores the covariance between assets, and the `x_i` array corresponds to the decision variables of the problem. At line 13 and 14, two variables are defined, the first one is used to facilitate the sum operations while the second one is the variable to be minimized within the cost function. Next, r is the expected return. At line 17, the instruction to solve the problem including the search strategy is stated. At line 20 and 24, the constraints corresponding to equation 2 and 3 are posted, respectively. Finally, the cost function is stated followed by an instruction to display the results. As can be seen, just an encoded representation of the mathematical model is needed to solve the problem.

```
1.  include "globals.mzn";
2.
3.  int: assets = 4;
4.  array[1..assets] of int: r_i = [7,8,9,10];
5.  array[1..assets, 1..assets] of int: covariance =
6.  array2d(1..assets, 1..assets,
7.      [40, 4, 6, 2,
8.        4, 60, 3, 1,
9.        6, 3, 85, 8,
10.       2, 1, 8, 100,]);
11.
12.  array[1..assets] of var 1..100: x_i;
13.  var int: total_1;
14.  var int: total_2; % to minimize
15.  int: r = 11;
16.
17.  solve :: int_search(x_i, first_fail, indomain_split, complete)
18.  minimize total_2;
19.
20.  constraint
21.      total_1 = sum(i in 1..assets) ( x_i[i]*r_i[i] )
22.      /\ total_1 >= 0 /\ total_1 >= r;
23
24.  constraint
25.      sum(x_i) = 100;
26.
27.  constraint
28.    total_2 = sum(i,j in 1..assets)( covariance[i,j] *
29.      x_i[i] * x_i[j]) /\ total_2 >= 0;
30.
31.  output [
32.      "total_2: " ++ show(total_2) ++ "\n" ++
33.      "x       : " ++ show(x_i) ++ "\n"
34.  ]
35.  ++ ["\n"];
```

Fig. 1. The PSP modeled in MiniZinc

4 Conclusion

In this paper, we have illustrated how to model and solve and important problem from finance, namely the portfolio selection problem, with CP via the MiniZinc language. We have illustrated the main difference of CP with respect to metaheuristics from a usability point of view. In CP, it suffices to encode the mathematical model in the language of the solver, while when metaheuristics are used it is necessary to implement a specific algorithm to solve the problem.

A permanent direction of research in CP is about facilitating the user modeling task, for instance to propose new modeling languages [13,18], new modeling techniques [2], and/or new modeling components [17,16,3] in order to provide expressiveness and easy problem-solving.

References

1. Bienstock, D.: Computational study of a family of mixed-integer quadratic programming problems. Mathematical Programming 74(2), 121–140 (1996)
2. Chenouard, R., Granvilliers, L., Soto, R.: Model-Driven Constraint Programming. In: Proceedings of the 10th International ACM SIGPLAN Conference on Principles and Practice of Declarative Programming (PPDP), pp. 236–246 (2008)
3. Chenouard, R., Granvilliers, L., Soto, R.: High-Level Modeling of Component-Based CSPs. In: da Rocha Costa, A.C., Vicari, R.M., Tonidandel, F. (eds.) SBIA 2010. LNCS, vol. 6404, pp. 233–242. Springer, Heidelberg (2010)
4. Crama, Y., Schyns, M.: Simulated annealing for complex portfolio selection problems. European Journal of Operational Research 150(3), 546–571 (2003)
5. Rossi, F.: Handbook of Constraint Programming. Elsevier (2006)
6. Di Gaspero, L., di Tollo, G., Roli, A., Schaerf, A.: Hybrid local search for constrained financial portfolio selection problems. In: Van Hentenryck, P., Wolsey, L.A. (eds.) CPAIOR 2007. LNCS, vol. 4510, pp. 44–58. Springer, Heidelberg (2007)
7. Di Gaspero, L., di Tollo, G., Roli, A., Schaerf, A.: Local search for constrained financial portfolio selection problems with short sellings. In: Coello, C.A.C. (ed.) LION 2011. LNCS, vol. 6683, pp. 450–453. Springer, Heidelberg (2011)
8. Golmakani, H.R., Fazel, M.: Constrained portfolio selection using particle swarm optimization. Expert Syst. Appl. 38(7), 8327–8335 (2011)
9. Fazel, M., Golmakani, H.: Constrained portfolio selection using particle swarm optimization. Expert Syst. Appl. 38(7), 8327–8335 (2011)
10. Di Gaspero, L., Tollo, G., Roli, A., Schaerf, A.: Hybrid metaheuristics for constrained portfolio selection problems. Quantitative Finance 11(10), 1473–1487 (2011)
11. Markowitz, H.: Portfolio selection. Journal of Finance 7(1), 77–91 (1952)
12. Markowitz, H.: The optimization of a quadratic function subject to linear constraints. Naval Research Logistics Quarterly 3(1-2), 111–133 (1952)
13. Nethercote, N., Stuckey, P.J., Becket, R., Brand, S., Duck, G.J., Tack, G.R.: MiniZinc: Towards a Standard CP Modelling Language. In: Bessière, C. (ed.) CP 2007. LNCS, vol. 4741, pp. 529–543. Springer, Heidelberg (2007)
14. Schaerf, A.: Local search techniques for constrained portfolio selection problems. Computational Economics 20(3), 177–190 (2002)

15. Soleimani, H., Golmakani, H.R., Salimi, M.H.: Markowitz-based portfolio selection with minimum transaction lots, cardinality constraints and regarding sector capitalization using genetic algorithm. Expert Syst. Appl. 36(3), 5058–5063 (2009)
16. Soto, R.: Controlling search in constrained-object models. In: Kuri-Morales, A., Simari, G.R. (eds.) IBERAMIA 2010. LNCS, vol. 6433, pp. 582–591. Springer, Heidelberg (2010)
17. Soto, R., Crawford, B., Monfroy, E., Paredes, F.: Syntax Extensions for a Constrained-Object Language via Dynamic Parser Cooperation. Studies in Informatics and Control 21(1), 41–48 (2012)
18. Soto, R., Granvilliers, L.: The Design of COMMA: An Extensible Framework for Mapping Constrained Objects to Native Solver Models. In: Proceedings of the 19th IEEE International Conference on Tools with Artificial Intelligence (ICTAI), pp. 243–250 (2007)

Adaptive and Multilevel Approach for Constraint Solving

Claudio León de la Barra[1], Broderick Crawford[1,2], Ricardo Soto[1,3], and Eric Monfroy[4]

[1] Pontificia Universidad Católica de Valparaíso, Chile
[2] Universidad Finis Terrae, Chile
[3] Universidad Autónoma de Chile, Chile
[4] CNRS, LINA, Université de Nantes, France
{claudio.leondelabarra,broderick.crawford,ricardo.soto}@ucv.cl,
eric.monfroy@univ-nantes.fr

Abstract. For many real world problems, modeled as Constraint Satisfaction Problems, there are no known efficient algorithms to solve them. The specialized literature offers a variety of solvers, which have shown satisfactory performance. Nevertheless, despite the efforts of the scientific community in developing new strategies, there is no algorithm that is the best for all possible situations. Then, several approaches have emerged to deal with the Algorithm Selection Problem. Here, we sketch the use a Choice Function for guiding a Constraint Programming solver exploiting search process features to dynamically adapt it in order to more efficiently solve Constraint Satisfaction Problems. To determine the best set of parameters of the choice function, an upper-level metaheuristic is used. The main novelty of our approach is that we reconfigure the search based solely on performance data gathered while solving the current problem.

Keywords: Algorithm Selection Problem, Constraint Solving, Constraint Satisfacion Problems, Autonomous Search.

1 Introduction

Optimization problems can be solved by different algorithms, with varied performance for different problem characteristics. Although some algorithms are better than others on average, there is not the best algorithm for all the possible instances of a given problem. To address this concern, recent work has focused on creating algorithm portfolios, which contain a selection of state of the art algorithms. To solve a particular problem with this portfolio, a pre-processing step is run where the suitability of each algorithm for the problem at hand is assessed. It is the same in Constraint Programming (CP), where the selection of an enumeration strategy is crucial for the performance of the resolution process, a correct selection can dramatically reduce the computational cost of finding a solution. However, it is well-known that deciding a priori the correct heuristic

C. Stephanidis (Ed.): Posters, Part I, HCII 2013, CCIS 373, pp. 650–654, 2013.

is quite difficult, as the effects of the strategy can be unpredictable. In recent years, different efforts have been done to determine good strategies based on the information generated through the resolution process. However, deciding what information must be measured and how to redirect the search is an ongoing investigation [1].

Here, we propose a hyperheuristic approach to manage a portfolio of enumeration strategies. A hyperheuristic is a heuristic that operates at a higher level of abstraction than the solver. The hyperheuristic has no problem-specific knowledge, at any given time the hyperheuristic must choose which enumeration strategy to call. To allow the hyperheuristic to operate, we define a choice function which adaptively ranks the enumeration strategies monitoring indicators of the search process. An analogy can be done with the well-known work methodology called Balanced Scorecard (BSC) [12]. Such a business approach aims at helping organizations to translate the strategy in terms of measures. In that way, the behavior and performance of the organization is driven towards the achievement of the strategic objectives. BSC involves concepts such as indicators, measures, strategic objectives and introduces the concept of "means", which refers to actions and initiatives that must be carried out for achieving the organization objectives. Such concepts can be seen as the inspiration of this research, and they are closely related to the actions to follow once we decide to replace the strategy in the CP solver.

2 Constraint Programming

Constraint Programming is a powerful software technology devoted to the efficient resolution of constraint-based problems. It smartly interbreeds ideas from different domains such as Operations Research, Artificial Intelligence, Graph Theory and Programming Languages. Currently, CP is largely used in different application domains. The principle behind CP is simple: the user states the problem and the system solves it.

The solving process demands two main phases: modeling and search. In the modeling phase, the user expresses the problem as a Constraint Satisfaction Problem (CSP), which in general terms corresponds to a sequence of variables lying in a domain and a set of constraints. In the search phase, the CSP is launched in a solving engine, commonly called *solver*, which is a black box composed of a set of powerful search algorithms. Such algorithms are responsible for finding a solution, that is, a variable-value assignment that satisfies the complete set of constraints.

Both phases are essential for an efficient CSP resolution. From a modeling standpoint, a main element is the language. It provides the expressiveness and the semantics for modeling the problems. From a search point of view, the efficiency of search algorithms is the key. The idea is to build a tree data structure holding the potential solutions and to perform a search process by interleaving two phases: constraint propagation and enumeration.

Constraint propagation can be seen as a filtering mechanism. It is able to prune the search tree by deleting those values that do not lead to any solution.

The enumeration, also called labeling, is responsible for creating the branches of the tree by assigning a value to a variable from its domain. The common idea is to generate one branch for each variable-value assignment until a complete solution is reached. However, if a partial solution violates a constraint, the process backtracks, i.e., it returns to the most recently instantiated variable that still has chance to reach a solution. This phase requires selecting the variable to be enumerated and then the value to be assigned; we refer to these steps as the variable and value selection heuristics.

3 The Enumeration Strategy Challenge

Jointly, a variable selection heuristic and a value selection heuristic constitute what is known as the enumeration strategy [1]. Such a pair of decisions is crucial in the performance of the resolution process, where a correct selection can dramatically reduce the computational cost of finding a solution. For instance, consider the simple case of choosing the right value on the first try for each variable: a solution could be found without performing backtracks.

For a simple CSP problem, a good enumeration strategy goes directly to a solution performing a few enumerations without backtracking. However, a bad strategy can perform a lot of backtracks before reaching a solution. Obviously strategies have drastically different efficiencies, often several orders of magnitude, and thus it is crucial to select a good one that unfortunately cannot be predicted in the general case. We are interested in making good choices for enumeration, i.e., selection of a variable and a value.

There exist various studies about enumeration strategies [3–5], some centered in defining general criteria, e.g., the smallest domain for variable selection, and its minimum, maximum, or a random value for value selection. As opposed to this idea, some research works have proposed strategies for a given class of problems, e.g., for job shop scheduling [14, 15], as well as for configuration design [6]. We can also find research focused on determining the best strategy based in some static criterion [2, 3, 16], i.e., the selection heuristic is determined only once before starting the resolution process, remaining unchangeable during the whole process. However, deciding a priori the correct heuristics is quite hard, as the effects of the strategy can be unpredictable.

We proposed techniques allowing the identification and measurement of indicators for the resolution process. The main goal is to make possible the classification of the execution process state, considered as the resolution progress, and in that way be able to determine if the current strategy exhibits a poor performance and whether it is necessary to replace it with a better one. Such an evaluation procedure is not carried out for improving the resolution of a single problem. We address our approach to efficiently find solutions for different problems. This can be done by exploiting search process features to dynamically adapt a CP solver changing the enumeration strategy in use when the other strategy looks more promising in order to solve the CSP at hand. The main novelty of our approach is that we reconfigure the searching based solely on performance data gathered while solving the current problem performing a general, correct, and opportune indicator-based detection. Becoming our solver in an Autonomous Search (AS) system [11].

4 Adaptive and Multilevel Approach for Constraint Solving

As mentioned above, this work addresses dynamic selection of enumeration strategies for solving constraint satisfaction problems. We focus our research in reacting on the fly, allowing an early replacement of bad performance strategies without waiting the entire solution process or an exhaustive analysis of a given class of problems. We make profit of indicators that gather performance data during the resolution process. Regarding this issue, we use AS mechanisms where a choice function adaptively ranks the enumeration strategies and the problem of determining the best set of parameters of the choice function is tackled using a metaheuristic (Genetic algorithm, Particle swarm ...).

Our solver is able to detect inefficiencies and, as a result, replace the enumeration strategy with a better one. To achieve this goal, we perform an indicator based observation during the solving process. The main purpose of indicators is to proportion the relevant information about the behavior of the resolution process. They must reflect the real state of progress in the problem resolution. In this way, we are able to elaborate a correct judgment about the search performance. To this end, we define simple and quantitative indicators, which can be used different times as well as percentage combinations of them depending on the used techniques and/or the problem to solve.

Our research focuses on developing solvers for CSPs. We are concerned with the design of hybrid resolution approaches including constraint programming and metaheuristics. We have been working on that area during the last years, exploring the different issues –from software engineering and optimization– involved in algorithm design, implementation, tuning and experimental evaluation. The details of our related work are in [7–10, 13].

5 Conclusions

Among the main contributions of our work we can state the design and implementation of a solver that is able to measure the search process (using some basic indicators) in order to perform an on the fly replacement of enumeration strategies (using a portfolio of basic enumeration strategies). The solver is based on enumeration strategies of different natures (based on the size of variable domains, on the number of occurrences of the variables in the constraints) and some indicators on the resolution progress (backtracks, visited nodes, variables fixed, shallow backtracks, deep of the search tree, ...). In our approach the replacement of the enumeration strategies is performed depending on a quality rank (priority), which is computed by means of a choice function fine-tuned by a metaheuristic.

References

1. Apt, K.R.: Principles of Constraint Programming. Cambridge University Press (2003)
2. Beck, J.C., Prosser, P., Wallace, R.J.: Trying again to fail-first. In: Faltings, B.V., Petcu, A., Fages, F., Rossi, F. (eds.) CSCLP 2004. LNCS (LNAI), vol. 3419, pp. 41–55. Springer, Heidelberg (2005)
3. Beck, J.C., Prosser, P., Wallace, R.J.: Variable ordering heuristics show promise. In: Wallace, M. (ed.) CP 2004. LNCS, vol. 3258, pp. 711–715. Springer, Heidelberg (2004)
4. Christopher Beck, J., Prosser, P., Wallace, R.J.: Toward understanding variable ordering heuristics for constraint satisfaction problems. In: Fourteenth Irish Artificial Intelligence and Cognitive Science Conference (AICS), pp. 11–16 (2003)
5. Castro, C., Monfroy, E., Figueroa, C., Meneses, R.: An Approach for Dynamic Split Strategies in Constraint Solving. In: Gelbukh, A., de Albornoz, Á., Terashima-Marín, H. (eds.) MICAI 2005. LNCS (LNAI), vol. 3789, pp. 162–174. Springer, Heidelberg (2005)
6. Chenouard, R., Granvilliers, L., Sebastian, P.: Search heuristics for constraint-aided embodiment design. AI EDAM 23(2), 175–195 (2009)
7. Crawford, B., Castro, C., Monfroy, E.: Integration of Constraint Programming and Metaheuristics. In: Miguel, I., Ruml, W. (eds.) SARA 2007. LNCS (LNAI), vol. 4612, pp. 397–398. Springer, Heidelberg (2007)
8. Crawford, B., Castro, C., Monfroy, E., Soto, R., Palma, W., Paredes, F.: A Hyperheuristic Approach for Guiding Enumeration in Constraint Solving. In: Schütze, O., Coello Coello, C.A., Tantar, A.-A., Tantar, E., Bouvry, P., Del Moral, P., Legrand, P. (eds.) EVOLVE - A Bridge Between Probability, Set Oriented Numerics, and Evolutionary Computation II. AISC, vol. 175, pp. 171–188. Springer, Heidelberg (2012)
9. Crawford, B., Soto, R., Monfroy, E., Palma, W., Castro, C., Paredes, F.: Parameter tuning of a choice-function based hyperheuristic using particle swarm optimization. Expert Syst. Appl. 40(5), 1690–1695 (2013)
10. de la Barra, C.L., Crawford, B.: Fostering Creativity Thinking in Agile Software Development. In: Holzinger, A. (ed.) USAB 2007. LNCS, vol. 4799, pp. 415–426. Springer, Heidelberg (2007)
11. Hamadi, Y., Monfroy, E., Saubion, F.: What is autonomous search? Technical Report MSR-TR-2008-80, Microsoft Research (2008)
12. Kaplan, R.S.: Conceptual Foundations of the Balanced Scorecard. SSRN eLibrary (2010)
13. Monfroy, E., Castro, C., Crawford, B.: Adaptive enumeration strategies and metabacktracks for constraint solving. In: Yakhno, T., Neuhold, E.J. (eds.) ADVIS 2006. LNCS, vol. 4243, pp. 354–363. Springer, Heidelberg (2006)
14. Sadeh, N.M., Fox, M.S.: Variable and value ordering heuristics for the job shop scheduling constraint satisfaction problem. Artif. Intell. 86(1), 1–41 (1996)
15. Smith, S.F., Cheng, C.: Slack-based heuristics for constraint satisfaction scheduling. In: AAAI, pp. 139–144 (1993)
16. Sturdy, P.: Learning Good Variable Orderings. In: Rossi, F. (ed.) CP 2003. LNCS, vol. 2833, p. 997. Springer, Heidelberg (2003)

Biological Objects Data Registration Algorithm for Modal (Low Dimensional) Analysis

Michal Rychlik, Witold Stankiewicz, and Marek Morzynski

Poznan University of Technology, Department of Virtual Engineering,
Piotrowo 3, 60965 Poznan, Poland
Michal.Rychlik@put.poznan.pl

Abstract. Principal Component Analysis, a statistical tool allowing to create a low dimensional subspace basing on input data, finds many applications in biomechanics. The PCA requires the same topology (mesh connectivity, number of nodes) for all objects in database. To achieve this, each new object added to database must be registered. In this article the finishing registration procedure, based on own software and created especially for biological data sets, is presented. The study of registration process for 3D input data (faces and hands) for PCA is discussed.

Keywords: 3D geometry reconstruction, data registration, low-dimensional model, modal analysis, Principal Component Analysis (PCA).

1 Introduction

Advanced numerical tools significantly increase the possibilities of existing methods of data analysis and give new potential in disciplines like bioengineering or biometrics. In biometrics the identification of people might be based on different input data, like the shape of the face [2, 13], hand [4, 14], or whole human body [1].

Facial identification reads the peaks and valleys of facial features, known as nodal points. In a human face there exist 80 points, but usually only 15-20 of them, known as „Golden triangle", are used for identification.

In the case of hand-based verification of individuals, usually overall structure, 2D shape (silhouette) and proportions of the hand (length, width and thickness of hand, fingers and joints) [10] are measured and analyzed. Hand geometry biometrics systems, measuring up to 90 parameters in 2D space.

Insufficient reliability of the currently used 2D recognition techniques (photos contain less information then the 3D surface) stimulates interest in 3D techniques.

Rapid increase of the amount of data to be analyzed leads to the need for modal analysis methods. These methods are used to simplify and minimize the number of parameters which describe objects. The kind of used modal method: mathematical, physical or empirical (PCA / POD), has a fundamental influence on the results [7, 8].

C. Stephanidis (Ed.): Posters, Part I, HCII 2013, CCIS 373, pp. 655–659, 2013.

2 PCA Analysis and 3D Input Data Acquisition of Biological Objects

For reconstruction of the 3D geometry, decomposition based on Principal Component Analysis (PCA) can be used. PCA provides a "relevant" set of basis functions, which allows construction of a low-dimensional subspace. PCA modes are optimal from viewpoint of information included inside of the each modes. The shape of each object is represented in the data base as the set of 3D polygonal surface and stored as a vector. PCA consists in centering of objects (by subtracting the average geometry) and the calculation of the covariance matrix [3]. Eigenvectors of this matrix (PCA modes) represent the geometrical features (shape) of the object, as well as additional information like physical features (density), texture or temperature map [9]. Only a small number of first modes carry most information, therefore each original object can be reconstructed by a mode basis truncated to the most dominant principal components.

The data input for numerical experiment was obtained by using the 3D structural light scanner. The two groups of biological models were measured: set of human faces and set of human hands. Each input object was scanned and 3D surface model (50k triangles mesh) was computed. During measurements of hand geometry the special hand holder (for the appropriate and repeatable fingers positioning) was used. The shape of the hand holder was comparable as used in hand silhouette 2D scanners [4]. In this work 100 faces of different persons (age: 22-24) with neutral expression and 100 human hands was acquired.

3 Biological Objects Data Registration Algorithms

The registration process used for the 3D model of face is performed in three stages.

First stage – preliminary registration – involves making a series of affine transformations (shift, rotation and scaling) on scanned face so that its position in a coordinate system is analogous as the reference face (fig. 1. a).

The second stage – elastic registration – consists of five steps:

1. detection of edge elements lying on the boundary of the face (fig. 1. b).
2. automatic detection of 16 specific points on the surface of the registrant (placed on the base) face (Fig. 1. c) defining: eyes, nose, mouth, beard / chin, basic on the curvature of the selected cross-sections of the 3D model.
3. The displacement of boundary curve points of reference grid onto new position on registrant grid, holding relative distance from the beginning of the curve.
4. Displacement of characteristic points of the reference grid in the corresponding position on the registrant grid.
5. Interpolation of the position of other nodes on reference grid basing on the known boundary conditions - steps 3); 4) - using the method of Shepard (Inverse Distance Weighting) [11].

The third stage – finishing registration – is the transfer of all the nodes in the reference grid to the position defined by the points lying on the registered grid. For each node (deformed in the second stage) reference grid is searched the next node on the registration grid - whose coordinates are assigned to the reference grid node (Fig. 1. d). In the case of the face registration this step leads to a better fit mesh in areas which are not described by the characteristic points and between of them (such as the cheeks and forehead, the curvature of the nose). The developed own numerical tool is based on kd-tree searching algorithm [5].

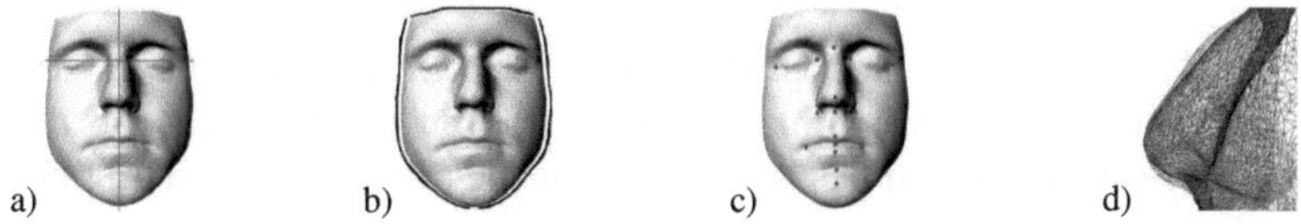

Fig. 1. Face elastic registration: a) origin point, b) detection of the edges curves, c) detected points, d) surface triangle grids: of elastic *(black)* and finishing registration *(light gray)*

The result of the applied registration is description of all faces in data base by the same (in topological meaning) surface mesh. The value of standard deviation between source and registered faces was 0.054mm and average distance 0.008mm.

For the 3D hands models, the special rigid registration software was eliminated. This step was done by using special hardware – hand holder.

The first step of non-rigid registration consists of the adjustment of the positions of fingers (phalanges and metacarpals). The skeleton nodes' positions are modified by genetic algorithm [12], resulting in a population with varying genotype (positions of skeleton nodes). For each individual (deformed skeleton) solid mesh representing base geometry is deformed using Finite Element System solving Hooke's law. Resulting deformed meshes are compared with respect to the new mesh being registered, and the objective functions, based on error measure, are computed. The whole process is depicted in Fig. 2.

After the adjustment of finger positions the widths and lengths are to be changed.

This process is done using in-house CFD (computational fluid dynamics) solver. The governing equation (1) is incompressible Navier-Stokes equation in penalty formulation [6] with additional volume forces, discretized using Finite Element Method. The forcing (source segment) depends on the difference between two monochrome slices – from registered and base meshes [8]:

$$\dot{V}_i + V_{i,j} V_j - \frac{1}{\mathrm{Re}} V_{i,jj} + \frac{\varepsilon - \lambda}{\rho} V_{j,ji} + (f - g) f_{,i} = 0 \tag{1}$$

where ρ is fluid density, V_i - velocity component, Re - Reynolds number, λ - bulk viscosity. The parameters ε and λ are used to control the fluid compressibility, f is the base object and g is the target object (input model). The CFD registration is performed on a set of equidistant slices perpendicular to the first principal axes of the phalanges and a set of slices through the metacarpus perpendicular to the x axis.

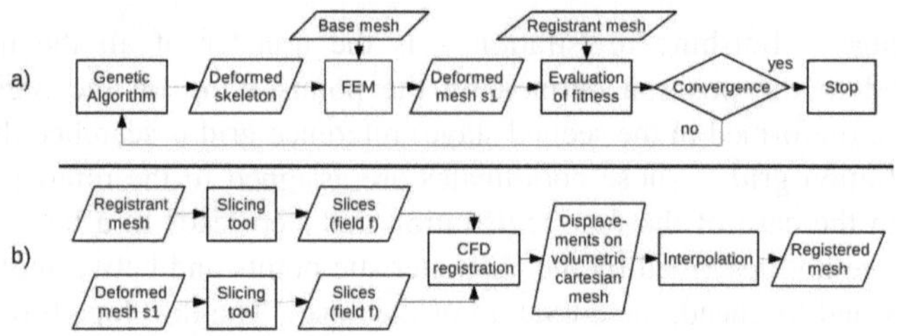

Fig. 2. Algorithm of the hand registration: a) skeleton based registration, b) fluid registration

The final step is the interpolation of displacements from CFD structured (Cartesian) mesh onto the (deformed) base mesh. The value of standard deviation between source and registered hands was 0.83mm and average distance 0.11mm.

4 Principal Component Analysis of 3D Biological Objects

For prepared databases of human faces and hands the PCA was performed. The result of this operation is the mean object, modes and coefficients values. To reconstruct 90% of information about decomposed geometry, first 19 modes for faces (Fig. 3 top) and first 10 modes for hands (Fig. 3 bottom) have to be used.

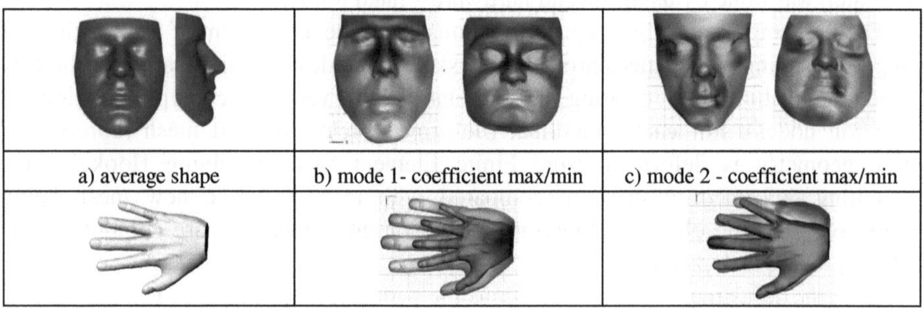

Fig. 3. Visualization of the average value and first two empirical modes of faces and hands

5 Summary

The quality of the registration process has a fundamental importance onto results obtained in modal analysis. In the article authors present two specialized algorithms – based on own software code – for three-dimensional registration of biological objects: faces and hands.

For 3D faces three-step registration process allows obtaining very precise final model. In the case of faces described in this article accuracy of registration was better than accuracy of 3D scanning (0.05mm) used for data acquisition.

For 3D hands skeleton-based and CFD registration were performed. The lower accuracy obtained in this case is due to lower quality of input data from 3D scanner. For evaluation of registered databases the brief results of PCA was shown.

Acknowledgments. The part of this work was supported under research grant no: N518 496039 from the Polish Ministry of Science 2010-2013.

References

1. Brett, A., Curless, B., Popović, Z.: The space of human body shapes: reconstruction and parameterization from range scans. ACM Transactions on Graphics (TOG) 22(3) (2003)
2. Bruce, D.A., et al.: Recognizing faces with PCA and ICA. Computer Vision and Image Understanding 91(1), 115–137 (2003)
3. Holmes, P., Lumley, J.L., Berkooz, G.: Turbulence, Coherent Structures, Dynamical Systems and Symmetry. Cambridge University Press, Cambridge (1998)
4. Jain, A.K., et al.: A prototype hand geometry based verification system. In: Proc. 2nd Int. Conf. Audio- and Video-Based Biometric Person Authentication, pp. 166–171 (1999)
5. Kennel, M.B.: KDTREE 2: Fortran 95 and C++ software to efficiently search for near neighbors in a multi-dimensional Euclidean space. Arxiv preprint physics/0408067 (2004)
6. Morzyński, M., Afanasiev, K., Thiele, F.: Solution of the eigenvalue problems resulting from global non-parallel flow stability analysis. Computer Methods in Applied Mechanics and Engineering 169, 161–176 (1999)
7. Rychlik, M., Stankiewicz, W.: Extraction of 3D Geometrical Features of Biological Objects with 3D PCA Analysis and Applications of Results. In: Naik, G.R. (ed.) Applied Biological Engineering – Principles and Practice, pp. 85–112. InTech (2012)
8. Rychlik, M., Stankiewicz, W., Morzyński, M.: Application of modal analysis for extraction of geometrical features of biological objects set. In: BIODEVICES 2008: Proc. 1st Int. Conf. Biomed. Electronics and Devices, vol. 2, pp. 227–232 (2008)
9. Rychlik, M., Stankiewicz, W., Morzynski, M.: Numerical Analysis of Geometrical Features of 3D Biological Objects for Three Dimensional Biometric and Anthropometric Database. In: Stephanidis, C. (ed.) Universal Access in HCI, Part II, HCII 2011. LNCS, vol. 6766, pp. 108–117. Springer, Heidelberg (2011)
10. Sanchez-Reillo, R., Sanchez-Avila, C., Gonzales-Marcos, A.: Biometric Identification Through Hand Geometry Measurements. IEEE Transactions on Pattern Analysis and Machine Intelligence 22(10), 1168–1171 (2000)
11. Shepard, D.: A two-dimensional interpolation function for irregularly-spaced data. In: Proceedings of the 1968 ACM National Conference, pp. 517–524 (1968)
12. Stankiewicz, W., Roszak, R., Morzynski, M.: Genetic Algorithm-based Calibration of Reduced Order Galerkin Models. Math. Mod. Anal. 16(2), 233–247 (2011)
13. Xuerong, C., Jing, Z., Xiao, G.: Nonlinear fusion for face recognition using fuzzy integral. Comm. Nonlin. Science and Num. Sim. 12(5), 823–831 (2007)
14. Yörük, E., Dutağaci, H., Sankur, B.: Hand biometrics. Image and Vision Computing 24(5), 483–497 (2006)

A GUI for Modeling Regular Constraints

Ricardo Soto[1,2], Broderick Crawford[1,3], Diego Riquelme[1], and Eric Monfroy[4]

[1] Pontificia Universidad Católica de Valparaíso, Chile
[2] Universidad Autónoma de Chile, Chile
[3] Universidad Finis Terrae, Chile
[4] CNRS, LINA, Université de Nantes, France
{ricardo.soto,broderick.crawford}@ucv.cl
diego.riquelme.a@mail.ucv.cl, eric.monfroy@univ-nantes.fr

Abstract. In constraint programming, a regular constraint is a special global constraint very useful in scheduling, in particular for the easy modeling of rostering problems. This constraint enforces a sequence of variables to take a value defined by a deterministic finite automaton. In practice, when the user models the problem, regular constraints are programmed in the language of the solving engine, which is in most cases a proprietary language or a classic programming language. However, there exists several modeling languages and very different encoding patterns for the regular constraint, turning the modeling into a tedious task. In this paper, we present a simple GUI for modeling regular constraints that clearly increases the usability for end-users. The tool allows to easily draw finite automata, which are automatically translated to the corresponding code of the regular constraint for the target solving engine.

Keywords: Constraint Modeling, Regular Constraint, Constraint Satisfaction.

1 Introduction

Constraint Programming (CP) is an efficient software technology for solving Constraint Satisfaction Problems (CSP). A CSP is a formal problem representation that mainly consists in a sequence of variables and a set of constraints. Solving a CSP implies to firstly model the problem and then to launch it in a solving engine –commonly called solver– which is responsible for search a result. In CP, a regular constraint is a special global constraint very useful in scheduling, in particular for the easy modeling of rostering problems. This constraint enforces a sequence of variables to take a value defined by a deterministic finite automaton.

In practice, when the user models the CSP, regular constraints are programmed in the solver language, which is in most cases a proprietary language or a classic programming language such as C, Java, or Prolog. However, there exists several languages for modeling CSPs, and the modeling of regular constraints is not standard. In fact, they follow very different encoding patterns. We can find various representations, for instance by using data structures such as list,

C. Stephanidis (Ed.): Posters, Part I, HCII 2013, CCIS 373, pp. 660–663, 2013.

matrices, and vectors; or also by using logic predicates, methods, or functions, depending on the programming paradigm of the solver language. Hence, modeling the regular constraint is commonly a tedious task, even more when the size of the constraint increases.

The aim of this work is to facilitate the task of CSP modelers. To this end, we provide a simple GUI for modeling regular constraints that clearly increases the usability for end-users. The tool allows to easily draw the finite automaton, which is automatically translated to the corresponding code of the regular constraint for the target solver. Currently, regular constraints can be translated to four solvers, being possible to fastly add new ones. The tool is publicly available under GNU license at [1].

2 The Tool

In order to illustrate the application of the proposed tool let us employ as example the nurse rostering problem. Nurse rostering aims at organizing an schedule of shifts for nurses in a given period of time. Consider that in a given health center there exist two kind of shifts: day (D), night (N); and we use (O) for day-off. In each period of 4 days a nurse must have at least one day-off, moreover a nurse cannot have three consecutive N shifts. This can be represented by the deterministic finite automaton (DFA) depicted in Figure 1. Table 1 describes the corresponding transitions.

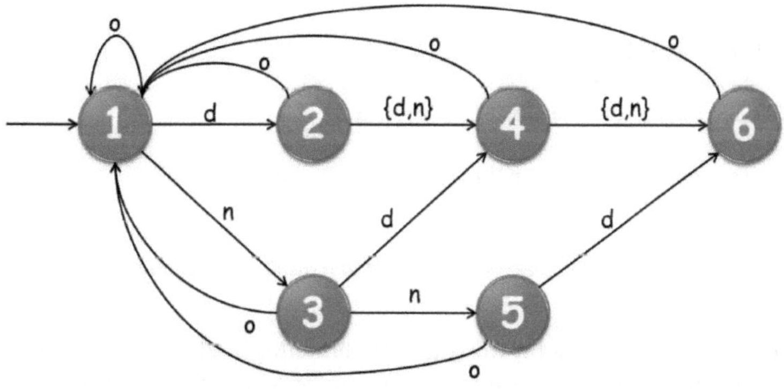

Fig. 1. DFA illustrating the shift nurses

Then, for instance to model the regular constraint in MiniZinc [4], which is a well-known CP language, it is necessary the portion of code depicted in Figure 2. The predicate representing the regular constraint is called `regular` and it is stated at the end. This constraint ensures that the sequence of values in the `roster` array is accepted by a given DFA, where `Q` is the number of states,

`1..S` corresponds to the DFA input, the array `t` defines the transitions of the DFA, `q0` is the initial state, and `STATES` represents the accepting states.

Table 1. Transition table for DFA

	D	N	O
1	2	3	1
2	4	4	1
3	4	5	1
4	6	6	1
5	6	0	1
6	0	0	1

```
int: num_days;
set of int: DAYS = 1..num_days;
...
int: S = 3;
int: Q = 6;
int: q0 = 1;
set of int: STATES = 1..Q;
...
array[STATES,SHIFTS] of int: t =
[| 2, 3, 1 % state 1
 | 4, 4, 1 % state 2
 | 4, 5, 1 % state 3
 | 6, 6, 1 % state 4
 | 6, 0, 1 % state 5
 | 0, 0, 1|]; % state 6
array[NURSES,DAYS] of var SHIFTS: roster;
...
regular( [roster[i,j] | j in DAYS], Q, S, t, q0, STATES)
```

Fig. 2. Using the regular constraint in MiniZinc

Hence, the idea is to facilitate the user modeling task by providing a simple tool that automatically generates the solver code from the DFA. The tool is called IGMRC, which corresponds to the Spanish acronym for graphical user interface for modeling regular constraints. The tool allows to easily translate DFAs to four solvers (Eclipse, Gecode, Google CP Solver, and MiniZinc) as well as for LaTeX. A screenshot of the tool is depicted in Figure 3.

3 Conclusion

In this paper, we have presented a simple GUI for the easy modeling of regular constraints. We have illustrated its application through a well-known rostering problem. A continue research direction in CP is about facilitating the user modeling tasks, for instance to propose expressive modeling languages [4,7], new modeling techniques [2], and/or new modeling components [6,5,3].

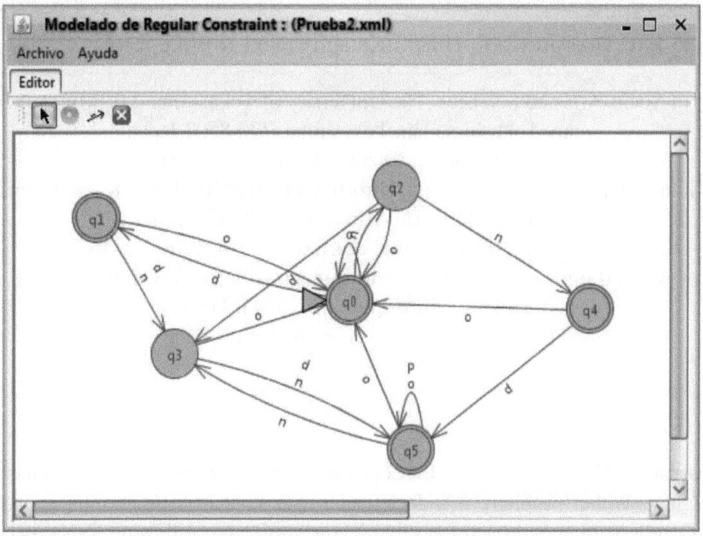

Fig. 3. A screeshot of the IGMRC Tool

References

1. IGMRC Proyect, `http://igmrc.diegoriquelme.cl/` (visited April 2013).
2. Chenouard, R., Granvilliers, L., Soto, R.: Model-Driven Constraint Programming. In: Proceedings of the 10th International ACM SIGPLAN Conference on Principles and Practice of Declarative Programming (PPDP), pp. 236–246 (2008)
3. Chenouard, R., Granvilliers, L., Soto, R.: High-Level Modeling of Component-Based CSPs. In: da Rocha Costa, A.C., Vicari, R.M., Tonidandel, F. (eds.) SBIA 2010. LNCS, vol. 6404, pp. 233–242. Springer, Heidelberg (2010)
4. Nethercote, N., Stuckey, P.J., Becket, R., Brand, S., Duck, G.J., Tack, G.: MiniZinc: Towards A Standard CP Modelling Language. In: Bessière, C. (ed.) CP 2007. LNCS, vol. 4741, pp. 529–543. Springer, Heidelberg (2007)
5. Soto, R.: Controlling search in constrained-object models. In: Kuri-Morales, A., Simari, G.R. (eds.) IBERAMIA 2010. LNCS, vol. 6433, pp. 582–591. Springer, Heidelberg (2010)
6. Soto, R., Crawford, B., Monfroy, E., Paredes, F.: Syntax Extensions for a Constrained-Object Language via Dynamic Parser Cooperation. Studies in Informatics and Control 21(1), 41–48 (2012)
7. Soto, R., Granvilliers, L.: The Design of COMMA: An Extensible Framework for Mapping Constrained Objects to Native Solver Models. In: Proceedings of the 19th IEEE International Conference on Tools with Artificial Intelligence (ICTAI), pp. 243–250 (2007)

An Interactive Approach with Four Criteria for Stochastic Weighted Weber Problems

Takeshi Uno[1], Hideki Katagiri[2], and Kosuke Kato[3]

[1] Institute of Socio-Arts and Sciences, The University of Tokushima, 1-1, Minamijosanjima-cho, Tokushima-shi, Tokushima, 770-8502 Japan
uno.takeshi@tokushima-u.ac.jp
[2] Graduate School of Engineering, Hiroshima University, 1-4-1, Kagamiyama, Higashihiroshima-shi, Hiroshima, 739-8527, Japan
katagiri-h@hiroshima-u.ac.jp
[3] Faculty of Applied Information Science, Hiroshima Institute of Technology, 2-1-1, Miyake, Saeki-ku, Hiroshima, 731-5193, Japan
k.katoh.me@it-hiroshima.ac.jp

Abstract. This paper considers an optimal location problem, called stochastic weighted Weber problem. It is formulated to a stochastic programming problem, and common approach for solving is to utilize the following four criteria: expectation of its objective function value, its variance, achievement probability for a given goal value by the decision-maker, and its fractile. It can be reformulated to a deterministic programming problem, if the locater can give her/his criterion in the above criteria or their highbred type. However, it is often hard to decide her/his criterion. This paper proposes to consider all the four criteria simultaneously. Then, it can be reformulated to four-objective deterministic programming problem, whose objective functions are corresponded to the above four criteria. Since multiobjective programming problems generally have too many Pareto optimal solution, this paper proposes an interactive solution approach for finding a satisficing location for her/him among the set of Pareto optimal solutions.

Keywords: Weber problem, stochastic programming, multiobjective programming, interactive approach, satisficing solution.

1 Introduction

Weber problem is an optimal location problem, which is to find a facility location for minimizing the sum of distances from all considering points. If the points have weights, the Weber problem is extended to a weighted Weber problem, to minimize the sum of weighted distances. Real world examples of Weber problem are to locate delivery center, fire station, and so on. Weber problems and their weighted version have been considered by many researches, and its recent studies are published by Pilotta and Torres [1], Canbolat and Wesolowsky [2], and so on.

C. Stephanidis (Ed.): Posters, Part I, HCII 2013, CCIS 373, pp. 664–668, 2013.

In this paper, we extend a weighted Weber problem to the problem with stochastic weights. We show a significance of extension by using the above first example, to locate delivery center. For this example, weights on points represent demands to deliver some goods to shops, store, and so on. An objective of locating delivery centers is to deliver efficiently, and then we can regard the objective as to minimize the sum of distances to addresses for delivery. Hence the location problem can be regarded to an ordinary Weber problem if the demands of delivery can be estimated accurately. However, since it is usually hard to estimate it, we suggest to representing the weights as stochastic variables. We call it stochastic weighted Weber problem.

For consider the extended Weber problem mathematically, we formulate it to a stochastic programming problem. A common approach for solving stochastic programming problems is to utilize the following four criteria: (i) expectation of its objective function value, (ii) its variance, (iii) achievement probability for a given goal value by the decision-maker, and (iv) its fractile. For the details of stochastic programming, the reader can refer to the book of Kall and Wallace [3]. Then, it can be reformulated to a deterministic programming problem, if the locater can give her/his criterion in the above criteria or their highbred type. However, it is often hard to decide her/his criterion.

In this paper, we propose to consider all the four criteria simultaneously. Then, it can be reformulated to four-objective deterministic programming problem, whose objective functions are corresponded to the above four criteria. Since multiobjective programming problems generally have too many Pareto optimal solution, this paper proposes an interactive solution approach, original idea is proposed by Nakayama [4], for finding a satisficing location for her/him among the set of Pareto optimal solutions.

2 Formulation of Stochastic Weighted Weber Problem

In this paper, we consider facility location on space R, e.g. plain and line segment, including m points. For i-th point, $i = 1,2,\dots,m$ its site and weight are given by $v_i \in R$ and $\overline{w}_i$, respectively. In this study, we represent $\overline{w}_1, \overline{w}_2, \dots, \overline{w}_m$ as stochastic variables. Let $\boldsymbol{v} = (v_i, v_i, \dots, v_i)$

There are n facilities locating on R, whose sites are denoted by $x_1, x_2, \dots, x_n \in R$. These are regarded as decision variables for the formulated stochastic weighted Weber problem, and let $\boldsymbol{x} = (x_1, x_2, \dots, x_n)$.

Next we define the distance $d(y_1, y_2)$ between any two points $y_1, y_2 \in R$, such as Euclidean distance, Manhattan distance, and so on. In this problem, we assume that the distance from facilities and any point is represented as the minimum of all distances, that is, for point $i = 1,2,\dots,m$,

$$d(\boldsymbol{x}, v_i) = \min_{j=1,2,\dots,n} d(x_j, v_i) \tag{1}$$

As the example of delivery center, it is rational to any address for delivery from its nearest facility.

Therefore, stochastic weighted Weber problem can be formulated as the following mathematical programming problem:

$$\left.\begin{array}{ll} \text{minimize} & \bar{W}(\boldsymbol{x}) = \sum_{i=1}^{m} \bar{w}_i \cdot d(\boldsymbol{x}, v_i) \\ \text{subject to} & \boldsymbol{x} = (x_1, x_2, \ldots, x_n) \in R^n \end{array}\right\} \quad (2)$$

Note that $\bar{w}_i$ is a stochastic variable for any point i, objective function of (2) is also represented as a stochastic variable. This means that (2) is a stochastic programming problem. Since objective function of (2) returns a stochastic variable, we cannot solve (2) directly. In the next section, we reformulate (2) to a deterministic multiobjective programming problem.

3 Reformulation to Multiobjective Programming Problem

First we show the following four criteria for evaluating stochastic variables.

(i) Expectation criterion: objective function of (2) is evaluated through its expectation, denote by $E(\boldsymbol{x})$. An objective of the locater is to minimize it.

(ii) Variance criterion: objective function of (2) is evaluated through its variance, denote by $V(\boldsymbol{x})$. An objective of the locater is to minimize it.

(iii) Probability criterion: objective function of (2) is evaluated through the probability that the objective function value is equal or less than a given value, denoted by W_0. We represent the probability as follows:

$$P(\boldsymbol{x}) = \Pr\left[\bar{W}(\boldsymbol{x}) \leq W_0\right] \quad (3)$$

Here Pr [·] is a probability. An objective of the locater is to maximize it.

(iv) Fractile criterion: objective function of (2) is evaluated through its fractile, which is the value that objective function achieves with more than a given probability, denoted by σ. We represent the fractile as follows:

$$F(\boldsymbol{x}) = \min\{ W_0 \mid \Pr\left[\bar{W}(\boldsymbol{x}) \leq W_0\right] \geq \sigma \} \quad (4)$$

An objective of the locater is to minimize it.

By considering the above four criteria simultaneously, we can reformulate (2) to the following four-objective deterministic programming problem:

$$\left.\begin{array}{ll} \text{minimize} & E(\boldsymbol{x}) \\ \text{minimize} & V(\boldsymbol{x}) \\ \text{maximize} & P(\boldsymbol{x}) \\ \text{minimize} & F(\boldsymbol{x}) \\ \text{subject to} & \boldsymbol{x} = (x_1, x_2, \dots, x_n) \in R^n \end{array}\right\} \quad (5)$$

4 Interactive Solution Method

First we introduce the definition of Pareto optimal solution for (4).

Pareto optimal solution: $\boldsymbol{x}$ is called a Pareto optimal solution if $\boldsymbol{x}$ holds the following condition: "If another solution is superior to $\boldsymbol{x}$ for one of four objective functions of (4), it is inferior to $\boldsymbol{x}$ for another objective function."

Since multiobjective programming problems generally have too many Pareto optimal solutions, we propose an interactive solution approach for finding a satisficing location for her/him among the set of Pareto optimal solutions, based on the satisficing trade-off method that was originally proposed by Nakayama [4].

Suppose that the locater gives her/his aspiration levels for objective functions as $\hat{E}$, $\hat{V}$, $\hat{P}$, and $\hat{F}$, respectively. Then, the Pareto optimal solution which is the nearest to the aspiration level vector is found by solving the following problem:

$$\left.\begin{array}{ll} \text{minimize} & \max\left\{\dfrac{E(\boldsymbol{x})-\hat{E}}{E^{nad}-E^{ide}}, \dfrac{V(\boldsymbol{x})-\hat{V}}{V^{nad}-V^{ide}}, \dfrac{\hat{P}-P(\boldsymbol{x})}{P^{ide}-P^{nad}}, \dfrac{F(\boldsymbol{x})-\hat{F}}{F^{nad}-F^{ide}}\right\} \\ \text{subject to} & \boldsymbol{x} = (x_1, x_2, \dots, x_n) \in R^n \end{array}\right\} \quad (6)$$

Here, $E^{nad}, V^{nad}, P^{nad}, F^{nad}$ are nadir values for corresponding objective function, and $E^{ide}, V^{ide}, P^{ide}, F^{ide}$ are their ideal values. These values can be calculated as follows:

$$E^{ide} \le E(\boldsymbol{x}^E), V^{ide} \le V(\boldsymbol{x}^V), P^{ide} \ge P(\boldsymbol{x}^P), F^{ide} \le V(\boldsymbol{x}^F), \quad (7)$$

$$E^{nad} = \max\{E(\boldsymbol{x}^V), E(\boldsymbol{x}^P), E(\boldsymbol{x}^F)\}, V^{nad} = \max\{V(\boldsymbol{x}^E), V(\boldsymbol{x}^P), V(\boldsymbol{x}^F)\}, \quad (8)$$

$$P^{nad} = \min\{P(\boldsymbol{x}^E), P(\boldsymbol{x}^V), P(\boldsymbol{x}^F)\}, F^{nad} = \max\{F(\boldsymbol{x}^F), F(\boldsymbol{x}^V), F(\boldsymbol{x}^P)\}, \quad (9)$$

where, $\boldsymbol{x}^E$ and $\boldsymbol{x}^V$ be the minimizer of Ex $[\overline{W}(\boldsymbol{x})]$ and Va $[\overline{W}(\boldsymbol{x})]$, respectively, $\boldsymbol{x}^P$ the maximizer of $\Pr[\overline{W}(\boldsymbol{x}) \le W_0]$, and $\boldsymbol{x}^F$ the minimizer of F.

Moreover, we introduce four parameters δ^E, δ^V, δ^P, and δ^F in (5). Then, we consider the following problem:

$$\left.\begin{array}{ll}\text{minimize} & \gamma+\rho\cdot S(\boldsymbol{x}) \\ \text{subject to} & \dfrac{E(\boldsymbol{x})-\hat{E}}{E^{nad}-E^{ide}}\leq\delta^{E}\gamma \\ & \dfrac{V(\boldsymbol{x})-\hat{V}}{V^{nad}-V^{ide}}\leq\delta^{V}\gamma \\ & \dfrac{\hat{P}-P(\boldsymbol{x})}{P^{ide}-P^{nad}}\leq\delta^{P}\gamma \\ & \dfrac{F(\boldsymbol{x})-\hat{F}}{F^{nad}-F^{ide}}\leq\delta^{F}\gamma \\ & \boldsymbol{x}=(x_1,x_2,\ldots,x_n)\in R^n\end{array}\right\} \tag{10}$$

Here, ρ is a sufficiently small positive number, say 10^{-6}, and $S(\boldsymbol{x})$ is the sum of four fractions in the left side of constraints. By updating the above eight parameters and solve (9), we can find a satisficing solution of the locater in set of Pareto optimal solutions.

Therefore, our proposing interactive solution method is described as follows:

4.1 Algorithm: Interactive Solution Method

Step 1. Calculate nadir values $E^{nad}, V^{nad}, P^{nad}, F^{nad}$, and give ideal values $E^{ide}, V^{ide}, P^{ide}, F^{ide}$.

Step 2. Set initial values for parameters $\hat{E}$, $\hat{V}$, $\hat{P}$, $\hat{F}$, δ^E, δ^V, δ^P, and δ^F.

Step 3. For the current values of parameters, solve (9).

Step 4. The DM is supplied with the corresponding Pareto optimal solution. If she/he is satisfied with the current location, then the algorithm is terminated. Otherwise, ask the DM to update the parameters $\hat{E}$, $\hat{V}$, $\hat{P}$, $\hat{F}$, δ^E, δ^V, δ^P, and δ^F. Return to Step 3.

References

1. Pilotta, E.A., Torres, G.A.: A Projected Weiszfeld Algorithm for the Box-Constrained Weber Location Problem. Applied Mathematics and Computation 218, 2932–2943 (2011)
2. Canbolat, M.S., Wesolowsky, G.O.: On the Use of the Varignon Frame for Single Facility Weber Problems in the Presence of Convex Barriers. European Journal of Operational Research 217, 241–247 (2012)
3. Kall, P., Wallace, S.W.: Stochastic Programming. Wiley, New Jersey (1994)
4. Nakayama, H.: Aspiration Level Approach to Interactive Multi-Objective Programming and its Applications. In: Pardalos, P.M., Siskos, Y., Zopounidis, C. (eds.) Advances in Multicriteria Analysis, pp. 147–174. Kluwer, Dordrecht (1995)

Quality Performance Monitor: A Server Performance Visualization Tool

Ziyuan Zhang[1] and Haoran Guo[2]

[1] Peking University, School of Software and Microelectronics, China
zhangziyuan@pku.edu.cn
[2] Nanyang Technological University, Wee Kim Wee School of Communication and Information, Singapore
hguo004@e.ntu.edu.sg

Abstract. Thousands of companies have deployed servers and it is necessary to measure, analyze and evaluate the performance of the servers through performance test. Generally, we mainly analyze performance data by drawing different performance charts. First, performance test is time-consuming, including calculating and drawing chart. And it is difficult to combine new performance data with history performance data to draw chart for analysis. Besides, various mistakes may be made by analyzing huge amount of performance data. Another challenge is to support performance test of every new projects and collaborative work in different teams like QA, Development and DBA in the companies. This paper presents a web-based tool called Quality Performance Monitor (QPM) for server performance monitor, supporting visualization of performance test, and demonstrates its superiority to traditional performance test.

Keywords: Performance test, Visualization, Functional Design, Data Analysis.

1 Introduction

The goal of performance test now is concrete and extraordinary quality analysis tools to improve the quality of the software rather than simply develop basic research prototypes [1]. Data visualization has lagged its sister disciplines including the automated extraction of information from feature models [2].

And usability of web-based tool now is lack of understanding about how users search for information. For functional testing, a test suite [3] and automated test data generator [4-5] that can detect fault in analysis are presented.

2 The Approach to the Research

2.1 Layout and Functional Design

Annotated line chart part (Figure 1):

C. Stephanidis (Ed.): Posters, Part I, HCII 2013, CCIS 373, pp. 669–672, 2013.

- "Annotated line chart" displays the lines of default attributes (the most important attributes).
- "Group drop list" lists group list.
- "Compare drop list" lists all the sever names of specified group.
- "Attribute drop list" lists all the attributes of specified group.
- Click "Refresh" button to display chosen data in annotated line chart.

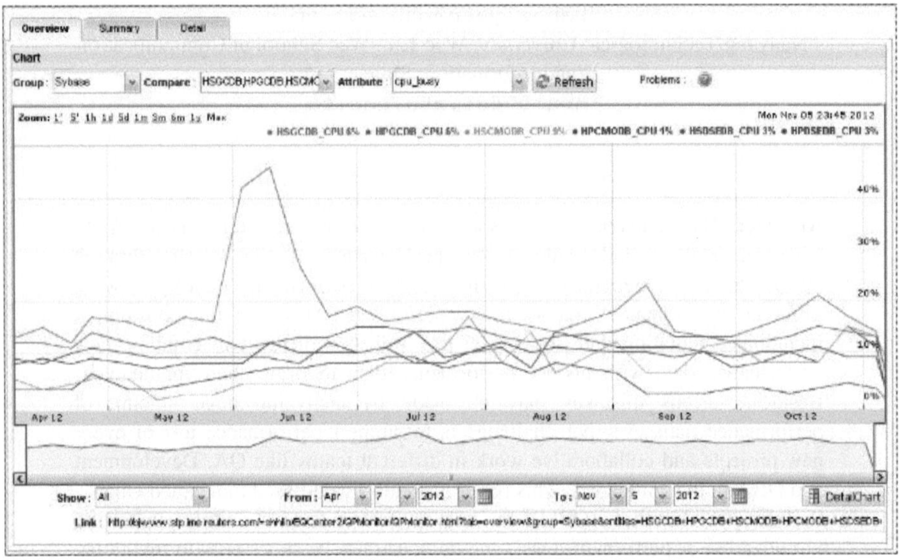

Fig. 1. Quality Performance Monitor

2.2 Working Principle

We mainly used SmartGWT and annotated time chart of GWT Visualization to develop web page component and chart component respectively as front end. And we used Perl, CGI to develop scripts and JSON formatted configuration files and related tables as back end (Figure 2).

2.3 Script to Fetch and Parse Log

The script will firstly read the configuration file to load setting information. Then it will automatically connect to log server and download logs to local server. Then script will read log line by line to check if it matches one of the regular expression statements. After finishing fetching data of each loop, it will write performance data to BCP file. It is easy to use the BCP data either by excel or import into database.

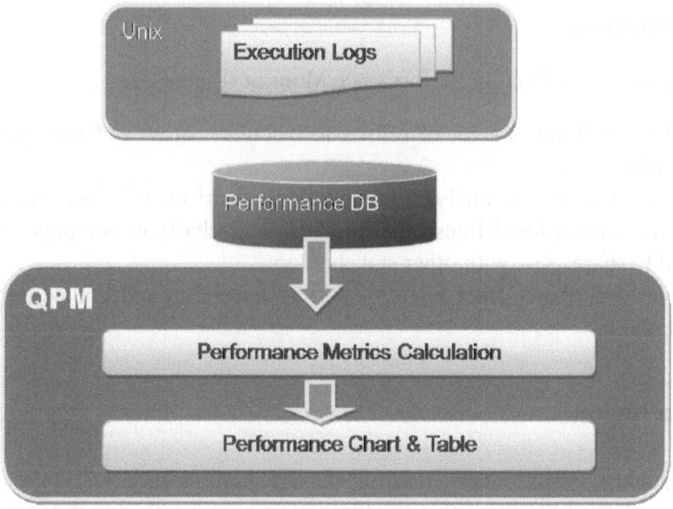

Fig. 2. Working Principle of Quality Performance Monitor

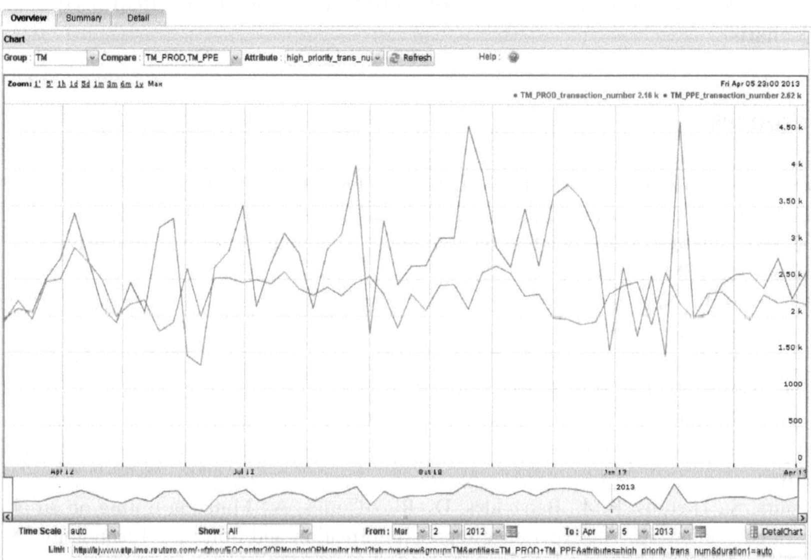

Fig. 3. Comparison of Transactions

2.4 Data Filter

There may be dirty or not complete record because of exception or error. And after we get the performance data, we will run an exception checking script to remove the record and summarize error information in error log. This will also assist us to find and examine the reason of error.

2.5 Key Features

The key features of the Quality Performance Monitor (Figure 3).

- Effort released: it saves a lot of efforts to calculate, draw and tack performance data manually.
- Easy to use: it is easy to analyze, compare and share view by user friendly web-based charts with colored lines, multiple attributes charts in one page and link to view used to share view with other stakeholders.
- Extendable: it supports other kinds of performance data and update performance data by daily.

3 Conclusion

We used Quality Performance Monitor in one performance test to explore the usability of tool. And we show that the there is an obvious change in the cost saving including time and headcount. Within TM performance test, only one tester completed 14 rounds of tests on 2 servers (10h per round) rather than used 2 tables and 5 charts.

References

1. Segura, S., Galindo, J.A., Benavides, D., Parejo, J.A., Ruiz-Cortés, A.: BeTTy: benchmarking and testing on the automated analysis of feature models. In: Proceedings of the Sixth International Workshop on Variability Modeling of Software-Intensive Systems, pp. 63–71. ACM (2012)
2. Benavides, D., Segura, S., Ruiz-Cortés, A.: Automated analysis of feature models 20 years later: A literature review. Information Systems 35(6), 615–636 (2010)
3. Segura, S., Benavides, D., Ruiz-Cortés, A.: Functional testing of feature model analysis tools: a test suite. IET Software 5(1), 70–82 (2011)
4. Segura, S., Hierons, R.M., Benavides, D., Ruiz-Cortés, A.: Automated metamorphic testing on the analyses of feature models. Information and Software Technology 53(3), 245–258 (2011)
5. Segura, S., Hierons, R.M., Benavides, D., Ruiz-Cortés, A.: Mutation testing on an object-oriented framework: An experience report. Information and Software Technology 53(10), 1124–1136 (2011)

Part X
Product Design, Marketing and Advertisment

Gesture-Based Human-Machine Interface: A Case Study Comparing the Realism of Furniture Products in E-Commerce

Kuen-Meau Chen*

Department of Industrial Design, National United University,
1 Lien Da, Kung-Ching Li, Maioli 36003, Taiwan
kmchen0721@gmail.com

Abstract. This paper presents a gesture-based augmented reality system, which enables users to adjust the size, coordinates, rotation angles, and other parameters via hand gestures. The proposed approach significantly enhances accuracy in identifying hand gestures and labels. To assess the accuracy of product representation, we compared the presentation of products in the forms of internet pictures (IP), augmented reality (AR), full-sized augmented reality (FSAR), and physical product (PP) demonstration. It was found that, in the example of furniture evaluation, augmented reality provided more three-dimensional information than internet pictures; however, internet pictures proved superior in terms of ease of operation and manufacturing. Despite 3D rendering integrated within a real-world environment, augmented reality failed to match the demonstration of physical products with regard to the accuracy of representation.

Keywords: Interactive Design, Form Perception, Realism, Gesture Recognition, Augmented Reality.

1 Introduction

Advances in computer technology have gradually shifted business models from traditional shopping malls to internet platforms. The main difference lies in the presentation of products, which has changed from physical to virtual. The demonstration of physical products enables consumers to feel the size, scale, texture, design, and color, while actually performing product functions and experiencing the sense of comfort provided by the product. Nonetheless, this kind of demonstration requires considerable floor space, which results in high rental costs. Virtual products can be presented using 2D digital images and 3D digital models, which dramatically reduces interaction with the products through vision and touch, while all but eliminating interaction with the physical environment. The internet precludes anything more than a cursory degree of interaction between products and consumers, which prevents consumers from experiencing product features and operations. In addition, the accuracy of product representation depends heavily on the actual size of products and their integration

* Corresponding author.

C. Stephanidis (Ed.): Posters, Part I, HCII 2013, CCIS 373, pp. 675–679, 2013.

with the environment.This study built a gesture-based augmented reality system, in which users control virtual images by moving their fingers. Model parameters, such as size, coordinates, and rotation angle are adjusted by triggering virtual buttons using hand gestures. This approach enhanced the accuracy of identifying hand gestures and labels. We then applied the proposed system to the representation of furniture in order to compare the accuracy with other rendering schemes. Our results revealed the accuracy representing products on printed images, in augmented reality and full-sized augmented reality as well as with physical products.

2 Literature Review

Augmented reality uses labels to enable interaction with users. For example, FingARtips uses the interaction between labels to enable the control of virtual models within a scene [1]. Many researchers have developed gesture-based augmented reality systems, which are fully interactive [1-3]. Augmented reality has attracted considerable attention because it dramatically changes the operating environment in which users function. Interacting with objects in a virtual PC environment has shifted toward augmented reality, in which users exist within an interactive space and any information absent from the environment can be provided by augmented reality. E-commerce applications have shifted from 2D interfaces to virtual reality for the presentation of products and user input [4]. E-commerce websites based on augmented reality provide more detailed information than 2D interfaces and frees users from the need to formulate how an object actually appears in 3D from a 2D image. Augmented reality allows allowing users to interact with objects intuitively through rotation and zooming and provides a shopping experience closer to physical reality. Smartphones are now ubiquitous and mobile e-commerce services are booming [5]. With the gradual maturing of the internet shopping as a business model, efficiency in the presentation of products is becoming increasingly important.

3 Research Methods

This paper compared the presentation of products on internet platforms in a variety of forms, including printed images, augmented reality, full-sized augmented reality, and physical demonstrations. Two modes were established for comparison: interactive operations and the accuracy of product representation. This study established an interactive environment based on augmented reality for the assessment of virtual products with regard to performance in satisfying user needs. Task analysis was conducted to identify the tasks that users must complete and a model interface was designed according to these results. The model was then tested on users to finalize the operating modes for this study. The virtual model in this paper included all possible operating modes within an environment based on augmented reality. Every possible interaction with the virtual objects was also evaluated, including the selection of models, zooming in/out models, rotating models (X/Y/Z axes), moving models (X/Y/Z axes), and zooming in/out views (Fig.1).

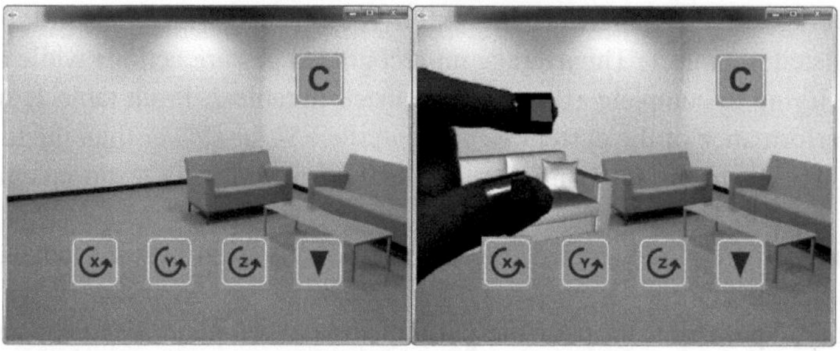

Fig. 1. Operation of Augmented Reality and Adding Model in the environment

This study conducted interviews with experts to reveal the major factors that influence the representation of products, including shape, overall presentation. Experiments on the shape and overall effect were conducted to help users understand the difference between each model's realism.

4 Results and Discussion

Before the experiment, each participant was given a tutorial on how to use the PinchAR system. Most of the participants were able to memorize the gesture set in few seconds and familiarize themselves with the gesture interface and AR system within 20 minutes. The collected experiment data is shown in Table 1 and Table 2.

Table 1. Average completing time for 10 repeated actions

	Click	Double click	Drag
Gesture	28.8 sec	42.35	102.16 sec
Touch panel	6.08 sec	7.63 sec	15.8 sec

Table 2. Average errors for 10 repeated actions

	Click	Double click	Drag
Gesture	4	3.9	2.8
Touch panel	0	0.2	1.6

Table 3. Recognition rate

	Click	Double click	Drag
Gesture	71.43%	71.94%	78.13%

The average time required to successfully complete 10 recognized designate actions are listed in table 1. The average un-recognized gesture actions while the participants are trying to complete 10 actions are listed in table 2. From table 1, we can see that the performance of the current gesture interface is far slower than the touch panel interface. To obtain the recognition rate, we used formula (1) to do calculation and listed the result in Table 3.

Recognition rate = recognized action times / recognized action times + unrecognized action time (1)

After the experiment, most of the participants do complain about the recognition rate of the gesture action and the slow tempo of the gesture that can be recognized by the system. However, they all agree that the gesture set we proposed is easy to be memorized and easy to use. Most of the participants are excited when they are being able to manipulate the virtual model in an AR environment. This new experience slightly alleviate the longer control time feeling for every single action. This might be because that the participant did not need to repeat the same action for large amount of times.

Table 4. Multi-comparison of significances of shape attribute

Dependent Variable	(I) type	(J) type	Mean Difference	Std.	Sig.
Shape attribute	IP	AR	.4417	.119	.001 (*)
	AR	FSAR	-.5048	.121	.000 (*)
	FSAR	IP	0.063	.119	.857

* $p<0.05$; internet pictures (IP), augmented reality (AR), full-sized augmented reality (FSAR)

Table 5. Multi-comparison of significances of overall effect attribute

Dependent Variable	(I) type	(J) type	Mean Difference	Std.	Sig.
Overall effect attribute	IP	AR	.5335	.132	.000 (*)
	AR	FSAR	-.2649	.135	.120
	FSAR	IP	-.2687	.132	.105

* $p<0.05$; internet pictures (IP), augmented reality (AR), full-sized augmented reality (FSAR)

Our results revealed considerable differences between internet pictures and reduced-size augmented reality with regard to product shape. The difference between reduced-size and full-size augmented reality was also significant. A significant difference was observed between internet pictures and reduced-size augmented reality with regard to form attribute and overall representation, as shown in Table 4,5. Initial analysis demonstrated that despite the reduced scale of internet pictures, they were still superior to reduced-size augmented reality in the evaluation and selection of furniture.

Internet pictures also outpaced the models with regard to ease of operation and manufacturing. Augmented reality can provide 3D representations integrated within the physical environment. If full-size augmented reality could provide a better effect than internet pictures, the technology could play a key role in ensuring the accuracy of product representation because it can demonstrate products on e-commerce platforms in full size. However, the demonstration of physical products still provides product representation with accuracy outpacing that of full-sized augmented reality.

5 Conclusion

This paper proposes a gesture-based interface based on the ARTookKits augmented reality system, in conjunction with a graphic interface for manipulating virtual objects in the environment. The design of the interface prevented the hands of users from covering labels during interaction, which significantly enhanced the usability and performance of the model. In the future, more instinctive operations based on the interaction between labels and the virtual model could be devised to further increase operational convenience and realism of the product. Nonetheless, the presentation of objects in full size will still have a considerable impact on the accuracy of product representation.

Acknowledgements. This study is supported by National Science Counsel, Taiwan, with project number NSC-100-2410-H-239-013-MY2.

References

1. Buchmann, V., Violich, S., Billinghurst, M., Cockburn, A.: FingARtips: gesture based direct manipulation in Augmented Reality. In: Proceedings of the 2nd International Conference on Computer Graphics and Interactive Techniques, pp. 212–221. ACM, New York (2004)
2. Lee, B.-J., Park, J.-S., Sung, M.Y.: Vision-Based Real-Time Camera Matchmoving with a Known Marker. In: Harper, R., Rauterberg, M., Combetto, M. (eds.) ICEC 2006. LNCS, vol. 4161, pp. 193–204. Springer, Heidelberg (2006)
3. Storring, M., Moeslund, T.B., Liu, Y., Granum, E.: Computer Vision-based Gesture Recognition for an Augmented Reality Interface. In: 4th IASTED International Conference on Visualization, Imaging, and Image Processing, Marbella, Spain, pp. 766–771 (2004)
4. Chittaro, L., Ranon, R.: Adding Adaptive Features to Virtual Reality Interfaces for E-Commerce. In: Brusilovsky, P., Stock, O., Strapparava, C. (eds.) AH 2000. LNCS, vol. 1892, pp. 86–97. Springer, Heidelberg (2000)
5. Lee, Y.E., Benbasat, I.: Interface Design for Mobile Commerce. Communications of the ACM 46(12), 48–52 (2003)

Designing a Service Innovation Measurement of SMEs

Yen-Hao Hsieh

Tamkang University, New Taipei City, Taiwan
yhhsiehs@mail.tku.edu.tw

Abstract. Enterprises have to increase their competency and ability to respond to the market variation and customer needs. Maintaining long term sustainability for enterprises has been an important topic, especially for traditional manufacturing businesses. With the attention of service around the world, many manufacturing enterprises gradually transform the product-driven business into the service-driven business. Service innovation is an important notion for manufacturing enterprises to apply. Developing a successful process of service innovation is an important event for enterprises. However, although there have been a lot of studies emphasizing the importance of service innovation, there is less research focusing on measuring service innovation. It is difficult for enterprises to systematically measure the effects and performances because different levels of enterprises have diverse choices of the service innovation categories. Consequently, this study is to analyze and define the critical factors of service innovation and build a systematical and quantitative service innovation measurement model by adopting system thinking.

Keywords: Design, service innovation, system thinking, SMEs.

1 Introduction

The service industry has been paid attention to by the governments in the world. The service industry in the Organization for Economic Cooperation and Development (OECD) countries performs main economic activities and generates high percentage of GDP. Accordingly, many large-scale enterprises transform the manufacturing orientation business to the service orientation business. These enterprises propose novel service concepts and define new value provision to customers based on service-dominant logic [7]. Customers can have unique experiences and gather specific values when they perceive delivered services from the new "service" enterprises.

In order to increase the core competence and business advantage, enterprises have to understand the importance and impact of "services" and also adopt "service concept and provision" as business strategies. Consequently, service innovation should be a critical way for enterprises to become a service companies and perform service activities [11], especially for the manufacturing enterprises. Service innovation is to leads enterprises to adopt innovative idea in the processes of service design, service marketing, service management and service delivery for the novel values co-creation with customers.

C. Stephanidis (Ed.): Posters, Part I, HCII 2013, CCIS 373, pp. 680–684, 2013.

Small and medium enterprises (SMEs) are the core businesses in many developed countries, although the large-scale enterprises lead and dominate the market trend. SMEs focus on the traditional manufacturing businesses that still play an essential role to have significant effects on the economic profits. However, SMEs face much more difficulties than large-scale enterprises to transform the manufacturing orientation business to the service orientation business. This study plans to conduct small and medium enterprises as examples to demonstrate the feasibility of the service innovation measurement model. The objective of this study is to investigate the key factors which could influence the success of SMEs to implement service innovation. We can apply the service innovation measurement model into potential SMEs for creating values during managing the service innovation process.

2 Service Innovation

Innovation has been an important concept for enterprises to design and create innovative products or services. Within the service-dominant logic, innovation in service sectors becomes a broad and essential topic for academic and practical fields gradually. Service innovation research composed many perspectives and aspects. Several important topics of service innovation include service innovation management [10], service innovation implementation [6], customer involvement [12], new service development [9] and service performance [8].

Service innovation can be considered as a catalytic element to create novel services and shape new markets for manufacturing enterprises to co-create values with customers. However, service innovation is also a complex and evolutionary process which is interactive, local, unpredictable and emergent [2]. Not only service sectors but also manufacturing businesses have to focus on how to adopt service innovation to increase their competitive advantages [3]. Finding the key factors of successful service innovation is a critical issue for enterprises to increase service performances [3, 4].

3 Method

3.1 System Thinking

System thinking is an appropriate approach to investigate the problems of real phenomena and advance the capability of dealing with problems [5, 13]. Besides, system thinking is to use the "macro" viewpoint to examine the casual relationships and performances among many variables of a system. System thinking provides a helpful approach to understand the structure responsible for designing a service innovation measurement model. According to different levels of managing the process of service innovation, it is a feasible way to measure the effects of service innovation based on the notion of system thinking.

3.2 Conceptual Framework Development

There has been a lot of pioneer research discussing the management of service innovation process. A novel innovation for service enterprises should be created by a design thinking way which is composed of inspiration, ideation and implementation [1]. Besides, according to [14], there are four main phases of the innovation process including idea generating, transformation into an innovation project, development and implementation. Dörner et al. (2011) divided the process of service innovation into three steps including defining new services, developing new services and launching new services [3]. These literatures give us a clear clue to the understanding of the key phases of service innovation. This study also summarizes and defines the main phases of service innovation including service concept and value definition, service development and service implementation based on the previous research (as shown in figure 1).

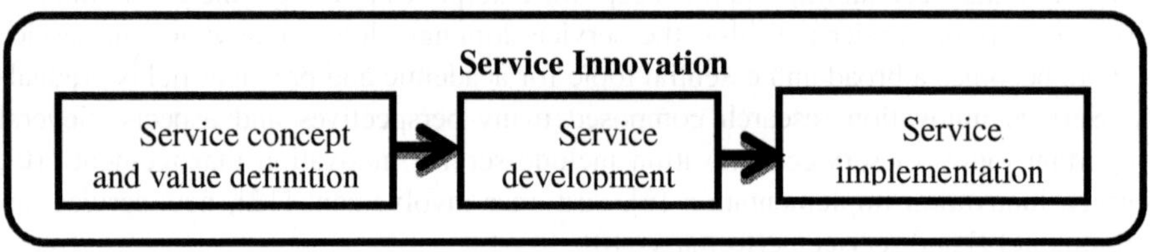

Fig. 1. The main phases of service innovation

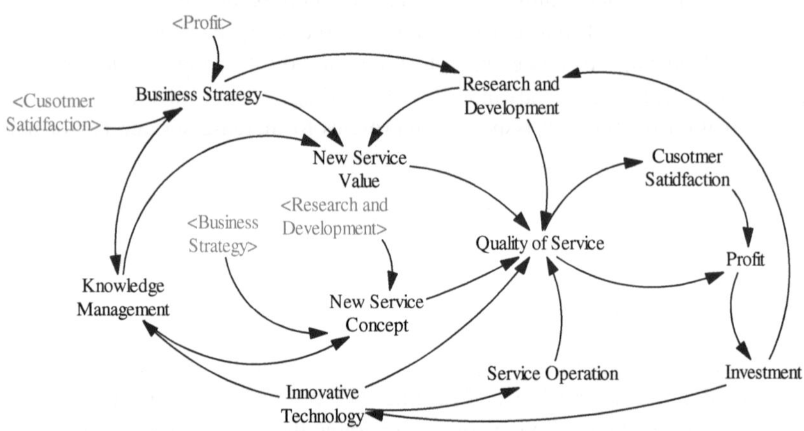

Fig. 2. The conceptual framework of service innovation

This study tries to build a conceptual framework of service innovation based on the proposed main phases by adopting the concept of system thinking (as depicted in figure 2). In the phase of service concept and value definition, new service values and new service concepts are defined as the main output. Quality of service can be considered as the evaluation indicator of service development phase which is affected by new service values and new service concepts. In the final phase, this study applies customer satisfaction and service profits to estimate service implementation which is also influenced by quality of service. Hence, figure 2 shows the causal loop diagram of service innovation. Business strategies, knowledge management and research and development of the SMEs can directly influence the numbers and results of new service concepts and values. Then, the SMEs can employ innovative technology, research and development and appropriate service operations to increase quality of services in order to have high customer satisfaction and service profits. Therefore, when the SMEs can gain a lot, they can invest on research and development and innovative technology continuously. Meanwhile, high customer satisfaction and service profits can alter SMEs to select proper business strategies. Besides, business strategies also directly affect the strategies of knowledge management and research and development.

4 Conclusion

Service innovation for SMEs is a critical and complex issue which can be regarded as a complex system. There are many important factors to influence the success of service innovation. This study tries to apply system thinking to analyze the key indicators within SMEs for proposing a conceptual framework of service innovation. Further research should continuously build stock and flow diagrams to simulate and implement policies testing based on the proposed framework of the causal loop diagram.

References

1. Brown, T.: Design thinking. Harvard Business Review 86, 84–92 (2008)
2. Chae, B.: An evolutionary framework for service innovation: Insights of complexity theory for service science. International Journal of Production Economics 135, 813–822 (2012)
3. Dörner, N., Gassmann, O., Gebauer, H.: Service innovation: why is it so difficult to accomplish? Journal of Business Strategy 32(3), 37–46 (2011)
4. Droege, H., Hildebrand, D., Heras Forcada, M.A.: Innovation in services: present findings, and future pathways. Journal of Service Management 20, 131–155 (2009)
5. Forrester, J.W.: System dynamics, systems thinking, and soft OR. System Dynamics Review 10, 245–256 (1994)
6. Kindström, D., Kowalkowski, C., Sandberg, E.: Enabling service innovation - a dynamic capabilities approach. Journal of Business Research 20, 156–172 (2012)
7. Lusch, R.F., Vargo, S.L.: The service-dominant mindset. In: Hefley, B., Murphy, W. (eds.) Service Science Management and Engineering: Education for the 21st Century, pp. 89–96. Springer (2008)
8. McDermott, C.M., Prajogo, D.I.: Service innovation and performance in SMEs. International Journal of Operations & Production Management 32, 216–237 (2012)
9. Menor, L.J., Tatikonda, M.V., Sampson, S.E.: New service development: areas for exploitation and exploration. Journal of Operations Management 20, 135–157 (2002)

10. Oke, A.: Innovation types and innovation management practices in service companies. International Journal of Operations & Production Management 27, 564–587 (2007)
11. Ordanini, A., Parasuraman, A.: Service Innovation Viewed Through a Service-Dominant Logic Lens: A Conceptual Framework and Empirical Analysis. Journal of Service Research 14, 3–23 (2011)
12. Rubalcaba, L., Michel, S., Sundbo, J., Brown, S., Reynoso, J.: Shaping organizing rethinking service innovation multidimensional framework. Journal of Service Management 23, 696–715 (2012)
13. Senge, P.M.: The fifth discipline: The art and practice of the learning organization. Random House, London (1990)
14. Sundbo, J.: Management of Innovation in Services. The Service Industries Journal 17, 432–455 (1997)

Collaborative Design Support System Based on Interactive Genetic Algorithm (IGA)

Yasufumi Inoue[1], Takashi Inoue[1], and Masataka Tokumaru[2]

[1] Graduate School of Kansai University
3-3-35 Yamate-cho, Suita-shi, Osaka 564-8680, Japan
[2] Kansai University, 3-3-35 Yamate-cho, Suita-shi, Osaka 564-8680, Japan
{k863806,k008376,toku}@kansai-u.ac.jp

Abstract. In this paper, we propose a system that facilitates collaborative design by multiple users of on the basis of Interactive Evolutionary Computation (IEC). Further, we conduct numerical simulations in order to analyze the optimized performance of the proposed system. In the simulations, multiple evaluation agents with bit strings are used to evaluate the design plans, instead of real users. The simulation results confirm that the proposed system provides satisfactory optimized performance in order to create a collaborative design.

1 Introduction

Recent years have witnessed growing opportunities for collaborative work in product development processes such as design creation. In other words, there are more opportunities for argument and discussion. However, it is not easy to summarize people's opinions and to arrive at a consensus. A previous study had investigated collaborative design support systems [1]; however, such systems facilitate only one-on-one interaction between a user and the system.

In this paper, we propose a system that facilitates collaborative design by multiple users. The proposed system consists of a server and some clients, where multiple users interact through each client. Our objective is to achieve collaborative design via interactions between multiple users and the clients. The server communicates with the clients and modifies the design for each of them. We implement these novel mechanisms using Interactive Evolutionary Computation (IEC) [2]. Thus, the proposed system can create a design that reflects the opinions of all users. Moreover, it can be potentially employed in various fields as a collaborative design support system based on human computer interaction involving multiple users. Finally, we conduct numerical simulations in order to analyze the optimized performance of the proposed system.

2 Proposed System

Figure 1 shows an overview of the proposed system; specifically, it shows the situation in which a user designs running shoes using the proposed system. The

C. Stephanidis (Ed.): Posters, Part I, HCII 2013, CCIS 373, pp. 685–689, 2013.

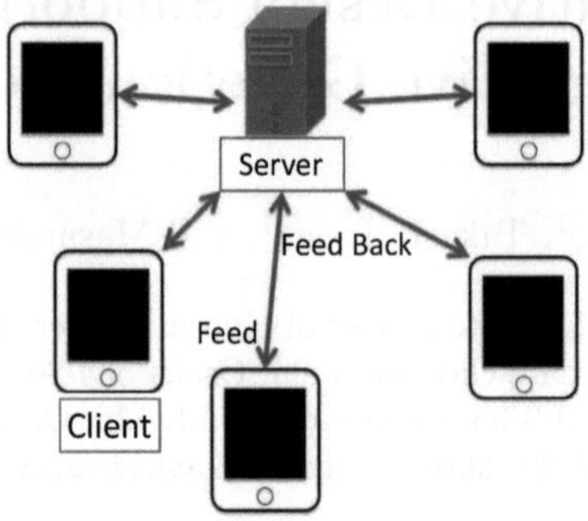

Fig. 1. Overview of the proposed system

proposed system consists of a server and some clients. Each client conducts a one-on-one interaction with each user, while the server summarizes the design plans from each client . In other words, each client creates design plans automatically and proposes them to the user. The users may evaluate the proposed design plans and sort them according to their preferences. Then, the client creates new design plans based on the users' evaluation. In other words, the users evaluate the design plans, and accordingly, the client evolves the designs using a Genetic Algorithm (GA) [3]. Then, each user feeds his/her favorite design plan to the server. The server modifies the design plans such that they reflect the opinions of all the users and feeds them back to each client.

In design creation using IEC, the system expresses a design using bit strings. In other words, the system creates various designs by changing the values of the bit strings. Therefore, such a system can be employed to process various things, such as images and sounds.

3 Design Example

In this section, we present a design example, i.e., a design running shoes. Figure 2 shows the gene coding of the running shoes design. This design consists of five parts: sole, base, toe, line, and shoelace. Further, each part has eight designs that are expressed using a 3 bit gray code. Therefore, the gene length is 15 bits. This design can generate 32,768 (= 2^{15}) patterns. The running shoes designs are generated by combining the shoe parts.

4 Simulation

4.1 Summary of Simulation

We conducted some numerical simulations in order to analyze the optimized performance of the proposed system; multiple evaluation agents with bit strings

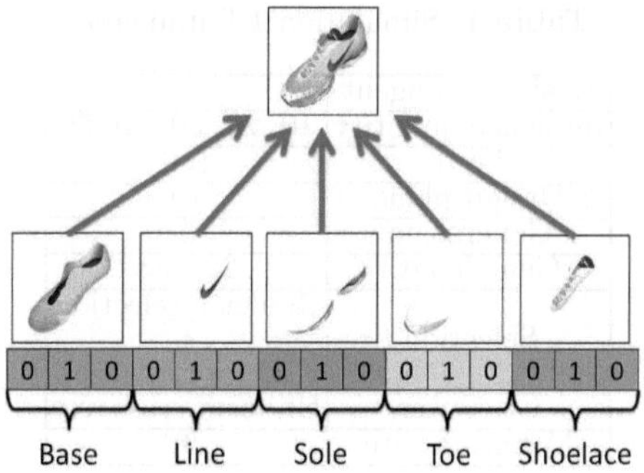

Fig. 2. Design example

were used to evaluate the design plans, instead of real users. The bit string patterns express the evaluation agents' preferences; each evaluation agent has a particular preference.

Accordingly, all evaluation agents were built such that the Hamming distance between any two evaluation agents is 40% of the bit string length. We used five evaluation agents in this simulation. An evaluation agent sorts the design plans and gives an absolute evaluation value by comparing the Hamming distance of the design plans. In other words, the absolute evaluation value expresses the design satisfaction of the evaluation agent.

Whenever each agent feeds a design plan to the sever, the server's new design plans are evaluated by all the evaluation agents. When the total of the absolute grading values from each evaluation agent is maximum, its design plan is assumed to be unanimously agreed upon. Equation (1) represents the absolute grading value fitness of each evaluation agent.

$$fitness = \frac{L - l}{L/10} \tag{1}$$

Here, L denotes the gene length of the design plans and l denotes the Hamming distance between the evaluation agent and the design plans that are evaluated. The absolute grading value of the simulation result is the average of the absolute grading values of all the evaluation agents for consensus. Moreover, each evaluation agent's highest absolute grading value is 10, and the highest average of the absolute grading values of all the evaluation agents for consensus is 7.5.

In the simulation, we analyzed the optimized performance of the design plans provided by the proposed system by varying the influence quantity from 10% to 50% (simulation 1) and the number of design plans from 2 to 10 (simulation 2). The influence quantity is a ratio that reflects the opinion of the evaluation agent.

4.2 Result of Simulation 1

Table 1 lists the parameters used in this simulation. Figure 3 shows the results of simulation 1. The results indicate that the initial convergence of the absolute

Table 1. Simulation 1 Parameters

Evaluation agent	5
Influence quantity	10, 20, 30, 40, 50
Feed	100
Design plans	10
Generation	5
Gene length	20 bits
Selection	Roulette selection + Elite preservation
Crossover	Uniform crossover
Mutation rate	1

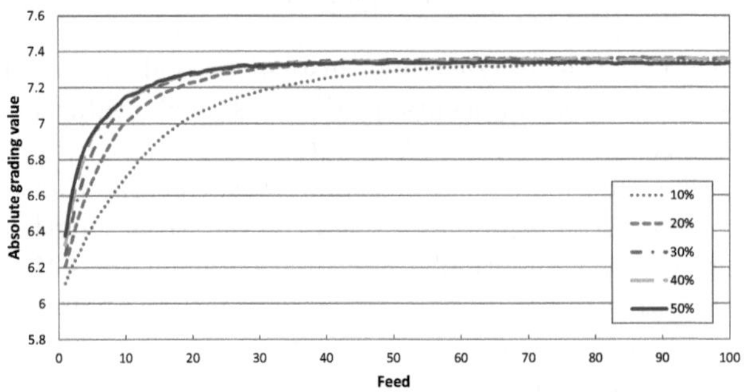

Fig. 3. Result of simulation 1

evaluation value improved as the influence quantity increased. However, the final converged absolute evaluation value degraded, even when the influence quantity was high. We assume an effective influence quantity of 30% to achieve a trade-off between the evolution performance and the initial convergence characteristics of the design plans.

4.3 Result of Simulation 2

Table 2 lists the parameters used in this simulation. Figure 4 shows the results of simulation 2. The results show the absolute evaluation value increased with the number of design plans. However, the evaluation load of real users can increase with the number of design plans. We assume an effective number of design plans for a system operated by real users to be 6.

5 Conclusion

In this paper, we proposed a system that facilitates collaborative design by multiple users, and we investigated its effectiveness via numerical simulations. The simulation results confirmed that the proposed system provides satisfactory optimized performance in order to create a collaborative design.

Table 2. Simulation 2 Parameters

Evaluation agent	5
Influence quantity	30
Feed	100
Design plans	4, 6, 8, 10
Generation	5
Gene length	20 bits
Selection	Roulette selection + Elite preservation
Crossover	Uniform crossover
Mutation rate	1

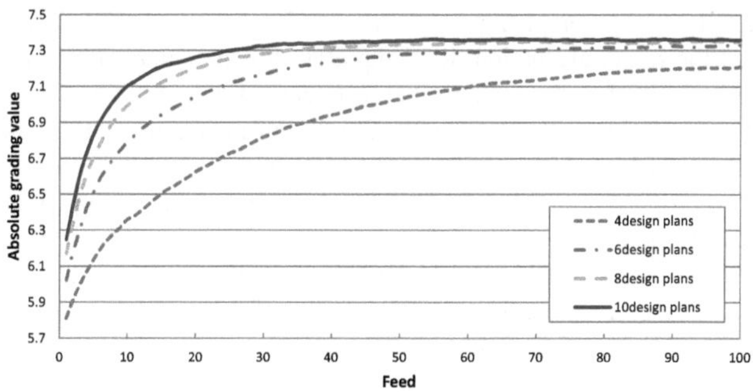

Fig. 4. Result of simulation 2

In the future, we plan to further enhance the proposed system. In addition, we plan to analyze the proposed system with real users and verify its effectiveness in real-life applications.

Acknowledgement. This work was supported by MEXT.KAKENHI (24500264).

References

1. Kubota, F., Inamori, Y., Nakano, M., Mitsuyuki, K., Yura, Y.: Navigation of Collaborative Manufacturing System Design Based on Dpio-Model. Journal of the Society of Project Management 9(6), 28–33 (2007)
2. Takenouchi, H., Tokumaru, M., Muranaka, N.: Tournament Evaluation System Considering Multiple People's Kansei Evaluation. Journal of Kansei Engineering International 9(2), 43–50 (2010)
3. Miki, M., Orita, H., Hiroyasu, T.: Design of Sign Sounds using Interactive Genetic Algorithm. In: Proc. IEEE Int. Conf. on Systems, Man, and Cybernetics, pp. 93–98 (2006)

Development of Brand Selection Model Considering Customer Service

Hiroki Kageyama, Fumiaki Saitoh, and Syohei Ishizu

Aoyama Gakuin University 5-10-1, Fuchinobe, Sagamihara City, 252-5258, Japan
kagetuncar@gmail.com, {saitoh,ishizu}@ise.aoyama.ac.jp

Abstract. In many companies, customer service becomes one of the critical factors of the brand evaluation. It is important for the companies to know the customer's utility functions about the customer service and repurchase of the products considering customer service. One of our main aims of this study is to develop brand selection model which considering utility of the customer service in order to propose promotion method for customer service of the company. In this study, we add some types of the customer services to utility in the models, and develop brand selection models. By the use of the questionnaire survey for the real companies, we confirm the adaptability of the proposed model, and we show the importance of the customer service.

Keywords: Brand selection model, customer service, customer satisfaction, maximum likelihood estimation, utility function.

1 Introduction

Companies that manufacture electronic device such as digital cameras and television provide customer service to assure customer satisfaction after purchase. Where the customer service means all activities served by the company to the customers after purchase the product, e.g. customer inquiry at call center, repairing the products etc. If the consumers are satisfied by the customer service, then customers will purchase the product of the same company again. It will be contribute to future sales of the company. It is important for the companies to know the customer's utility functions about the customer service and repurchase of the products considering customer service.

There are some studies about brand selection model which analyze to select products. Choice probability of the products was formulated by Multinomial logit model on the assumption that consumers choose brands whose utility was the highest [1]. Brand selection models evaluating the effects of the price promotion were proposed [2], [3], [4]. Brand selection models for evaluating the customer satisfaction was also proposed [5]. These studies mainly concern the price at the purchase of the products. But in the brand selection model, the utility of the customer service is not considered. Since all customers may not receive the customer service, whether the customers receive the customer service or not is a very important factor for brand selection

C. Stephanidis (Ed.): Posters, Part I, HCII 2013, CCIS 373, pp. 690–694, 2013.

model. One of our main aims of our study is to develop a brand selection model which considering utility of the customer service in order to propose a promotion method for customer service of the company. In this study, we add the customer services to utility model, and develop a brand selection model for products created by companies and customer service received by customer. By the use of the questionnaire survey for the real products, we confirm the adaptability of the proposed model, and we show the importance of the customer service.

2 Brand Selection Model

A feature of this study is that bland selection model considers after purchase utility depending to the situation whether received customer service or not. Here we develop a brand selection model using a maltinomal logit model. We then consider the utility of each brand. The following is the definition of the utility U_{it}^{n}, when consumer n selects brand i at the term t.

$$U_{it}^{n} = V_{it}^{n} + \varepsilon_{it}^{n} \tag{1}$$

Where V_{it}^{n} is the settled part of U_{it}^{n}, and ε_{it}^{n} is the probability part of U_{it}^{n}.

We assume that each ε_{ij}^{n} obeys the same double exponential independent distribution. Then, the following is the definition of the probability in which a consumer n will selects a brand i at the term t.

$$P_i^n(i) = \frac{\exp(V_{ij}^{n})}{\sum_k \exp(V_{ij}^{n})} \tag{2}$$

3 Brand Selection Model Considering Customer Service

3.1 Market Data

In order to develop a brand selection model considering customer service, we use the following market data about the digital camera. The attributes of the market data is shown in Table 1. We use the customer satisfaction data about the customer service (CS) (Copyright(C) 2011 and 2012 Nikkei BP Consulting, Inc.), and the product quality (PQ) data researched by kakaku.com. In Table 1, CS2011 means the customer satisfaction data about customer service of each company at fiscal year 2011.

PS 2011 means the customer satisfaction data about product quality of each company at fiscal year 2011. Customer satisfaction data involve the selected product numbers and repurchase intention of each company.

Table 1. Market data

Brand name	CS 2011	CS 2012	PQ 2010	PQ 2011	PQ 2012	Selected number	Repurchase intention
A	****	****	****	****	****	****	****
B	****	****	****	****	****	****	****
C	****	****	****	****	****	****	****

3.2 Model Development

In this paper we introduce 3 types of the brand selection models (Table 2). We follow the definitions (1) and (2). The difference of the models is the difference of the definitions of the settled part of utility V_{it}^{n} . First model is the following model considering reference satisfaction of product quality only and shown by the RS model in Table 2.

$$V_{it}^{n} = \alpha_i + \beta \, RS_{it}^{n} \tag{3}$$

Where RS_{it}^{n} means reference satisfaction of the product quality and is defined by equation (4).

$$RS_{it}^{n} = \sigma \, PS_{i(t-1)}^{n} + (1-\sigma) RS_{i(t-1)}^{n} \tag{4}$$

Second model is the model considering customer service and shown as CS model in Table 2.

$$V_{it}^{n} = \alpha_i + w_{it}^{n} \gamma CS_{it}^{n} \tag{5}$$

Where w_{it}^{n} is a dummy variable for customer service. If the customer n receive a customer service of brand i in the term t then w_{it}^{n} is 1, and otherwise w_{it}^{n} is 0.

We propose the following third model which considering both the product quality and customer service.

$$V_{it}^{n} = \alpha_i + \beta \, RS_{it}^{n} + \gamma * w_{it}^{n} CS_{it}^{n} \tag{6}$$

Table 2. Brand selection models

	Mode name	Definition of utility
1	2013-RS	$V_{it}^{n} = \alpha_i + \beta \, RS_{it}^{n}$
2	2013-CS	$V_{it}^{n} = \alpha_i + \gamma \, CS_{it}^{n}$
3	2013-RSCS	$V_{it}^{n} = \alpha_i + \beta \, RS_{it}^{n} + \gamma \, CS_{it}^{n}$

3.3 Estimation Method

We used the maximum likelihood estimation as the estimation method. The following equation shows the likelihood function L.

$$L=\prod_{i}^{I}\prod_{t}^{T}\prod_{n}^{N}P_t^n(i)^{y_{it}^n} \tag{7}$$

y_{it}^n is a dummy variable for representing the customer's brand selection. If a consumer n selects brand i then y_{it}^n is 1, otherwise y_{it}^n is 0.

The following is the equation for the logarithm likelihood function.

$$\ln L=\sum_{i}^{I}\sum_{j}^{J}\sum_{n}^{N}y_{it}^n\left[\exp(V_{it}^n)-\ln\left[\sum_{k=1}\exp(V_{kt}^n)\right]\right] \tag{8}$$

We will estimate model parameters α_i, β, γ, σ where the logarithm likelihood function is maximized. For parameter estimation, we use Mathematica.

4 Application of Brand Selection Model

4.1 Estimation of the Parameters in the Models

Table 3 shows the estimated parameters of RSCS model. AIC in Table 3 is an index of model fitness, and the lower AIC model means better fitness model to the real data. In this sense, the proposed model 2013-RSCS is the best model within the 3 models. The parameters β, γ, are weight parameters of product quality and customer service, and the ratio is 0.1737=0.62/3.57. This means the importance of the customer service is 17.37% of product quality.

Table 3. Estimated parameters in each model

Parameters	2013-RS	2013-CS	2013-RSCS
α_1	2.51	1.80	3.05
α_2	1.21	0.59	1.66
α_3	0.84	0.42	1.08
β	1.27	no	3.57
γ	no	0.59	0.62
σ	0.88	no	0.69
AIC	-2321.80	-1106.43	-3011.58

By the use of this model, we can easy to predict the utility and the selection probability as shown in Table 4. The prediction errors are 0, and the model 3 is well fit for the prediction of the real share of the companies.

Table 4. Estimation of utility and selection probability

Company	Utility	Selection probability	Prediction error
A	5.29	64.49%	0.00
B	4.07	19.14%	0.00
C	3.91	16.36%	0.00

4.2 Customer Service Promotion

Table 5 shows the growth rate of market share when customer satisfaction index of customer service increase 1 point, where customer satisfaction index of customer service is scored by 1 to 5 degree. In company B and C, the growth rate increase more than 10%. As shown in Tables 4 and 5, the selection probability of company C is smaller but the growth rate of company C is greater than company A and B.

Table 5. Growth rate of market share

Company	Growth rate
A	4.21%
B	10.55%
C	10.97%

5 Conclusion

We developed brand selection model by considering customer service and we estimate model parameters by the use of the market data of questionnaires related to purchasing, and we confirm the adaptability of the proposed model. From the estimated parameters, we show that customer service effects 17.37% in the whole brand utility. By the model we can estimate the market share of each brand according to the improvement of the customer service. This paper will contribute the brand planning considering appropriate balance among product quality and customer service. In this way, we consider promotion by comparing each company's utility. We hope that this knowledge contributes to the performance of customer service for companies.

References

1. McFadden, D.: Conditional Logit Analysis of Qualitative Choice Behavior. In: Zarembka, P. (ed.) Frontiers in Econometrics, pp. 105–142. Academic Press, London (1974)
2. Briesch, R.A., Lakshman, K., Mazumdar, T., Raj, S.P.: A Comparative Analysis of Reference PriceModels. Journal of Consumer Research 24(2), 202–214 (1997)
3. Hotta, S., Ishizu, S., Nagai, Y.: Development of price promotion model for online store selection. In: Salvendy, G., Smith, M.J. (eds.) HCII 2011, Part II. LNCS, vol. 6772, pp. 246–252. Springer, Heidelberg (2011)
4. Kiuchi, T.: A Brand Choice Model with the Price Acceptability. In: JAMS Proceedings of the Conference of the National, vol. 39, pp. 212–213 (2007) (in Japanese)
5. Abe, T.: What is Service Science? The Fujitsu Research Institute Economic Research Center, 1–27 (2005) (in Japanese)

Mobile In-App Advertising for Tourism: A Case Study

Tek Yong Lim, Teck Lun Tan, and Geoffrey Emeka Jnr Nwonwu

Faculty of Computing and Informatics, Multimedia University,
Jalan Multimedia, 63100 Cyberjaya, Selangor, Malaysia
tylim@mmu.edu.my, alecteck@gmail.com, mekkzy@yahoo.com

Abstract. A successful tourism advertisement can attract tourists to a certain country. This paper explored the effective ways of incorporating ads in mobile app for tourism industry. My Travel Malaysia was selected as a case study. A mobile advertising guideline was used for creation of mobile in-app banner ad. A mobile app prototype was developed and embedded with four different ads. A usability testing was carried out with ten participants and all were asked to find a particular hotel room rate. The results revealed that participants were able to recall images banner ad compare to text banner ad but they were also more likely to perceive large image banner ad as app content. However, all participants did not click on these banner ads because not relevant to their tasks.

Keywords: In-App Advertising, Mobile Tourism, Usability Testing.

1 Introduction

Tourism is mainly giving services to travelers such as transportation, hospitality, entertainment venues, travel agencies, tour operator and other related services. In short, tourism is about selling dreams to people and promotion such as advertising plays an important role in tourism. Previous studies showed that a successful advertisement could attract tourists to a certain country [1]. In 2011, travel and tourism industries spent $2.4 billion and were ranked as the third spenders on Google AdWords [2]. The tops five companies that spent million on Google advertising were Booking.com, Expedia, Kayak, Marriott and Priceline.com.

[3] estimated that there were 6.8 billion mobile subscriptions in 2013 and more than half of subscribers in the Asia-Pacific region. A recent study by [4] indicated that 51% of smart phone owners accessed travel information on their devices while planning a trip or traveling. This included air travel related activity (e.g. check airfare price) and hotel related activity (e.g. look up hotel direction). This is an opportunity for advertisers to reach out their potential mobile travelers. There were many advertising strategies employed on mobile device. For example, ads were displayed in mobile app, mobile web, mobile video, text messaging, and multimedia messaging. [5] predicted that mobile advertisement would generate $24.5 billion for app developers in 2016. Thus, this paper explored the effective ways of incorporating ads in mobile app for tourism industries.

C. Stephanidis (Ed.): Posters, Part I, HCII 2013, CCIS 373, pp. 695–699, 2013.

2 Literature Review

There are various definitions of advertising. [6] suggested that advertising is defined as a communication designed to entice an audience to take some action, either instantly or in the near future. The advertisement is usually paid from an identifiable source and can be conveyed through print, electronics and other methods.

Newspaper and magazine are considered the common venues for advertisers. Unlike the traditional advertising, online advertisers were able to display interactive and more personalized ad content for each individual [7]. Web developers would specify an ad unit (usually a rectangle space allocated for displaying ads) in their web page. Although the online ad goals were to build a product image and stimulate direct purchase, but previous studies revealed that many users rated negatively on their experience with online ads. The following were examples of bad ad design element: pop-up window, taking long time to load, attempt to deceive user into clicking on it, disappearance of close button, doesn't tell its purpose, content being shifted, and others [8]. In addition, [9] found that ad banners also decreased user search performance. Thus, a guideline was provided to design a good online ad. The ad should inform what will happen if user click on it, relate with user current online task, identify itself as advertisement, tell the advertising purpose, and supply additional information without leaving the current page [8].

In mobile setting, developers need to understand the user behavior and hardware limitation. Mobile users would use their mobile device for two main tasks, namely to save time and to fill time [10]. In time saving situation, user would search quick information on the fly and then return to what they were doing. In time filling situation, user would engage with entertaining app to fill short moments in the day. Besides that, developers also need to support wide spectrum of different mobile devices on the market that varied in term of user interfaces, processor capabilities, storage size and display resolution. Therefore, [11] established a standard guideline on mobile advertising. This guideline proposed different ways displaying ads in mobile app such as in-app display advertising unit, integrated ad, branded mobile app, and sponsored mobile app. There were relatively few studies on user experience of mobile in-app advertising and how these mobile ads affect the users.

3 Design of Mobile In-App Banner Ad

There is a need to design effective mobile in-app banner ad for promoting Malaysia because Malaysia became the ninth most visited country in term of the number of international travelers in year 2011. My Travel Malaysia is a free mobile app available in iTunes store and one of the Top 10 Malaysia Travel Apps. Thus, this app is selected as a case study. Mobile travelers can search specific destination by typing in the location name (see Figure 1). If mobile travelers are unfamiliar with the local places, they can still find nearby attractions and hotels by using their current mobile global positioning system (GPS). Mobile travelers can save an attraction or hotel by adding it to favorites and share it with friends via email.

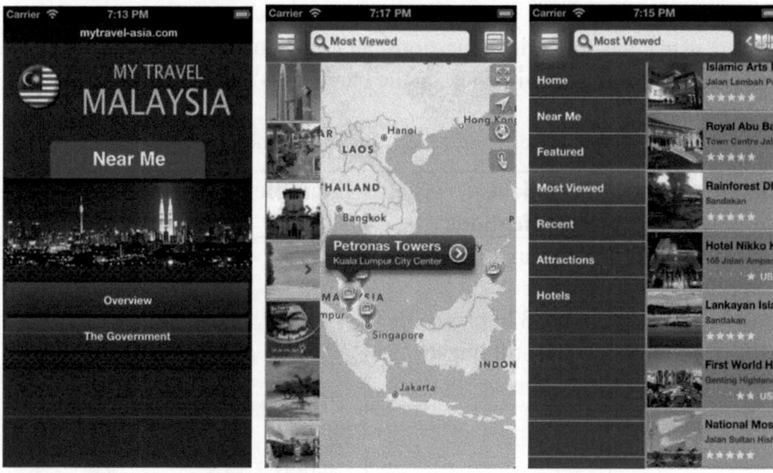

Fig. 1. Screenshots of My Travel Malaysia app

Mobile advertising guidelines by [11] is used for designing mobile in-app banner. Mobile in-app banner ad is defined as a color image ad unit appears within a mobile application. This banner ad can be display in the form of a still image, text or both. This banner ad can be placed anywhere within the mobile app such as main menu and content page. Mobile user can click on the banner ad. A low fidelity prototype based on My Travel Malaysia app was developed. This mobile app prototype was embedded with four different banner ads (Ad 1, Ad 2, Ad 3 and Ad 4). Three banner ads were still images in JPG format but with different heights and widths (see Table 1). The images were taken from Malaysia Airline System and Sabah Tourism Board. The fourth banner ad was a white text tagline with black background. Ad 1 was placed below "Overview" content page. Ad 2 and Ad 4 were placed below "Main menu" page. Ad 3 was placed within "Hotels" listing. All banner ads were visible on screen and user would receive additional information from advertiser when clicking on the ads. User can return to the previous page in the app prototype by clicking back button.

4 Usability Testing

The purpose of this usability testing was twofold: (1) to assess user memory for mobile in-app banner ad and (2) to find out why user ignore or interact with the banner ad. Ten participants (5 males and 5 females) volunteered to take part in this testing and all gave informed consent. Seven participants were Malaysian and the remaining were foreigners. All participants had computer experience and had used mobile travel app.

The usability testing was conducted in a controlled setting. First, each participant was asked to fill out a short survey. Then, the participant was given a brief introduction to mobile app prototype and was asked to find the room rate of *Glenmarie Hotel, Selangor* using the app prototype. Participants were encouraged to think aloud while performing the task. After the participant completed his/her task, each participant was interviewed using the following questions: (1) How many banner ads did you noticed? (2) Do you think you will click on the banner ads? If not, why?

Table 1. Design of Mobile In-App Banner Ad Units

Ad Design	**Technical Specifications**	**Example (approx. dimension)**
Ad 1 (MAS, Fly Me There)	XX-Large Image Banner 320 x 320 pixels JPEG still image	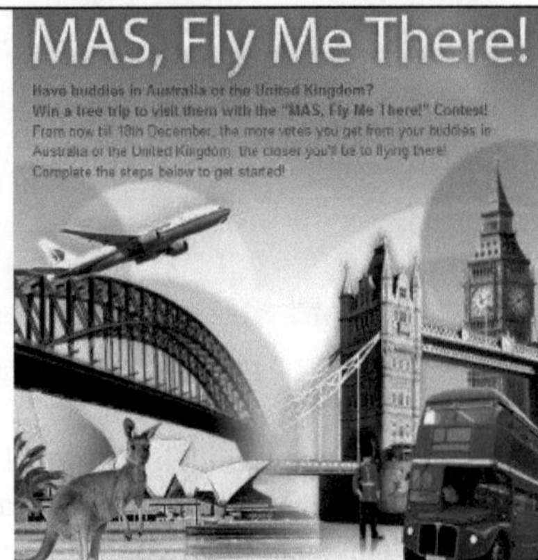
Ad 2 (Sabah Tourism Board)	X-Large Image Banner 300 x 75 pixels JPEG still image	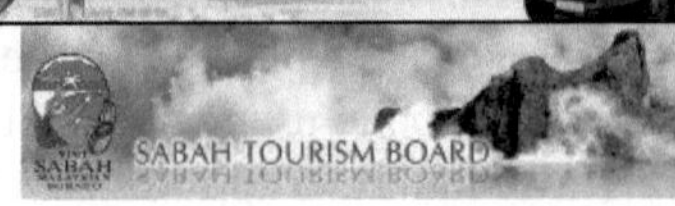
Ad 3 (Super Sales Malaysia)	Large Image Banner 216 x 36 pixels JPEG still image	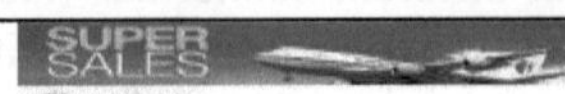
Ad 4 (*Sipadan* Travel Package)	Text Tagline 22 characters	Sipadan Travel Package

The findings revealed that all participants completed the task successfully. All participants were able to recall the Ad 2 due to its prominent colorful visual and location on main page. Eight participants recalled the Ad 3. However, only one participant recalled the Ad 4 because most participants ignored the bottom part of main page. There is only one participant able to recall the Ad 1 because most participants thought the large image was part of the app content instead of banner ad. However, all participants did not click on any of these mobile in-app banner ads because these banner ads were not relevant to the task given.

5 Discussion and Conclusion

The results revealed that participants experienced text ad blindness in mobile setting because they tend to miss information in text banner ad compare to image banner ad. This is especially true when participants are searching for specific information [12].

On the other hand, they were also more likely to perceive xx-large image banner ad as app content. This is considered as unethical because the ad can mislead participants and resulted negative impact on business [13]. Having an image banner ad in mobile app can be a double-edged sword.

In conclusion, this paper showed that the current mobile advertising guideline was good for ensuring advertisements being display effectively across different mobile devices. However, [14] suggested that advertisements only work if an ad fit with the user's goal. Future work will concentrate on matching relevant banner ad to in-app content and evaluate the banner ad effectiveness based on user click.

References

1. Brida, J.G., Schubert, S.F.: The Economic Effects of Advertising on Tourism Demand. Economics Bulletin 6(45), 1–16 (2008)
2. Kim, L.: What Industries Contributed to Google's $37.9 Billion in 2011 Revenues, http://www.wordstream.com/blog/ws/2012/01/23/google-revenues
3. International Telecommunication Union The World in 2013 ICT Facts and Figures, http://www.itu.int/ITU-D/ict/facts/material/ICTFactsFigures2013.pdf
4. Radwanick, S.: Smart Travel: Majority of Smartphone Owners Now Access Travel Information on their Devices, http://www.comscore.com/Insights/Press_Releases/2012/4/Majority_of_Smartphone_Owners_Now_Access_Travel_Information_on_their_Devices
5. Baghdassarian, S., Frank, A.: Forecast: Mobile Advertising, Worldwide (2009-2016), http://www.gartner.com/resId=2247015
6. Richards, J.I., Curran, C.M.: Oracles on "Advertising": Searching for a Definition. Journal of Advertising 31(2), 63–77 (2002)
7. Park, T., Shenoy, R., Salvendy, G.: Effective Advertising on Mobile Phones: A Literature Review and Presentation of Results from 53 Case Studies. Behaviour and Information Technology 27(5), 355–373 (2008)
8. Nielsen, J.: The Most Hated Advertising Techniques, http://www.nngroup.com/articles/most-hated-advertising-techniques/
9. Burke, M., Hornof, A., Nilsen, E., Gorman, N.: High-Cost Banner Blindness: Ads Increase Perceived Workload, Hinder Visual Search, and Are Forgotten. ACM Transactions on Computer-Human Interaction 12(4), 423–445 (2005)
10. Interactive Advertising Bureau: A Mobile Advertising Overview, http://www.iab.net/media/file/moble_platform_status_report.pdf
11. Mobile Marketing Association: Mobile Advertising Guidelines, Version 5.0, http://www.mmaglobal.com/files/mobileadvertising.pdf
12. Owens, J.W., Chaparro, B.S., Palmer, E.M.: Text Advertising Blindness: The New Banner Blindness? Journal of Usability Studies 6(3), 172–197 (2011)
13. Spizziri, M.: Ethical Issues in Online Advertising: Rules for Online Ads, http://advertising.about.com/od/onlineadvertising/a/guestethicalads.htm
14. Nielsen, J., Norman, D.: Making Web Advertisements Work, http://www.nngroup.com/articles/making-web-advertisements-work/

The GUI Design for the Products of Business Use by Using the Business User Model

Toru Mizumoto[1] and Toshiki Yamaoka[2]

[1] Graduate School of Systems Engineering, Wakayama University, 930 Sakaedani, Wakayama-shi, Wakayama 640-8510, Japan
[2] Faculty of Systems Engineering, Wakayama University, 930 Sakaedani, Wakayama-shi, Wakayama 640-8510, Japan
Mizumoto.Toru@sysmex.co.jp, Tyamaoka6@gmail.com

Abstract. The products of business use mean the instruments for office work, the machine tools, the medical instruments and the other instruments for professional use that are delivered to offices, factories, hospitals and other facilities. Because the user uses it for occupation, the context of use is confined or restricted. If we would like to design the GUI with good usability logically, we have to specify the context of use of the products of business use. Therefore, we propose the method to clarify the context of use by using the Business User Model (the persona for the products of business use).

Keywords: GUI, Persona, Business use.

1 Background

The products of business use mean the instruments for office work, the machine tools, the medical instruments and the other instruments for professional use that are delivered to offices, factories, hospitals and other facilities. The user of the products of business use uses the instruments for occupation. Therefore the context of use is confined or restricted.

For example, in the case of the electronic medical records (EMR), there is the context of use such as "The doctors look at the screen carefully about five hours each day in the examination room of the hospital". When we consider the GUI design of the EMR, the designer designs the GUI and we make the checklist (Ex. Structured Heuristic evaluation method [1]) for usability evaluation. After the design of GUI, we try to find usability issues on the GUI by using the checklist.

The checklist is very useful to evaluate the usability of the GUI design of products of consumer use that are not specific the context of use. But, it is difficult to find problems of the products of business use by using the general usability evaluation method. Because the user uses instruments only for their works, the context of use is confined or restricted.

For example, the doctors look the EMR screen carefully for a long time. If we use the generally checklist for usability evaluation such as "Contrast is too low?",

C. Stephanidis (Ed.): Posters, Part I, HCII 2013, CCIS 373, pp. 700–704, 2013.

"Characters are too small?" and "A step-by-step guide appear?". The general usability evaluation method judges the low contrast screen have bad usability. And, we will select the screen that separated by vivid color. But, does the high contrast screen really have good usability for doctors? With such a design, doctors will feel the pain in their eyes.

If we sale the products that have such a problem, user will say the claim to us. So, customer satisfaction will be down and we have to change the design of the products by using our man-power and cost. That is big demerit for company that develops the products of business use.

2 Purpose

In this way, we cannot improve the usability of GUI design by using generally checklist for usability evaluation. If we would like to improve the usability of GUI design of the products of business use, we have to clarify the context of use such as "User looks at the screen long time". If we understand the context of use, then we will not select the screen that distinguished by color. Therefore, we propose the method for select the GUI logically by using the context of use of the products of business use in this paper.

3 Issue for Clarification of the Context of Use of the Products of Business Use

We have to consider the method in order to clarify the context of use. The "Persona" is the concrete person image which set up name, mug shot, role, goal, etc. supposing a typical user of the products. The technique for planning and development of the products which satisfies the persona's goal by always using the persona is called "Persona method". The persona method is often published in technical books and magazines. Then, a lot of products planners and designers know the methodology and effectiveness of the persona method as very effective user centered design method to improve customer's satisfaction on their products. [2]

However, the examples shown in the technical books and magazines are almost only about the end user of the products of consumer use like home electronics, food, etc. Of course it is important that we understand the end user for the products of business use too. But, in the case of the products of business use that is purchased by facilities budget, there are additional important factors such as the relation between end users and purchasing decider, the stakeholders of the facility, etc. Thus, the persona for the products of consumer use is inapplicable to the products of business use. [3]

4 Construction of Persona for the Products of Business Use

We gathered the well-informed people of our company and carried out brainstorming to extract the user's peculiar to the products of business use. We show the example of the EMR. We were able to extract the following attributes. "place to use, way of the setting, doctor(end user), purchasing decider, nurse, patient, number of patient, how to learn, frequency to use, purpose to use, favorite design, etc." Then, we arranged the attributes and made the flow of the user interview. And, we investigated elements in every attribute by the user interview.

The model of the target user for the products of business use is completed by performing a classification of the result of the user interview by KJ method. This model is the new type of the persona for the products of business use. We call it the "Business User Model" in distinction from the conventional persona.

Table 1. Contents of the Business User Model

Item	Contents
Facility model	location, scale of facility, basic principle, culture, external environment, etc.
Organization model	scale of examination room, philosophy, role, the number of staffs, etc.
Personas	doctor, nurse, patient
Communication flow	flow of examination, consultation between employees, etc.
Communication scenarios	events of each communication

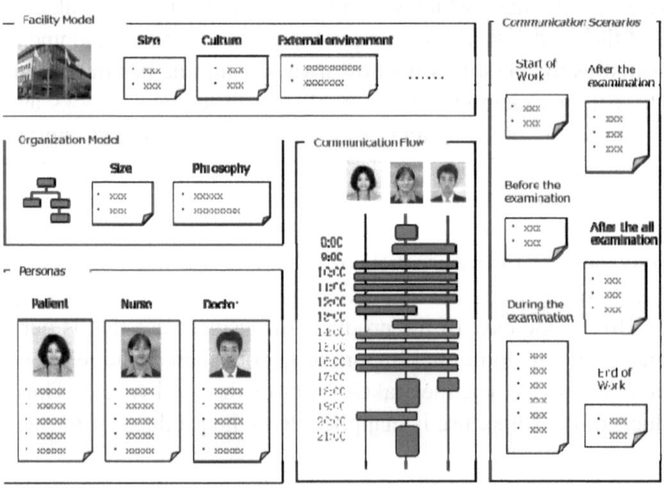

Fig. 1. The Business User Model

5 Clarification of the Context of Use by the Business User Model

We clarify the context of use by background information obtained from the Business User Model and issue of user obtained from the voice of user such as results of the user interview, claim, etc.

Table 2. The Business User Model + The voice of user = The context of use

No.	The Business User Model	The voice of user	The context of use
1	Communication flow: The doctors use 5 hours total to patient examination	I want to explain the results carefully to the patient.	The doctors look carefully the EMR screen for a long time.
2	Organizational model: Philosophy of hospital accountable to the patient. Communication scenario: The nurse attends a medical examination.	When I show a test result and a policy of the medication on the EMR screen, I am hard to talk with a patient.	The doctors operate the EMR screen while talking with a patient. A patient and a nurse varying in quantity of knowledge about the medical care watch the EMR screen at same time.

6 The Logical Design of the GUI

We consider the GUI design with good usability by clarified context of use by the Business User Model. If there is context of use such as "The doctors look carefully the EMR screen for a long time.", we can understand that the screen elements separated by group boxes or space is better than screen elements separated by high contrast.

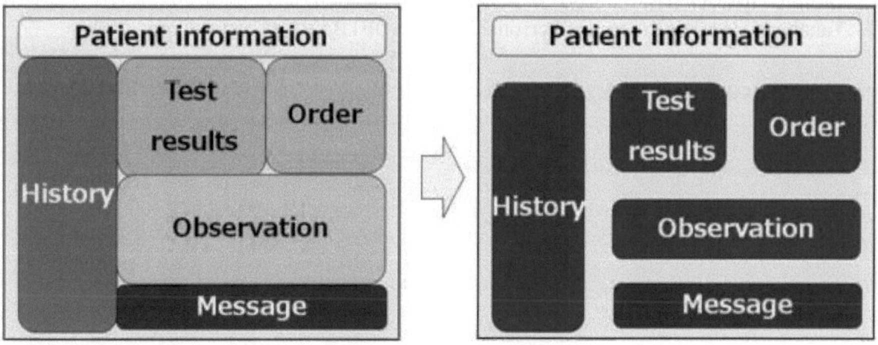

Fig. 2. Case studies - 1

And, if there are contexts of use such as "The doctors operate the EMR screen while talking with a patient.", "A patient and a nurse varying in quantity of knowledge about the medical care watch the EMR screen at same time.", we can understand that the EMR displays the information on screen in parallel is better than the EMR displays the information on screen consecutively.

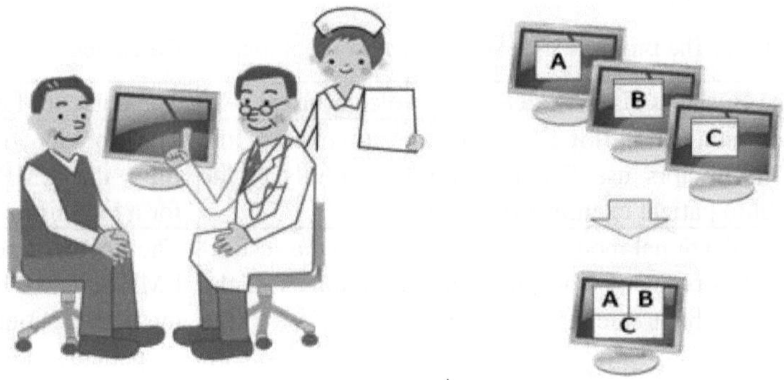

Fig. 3. Case Studies - 2

7 Conclusion and Perspectives

If we clarify the context of use by the Business User Model, we can design the GUI with good usability logically. In the next step, we will collect more examples and we would like to show the relationship between the context of use and the GUI design.

References

1. Kurosu, M., Matsuura, S., Sugizaki, M.: Categorical Inspection Method - Structured Heuristic Evaluation (sHEM). IEEE SMC (1997)
2. Pruitt., J.S., Adlin, T.: The Persona Lifesycle Keeping People in Mind Throughout Products Design. DIAMOND, Inc. (2007)
3. Tanahashi, H.: The Process of Persona Design. SOFTBANK Creative Corp. (2008)

Modeling Relationship between Visual Impression of Products and Their Graphical Features

Shimon Niwa and Toshikazu Kato

Faculty of Science and Engineering, Chuo University, 1-13-27 Kasuga, Bunkyo-ku, Tokyo, 112-8551, Japan
a09.834a@g.chuo-u.ac.jp, kato@indsys.chuo-u.ac.jp

Abstract. Consumers feel heavy burden to find products suited individual preferences owing to large quantity of them on the Web. Therefore, it is necessary to classify products based on subjective preferences. This paper describes the method to model the relationship between subjective visual impressions and objective graphical features through machine learning for each user. The way to describe the visual impression is to use adjectives used by the professional photographers. As graphical feature vectors, we compute Lab color histogram and SURF from product photos. We estimate the subjective visual impression of products and classify them by constructing classifiers for the impression groups using Random Forests. As a result of the experiment, the proposed method achieved 80.1% accuracy on average.

Keywords: Modeling, Subjective Visual Impression, Machine Learning, Graphical Features.

1 Introduction

Recently, consumers have the opportunity to look at products on the Web frequently. However, consumers feel heavy burden to find products suited individual preferences owing to large quantity of them on the Web. Therefore, it is necessary to classify products based on subjective preferences.

This paper describes the method to model the relationship between subjective visual impressions and objective graphical features through machine learning for each user [1][2]. Thus, our method can estimate the visual impression of product photos and classify them based on individual subjectivity by the model.

2 Representation of Visual Impression

The way to describe the visual impression of products is to use four adjectives (which we call impression words) used by the professional photographers. Impression words

C. Stephanidis (Ed.): Posters, Part I, HCII 2013, CCIS 373, pp. 705–708, 2013.

we use are "Wild", "Sharp", "Fresh", and "Natural". According to the subjective visual impression, a user classifies training examples into groups labeled by impression words.

3 Graphical Features

Product photos giving us similar visual impression would have similar graphical features. To quantitatively represent product characteristics, we compute graphical feature vectors of product photos.

Visual perception system of human beings has photoreceptors, which extract features of colors and brightness. Then, by integrating and selecting features extracted by photoreceptors, human beings perceive shapes [3]. Colors and shapes greatly affect the impression of objects. Therefore, we compute their graphical feature vectors from product photos.

3.1 Color Features

As the color graphical features, we calculated values of the color histogram in Lab color space. Unlike the RGB and CMYK color models, Lab color space (with ranges [0,100], [0,255], [0,255], respectively) is designed to approximate the visual perception system of human beings. Although many colors can be defined in computer system, the colors that can be recognized by human beings are limited. Thus, we calculated the 64 bins color histogram.

3.2 Shape Features

As the shape graphical features, we calculated SURF (Speeded Up Robust Features) [4]. SURF is a robust local feature detector that is used in computer vision tasks such as object recognition. We can describe the shape and structure of parts using SURF feature vectors. We construct the bag of features by K-means clustering algorithm ($K = 500$), quantize the SURF descriptors according to the bag of words. Thus, product photos can be represented as the histograms of the visual words that are the features vectors of them.

4 Estimation of Subjective Visual Impression

To estimate the subjective visual impression of products and classify them, by constructing classifiers for the impression groups using Random Forests [5], we model the relationship between impression words given by each user and their graphical feature vectors. Random Forests gives estimations of what variables are important in the classification. The variable importance is based on the Gini gain.

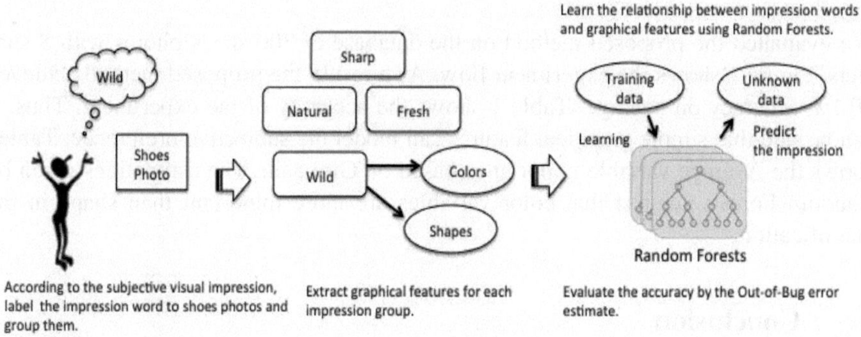

Fig. 1. Experiment flow chart

Table 1. Experiment accuracy

Subject	Impression words				
	Wild	Sharp	Fresh	Natural	All
1	85.1%	89.1%	85.9%	80.2%	84.7%
2	83.5%	76.4%	38.5%	91.3%	78.7%
3	82.5%	91.5%	49.0%	85.7%	80.0%
4	86.7%	76.8%	85.7%	79.1%	82.7%
5	78.8%	64.0%	81.8%	78.8%	77.0%
6	66.7%	79.8%	69.5%	65.1%	70.7%
7	85.1%	84.6%	85.3%	75.6%	82.7%
8	83.3%	92.6%	88.9%	68.9%	84.3%
Average	81.5%	81.9%	73.1%	78.1%	80.1%

Table 2. Average Variable Importance (Gini gain)

Subject	1	2	3	4	5	6	7	8
Color Importance	2.42	2.49	2.86	2.26	2.39	2.69	2.29	2.38
Shape Importance	0.32	0.32	0.31	0.33	0.32	0.32	0.34	0.33

5 Experimental Result

We evaluated the proposed method on the database of 300 shoes photos with 8 subjects. Figure 1 shows the experiment flow. As a result, the proposed method achieved 80.1% accuracy on average. Table 1 shows the accuracy of the experiment. Thus, it can be said that simple graphical features can model the subjective preference. Table2 shows the Average variable importance based on Gini gain. The estimations given by Random Forests suggest that color variables are more important than shape in the classification.

6 Conclusion

To classify product photos on the Web based on subjective preferences, this paper describes the method to model the relationship between subjective visual impressions using impression words and objective graphical features through Random Forests for each user. The experimental result suggested that simple graphical features could model the subjective preference. In addition, it is found that color variables are more important than shape in the classification. In our future work, we intend to design low dimensional graphical features to describe the features more clearly.

References

1. Tada, M., Kato, T.: Visual Impression Modeling Using SVM for Automatic Image Classification. In: 2006 IEEE International Conference on Systems, Man and Cybernetics, pp. 872–877. IEEE (2006)
2. Uesaka, S., Yasukawa, K., Kato, T.: Kansei Modeling on Visual Impression from Small Datasets. In: Stephanidis, C. (ed.) Posters, Part I, HCII 2011. CCIS, vol. 173, pp. 605–609. Springer, Heidelberg (2011)
3. Spillman, L., Werner, J.S.: Visual Perception: The Neurophysiological Foundations. Academic Press (1990)
4. Bay, H., Tuytelaars, T., Van Gool, L.: SURF: Speeded up robust features. In: Leonardis, A., Bischof, H., Pinz, A. (eds.) ECCV 2006, Part I. LNCS, vol. 3951, pp. 404–417. Springer, Heidelberg (2006)
5. Breiman, L.: Random Forests. Machine Learning 45, 5–32 (2001)

Estimation of Dominant Attributes of Product for Each Customer through Behavior Observation of Shopping

Mika Okuzawa[1] and Toshikazu Kato[2]

[1] Graduate School of Science and Engineering Chuo University
1-13-27 Kasuga, Bunkyo-ku, Tokyo, 112-8551 Japan
[2] Faculty of Science and Engineering Chuo University
1-13-27 Kasuga, Bunkyo-ku, Tokyo, 112-8551 Japan
kato@indsys.chuo-u.ac.jp

Abstract. Our purpose is to make a personalized shopping support system in a retail store. In this study, we estimated dominant attributes for each customer through behavior observation of shopping to collecting decision-making data of them with various kinds of products. The dominant attributes are estimated by conjoint analysis of the product attributes and the degree of interest in the product estimated from customer's behavior. In the experiment with a trial retail store, we achieved success about estimations of 3 of 4 customers. The products recommended by our system also were shown to be better suit for customers.

Keywords: Ubiquitous Sensing, Modeling of Customer Preference, Smart Shop, Online Shop.

1 Introduction

Current recommendation services are mostly based on social recommendation by collaborative filtering of huge number of shopping logs of many consumers. To perform personalized recommendation we need effective method for collecting decision-making data of each consumer with various kinds of products.

The purpose of our study is to quickly estimate the individual tastes of each consumer on products through observation of shopping behavior in a shop equipped with ubiquitous sensors. Personal taste can be described with dominant attributes and their attribute values.

2 System and Implementation

2.1 Smart Shop

We built an experimental shop, Smart Shop, with ubiquitous sensors to capture the passive observation of the each consumer's behavior such as "look", "touch", and "take" action to products [1]. The installed sensors are RFID readers and tags attached to customer cards and shirts and web cameras. The former is to locate and identify the customer and to sense which shirt is taken, and the latter is to sense customer's action.

C. Stephanidis (Ed.): Posters, Part I, HCII 2013, CCIS 373, pp. 709–713, 2013.

Our Smart Shop also has digital signage devices with web camera for active observation of consumer's gaze as "watch" action to the computer coordinated signage.

2.2 Estimation of Dominant Attributes

We adopt conjoint analysis as to find the dominant attributes [2]. The sample products for the method are provided based on an orthogonal array. We analyze these products with quantification methods 1. The explanatory variables are the product attributes and the response variables are the degree of taste to the products estimated by the Smart Shop. As the result of the multiple regression analysis, the maximum |t| value of each attributes are considered as the degree of dominant attributes and the maximum degree is considered as the best dominant attribute.

2.3 Method of Recommendation Considering Dominant Attributes

The Smart Shop recommends products based on each customer's taste when they stand in front of a digital signage device. They are recommended by order having high score as follows:

$$Score_p = \sum_{(a,v)\in p} \frac{V_a \times S_v \times D_a}{S \times N_v},$$

where p, a, and v are a product, an attribute, and an attribute value. V_a is a number of total attribute values the attribute a has. S_v is a number of times a customer chose products which has the attribute value v. D_a is a degree of dominant attributes of the attribute a. S is a total number of times a customer chose products. N_v is a number of products which have attribute value v. The taste degrees of each attribute value are obtained by D_a and the number of times a customer chose v. The scores of each product p are obtained by the total of the taste degree of each attribute falling under p.

3 Experiment

We conducted an experiment to compare our implicit method by Smart Shop and previous explicit one by questionnaire. Subjects were 4 male students. The process is as follows:

1. A subject did shopping in Smart Shop. The products were 18 t-shirts selected randomly. The Smart Shop analyzed the subject's action data and estimated a formula of subject's action pattern.
2. The subject also did shopping in the Smart Shop. However the products were 18 t-shirts selected based on an orthogonal table. The Smart Shop estimated the taste degree of products and the degree of dominant attributes based on the action pattern formula.
3. The subject answered survey questions to evaluate the preference to the products with 5 phases (+2, +1, 0, -1, -2). We also estimated the degree of dominant attributes based on the answer.

4. Each recommendation products of the Smart Shop and the questionnaire data obtained by the degree of dominant attributes. Digital signage devices showed 5 of them based on the subject action for products. The subject evaluated the preference to the 5 recommendation products with 5 phases. This recommendation step was repeated 3 times and we got 15 product evaluations in total.

4 Results and Discussion

Table 1 shows the rates which evaluations estimated by Smart Shop was matched with another estimated by questionnaire. The evaluations were divided into likes and dislikes. We showed 2 cases that 0 is likes or dislikes because an evaluation is 0 on questionnaire may differ depending on subjects. The estimation accuracies of subject A and B were more than 61% in both case, however, it of subject C and D were less than 50% in case that 0 is likes.

Table 1. Estimated rate of taste by Smart Shop's behavior observation

Subject	Like: +2 ~ 0 Dislike: -1 ~ -2	Like : +2 ~ +1 Dislike : 0 ~ -2
A	0.722	0.722
B	0.611	0.833
C	0.389	0.667
D	0.500	0.833
Average	0.556	0.764

Table 2 shows the degree of dominant attributes estimated by Smart Shop or with questionnaire. The dominant attribute estimated by Smart Shop were matched with another estimated with questionnaire about subject A and B. Particularly about subject A, the order of dominance were also matched with another. The decimal place's difference about subject B suggests that Smart Shop can estimate the degree of dominant attributes more correctly than questionnaire. However, the dominant attributes of 2 methods were matched about subject C and D. These results may be caused by Smart Shop's estimation or questionnaire.

Table 2. Dominant attribute rates of each subject (|t| value)

Subject	Method	Color	Design	Shape
A	Smart Shop	0.434	**2.288**	1.929
	Questionnaire	0.569	**3.128**	2.560
B	Smart Shop	1.691	**2.938**	1.756
	Questionnaire	3.232	**3.555**	3.232
C	Smart Shop	**2.084**	0.849	1.443
	Questionnaire	2.410	2.410	**8.677**
D	Smart Shop	2.932	**4.962**	2.039
	Questionnaire	6.978	3.806	**8.881**

Table 3 shows the ratio which subjects liked the recommended products. All subject's results were more than 60%. The results suggest Smart Shop with this study's method can provide stable satisfaction to each subject.

Recommended Products for subject A and B by Smart Shop were the same as another by questionnaire because both estimated dominant attributes were the same. On the other hand, those for subject C and D were not the same as another. Subject C rated the products recommended by Smart Shop less by 30% than another although subject D rated them more by 6.7%. These results indicate the need for review of the action pattern formula by Smart Shop.

Table 3. Good evaluation rate in the recommendation

Subject	Smart Shop	Questionnaire
A	0.800	0.800
B	0.667	0.667
C	0.333	0.600
D	0.667	0.600

Table 4. Regression equation of shopping behavior

Subject		Formula $(y_{Item} = \cdots)$	Adjusted R-square
A	Before	$-1.796 + 0.087x_{Look} + 0.618x_{Touch} - 0.007x_{Take}$	0.430
	After	$-1.274 + 0.587x_{Touch}$	0.505
B	Before	$-2.720 + 0.622x_{Look} + 0.626x_{Touch} + 0.0237x_{Take}$	0.497
	After	$-2.818 + 0.656x_{Look} + 0.682x_{Touch}$	0.532
C	Before	$-1.868 + 0.195x_{Look} + 0.109x_{Touch} + 0.219x_{Take}$	0.722
	After	$-1.952 + 0.221x_{Look} + 0.248x_{Take}$	0.741
D	Before	$0.202 - 0.216x_{Look} + 0.466x_{Touch} + 0.123x_{Take}$	0.712
	After	$0.202 - 0.216x_{Look} + 0.466x_{Touch} + 0.123x_{Take}$	0.712

Table 5. Dominant attribute rates of each subject (re-estimate)

Subject	Method	Color	Design	Shape
A	Smart Shop	0.283	**1.794**	**1.794**
	Questionnaire	0.569	**3.128**	2.560
B	Smart Shop	1.693	**3.093**	1.685
	Questionnaire	3.232	**3.555**	3.232
C	Smart Shop	1.659	0.857	**1.671**
	Questionnaire	2.410	2.410	**8.677**
D	Smart Shop	2.932	**4.962**	2.039
	Questionnaire	6.978	3.806	**8.881**

Therefore we reviewed and optimized the action pattern formula of all subjects to maximize adjusted R-square. Some of the formulas have had unnecessary variables. The action pattern formulas before and after the optimization are shown in Table 4.

Table 5 shows the degree of dominant attributes estimated with optimized formulas of Smart Shop. The optimized formula of subject C made his dominant attributes, estimated by Smart Shop, agree with another by questionnaire. Those of subject A, B and D were not changed. We can consider the product recommendation by Smart Shop is able to satisfy subject C well as another by questionnaire.

Finally, these results presented Smart Shop with our method attained implicit estimation of dominant attributes in 3 of 4 subjects. These also presented that, in the case of estimated dominant attributes by Smart Shop and another by questionnaire did not fit, it satisfied a subject better than modeling by questionnaire.

5 Conclusion

We suggested the estimation method of product dominant attributes for each customer through behavior observation in a retail store. Also, we implemented the product recommendation system for experiments which recommends products based on each customer's dominant attribute estimated using Smart Shop. The purpose was this system recommends more satisfactory products for each customer than another by questionnaire with 5 phases. Experiment led to a result this system accuracy is equal to or better than another by questionnaire. In addition, the result suggested the formula of each customer's action pattern needs optimization before attribute analysis.

A hypothesis in this paper was each customer's dominant attribute are fixed. However, Smart Shop needs to understand each customer's taste changing actively. Further consideration will be needed to yield any findings about method Smart Shop analyzes a dominant attribute which is not fixed.

Acknowledgements. This work was partially supported by JSPS KAKENHI grants, "Effective Modeling of Multimodal KANSEI Perception Processes and its Application to Environment Management" (No. 24650110), "Robotics modeling of diversity of multiple KANSEI and situation understanding in real space" (No. 19100004) and TISE Research Grant of Chuo University, "KANSEI Robotics Environment".

References

1. Ogino, A., Kobayashi, T., Iida, Y., Kato, T.: Smart Store Understanding Consumer's Preference through Behavior Logs. In: Rau, P.L.P. (ed.) IDGD 2011. LNCS, vol. 6775, pp. 385–392. Springer, Heidelberg (2011)
2. Yomo, A., et al.: Estimation of Important Attributes of Items in Purchase Process for Personalized Recommendation Service. IPSJ SIG technical reports 2012-HCI-147 (20), 1–8 (2012) (in Japanese)
3. Inoue, K., et al.: Application of Rough Set to Kansei Engineering. Kaibundou, Japan (2009) (in Japanese)

Free Design Bank

Case Study of Design Action to Alleviate Poverty

Nélida Ramírez[1,2], Manuel Lecuona[2], and John Cardozo[1,2]

[1] Universidad Nacional de Colombia
{nyramirezt,jjcardozov}@unal.edu.co
[2] Universidad Politécnica de Valencia
mlecuona@dib.upv.es

Abstract. This paper illustrates how industrial design implementation can be a tool of poverty alleviation, throughout a case study. According to Weis classification, design actions towards social development are: 1. Design for skills development, 2, Design for social enterprise, and 3. Design for development promotion. Based on the aforementioned this document fouses on the first category. The FREE DESIGN BANK (FDB) case is presented: FDB is an on-line platform, a communication instrument between craftsmen and design schools, supported by fair trade strategies. As a result the relationship between FDB and communities vulnerable by poverty is described, from the interaction among the design team and the community, and also the design process and the benefit obtained by the community.

Keywords: Industrial design, Poverty, Case Study.

1 Introduction

Poverty indicator referenced by the Caritas Internationalis Organization [1], warns that at the beginning of the 21st century a quarter of the world's population qualifies as extremely poor. "Fundamentally, poverty is a denial of choices and opportunities, a violation of human dignity. It means lack of basic capacity to participate effectively in society. It means not having enough to feed and clothe a family, not having a school or clinic to go to, not having the land on which to grow one's food or a job to earn one's living, not having access to credit. It means insecurity, powerlessness and exclusion of individuals, households and communities. It means susceptibility to violence, and it often implies living on marginal or fragile environments, without access to clean water or sanitation" -UN Statement, June 1998; signed by the heads of all UN agencies-, in [2]. Poverty require immediate attention in order to improve human wellbeing at world level [3], [4]. From design perspective, Papanek [5] proposed the enhancement of living conditions of particularly vulnerable communities (poverty, disabilities, age or health), Margolin [6] , argues that is required to assume a critical position along with professional practice, and in the same way, Maldonado, Ricard,

C. Stephanidis (Ed.): Posters, Part I, HCII 2013, CCIS 373, pp. 714–718, 2013.

Bonsiepe, Manzini and Fry, among others, assert that designers must take a more critical position with what they are doing, and act accordingly.

2 Reference Framework

Weis [7] , classifies the design activities to help people in poverty conditions establishing three categories:

- Design for skill development: It focuses on the selection of poor communities in order to perform handcrafted tasks, through cooperation programs. These programs aim to develop and commercialize products, by providing: basic education or training and job and/or income generation. For instance, Aid and Artisans is an organization with more than 33 years of operations and representation in more than 110 countries worldwide, and it follows this way of running business.
- Design for social Enterprise: It implies a mutual benefit among profit firms and poor communities. Those needs faced by the communities are researched, in order to understand them, and to set and inspire further development of business models and inclusive markets, with the purpose of create new opportunities and better life conditions. Firms such as IDEO and Catapulta Design are within this category.
- Design for development promotion: It has the goal to assist people, communities and organizations, through products and services. Within this category projects are developed in those aspects that the community might need and based in a great participation of the very community; partially because financial funds come from sponsors, donations, loans and personal aids. Engineers Without Borders – International (EWB-I), works under these guidelines.

3 Material and Methods

The current work is delivered under Case Study guidelines as qualitative research method. This research methodology, according with Pérez Aguilar en Sarabia [8, p. 227] , "is a good way to investigate unknown, very complex and dynamic events, or when elements of intangible nature or hardly observable take place". Yin [9, p. 4] defines case study as "An empirical inquiry about a contemporany phenomenon, set within its real -worldcontext- especially when the boundaries betwen phenomenon and context are not clearly evident".

The main goal is to know "how" FREE DESIGN BANK (FDB) develops its product design process and "which" strategies are implemented in order to help Vulnerable Communities by Poverty (VCP), having the following questions: ¿How is the interaction between FDB and the VCP?; ¿How design process is developed to favor the VCP?; ¿What is the benefit gained by the VCP?

Yin [10] , emphasizes the importance of establishing within the "study cases", the assessment unit, which in this research is: "design organizations for development to VCP".

Free Design Bank has been chosen among 35 cases of design focused in poverty alleviation, having as selection criteria: being part of the group "design for skills development", program development (representation in more than 10 countries and more than 10 years of experience), the availability of information and key sources of information. Data for construction were obtained through a protocol, which went through a review and approval process of eight research-on-design experts, through a focus group implementation. Data was collected via in-depth interviewing, applied to Professor Manuel Bañó [11] , website review [12] , and catalogues, in a 3 months period.

4 The Free Design Bank (FDB) "Case"

FREE DESIGN BANK is a university program created under the direction of Professor PhD. Manuel Bañó, at CEU - Cardenal Herrera University, in Valencia (CEU-UCH) Spain, with financial support of the Santander Group. Such initiative emerged in 1998 as a by-product of the project entitled Diseño para el Mundo Real (Design for the real world). It is an exchange website between craftsmen, design schools and fair trade organizations. It works along with NGO's and its scope is focused in developing nations such a Kenya, Tanzania, Ecuador, Peru, Sri Lanka, Colombia, Cuba, Philippines, Nepal, India or Senegal.

4.1 Interaction between the FREE DESIGN BANK (FDB) Team and the Vulnerable Communities by Poverty (VCP)

In FDB every interaction with a VCP, is in itself a unique experience with its own particularities and specific conditions (see Table 1.), given from culture, communication and existing skills among those members of the community.

Table 1. Interaction between FDB and VCP

N°	Criteria	Free Design Bank
1	Interaction definition	Assistance, help or cooperation.
2	Work driver	Enhancing skills and opportunities of communities.
3	Community selection	By request of the community; by previous awareness of the community; by a third party request.
4	Ways of engagement	Design; Job generation; Training, gender equality and environmental protection.
5	Communication with the community	Given by the fact of being in touch, either by physical ways or by telematics means. Physically can be done with the presence of a member of the FDB team member by at least 15 days within the influence zone. By telematics with virtual encounters on daily-basis. Communication is held in the native language of the community, (Spanish, English or French and in some cases with interpreters intervention, from instance Swahili to English)

Table 1. *(Continued.)*

6	People and interaction ways	The interaction takes places in meetings with community leaders and local authorities, then with craftsmen in general workshops.
7	Decisions. Projects to be developed	It is required a contact with the community, to identify and to know to what extent the skill or the dexterity has been developed; and to establish the complexity of the design to be implemented.
8	Frequency	Interaction frequency depends on the general framework of each project; nevertheless, there are minimum average work periods between 9 months and a year.

4.2 The Design Process

General sequence of the process followed by FDB to favor a VCP is developed in four stages (see Fig. 1).

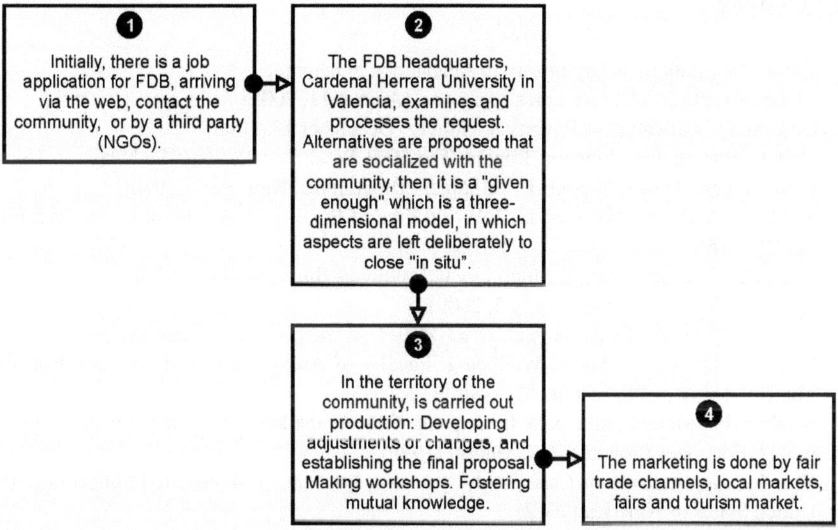

Fig. 1. FDB Design Process

4.3 Benefits for the Vulnerable Communities by Poverty (VCP)

Most of the work undertaken by Free Design Bank provides to the affected community social and economic benefits. Economically speaking, they are represented in jobs and incomes, training in a task, documentation and design standardization; whereas socially speaking they account for social cohesion, sense of belonging to the group, coexistence, common problem-solving and identity sense.

5 Conclusions

It is important that from a design perspective can emerge different stages directed to the alleviation of one of the biggest world problems, as so it is poverty. Initiatives such as the Free Design Bank, are very important because they help less fortunate people by bringing economic and social opportunities, making a continuous monitoring process via internet. As it is a university program, it involves and teaches future professionals to recognize realities different that the ones experienced by them, and to work with ethics and responsibility. Programs of this nature should be emulated worldwide, but they should develop and engage strong commercialization programs to achieve better results.

Acknowledgements. The authors of this paper wish to express their most sincere gratitude to professor Manuel Bañó, to the Free Design Bank work team and to Cardenal Herrera University of Valencia, for allowing the access to the required information and the permission to disclosure their experiences.

References

1. Caritas Internationalis Organization, Acabar con el hambre, http://mdg2015.caritas.org/es (August 11, 2005)
2. Gordon, D.: Indicators of Poverty & Hunger (December 12, 2005)
3. UNDP, Human Development Report. The Real Wealth of Nations: Pathways to Human Development, United Nations Development Programme, New York (2010)
4. World Bank Group, Working for a World Free of Poverty, World Bank Group, Washington DC (2006)
5. Papanek, V.: Diseño Para el Mundo Real, Ediciones Blum, Madrid (1977)
6. Margolin, V.: Foroalfa (February 2, 2009), http://foroalfa.org/articulos/el-disenador-ciudadano
7. Weis, E.: Design for Social Wellbeing, Faculty of Architecture, Building and Planning. The University of Melbourne, Melbourne (2010)
8. Sarabia, F.: Metodología para la investigaci6n en marketing y direcci6n de empresas, p. 227. Ediciones Pirámide S.A, Madrid (1999)
9. Yin, R.: Applications of Case Study Researh, 3rd edn., p. 4. SAGE Publications, Inc., United States of America (2012)
10. Yin, R.: Case Study Research. Design and Methods. SAGE, London (1994)
11. Bañ6, M.: Interview, Free Design Bank. Interview (November 27, 2012)
12. Universidad Cardenal Herrera, Free Design Bank (2000), http://www.freedesignbank.org/

Promoting Consumer Products with Fictional Stories

Mizuki Sakamoto, Tatsuo Nakajima, and Sayaka Akioka

Department of Computer Science and Engineering
Waseda University, Japan
{mizuki,tatsuo,akioka}@dcl.cs.waseda.ac.jp

Abstract. Our everyday consumer lifestyle has been enhanced by embedding stories in our daily life. The stories define the meaning of an artifact appeared in them. In Japan, promoting consumer products with fictional animation stories is recently very common. We believe that analyzing the stories gives us useful insights to design future ambient intelligent services that integrate virtual and real worlds. This paper discusses the analysis of several product promotions that use fictional Japanese animation movies, and presents guidelines for successful promotions. The insights presented in the paper are effective for designing future product promotions.

Keywords: Fictional stories, Product promotion, Reality, Alternate Reality Game, Transmedia storytelling.

1 Introduction

Our everyday consumer lifestyle is enhanced by embedding various stories. The stories tell us how to use products, and how they are effective or attractive in our daily life [2]. Recently, storytelling is an essential issue in the human computer interaction research community, and especially, using a fictional story to mix the fictional world and the read world is an important topic for integrating stories in our daily life. For example, alternate reality games (ARGs) [3] will be used in a variety of future product promotions for embedding fictional stories seamlessly in our dally life. Transmedia storytelling [1] will be a basic way to enhance the meaning of products for promoting technology enhanced products. However, design guidelines are necessary to mix fictional stories in our real world in a more seamless fashion. In Japan, fictional animation movies have been used for promoting commercial products and their brands. They make it possible to use mysterious artifacts, super human powers, futuristic scenes that do not exist in the real world to expand people's imagination and fantasy. Thus, they offer a feeling to increase human potentiality, and the effect can be used to provide strong impressions on our experiences in the real world. Recently, the promotion is broadcasted on public video streaming services such as Youtube and NicoNico Douga[1], and is advertized through social media like Twitter and Facebook. The reputation of the promotions becomes well know through a word of mouth

[1] http://www.nicovideo.jp/

C. Stephanidis (Ed.): Posters, Part I, HCII 2013, CCIS 373, pp. 719–723, 2013.

delivered in social media. This paper shows the analysis of existing promotion that uses Japanese animation movies. The analysis leads to design guidelines identifying why the promotions have been successful. Then, we present some case studies to show how the successful promotions fit the guidelines. The insights extracted from the analysis presented in the paper are useful to design future ambient intelligent services that integrate virtual and real worlds.

2 Promoting Products with Fictional Animation Stories

Using animation movies is very useful because it is easy to offer fictional worlds and characters. This makes us to offer empathetic fictional creatures and marvelous futuristic worlds to attract us easily. The animation story is easy to embed ideological messages that represent human dreams and expectation. Also, many Japanese animation stories are full of positive thinking, so the stories can increase our self-efficacy to overcome hard problems while enjoying the stories. Currently, typical product promotions use empathetic characters that are appeared in popular animation stories. For example, Pokémon[2] characters are widely used for promoting foods for kids like a retort-packed curry food and bread. The animation movie is very popular by most of Japanese kids so the promotion broadcasted within the animation television movie is effective to appeal the products to these kids. However, although the promotion makes it possible to increase their buying impulse, the promotions do not make them believe that the products are attractive. Thus, the products will be forgotten when they become adults.

3 Guidelines to Promote Products with Fictional Stories

In this section, we present four design guidelines for promoting commercial products by using fictional stories. The guidelines are extracted while discussing in workshops to watch several video animation movies for product promotions.

I. Offering the strong visual impact that makes us attract the products. Pepsi NEX uses Cyborg 009[3] for the product promotion, and Tiger & Bunny[4] uses several Japanese company logos such as Softbank and Bandai for promoting the company brands. In the Pepsi NEX promotion, cyborg heroes move very speedy so this becomes a metaphor of the Pepsi NEX's sharp taste. Also, a pretty heroine brings us an empathetic feeling on the products. In the story of Tiger & Bunny, justice and heroics are commercialized commodities. Some people choose to become costumed superheroes, and each is sponsored by a major present real-life company, which is featured as advertisements on the heroes' uniforms. These cool superheroes become metaphors that the companies are also cool. These vivid expressions in an unusual daily life

---

[2] http://www.pokemon.com/us/

[3] http://009.ph9.jp/pepsi-nex/

[4] http://tigerbunny.wikia.com/wiki/Tiger_%26_Bunny_Wiki

make it possible to offer people surprises that memorize strong impressions on target products.

II. Offering the non fictional story that makes us believe the promotion. TAISEI corporation promotes its brand image by using an animation movie[5]. In the movie, a lady is working on the construction of the Bosporus tunnel. The non fictional story presents that her work contributes to a amazing work that can be appeared in the world map. The movie shows the fact that the company has achieved the amazing work as trusted information so the audience of the movie can own the positive feeling on the company through amazingly realistic scenes of the tunnel. The promotion is very useful because most of us do not know that TAISEI corporation has built such amazing constructions all over the world.

III. Offering the reality that makes us believe the fictional story in the promotion. In the DOCOMO's promotion named Xi AVANT[6] to show the vision of the future mobile phone, the promotion movie uses the several realistic landscape scenes of present Barcelona. The reality of the background landscape scene offers a feeling that the vision told in the fictional story will be realized soon. The Tokyo Disney Resort's promotion[7] reminds each person's real memory that she visited to Tokyo Disney Resort before. So the story shows that she will enjoy to visit Tokyo Disney Resort even she becomes old. Therefore, we think that the happy memory in Tokyo Disney Resort will be inherited to our children.

IV. Offering the empathy that makes us attract the products in the promotion. This is a typical way to use animation characters in the promotion videos. As described previously, Pokémon characters are used for promoting various commercial products for kids. Also, Japan Racing Association uses characters and giant humanoids in Evangelion, which is a very popular animation movie that many Japanese young adults like[8]. The purpose of the promotion is to promote the horse racing to young adults. The animation stories are usually preferred in a wide generation in Japan, but each animation covers only specific target generation. Thus, the animation that is interested in a specific generation can be used to appeal to a different generation who may not have strong interests in the target products.

Toyota's Peace Eco Smile[9] promotes its brand by using an original animation story. In the movie of the story, a young male person who comes from an outer space tries to learn products and rules in our world. Especially, the story tells that the technologies developed by *Toyota* are very eco-friendly with his love story. However, the characters in the story are not enough empathetic. Also, the story does not give us enough information that the Toyota's technologies are superior. Also, the background scenes are not enough realistic, and there are a few impressive visual representations to give us metaphors showing *Toyota*'s excellence. Thus, the promotion that does not fit to these guidelines has not been successfully accepted from the most of audiences.

---

[5] https://www.youtube.com/watch?v=OKoCl-3E0Vw

[6] https://www.youtube.com/watch?v=IP5nAkG5lME

[7] https://www.youtube.com/watch?v=clFq7xwxV-Q

[8] https://www.youtube.com/watch?v=toEcz4inet8

[9] http://www.toytoyota.com/pes/

4 Case Study: Analyzing Advertisements with Original Animation Stories

This section analyzes three promotion movies that use original animation stories discussed in our *workshops*. The movies are successful to promote products and company brands. We consider how the movies fit to the guidelines explained in the previous section.

The first is the promotion movie for Meiji fruits gummi candy. The story is named Megumi and Taiyo Tweet Love Story[10]. In the story, a heroine Megumi eats a grape gummi candy when something needs to be considered deeply. The scene fits to guideline 1. When using a fictional story, it is not easy how the audiences feel the reality on the story in *accordance* with guideline 2. Tweet Love Story uses a social media, Twitter, to make us feel the reality of the story. The audience can talk with the story's hero Taiyo via Twitter. Taiyo gives us answers when we gave him some advices on how to get closer to Megumi. Megumi and Taiyo also talk with each other on Twitter so everyone can know their conversation. The audiences' advices have strong impacts on the conversation between Megumi and Taiyo. This means that the story changes its ending according to our advices to Taiyo, and the fact feels us that the story is realistic in our world.

Taiyo is working at a vineyard, and there are some scenes showing that grapes are healthy and delicious. This gives enough information showing the product's excellence in accordance with guideline 3. Finally, the story chooses a character designer whose characters are recently very popular in many media. Thus, the audience easily feels the empathy on the characters even though the story and its characters are original. Then, guideline 4 is satisfied.

The second is the promotion movie named Mercedes-Benz Next A-Class[11], which promotes Mercedes-*Benz's* new A-Class cars. In the story, the promoted car is depicted in a near future world. The speediness of the car is nicely shown in the movie. This fits to guideline 1. Also, the movie shows that the car offers very high performance that is fit to guideline 2.

In the animation movie, the presentation of the car is very realistic. Also, the story is just to catch a *legendary* ramen noodle shop. Finding a nice ramen noodle shop is very popular culture for Japanese young adults. Thus, the story is especially very realistic for the young adults who are target users for the A-Class cars. This fits to guideline 3.

Finally, the movie adopts a character designer of Evangelion, where most of young males know and like Evangelion. It is one of the most popular animations in Japan, and its characters are also well known. People who like Evangelion's characters also like the characters in Next A-Class. Thus, this fits to guideline 4.

The third is the promotion movie of Subaru, which is a Japanese automobile company. The promotion movie is named Wish Upon the Pleiades[12]. The promotion is

---

[10] `http://www.meiji.co.jp/sweets/candy_gum/fruits_gummi/part1/`

[11] `http://next-a-class.com/`

[12] `http://sbr-gx.jp/`

very interesting because a very few are promoted about Subaru in the movie. The name of the main heroine is *Subaru*, but the movie does not show any cars in the story. However, the characters in the story and the story itself offer strong attractiveness to many Japanese traditional animation fans. The story is based on magic girls' story, and many scenes in the movie are very typical in the magic girls' animation movie. Thus, the movie becomes very empathetic to many animation fans, and the characters in the movie become very famous in the geek animation communities.

The movie makes the name Subaru well known although the company name may not be popular in young adults. Also, the company has opens several public attractions using the *characters*. Many young adults having interests in the characters visited to the attractions, and learn more details about the company. The original story follows only guideline 1 and 4, but guideline 2 and 3 that do not satisfied in the story may be compensated by the reality offered in real world attractions. This shows the future possibility to use transmedia storytelling for effective promotions.

Original stories need not take into account the consistency with promoted products. Thus, there is a very big freedom for the promotion, but the cost to create the movie of an original story is high.

5 Conclusion and Future Direction

This paper presented design guidelines to promote products by using animation stories. We showed some case studies to discuss the analysis of the several promotion movies. The insights from the analysis are useful to design future ambient intelligent services. We are interested in to use the proposed guidelines to analyze a story fragmented on multiple media. In Japan, especially, animation movies are recently used to promote local regions that are used in the story. The region plans to attract people who like the story when visiting to the region for enjoying extra original new stories. The proposed guidelines are helpful to consider how the unsatisfied guidelines in the promotion movie are supplemented in regional real world attractions. Our approach is also useful to analyze the story to compose multiple existing stories. For example, MacDonald sells Happy Meal that gives us character goods in various stories. Currently, there is no interaction among the characters in different stories. On the other hand, our approach offers a promising way to enhance their consumers' experiences by consistently integrating stories of multiple characters.

References

1. Dena, C.: Transmedia Practice: Theorising the Practice of Expressing a Fictional World across Distinct Media and Environments, Dissertation Thesis, University Sydney (2009)
2. Mattila, A.S.: The Role of Narratives in the Advertising of Experiential Services. Journal of Service Research 3, 35–45 (2000)
3. McGonigal, J.: This Might Be a Game: Ubiquitous Play and Performance at the Turn of the Twenty First Century, Ph.D thesis U.C.Berkeley (2006)

Service Designs for Lifestyle Changes

Yasuhide Shimizu[1], Kazuma Obata[1], Leo Wakiya[1], Daichi Aoki[1], Kazuhiro Kimura[1], Eichi Shibata[1], Toshiya Sasaki[1], Kazuhiko Yamazaki[1], Tomonori Yazaki[2], and Kengo Fujita[2]

[1] Chiba Institute of Technology, Chiba, Japan
[2] KDDI R&D Laboratories, Inc., Saitama, Japan
yasuhide1113@yahoo.co.jp

Abstract. Purpose of this research is to propose design approach and method for service design with lifestyle change based on human centered design. In addition, another purpose is to propose new system and product for network system. For this purpose, user research for extreme user was done and creates idea beyond current thinking. After making scenario and storyboard, design concept was proposed with prototype and concept movie. Based on this prototype and video, user evaluation was done to evaluate design concept. They base proposed design approach on utilizing extreme user to find new thinking for lifestyle change and to evaluate idea. Result of this research, exercise application named "pinch hitter" for diet was proposed. To continue exercise this application helps user to show the animation of pinch hitter that will exercise instead of real user.

Keywords: User Centered Design, Storyboarding, Scenario, Persona.

1 Introduction

Recently, people have been eager about making a new product with new style of interface just like iphone effects. Therefore, we are thinking a new product with new interface not only for convenience but also it can apply to human centered design. The proposal of this research is about "Service Designs for life-style changes". Our processes and ideas are basic on HCD and discover the needs from users inside voice and desires.

2 Purpose and Research Methods

2.1 Service Designs for Life-Style Changes

The purpose of this research is basic on HCD and discovers the needs from users inside voice and desires.

2.2 Service Designs for Life-Style Changes

In order to make this research, we follow the steps from HCD design and we use these effects as the results.

C. Stephanidis (Ed.): Posters, Part I, HCII 2013, CCIS 373, pp. 724–728, 2013.

Process: following steps (1) Design process proof, (2) Results outcome, (3) Conclusion.

3 Design Process

3.1 Background and Purpose

Background and purpose: Explanations of Service Designs for life-style changes.

3.2 The Background of Product Design Process

Human centered design is an approach that integrates multidisciplinary expertise towards enhancing human well-being and empowering people. It leads to systems, machines, products, services and processes which are physically, perceptually, cognitively and emotionally intuitive to use. Therefore, our product processes are basic following this concepts and ideas.

3.3 Explanation of Product Design Process

Application of the proposal Service Designs for life-style changes steps are following.

1. Ideas from memories workshop
2. Idea analysis: making a topic
3. Result about observation
4. Ideas from observation and brain storming. Final idea
5. Developing the idea, making a scenario
6. Making a story board
7. Mock up
8. Pro-typed products
9. Story boarding
10. Video demonstration

4 Verification

Explanation of each process with detail.

4.1 Memories Workshop and Making A Topic

From this process, suppose we have a user. From his/her unique experience and memories about design, we can use that experience and memories to develop ideas. Probably, we could find out new ideas or now life style to make a new topic(Fig.1).

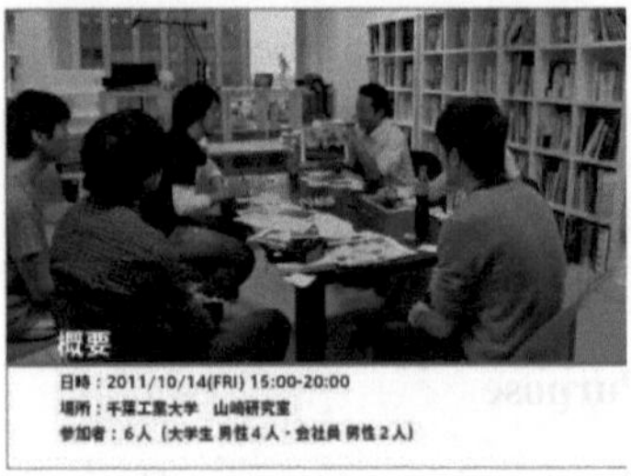
概要
日時：2011/10/14(FRI) 15:00-20:00
場所：千葉工業大学 山崎研究室
参加者：6人（大学生 男性4人・会社員 男性2人）

Fig. 1. Memories workshop

4.2 User Research

After setting a topic and we make researches which fit about our topic. However, we make some interviews to with some users (extreme users are included).

The questions about interview: users' basic information such as goal, hobbits, interests (Fig.2). The formation of the interview is about their lives in week day and weekend (fig.3).

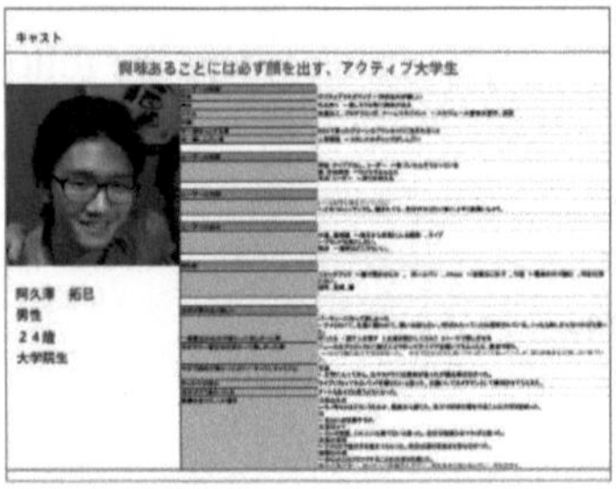

Fig. 2. Persona

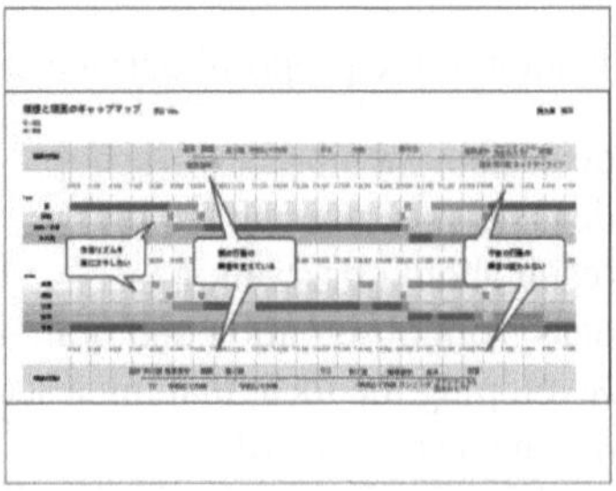

Fig. 3. Gap map whichi ideal life and an actual life

4.3 Idea Development

According the result from user researches, we are developing ideas from each topic scene. We make a vision map that basic on the result of interview. The contact of vision map is about comparison of ideal life and realistic life. We check out the result from research and make the development with each topic idea while the map is the key of making the scene.

4.4 Story Boarding

We make our ideas in to a scenario, for example, we put our life pictures and make them as episode series so that it is clear to the users (Fig.4).

1. We divided scenario by several micro scenarios
2. Around 5-10 micro scenarios
3. We make story boarding sheets from each micro scenario
4. We compose pictures with people and background
5. We use these pictures applying our products.
6. The contacts of story boards also included from what user dialogs.
7. We make sketches from each scene at beginning
8. After making sketches, we double check them and make some correction if they are necessary.

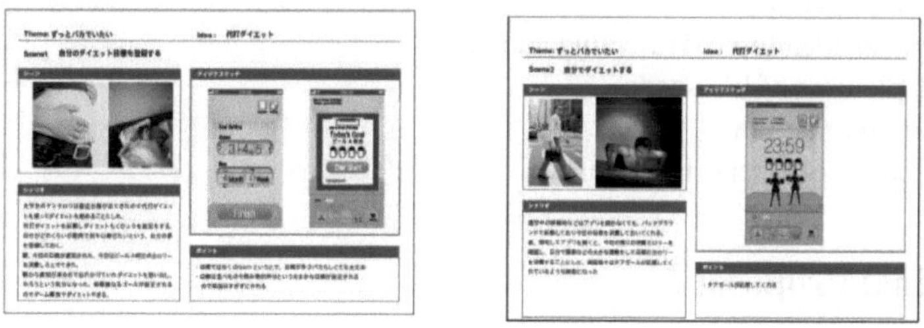

Fig. 4. Storyboard

4.5 Simple Product Pink

Before making the product, we start to work on interface, even the software is not done yet. We make several simulations to operate the interface. By using Adobe flash we update interface in they are necessary.

4.6 Response from Scenario and User Interface Valuation

We use story boards that we made before, and see how users' response. We let users operate the final product that we been made, and check the interaction between users and interface. While operating the products, we ask users to make valuation about product services.

Response from Scenario. While reading story board, users make their valuation. There are 4 levels of valuation sheet.

We make the valuation digitalization.

1. While reading story board, users make their valuation. There are 4 levels of valuation sheet. We make the valuation digitalization.
2. Interview with the items that user's concerned

Interaction valuations are the following:

1. Difficulty with scenario when seeing story board
2. Operation about scenario

3. There are 4 levels of valuation sheet including Satisfaction, understanding, and operation in each scene.

4.7 Final Proposal Movie

We made video about scenario that following with story boards. It includes user interface and interaction. We will make some reviews whether it is proper to expand the vision experience

1. Example of topic
2. Example of persona
3. Example of Idea topic with value added
4. Taking pictures of life scenes
5. Showing Interaction
6. Performance of Users' Experience

5 Final Proposal

Author have made a review of service over-view and in order to make the final proposal done, we also viewed the property of ideas. Main contact includes persona, story boards and final proposal movies. Result of this research, exercise application named "pinch hitter" for diet was proposed. To continue exercise this application helps user to show the animation of pinch hitter that will exercise instead of real user. And another result of this research is proposed design approach will be good for designer to proposed system and product for lifestyle change. Fig.5).

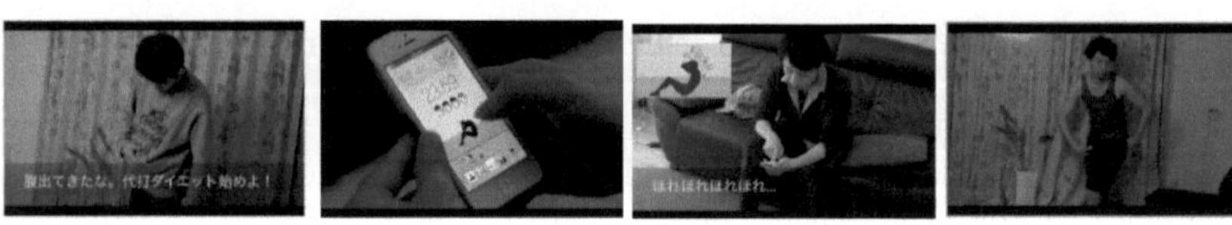

Fig. 5. Story movie

6 Conclusion

This research is about the process and technique of making a new service design by changing your life-style from user experience. The steps of making new design are basic on human-centered design that help us discover the potential needs from users and we are aiming for how accuracy of this. Author make new service design for life-style changes, and it have studied its characteristics in topic. This research had over-viewed our valuation by users with story boards and product operation. Therefore, we made this proposal connecting between user experiences and service value.

5. Hierarchy series connection.
6. Defuzzification: Convert fuzzy numbers to easy-comprehended definite values, this study adopts the center of gravity method to solve fuzzy numbers.
7. Sequencing: Sequence defuzzified criteria.

4 Case Study

The case company was established in 1983 and specializes in the field of Memory Card connectors. Table 1 shows the weights of green supplier assessment obtained by FAHP. Furthermore, application of the inspection exemption guideline based on the MIL-STD-1916 procedure, eight of the suppliers are certificated as inspection exemption suppliers. According to the inspection records of years 2009 and 2010, a reduction of 12.13% in material inspecting time for the case company can be saved.

Table 1. Weights of aspects and criteria for green suppliers assessment

Aspect	Aspect weight	Criteria	Criteria weight	Global priority	Ranking
Quality management	0.309	Raw material inspection report	0.119	0.037	14
		Promise of not using hazardous substance	0.137	0.042	12
		Management system verification	0.165	0.051	10
		Regulation restriction and customer request	0.315	0.097	2
		Quality system audit	0.264	0.082	3
Resource management	0.155	Raw material management	0.196	0.030	15
		Equipment environment	0.128	0.020	16
		Equipment procurement management	0.243	0.038	13
		Training	0.434	0.067	7
Design and Development management	0.280	Product innovation	0.169	0.047	11
		Green procurement	0.566	0.158	1
		Cleaning cost	0.265	0.074	5
Process management	0.257	Control of production process	0.241	0.062	8
		Control of nonconforming product	0.289	0.074	4
		Shipping management	0.269	0.069	6
		Product preservation	0.201	0.052	9

5 Conclusion

This research proposes a green suppliers assessment methodology through a modified Delphi method, and a Fuzzy Analytic Hierarchy Process. The top five assessment criteria determined are Green procurement, Regulation restriction and customer request, Quality system audit, Control of nonconforming product and Cleaning cost. After implementing these criteria to the material suppliers of the case company, eight of the suppliers are certificated as inspection exemption suppliers. A reduction of 12.13% in material inspecting time can be saved.

References

1. Buckley, J.J.: Fuzzy Hierarchical Analysis. Fuzzy Sets and Systems 17(3), 233–247 (1985)
2. Hu, A.H., Hsu, C.W., Kuo, T.C., Wu, W.C.: Risk evaluation of green components to hazardous substance using FMEA and FAHP. Expert Systems with Applications 36, 7142–7147 (2009)
3. International Electro technical Commission, IEC62321 CDV (111/95/CDV), IEC 62321, Ed.1: Procedures for the Determination of Levels of Regulated Substances in Electro technical Products (2005)
4. Kreng, V., Hsu, Y.L., Lee, C.H.: The application of Fuzzy Delphi Method and Fuzzy AHP in lubricant regenerative technology selection. Expert Systems with Applications 37(1), 419–425 (2010)
5. Laarhoven, P.J.M., Pedrycz, W.: A fuzzy extension of Sati's priority theory. Fuzzy Sets and System 11, 229–241 (1983)
6. Saaty, T.L.: The Analytic Hierarchy Process. McGraw-Hill, New York (1980)

Optimizing Product Interface Training Program for Older Adults-A Pilot Study

Wang-Chin Tsai[1,*], Chih-Sheng Chang[1], Kung-Chih Lo[1], and Chang-Franw Lee[2]

[1] Department of Product and Media Design, Fo Guang University
No.160, Linwei Rd., Jiaosi , Yilan County 26247, Taiwan (R.O.C.)
[2] Department of Industrial Design, National Yunlin University of Science and Technology
123 University Road, Section 3, Douliou, Yunlin 64002, Taiwan, (R.O.C.)
forwangwang@gmail.com

Abstract. This paper conducted a pilot experiment planning and compared the relative performance of two types of training method, two types of interface mode and high and low working memory levels of older adults in training to use a product interface. According to the cognitive learning theory and human knowledge system, two kinds of training method were developed. The procedural training method based on the procedural knowledge concept was provided to reduce working memory demands by telling participants which steps to perform and in which order. Generally, this training method was hypothesized to be better for older adults. The declarative training method from the declarative knowledge concept was designed to assist participants in properly allocating their attention but to require them to be more actively involved in determining the specific steps of the task. Although this type of training method might be most supportive of learning for older adults of high working memory level, it might too working-memory demanding for the older adults and hence be ineffective. The major findings were as follows: There was a significant effect of training methods on direct interface mode and hierarchical mode tasks. This study has shown evident relationships of performance as a result of the declarative training method versus the procedural training method in older adults with different cognitive attributes and ability levels.

Keywords: Training Method, Working Memory, Product Interface, Older Adults.

1 Background

As mentioned, the training materials do play an important role in the older adults' training issues. Likewise, the design of proper training method is equally important for older adults when interacting with product interface. Enabling older adults to interact with product interface efficiently is an important immediate and long-term goal for training research. Previous literature provides general guidance for the developing training program. General guidelines are available to enhance older

* Corresponding author.

C. Stephanidis (Ed.): Posters, Part I, HCII 2013, CCIS 373, pp. 733–737, 2013.

adults' ability to learn to use new product interface by providing training program (e.g., Czaja et al, 2012 ; Fisk et al., 2009 ; Rogers et al., 2010). However, numerous ambiguous questions regarding training program content remain to be unanswered in the context of aging and product interface. Lack of age-appropriate product interface training program has consistently been identified as a major obstacle to older adults' learning and use of products. Therefore, it is important to determine the type of training method, interface mode and the working memory ability limitation that works best for older adults, for immediate performance; and for learning. After understanding the issues of training materials for older adults' needs and requirement in the previous research(Tsai, Rogers, & Lee, 2012), this preliminary research continue to conduct a research to design two training methods to compare the effects of emphasizing different concepts during training of working memory difference on performance measures of product interface test. The purpose of this research is to provide insight into these unknown issues.

Figure 1 presents the overview of the experimental procedure used in the current study. Selected 80 older adults participated in this research. Participants in each working memory group received procedural training and declarative training in both interface task mode schedule. Participants began with working abilities testing and mouse training. They then began the training phase of either procedural or declarative training after which, participants moved into the assessment phase of the experiment. Interface performance was assessed using time on tasks participants conducted during test and tasks they were not trained on, the ability to incorporate interface goals, the ability to understand, and working memory for interface surface features.

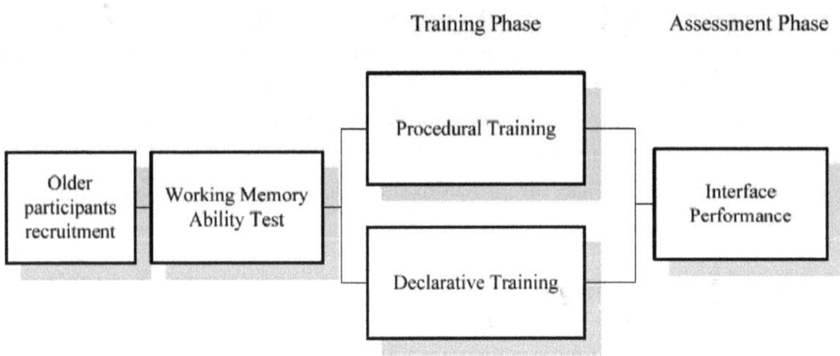

Fig. 1. Illustration of the experimental concept used in the current study

2 Methods

2.1 Participants

One hundred and twenty older adults were first recruited in this study. The protocol was explained and informed consent was obtained from each subject. First of all, participants completed a thirty minutes battery of working memory ability measures from the Wechsler adult intelligence scale test-3rd version (WAIS-III) (Wechsler, 1997).

The Digits Forward and Digits Backward tests (Wechsler, 1958), as well as the Daneman and Carpenter reading span test (1980) were used to test older adults' working memory. A compound latent factor score of working memory was calculated from these three measures. A higher compound latent factor score indicates higher working memory capacity. In addition to the working memory digit span measures, both near and far visual acuity were assessed using a Snellen eye chart, with the criterion set at 20/40 (corrected or uncorrected). Hearing was also assessed using an audiometer, there was no criterion set, and all participants were able to hear conversation between themselves and the experimenter with or without the assistance of a hearing device. There was no prior experience in using the experimental interface during the training conditions for the older adults. According to the digit span results, the scores of digit span selected ranged from 10 to 28 in the study, and the average value was 7.3 (SD = 3.2). The average value plus/minus fifty percentage of standard deviation was used as the dividing points for defining working memory levels. Low and high working levels were established respectively. The high working memory level group was composed of 40 older adults ranging in age from 65 to 72 years of age (SD = 6.8). The low working memory level group was made up of another 40 older adults ranging in age from 67 to 78 years of age (SD = 5.3). Older adults received $100 for their participation. The experiment lasted approximately 1 hour for two types of training method. Participants were pre-screened via the telephone and then mailed a home questionnaire. These measures included demographic and health questionnaires.

2.2 Materials-Development of Training Programs

Procedural Training Method. Procedural training instructions included minimum step-by-step directions to operate the product interface, but did not give information on what was to be completed in each step. Procedural training instructions only emphasized procedural information for the current interface state and tasks, therefore providing minimal conceptual information. During training, participants were given the goal and instructions on exactly what button to select; they were required to only follow the steps to complete the task.

Declarative Training Method. Dcclarativc training mcthods arc dcfincd as an abstract or generic ideas generalized from particular instances, which are task-independent procedures. Declarative training instructions consisted of generalized directions necessary to complete a task used in the product interface. Participants were given instructions on what to do to complete a task but not how to complete a task, the precise function selection was not provided. Declarative training instructions only emphasized general system information, and therefore provided minimal procedural (i.e. step-by-step) information. During training, participants were given the goal and general instructions on what is being performed during each step. They were required to extrapolate the exact button presses from the goal based on the given general instructions to complete the task. Just as with procedural training, to complete the task, participants had to read the problem statement to identify the appropriate tool, identify the value, and change the value. However, in declarative training, older participants were given the generalized hierarchical framework, identified through an interface analysis, needed to complete the task.

2.3 Materials-Interface Task Modes

In order to investigate learning to use a product interface, a computer simulated interface "Microsoft Media Player" was designed to emulate two types of interface tasks. The Microsoft Media Player was structured with a number of variables and functions that the user must take into account to produce a result. It provides the direct control mode tasks and hierarchical mode tasks. The direct control mode task is controlled from the basic level of the cognitive processing hierarchy, and may be characterized as "smooth, automated, and highly integrated" and takes place (critically) "without too much conscious attention or control". Effective direct control mode task performance relies on heavy feed forward control flows throughout, "depends upon a very flexible and efficient dynamic internal world model". The hierarchical mode tasks is controlled by the advanced level of the processing hierarchy, and may be characterized as consisting of "a sequence of subroutines in a familiar work situation", where the subroutines follow previously stored rules, again relying primarily on feed forward control. Users are required to use their higher knowledge and logical method to complete a task. Moreover, older adults' participants have not encountered similar simulated interface before. Therefore, the novelty, complexity, and unique nature of the Microsoft Media Player made it an appropriate product interface simulation for answering the previously stated research questions.

2.4 Procedure

In this study, the author use the Microsoft Media Player as a demonstration platform to train older adults of 40 minutes interface training for 10 tasks (including 5 direct control mode tasks and 5 hierarchical mode tasks). The training program taught each older adults group separately what to do or how to do it with hard copy tutorials designed by the researcher (Please follow the Appendix A for detailed content). The procedural training program told the participants how to operate the tasks but didn't explicitly tell them what they were doing. Otherwise, the declarative training method presented a conceptual paragraph for the interface task information, but didn't include detailed and sequenced instruction for using it to complete the task. That is, the declarative training method told participant what to do instead of how to do it. The detailed training program arrangement is shown as the Figure 4.5. After participant complete this assigned 40 minute training program, they were requested to perform another 6 tasks to differentiate the training performance and effectiveness.

3 Results

The improved performance of low working level older participants for task completion time and high working level older adults for task time indicates that these results pertain to task time where in accordance with the hypothesis that declarative training results in better performance on hierarchical mode tasks compared to performance of participants in the procedural training condition. This supports the notion that declarative training results in performance benefits in task speed for advanced or novel tasks, which may be due to a better understanding of the interface structure. Several conclusions can be drawn from these findings. However, examining one measure by itself gives an incomplete picture of effects of training on learning. Older participants in the declarative training condition performed hierarchical mode tasks faster than participants in the procedural training condition.

4 Summary and Implication

From a practical perspective, these results have clear implications for the development of training programs to optimize training for different working memory ability older adults learning to use a technology interface. If the goal is fast and efficient performance with training materials in view, then procedural training method is better, especially for low working memory older adults during training. If, however, the goal is to support learning to enable older adults to use product interface even when the training materials are not available, declarative training method is better.

Older adults are capable of learning to use new product interface. The optimal training method will likely involve a combination of specific training procedures. The present study makes clear the relative benefits of declarative versus procedural training for older adults of two different working memory levels and suggests how experts should incorporate these types of training into a training program. Finally, applying this research to the development of training programs may increase proper product usage of complex technological product interface for older adults. With the development of these types of interface occurring every day in domains such as medical care, communication, transportation, and entertainment, understanding the product interface structure may result in a better quality of life.

References

1. Tsai, W., Rogers, W.A., Lee, C.: Older adults' motivations, patterns, and improvised strategies of using product manuals. International Journal of Design 6(2), 55–65 (2012)
2. Czaja, S.J., Sharit, J.: Designing Training and Instructional Programs for Older Adults. CRC Press (2012)
3. Fisk, A.D., Rogers, W.A., Charness, N., Czaja, S.J., Sharit, J.: Designing for Older Adults-Principles and Creative Human Factors Approaches, 2nd edn. CRC Press, Boca Raton (2009)
4. Rogers, W.A., Fisk, A.D.: Toward a Psychological Science of Advanced Technology Design for Older Adults. Journal of Gerontology: Psychological Sciences 65B(6), 645–653 (2010)

The Changing Room
Multimedia Interactive Display System for Retail Stores

Ching-Yueh Tseng[1] and Chang-Chih Tseng[2]

[1] Department of Digital Multimedia Design, China University of Technology
[2] InnoCirque New Media Co.
jingyueh@cute.edu.tw, jasper@innocirque.com

Abstract. The Changing Room is a multimedia interactive display system. Digital media is used to make a projection on the walls, the ground and merchandise in the mall's display space, so customers can experience merchandise in the created context of digital images. Within the display space, the customers' various acts such as walking around, touching, and staying can trigger the sensors and then a variety of digital information will show up. For instance, directly projecting the relevant sales information around the merchandise, or producing a variety of different visual transition effects, to guide customers to participate in interaction and imagine the scenario or atmosphere by using this product.

Keywords: Interactive display system, shopping experience, projection.

1 Introduction

The majority of customers in retail stores, such as furniture and furnishings are often confused about what kinds of goods they should choose. This is mainly because they often cannot imagine the kind of scenario or atmosphere at home that will be created with those home supplies.

The Changing Room attracts customers by its visually interactive user interface. Through the display of a wide range of changing scenes and the instant availability of product details, customers can get sales information, and they can also immediately experience the related scenarios, further identifying their favorite goods and showing purchase intention. The digital content (including product information) can also be customized depending on the need of retailers in order to create miscellaneous experience spaces.

2 System Overview

The Changing Room is designed for the annual exhibition at Osaka University of Art and aims to guide people to experience a variety of interior design scenarios based on different themes (see Figure 1). The project proposes a simulation solution by projecting the images to physical space. The appearance of the items in all sizes such as walls, tables, chairs and tableware is all presented through the projector. Visitors are

C. Stephanidis (Ed.): Posters, Part I, HCII 2013, CCIS 373, pp. 738–741, 2013.

free to pick a projected scenario similar to their home or an interior design style they prefer, and specify the appearance and color of each item to more precisely determine whether the targeted products meet their requirements. The relevant design details are described as below.

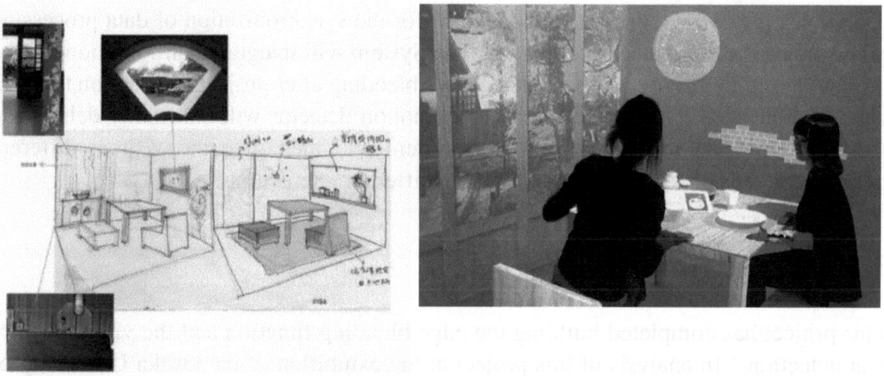

Fig. 1. From left to right - the concept image of Japanese elements oriented digital content display, completed works

2.1 System Architecture

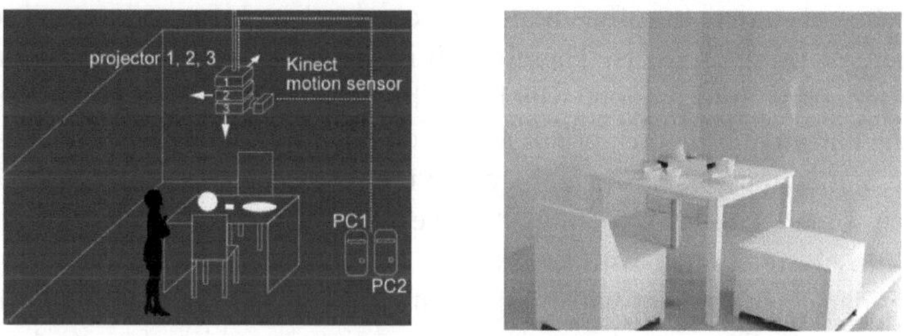

Fig. 2. From left to right - System Configuration, pure white colorless model

As Figure 2 shows, exhibition walls, tables and chairs and desktop objects are pure white colorless model before projection. The overall exhibition spatial configuration is 2.5 x 2.5 x 3 (L x W x H, unit: m); system devices contain three 5000 lumens (lm) of short-focus projector, two PCs, and one Microsoft Kinect motion sensor. The computer system's graphics card with multiple output functions allow three projectors to project images on the two walls, desktops and floors respectively. In addition, a Kinect motion sensor on the ceiling, by detecting the visitors' behaviors such as walking around, touching and staying, triggers the computer system to project a variety of interior design details and change the spatial scenarios.

2.2 Edge Blending and Motion Detection

As the exhibition space has three sides of the projection surface (walls on both sides and the desktop and the ground on the same side), the computer system needs to deal with the huge amount of image data, as well as motion detection functions. Therefore, during the virtual image projection, in order to reduce the workload of the display and detection operations, the two computers are connected for the synchronization of data processing to maximize the computer performance. The System will integrate configuration for the display of digital images, and then make edge blending after projecting them on the wall via different projectors. Further, the Kinect motion detector will constantly deliver the movements of the visitors back to the system and then give the visitors different projections of feedback content according to different interactions.

3 Future Work

This project has completed building the edge blending function and the visitors' "motion detection." In analysis of this project at the exhibition of the Osaka University of Arts in February 2013, with the experience of interaction with the visitors, this paper suggests that all goods information database should continue to be built and the function of customer image input provided.

3.1 Goods Information Database

The ultimate aim of The Changing Room is to provide retailers an exhibition and sales space in order to offer real-time commodity information and create the atmosphere of using products. Therefore, it is very crucial to build a database storing digital commodity information, which can be divided into three parts: the projected image, the narrative of goods, prices and stock quantity. For product images as shown in Figure 3, they must be designed based on the surface of the white projection model, so that customers can have feelings "on the spot." Commodity prices and inventory are also closely integrated with the system. For retailers with many stores, real-time inventory data management will bring great convenience for customers. In addition, the system must also provide product data maintenance interface to help retailers organize and input digital content that system can present in sequence.

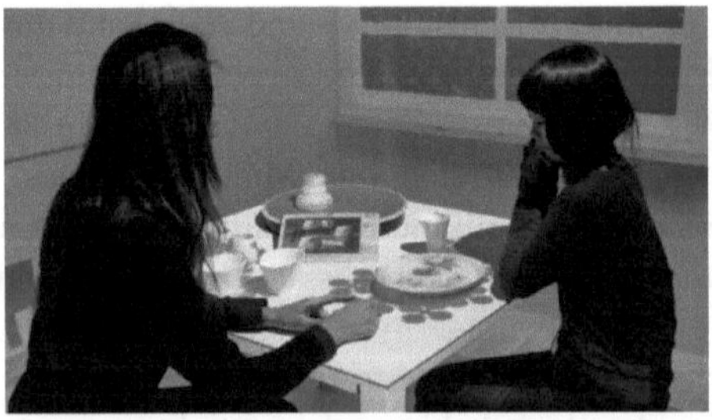

Fig. 3. Product digital images projected on the white model

3.2 Customers Input Information by Themselves

Web2.0 represents the content is produced due to the participation of each user; by participating in the platform, there will be more diverse content [1]. On the second stage, the system development will focus on the function design, where customers input their own images. The input function can do real-time input through community website platform, or at the exhibition spot. Customers can input their own images at home, allowing The Changing Room to provide more experience. In other words, by replacing the system's built-in indoor scenes with customers' photos provided by them, the home display tends to be more personalized, allowing customers to experience more accurate atmosphere of trial commodities.

4 Conclusion

Our society has entered an era of emotion-oriented business, and "purchase of goods" is no longer the sole purpose of the consumption process. Customers often pursue more psychological satisfaction and responses. For instance, " Factory tour" in combination of tourism and manufacturing, attracts a large number of crowds and bring business opportunities, which is exactly the specific marketing model of the commercialization of "experience in person." Therefore, whenever the company puts service on the stage, uses commodities as props and let customers emerge into the setting, the so-called "experience" has been done. To put it in another way, when customers buy the experience, they are spending time on enjoying the feeling "on the spot" offered by the company [2].

Through the exhibition space created by digital images, retailers shape the shopping process as an experience process and use information technology to make "product experience" available. Therefore, The Changing Room rearranges details of consumption process and recreates the customer's shopping experience aiming to encourage them to explore the new implication on consumption, shaping an "experience economy."

References

1. O'Reilly, T.: What Is Web 2.0, `http://oreilly.com/web2/archive/what-is-web-20.html`
2. Pine, B.J., Gilmore, J.H.: The experience economy: work is theatre & every business a stage. Harvard Business Press (1999)

Estimation of Dominant Features of Commodities Based on Shopping Behavior Analysis

Shungo Uchida[1] and Toshikazu Kato[2]

[1] Graduate School of Science and Engineering Chuo University
shungodesu77@gmail.com
[2] Faculty of Science and Engineering Chuo University 1-13-27 Kasuga, Bunkyo-ku, Tokyo, 112-8551 Japan
kato@indsys.chuo-u.ac.jp

Abstract. It is necessary to provide suitable assistance to each consumer in shopping to choose preferable commodities. Each consumer does shopping with checking dominant features of the commodities according to his own criteria [1]. For example, "I want a cloth of a good material", "I want a T-shirt in cool color", and so on. We have developed an experimental shopping space equipped with ubiquitous sensors such as cameras and RFID-tag readers. In our experiment, each subject freely walked around the shelves to find the preferable T-shirts. Our system observed typically the time of three actions, "Look at", "Touch" and "Take" a T-shirt. In this study, we have tried to estimate the dominant features with each consumer through suggest the approach to recommend information in consideration of personal dominant features from observation and analysis of shopping behavior to perform suitable assistance.

Keywords: Purchasing Behavior, Behavior Analysis, Dominant Features.

1 Introduction

In recent years, the choice to commodities of consumers spreads by the diversification of them in the store. However, it is the problem that consumers feel a burden to find them. So it is necessary that we provide the service that they don't feel a burden. There are shops that they are recommended information to show commodities on digital signage [1]. But it is thought that the consumers do shopping with dominant features [2]. For example, "I want good clothes of the material. I want T-shirt of cool color". The service by current digital signage cannot consider dominant features. In this study, we suggested the approach to recommend information in consideration of personal dominant features from purchasing behavior analysis.

2 Approach of Our Study

We focused on consumer's purchasing behavior to grasp their dominant features. We thought behaviors that are important for consumers are different each their dominant features. For example, the subject who has dominant features in colors compares

C. Stephanidis (Ed.): Posters, Part I, HCII 2013, CCIS 373, pp. 742–746, 2013.

clothes. Thus, we supposed that an action of "Look at" became important for them. We explain our past study here. We have developed an experimental shopping space equipped with ubiquitous sensors such as cameras and RFID-tag readers as shown in Fig.1. In our experiment, each subject freely walked around the shelves to find the preferable T-shirts. Table 1 shows the definition of three actions. Our system observed typically the time of three actions, "Look at", "Touch" and "Take" a T-shirt. Thus, we adopted three action times and preferable rate, like and dislike, to the T-shirt as explanatory variables and a response variable, respectively, and have applied multiple regression analysis [3]. The multiple regression types are as follows.

$$y = \alpha\, Look + \beta\, Touch + \gamma\, Take + \varepsilon \qquad (1)$$

Therefore, we focused on regression coefficient in this study. We can expect that the difference in important action appeared as difference in regression coefficient. We grasp their dominant features to compare the regression coefficients of each group of consumer and all them.

Table 1. The definition of three actions

Action	Definition
Look at	Action that a subject looks at commodities.
Touch	Action that a subject touches commodities to check feel of a material.
Take	Action that a subject takes commodities.

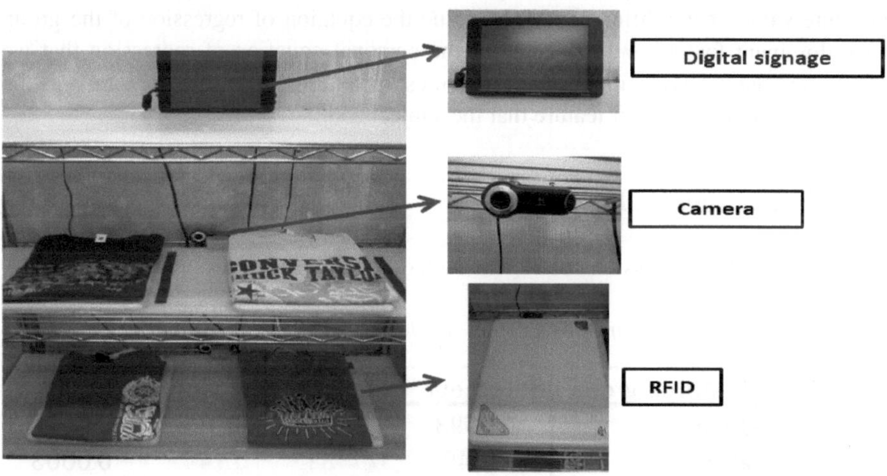

Fig. 1. Experiment space

3 Our Experiment

Experimental procedure is as follows. We had subjects answer a paired comparison question about element of dominant features, and we assumed the first place the dominant features that they have. Table 2 shows element of dominant features.

Table 2. Element of dominant features

Colors	Patterns	Materials	Shapes	Price	Bland	Size

(1) In experiment space, we had 20 subjects choose the favorite clothes in 24 pieces of T-shirts from doing purchasing behavior.
(2) We had 20 subjects evaluate the degree of the interest for 24 pieces of T-shirts in total by five phases of evaluations.

4 Analysis Method

Firstly, we assumed the subject with the same feelings the same group by a paired comparison. We adopted three action times and preferable rate, like and dislike, to the T-shirt as explanatory variables and a response variable, respectively, and have applied multiple regression analysis. We adopted that the grade of over 3 indicates interest of subjects about five phases of evaluations, and 1, 2 indicates not interest. We compared a difference of the size of the regression coefficient each dominant feature with size of the regression coefficient of all the subjects. And we grasped the behavior that is important for subjects each dominant features.

We evaluated the equation of regression each dominant feature. We substituted the behavior time by an experiment for the equation of regression of the group each dominant feature and the equation of regression of a subject. And we got the total of the absolute value of the difference of the value the equation of regression of the group each dominant feature and the value of the personal equation of regression that we substituted the behavior time. Therefore we estimated the value that the total was the smallest with the dominant feature that the subject had.

5 Experimental Result

Table 3 shows the regression coefficient each dominant feature group.

Table 3. Regression Coefficient Each Dominant Feature Group

dominant features group	Intercept	Look at	Touch	Take
Colors	−0.0593	0.1198	−0.1066	0.0535
Patterns	0.1149	0.1181	0.1447	0.0003
Materials	0.0672	0.1084	0.247	0.0122
Shapes	0.0868	0.0826	0.0299	0.0496
All subjects	0.1013	0.1021	0.0712	0.0265

The group which had dominant feature in colors had high ratio of "Look at" and "Take". Next, the group which had dominant feature in patterns had high ratio of "Look at" and "Touch". The group which had dominant feature in materials had high ratio of "Touch". Finally, the group which had dominant feature in shapes had high ratio of "Take". However, the group of price, brand and size were not different from the regression coefficient of all the subjects.

We estimated the dominant features of the subjects and evaluated whether the dominant features we estimated corresponded with dominant features they had. Table 4 shows estimated precision of each dominant feature.

Table 4. Estimated precision of each dominant feature

	Colors	Patterns	Materials	Shapes	All
Subjects who has dominant features	3	5	4	8	20
The number of people that an estimate proved right	2	2	3	5	12
Estimated precision(%)	66.7	40	75	62.5	60

The estimated precision each dominant feature exceeded 60% except patterns. The estimated precision of the pattern was 40%.

6 A Study

The reason that resulted in table 2 is thought about as follows. It is thought that a ratio of "Look at", "Take" became higher because the group which had dominant feature in colors compares the color of the T-shirt and takes to check an overall color. It is thought that a ratio of "Look at", "Touch" became higher because the group which had dominant feature in patterns looks at patterns of the T-shirt and Touch them. Next, it is thought that a ratio of "Touch" became higher because the group which had dominant feature in materials checks the feel of a material to touch T-shirts. Finally, it is thought that a ratio of "Touch" became higher because the group which had dominant feature in shapes takes to check the shape of T-shirts. Because 24 pieces of T-shirts made a little difference about price, brand, size, I thought that it was not different in regression coefficient.

We consider the reason the estimated precision of patterns had become 40% in table 3. A ratio of “Look at”, “Touch” was high in the group which had the dominant feature of patterns at first. However, because the group which had dominant feature in colors had high ratio of “Look at” and the group which had dominant feature in materials had high ratio of “Touch”, we thought the group which had dominant feature in patterns was estimated that it had dominant feature in colors or materials by mistake.

7 Conclusion

In this study, we revealed difference in regression coefficient each dominant feature to grasp them that consumers have by analyzing purchasing behavior. And as a result of having estimated dominant features by using a provided model type, the dominant features except patterns became the high estimated precision.

In future, we think the method to improve estimated precision and examine new analysis that reveals dominant features.

References

1. Digital signage of NEC, world's largest UNIQLO operation - ITmedia news, http://www.itmedia.co.jp/news/articles/1203/15/news065.html
2. An element to make much of when the customers choose the clothes. A man the "brand" "opinion of a family, the friend ", http://chosa.nifty.com/cs/catalog/chosa_report/catalog_120510000286_1.htm
3. Imamura, N., Ogino, A., Kato, T.: Pattern Analysis of Customer Behavior Using Ubiquitous Interface. In: Proceedings of the Annual Conference of JSKE, vol. 8(3), pp. 741–747 (2009)

A Study on Consumers' Emotions Evoked by Product Semantics

Che-Jue Wu, Tyan-Yu Wu, and Jean-Lon Chen

Chang Gung University, Taiwan
wyb0720@hotmail.com, tnyuwu@mail.cgu.edu.tw,
bigmac1479@gmail.com

Abstract. This study investigates consumers' emotions elicited by a product with different levels of semantics and their neural responses. Event-related potentials (ERPs) were used to collect emotional signals. As stimuli, products were distinguished into three Semantics categories (i.e. icon, index, and symbol) of possible referential associations.

Keywords: Products Semantics, Emotion, Event-related potentials (ERPs).

1 Introduction

Nowadays consumers expect products that not only providing functional and ergonomic satisfaction but also supply a pleasurable user experience (Jordan, 2000). In particular, products with cultural meanings can elicit pleasure if these meanings are understood (Krippendorff, 1994). This study attempts to argue that consumers' emotions (i.e. pleasure and arousal) can be elicited by a product with semantics and further to investigate if product semantics difference can affect consumers' emotions differently.

1.1 Product Emotion

Products not only perform the role of the object, they also made people feel happy, angry, proud, ashamed, peace of mind and anxiety (Marzano, 1998). Jordan (1998) investigated different sources of product pleasures: physiological, psychological, sociological, and ideological. Physiological pleasures involve bodily sensations; psychological pleasures are about achievements of the self; sociological pleasures are the pleasures of social interaction; and ideological pleasures are about intellectual stimulation. Norman (2004) also focused on the mental processing that gives rise to affective responses. He identified three levels of processing: a visceral level governing responses through direct perception, a behavioral level involving learnt but automatic affective responses, and a reflective level involving affective responses due to conscious thinking. In line with those levels, Norman proposed three design strategies:

C. Stephanidis (Ed.): Posters, Part I, HCII 2013, CCIS 373, pp. 747–751, 2013.

design for appearance (visceral design), for ease of use (behavioral design), and for reflective meaning (reflective design). This study focused on emotional responses evoked by product semantics. In this paper, we explore sociological pleasures, ideological and reflective meaning.

1.2 Product Semantics

Norman's (2004) reflective emotion is intellectually driven. It is influenced greatly by the knowledge, culture and experience of the user. Products often act as symbols for people, providing personal meaning and communicating the owner's personal characteristics to others. Emotions in using a product depend on what the product means or implies to the user. This is called product semantics (Krippendorff, 2006).

According to Peirce's theory (1935), product semantics were distinguished into three categories of possible referential associations. These three categories describe the formal relationship that can exist between signs and the objects that they represent. The three signs include icon, index, and symbol. Icon deals with needs to resemble that entity in some way. Index pertains to needs to be either causally related to, or spatio-temporally associated with the thing. Symbol pertains to links between the two phenomena and needs to be established by means of a convention, agreement, or culture.

1.3 Event-Related Potentials(ERP)

Emotional processing in the human brain is receiving increased attention. The millisecond temporal resolution of ERPs enables the assessment of neural responses to emotional events. Processing of emotional information can be assessed by analyzing amplitudes (size) and latencies (timing) of ERP components (Rugg and Coles, 1995). Thus, the ERP is used as a new tool for design assessment.

2 Method

2.1 Participants

Ten undergraduate students (5 male, 5 female; mean age= 23.5 years old) from Chang Gung University to participate in the experiment.

2.2 Stimuli

Stimuli covered four seasoning pots with gray tone (see Table 1). Four stimuli were designed by adopting Peirce's Icon, Index and Symbol which represented different levels of semantics, while Nature was constructed with geometric form indicating semantic freedom.

Table 1. Four stimuli, seasoning pots

Icon	Index	Symbol	Nature
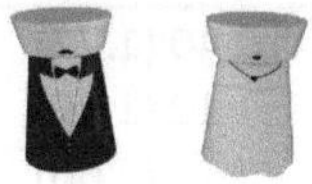	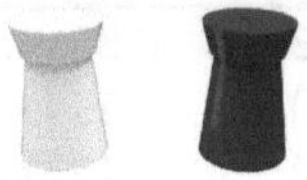	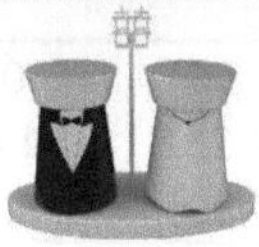	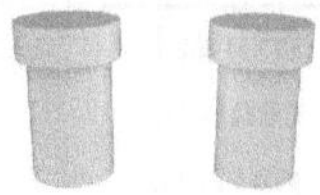

2.3 Procedure

Each trial began by showing a fixation point at the center of the screen for 500ms. After the fixation point disappeared, the prime image (i.e., Icon seasoning pot) was presented for 3000ms, followed by a fixation point presented for 500ms. After the prime image disappeared, a fixation point was presented. Each picture was repeated twenty times randomly. During this brief period, the participants judged whether the product was pleasant or not.

2.4 ERP Recording

EEG signals were recorded from International 10–20 system by NuAmpsTM, 19 of which were embedded in an elastic cap. Data were acquired from 19 electrode sites.

3 Result

3.1 Questionnaire

The results of questionnaire shows that the means of consumers' pleasure had the following descending order: Symbol (Mean= 3.10, SD=0.99) > Icon (Mean= 3.00, SD=0.81) > Nature (Mean= 1.70, SD=1.25). The results implied that products attached with symbolic and icon semantics have a greater chance to evoke users' emotions than nature and index do.

3.2 ERP Analysis

Repeated measures ANOVA tests were used to analyze ERP data. The ERPs were quantified by measuring the mean amplitudes over the P300 (300–500 ms) and the Slow wave (500-1000 ms) time period after stimulus onset. Data were included from the left frontal (F3), medial frontal (Fz), right frontal (F4), left central (C3),medial central (Cz), right central (C4), left parietal (P3), medial parietal (Pz,), and right parietal (P4) electrode sites.

P300 Window

In the P300 window, Picture Content modulated ERPs over frontal (F=2.630, P=0.053) and with Icon showing less positivity over frontal sites (Table 2). We found that the average amplitude of Icon was the strongest at frontal.

Table 2. Analysis Comparison Chart of the Mean voltage (standard error) of the ERP Wave Range in P300 with different product semantics

	Icon	Index	Symbol	Nature
frontal	0.95 (1.69)	-0.30 (2.23)	0.85 (1.94)	0.40 (1.77)
central	1.54 (2.15)	1.45 (1.48)	1.73 (1.65)	1.12 (1.26)
parietal	3.01 (1.90)	3.39 (2.00)	3.72 (2.69)	3.12 (2.00)

Slow Wave Window

In the Slow wave window, Picture Content modulated ERPs over parietal (F=2.628, P=0.054) and with Nature showing less positivity over parietal sites (Table 3). We found that the average amplitude of Nature was the strongest at parietal.

Table 3. Analysis Comparison Chart of the Mean voltage (standard error) of the ERP Wave Range in Slow wave with different product semantics

	Icon	Index	Symbol	Nature
frontal	0.24 (1.27)	-0.14 (1.31)	-0.01(1.28)	-0.05 (1.46)
central	0.47 (1.54)	0.55 (1.46)	0.38 (1.03)	0.23 (0.73)
parietal	0.05 (0.73)	0.22 (1.24)	0.62 (1.77)	-0.25 (0.94)

4 Discussions

Based on the results, it is obvious that the ERP amplitude of product semantics in the Icon is the strongest at frontal and that Nature is the strongest at parietal. Various researches have proposed that different emotional stimulations can be presented clearly because P300 has been verified as a credible testing wave range (Davidson, 2001). The Slow wave's amplitude increases corresponds to improved recognition memory performance, and the results can be interpreted as ERP memory formation effects for affective stimuli (Oloffsson et al, 2008).

References

1. Davidson, R.J.: Toward a biology of personality and emotion. In: Unity of Knowledge: The Convergence of Natural and Human Science, vol. 935, pp. 191–207 (2001)
2. Jordan, P.W.: Human factors for pleasure in product use. Applied Ergonomics Volume (1998)
3. Jordan, P.W.: Designing Pleasurable Products: An Introduction to the New Human Factor. Taylor & Francis, London (2000)
4. Krippendorff, K.: A recursive theory of communication. In: Crowley, D., Mitchell, D. (eds.) Communication Theory Today, pp. 78–104. Polity Press, Cambridge (1994)
5. Krippendorff, K.: The semantic turn: A new foundation for design. Taylor & Francis, Boca Raton (2006)

6. Marzano, S.: Suffusing design through the organization. Design Management Journal 11(1) (Winter 2000)
7. Norman, D.A.: Emotional design. Basic Books, New York (2004)
8. Olofsson, J.K., Nordin, S., Sequeira, H., Polich, J.: Affective picture processing: An integrative review of ERP findings. Biological Psychology 77(3), 247–265 (2008), doi:10.1016/j.biopsycho.2007.11.006
9. Peirce, C.S.: Collected papers of Charles Sanders Peirce. Belknap Press (1935)
10. Rugg, M.D., Coles, M.G.H. (eds.): Electrophysiology of Mind: Event-related Brain Potentials and Cognition. Oxford University Press, New York (1995)

Author Index

MIX
Papier aus verantwortungsvollen Quellen
Paper from responsible sources
FSC® C105338

FSC
www.fsc.org

If you have any concerns about our products,
you can contact us on
ProductSafety@springernature.com

In case Publisher is established outside the EU,
the EU authorized representative is:
Springer Nature Customer Service Center GmbH
Europaplatz 3, 69115 Heidelberg, Germany

Printed by Libri Plureos GmbH
in Hamburg, Germany